Exam Preparatory Manual for Undergraduates

PATHOLOGY

for Dental Students

Exam Preparatory Manual for Undergraduates

PATHOLOGY
for Dental Students

Ramadas Nayak MBBS MD
Professor and Head
Department of Pathology
Yenepoya Medical College
Yenepoya University
Mangaluru, Karnataka, India

Formerly, Professor and Head
Department of Pathology
Kasturba Medical College
Manipal University
Mangaluru, Karnataka, India

Foreword
Yenepoya Abdulla Kunhi

JAYPEE *The Health Sciences Publisher*
New Delhi | London | Philadelphia | Panama

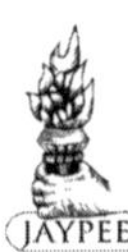

Jaypee Brothers Medical Publishers (P) Ltd

Headquarters

Jaypee Brothers Medical Publishers (P) Ltd
4838/24, Ansari Road, Daryaganj
New Delhi 110 002, India
Phone: +91-11-43574357
Fax: +91-11-43574314
Email: jaypee@jaypeebrothers.com

Overseas Offices

J.P. Medical Ltd
83 Victoria Street, London
SW1H 0HW (UK)
Phone: +44 20 3170 8910
Fax: +44 (0)20 3008 6180
Email: info@jpmedpub.com

Jaypee Medical Inc.
325 Chestnut Street
Suite 412, Philadelphia, PA 19106, USA
Phone: +1 267-519-9789
Email: jpmed.us@gmail.com

Jaypee-Highlights Medical Publishers Inc.
City of Knowledge, Bld. 237, Clayton
Panama City, Panama
Phone: +1 507-301-0496
Fax: +1 507-301-0499
Email: cservice@jphmedical.com

Jaypee Brothers Medical Publishers (P) Ltd
17/1-B Babar Road, Block-B, Shaymali
Mohammadpur, Dhaka-1207
Bangladesh
Mobile: +08801912003485
Email: jaypeedhaka@gmail.com

Jaypee Brothers Medical Publishers (P) Ltd
Bhotahity, Kathmandu, Nepal
Phone: +977-9741283608
Email: kathmandu@jaypeebrothers.com

Website: www.jaypeebrothers.com
Website: www.jaypeedigital.com

Inquiries for bulk sales may be solicited at: jaypee@jaypeebrothers.com

Exam Preparatory Manual for Undergraduates: Pathology for Dental Students

First Edition: **2016**

ISBN: 978-93-5250-118-2

Printed at Rajkamal Electric Press, Plot No. 2, Phase-IV, Kundli, Haryana.

Dedicated to

Students who inspired me,
Patients who provided the knowledge,
My parents and family members
who encouraged and supported me

Foreword

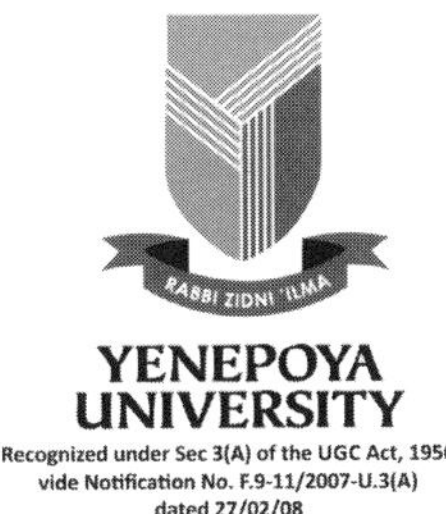

I am extremely delighted to write this foreword for *Exam Preparatory Manual for Undergraduates: Pathology for Dental Students* written by Dr Ramadas Nayak, Professor and Head, Department of Pathology, Yenepoya Medical College, a constituent institution of Yenepoya University, Mangaluru, Karnataka, India.

A professor par excellence, Dr Ramadas Nayak has over three decades of illustrious teaching experience with several publications, including over 82 scientific papers in both national and international journals, to his credit. Having held several key portfolios and having won several awards, including the "Good teacher award" on two occasions, his book must indeed be the "touchstone" of success for students in that stream.

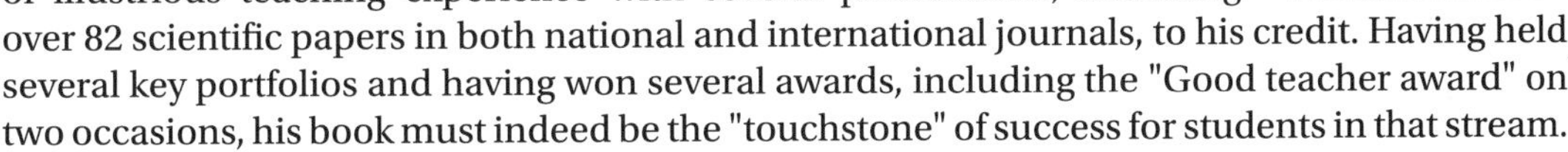

I am truly impressed by his zeal to improve the learning capabilities for his students by taking pains to come out with such a useful and highly innovative book. I know Dr Ramadas to be a highly motivated and enthusiastic person and I applaud his efforts in compiling this manual.

I am sure it will soon be the hands reference manual for many students in the region and beyond. I wish Dr Ramadas every success in this and all his future endeavors.

For the great teacher that Dr Ramadas is, I conclude with the wise words of William Arthur Ward:

"The mediocre teacher tells
The good teacher explains.
The superior teacher demonstrates.
The great teacher inspires."

Thank You

Yenepoya Abdulla Kunhi
Chancellor
Yenepoya University
Mangaluru, Karnataka, India

Preface

Pathology is a rapidly expanding and ever-changing field and lays the foundation for understanding diseases. This book is an endeavor to present the vast knowledge of pathology in a lucid manner for dental students. My aim is to provide a sound knowledge of pathology and hence give insight into etiology, pathogenesis, pathology and the disease course. Every attempt has been made to present information in a simplified text augmented with the use of illustrations.

Organization

This book consists of 22 chapters and is organized into two sections namely Theory and Practicals.

Section 1—Theory: It consists of pathology theory required for dental students and provides an overview of the basic pathologic mechanisms underlying diseases.

Section 2—Practicals: It deals with all the practical exercises with illustrations.

After many years (more than 35 years) of teaching undergraduates, I found that dental undergraduate students find it difficult to understand, remember and answer the questions during examinations, in a satisfying way. There are many pathology textbooks, but dental undergraduates face difficulty to refresh their knowledge during examinations. This encouraged me to write a book to fill the niche to provide basic information to dental undergraduates in a nutshell. The text provides all the basic information the student will ever need to know. Key words are shown in bold words so that students can rapidly go through the book on the previous day or just before the examination. Most students are fundamentally "visually oriented." As the saying "one picture is worth a thousand words", it encouraged me to provide many illustrations.

How to use this book

I recommend that this book to be used by all dental students for understanding the basic knowledge and refresh their knowledge during examinations. The readers are requested to give more emphasis on word in bold letters that represents the key words to be remembered.

About 161 illustrations, 21 gross photographs, 68 photomicrographs, 128 tables, 47 flowcharts and 3 X-rays photographs have been incorporated for easy understanding of the subject.

Ramadas Nayak

Acknowledgments

My sincere thanks to all my family members, especially my wife Smt Rekha Nayak, my daughter Ms Rashmitha Nayak and my son-in-law Mr Ramnath Kini, who have patiently accepted my long preoccupation with this work. A special thanks to my grandson Master Rishab Kini who kept me agile throughout the preparation of this book.

I am indebted to Mr Yenepoya Abdulla Kunhi, Honorable Chancellor, Yenepoya University, Mangaluru, Karnataka, India, for the inspiration and for writing the foreword.

I would like to express my gratitude to all my friends and colleagues who helped me in the different stages of preparing the manuscript; to all those who provided support, talked things over, read, offered comments and assisted in the editing, proofreading and designing.

- Dr Jagadish Rao PP MBBS MD DNB PGDCFS Dip. Cyber Law PGCTM MNAMS, District Medicolegal Consultant (Government Wenlock District Hospital), and Associate Professor, Department of Forensic Medicine and Toxicology, Kasturba Medical College (Affiliated to Manipal University), Mangaluru, Karnataka, India.
- Dr Sharada Rai MBBS MD, Associate Professor, Department of Pathology, Kasturba Medical College, Manipal University, Mangaluru.
- Dr Rakshatha Nayak, Tutor in Pathology, Yenepoya Medical College, Yenepoya University, Mangaluru.
- Dr Sonali Ullal, Associate Professor, Department of Radiodiagnosis, Kasturba Medical College (Affiliated to Manipal University), Mangaluru.
- Dr Krishnaraj Upadhyaya, Professor, Department of Pathology, Yenepoya Medical College, A constituent of Yenepoya University, Mangaluru.
- Dr Mahesh H Karigoudar, Professor, Department of Pathology, Shri BM Patil Medical College, BLDE University, Bijapur, Karnataka.
- A special thanks to Shri Jitendar P Vij (Group Chairman), Mr Ankit Vij (Group President), Mr Tarun Duneja (Director–Publishing), Ms Chetna Malhotra Vohra (Sr Manager, Business Development) of M/s Jaypee Brothers Medical Publishers (P) Ltd, New Delhi, India, for publishing the book in the same format as wanted, well in time. I am grateful to Shri Jitendar P Vij for unmasking my talent as an author.
- I would like to offer a huge appreciation to the wonderful work done by Ms Sunita Katla (Publishing Manager), Ms Samina Khan (Executive Assistant to Director–Publishing), Mr Rajesh Sharma (Production Coordinator), Mr Prasun Kumar (Proofreader), Mr Mohit Bhargava (Coordinator), Mr Rajesh Ghurkundi (Graphic Designer) and Mr Om Prakash Mishra (DTP Operator) of M/s Jaypee Brothers Medical Publishers (P) Ltd, New Delhi, India.
- I thank especially Mr Venugopal V (Bengaluru) and Mr Vasudev H (Mangaluru) of M/s Jaypee Brothers Medical Publishers (P) Ltd, Bengaluru Branch, Karnataka, for taking this book to every corner of Karnataka.
- Last but definitely not least, a thank you to all my undergraduate and postgraduate students. Without you, I would not write. You make all my books possible.

There are many more people I could thank, but space, and my modesty compel me to stop here.

Contents

SECTION 1: THEORY

SECTION 2: PRACTICALS

Plate 1

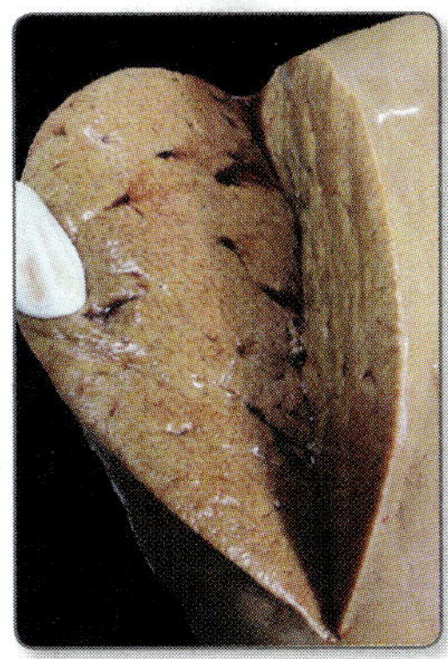

Fig. 2.13: Fatty liver showing a part of liver with yellow color and sharp border

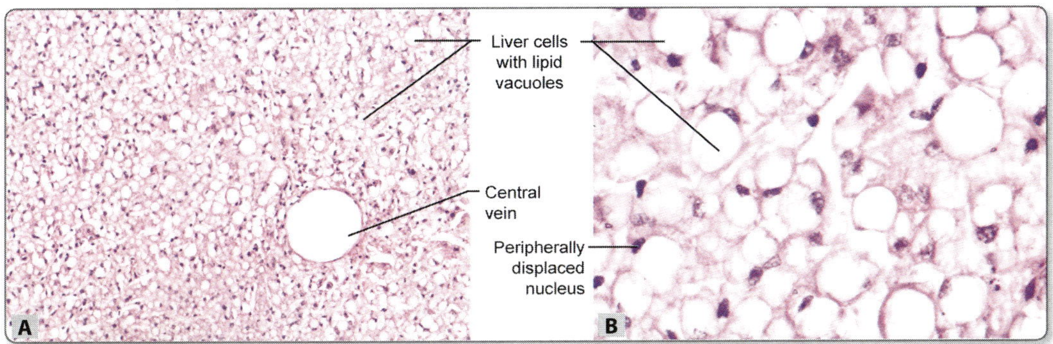

Figs 2.14A and B: A. Fatty liver in which the hepatocytes show accumulation of fat which appear as clear vacuole in the cytoplasm; B. Hepatocytes at higher magnification in which the nucleus is displaced to the periphery by accumulated fat

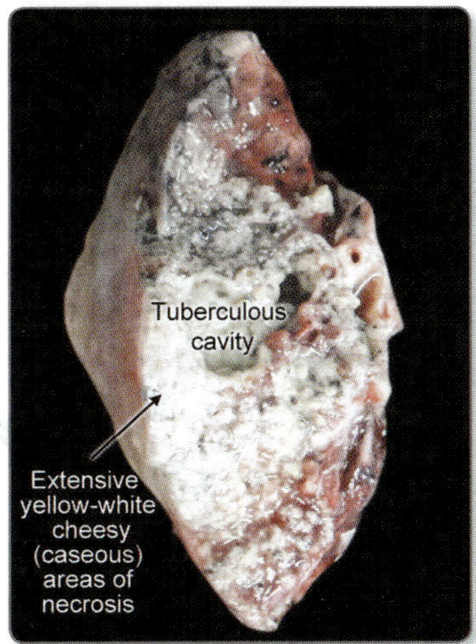

Fig. 2.18: Gross appearance of caseous necrosis. Lung shows cavity with caseous necrosis

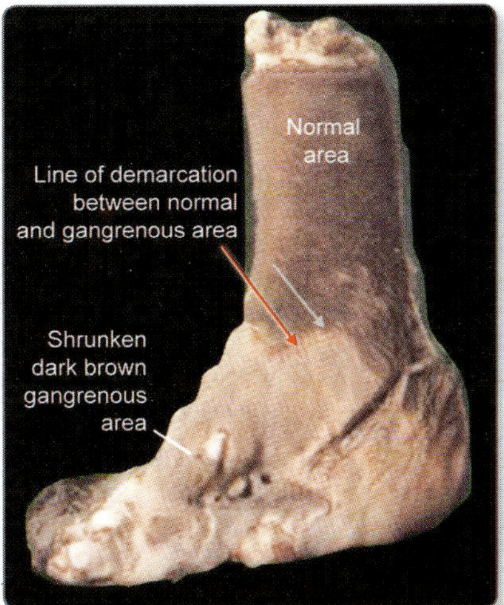

Fig. 2.21: Dry gangrene of left leg shows dry shrunken discolored gangrenous foot separated from adjacent normal area by a line of demarcation

Plate 2

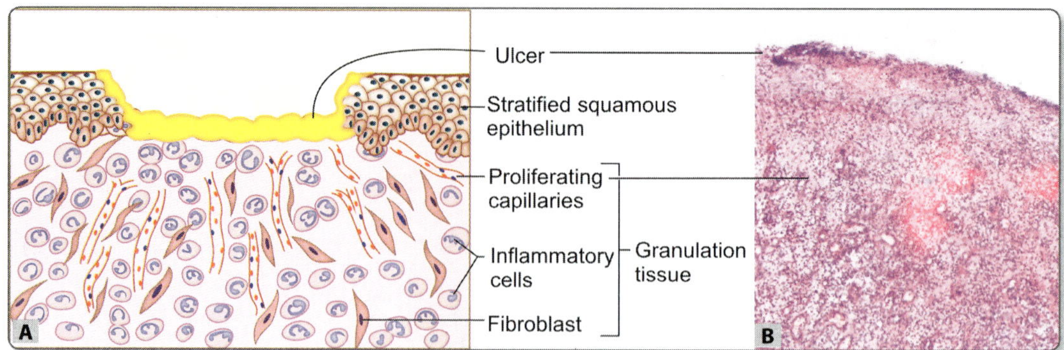

Figs 4.3A and B: Granulation tissue consisting of numerous blood vessels, fibroblasts and edema. A. Diagrammatic; B. Hematoxylin and eosin

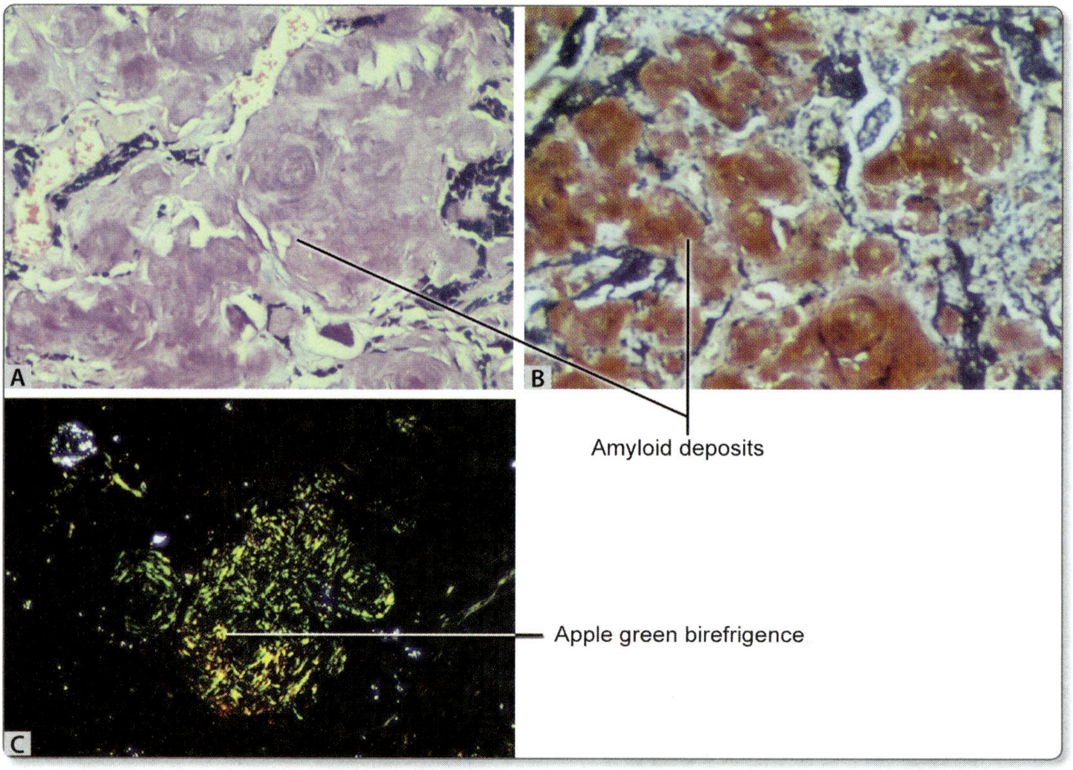

A
B
Amyloid deposits
C
Apple green birefrigence

Figs 5.17A to C: Amyloid deposits in medullary carcinoma of thyroid. A. Amyloid appear as extracellular, amorphous, eosinophilic substance under H and E stain. B. Congo red stain gives red color to the amyloid deposits. C. Congo red stain viewed under polarizing microscope gives apple-green birefringence to amyloid deposits

Plate 3

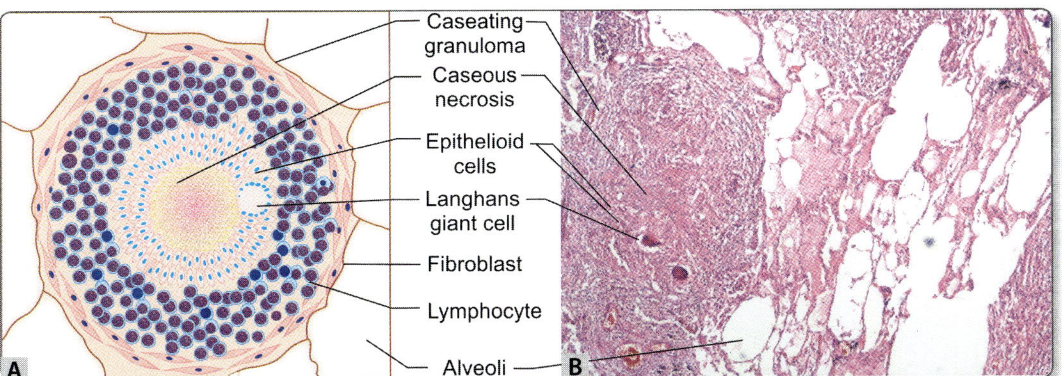

Figs 6.3A and B: Microscopic appearance of tuberculous of lung. A. (diagrammatic); B. (photomicrograph). Central area of caseation surrounded by epithelioid and multinucleated giant cells

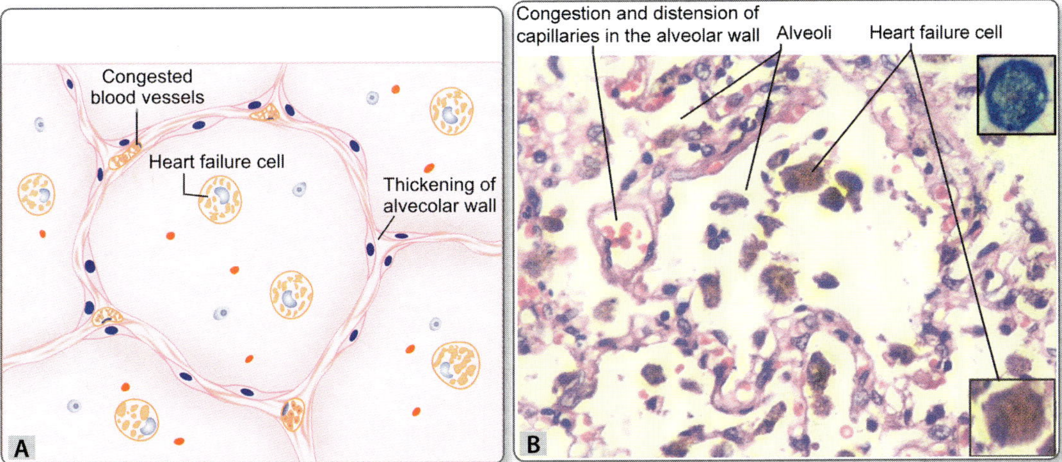

Figs 7.1A and B: Chronic venous congestion lung (A. diagrammatic and B. H and E) with thickened alveolar walls and hemosiderin laden macrophages (heart failure cells) in the alveolar lumen Inset of B, lower right-hemosiderin laden macrophage and upper left-Perl's stain imparting blue-black color to hemosiderin in the cytoplasm

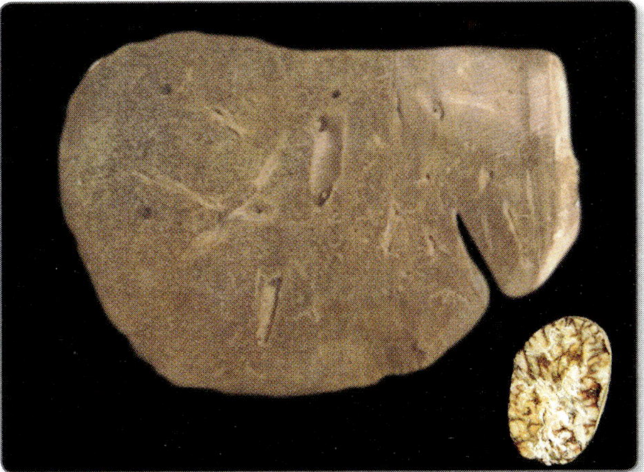

Fig. 7.2: Gross appearance of chronic venous congestion of liver, which shows alternate dark and light area and resembles the cut surface of a nutmeg (inset)

Plate 4

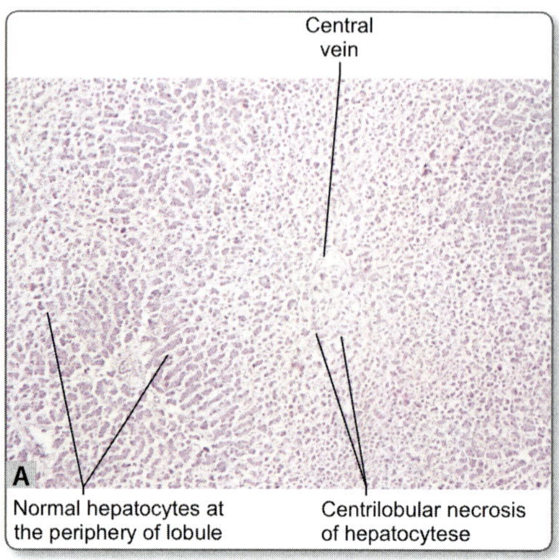

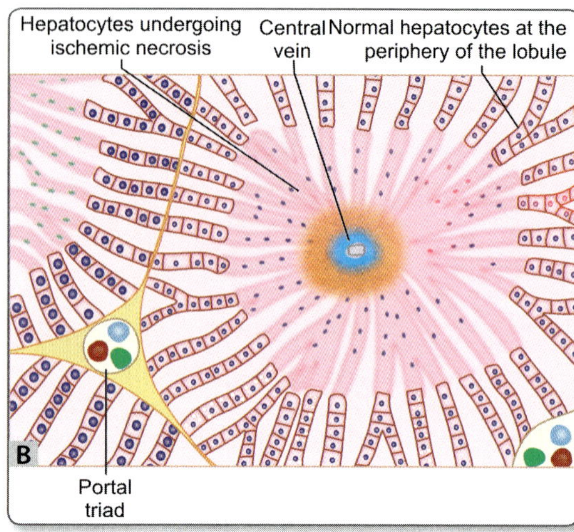

Figs 7.3A and B: Chronic venous congestion liver shows centrilobular necrosis with degenerating hepatocytes surrounded by apparently normal hepatic parenchyma in the periportal region. A. Photomicrograph; B. Diagrammatic

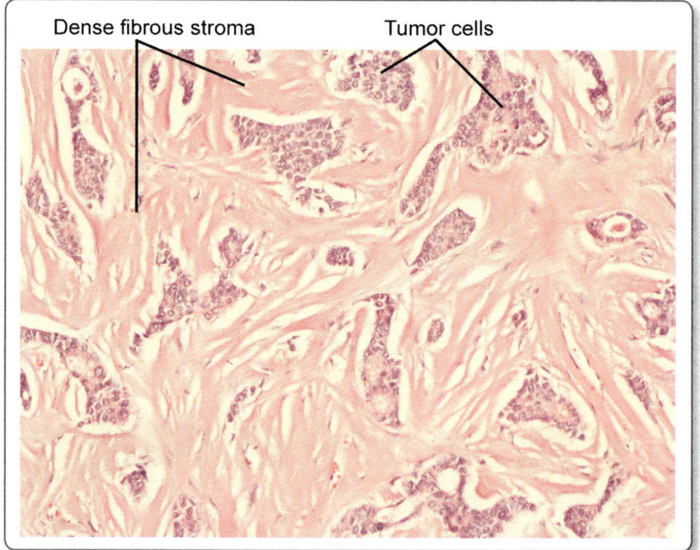

Fig. 11.1: Carcinoma of breast with abundant stroma separating malignant cells

Plate 5

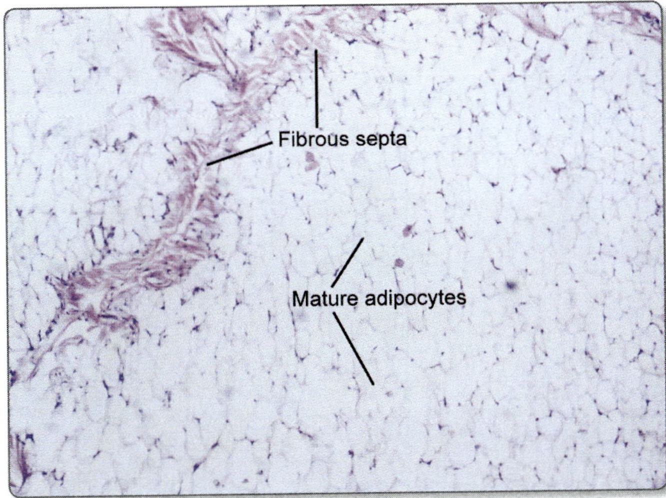

Fig. 11.4: Lipoma is a benign, well-differentiated tumor composed of lobules of fat cells that are identical in appearance to normal fat cells

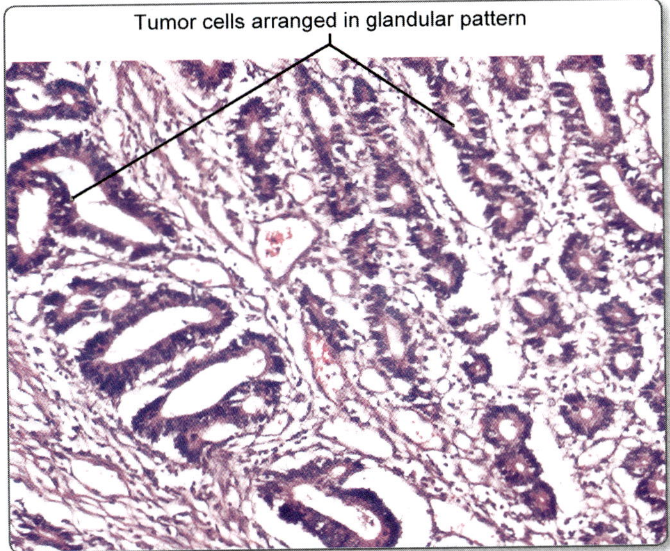

Fig. 11.5: Well-differentiated adenocarcinoma of the colon. It shows cancerous glands are irregular in shape and size invading the muscular layer of the colon

Plate 6

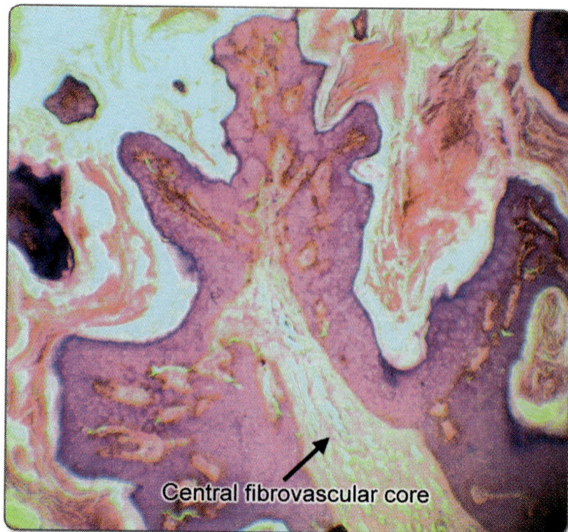

Fig. 11.20: Squamous papilloma composed of finger-like projections supported by central fibrovascular core and covered by an orderly stratified squamous epithelium.

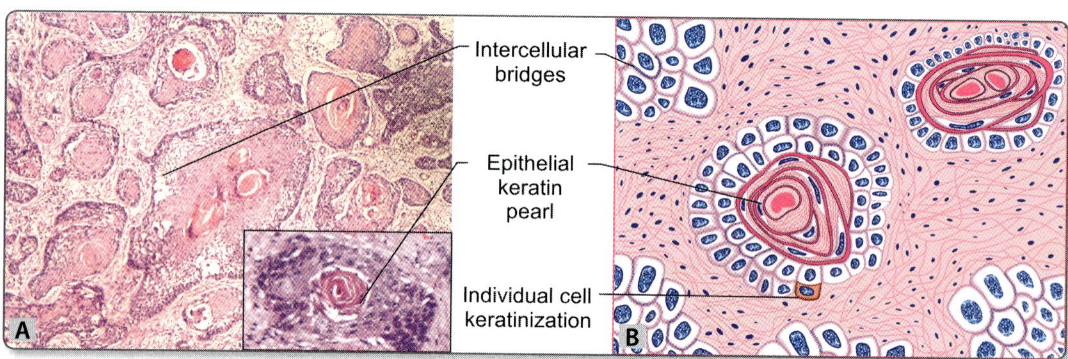

Figs 11.24A and B: A. Photomicrograph and B. Diagrammatic; Well-differentiated squamous cell carcinoma composed of polygonal squamous tumor cells arranged in orderly lobules and produce large amounts of keratin. Some of this keratin form epithelial or squamous pearls (inset of A)

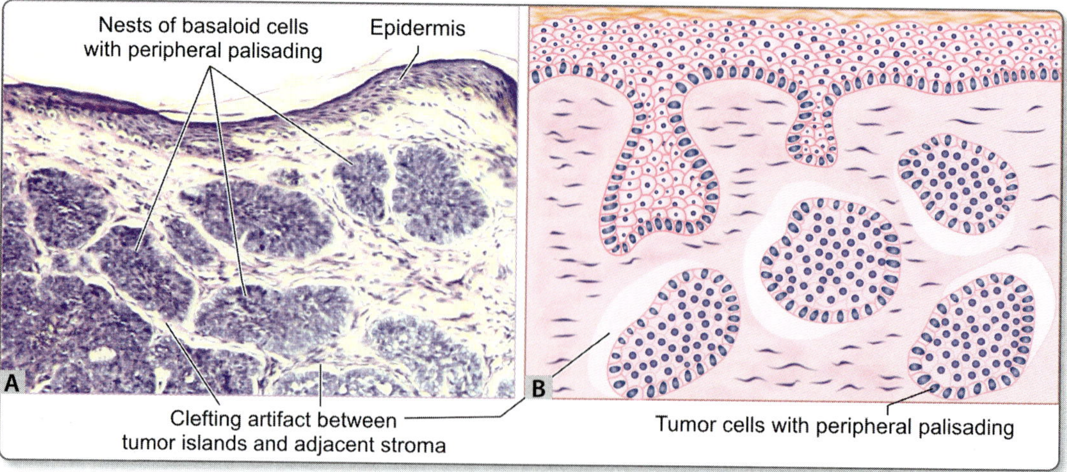

Figs 11.25A and B: Basal cell carcinoma. Composed of nests of uniformly atypical basaloid cells within the dermis, that are often separated from the adjacent stroma by thin clefts. A. Photomicrograph; B. Diagrammatic

Plate 7

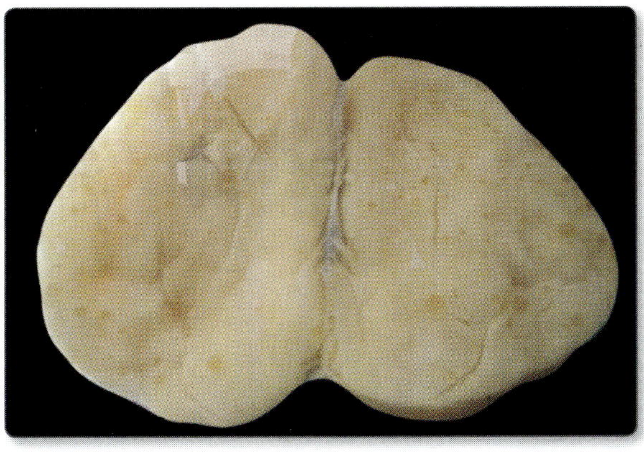

Fig. 11.31: Lipoma-well capsulated, lobulated and yellow benign tumor of fat..

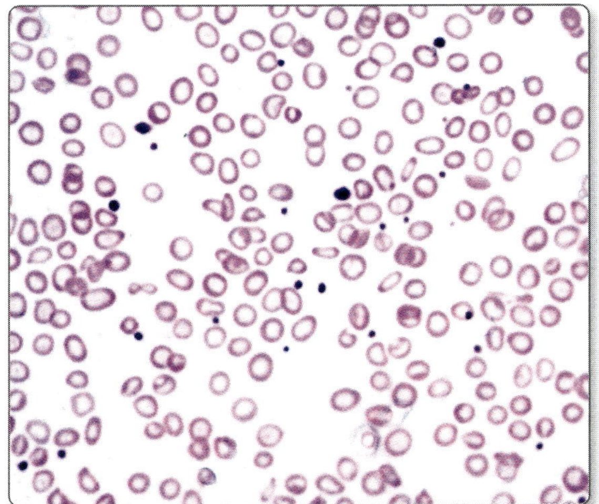

Fig. 12.1: Peripheral blood smear showing microcytic hypochromic red blood cells

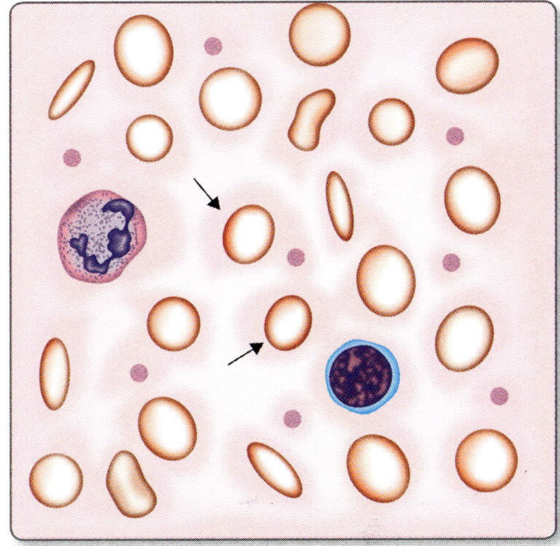

Fig. 12.2: Diagrammatic appearance of peripheral blood smear with microcytic hypochromic red blood cells (arrows)

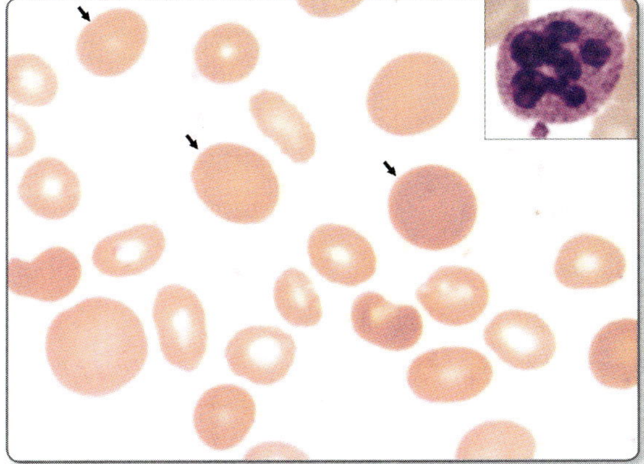

Fig. 12.3: Peripheral blood smear showing macro-ovalocytes (arrows) and hypersegmented neutrophil (inset)

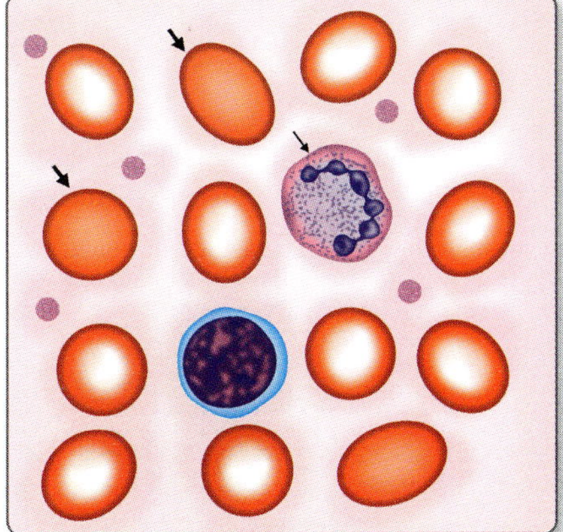

Fig. 12.4: Diagrammatic peripheral blood smear showing macro-ovalocytes (thick arrows) and hypersegmented neutrophil (thin arrow)

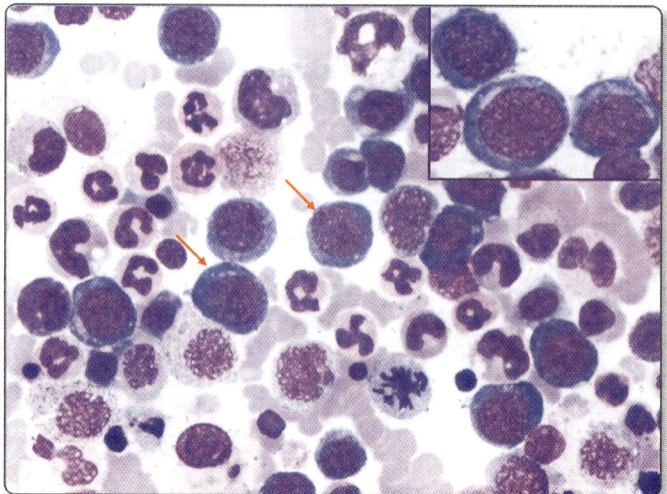

Fig. 12.6: Bone marrow aspirate showing megaloblastic precursors (arrows) in varying stages of maturation (inset shows early megaloblast)

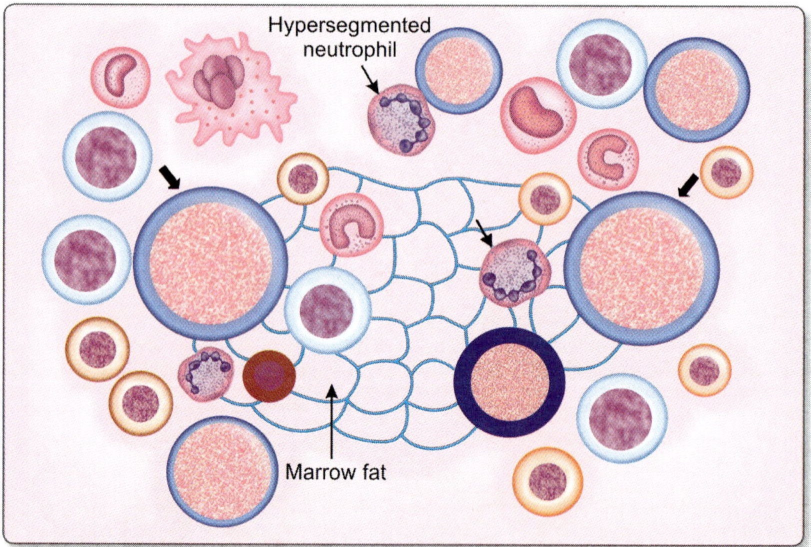

Fig. 12.7: Diagrammatic picture of bone marrow aspirate showing megaloblastic precursors (thick arrows) in varying stages of maturation

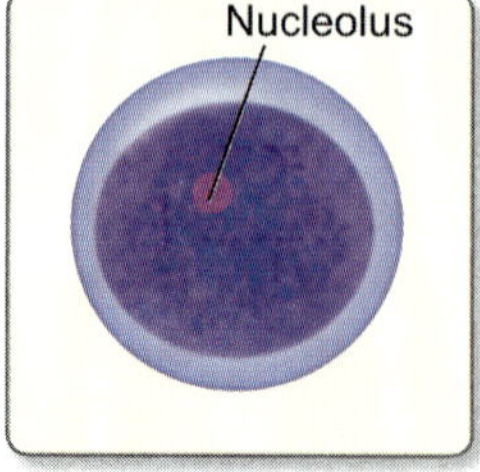

Fig. 12.18: Diagrammatic appearance of lymphoblast

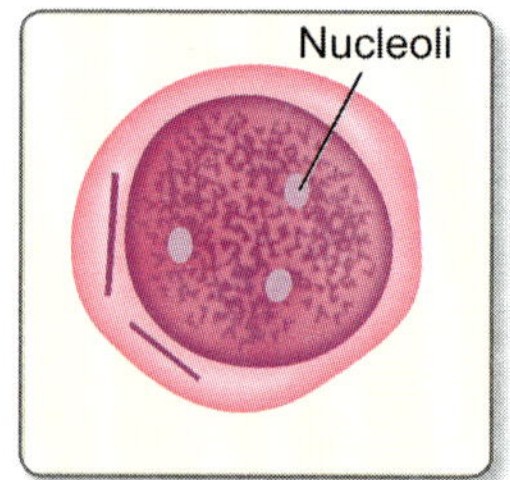

Fig. 12.19: Diagrammatic appearance of myeloblast

Plate 9

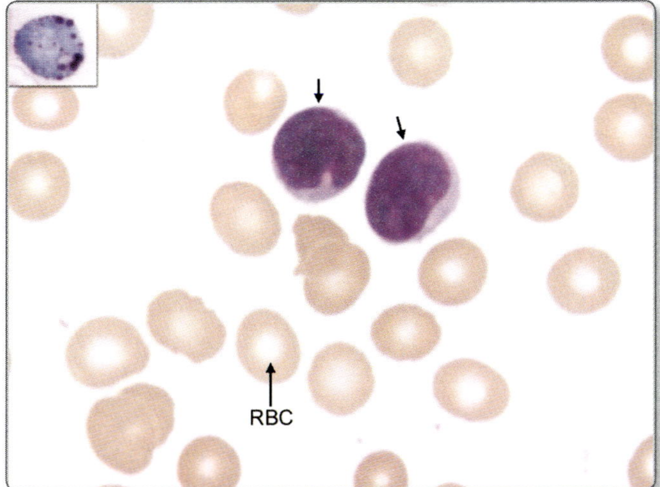

Fig. 12.20: Peripheral blood smears in acute lymphoblastic leukemia showing lymphoblasts (arrows). Inset shows lymphoblast with block positivity with PAS stain

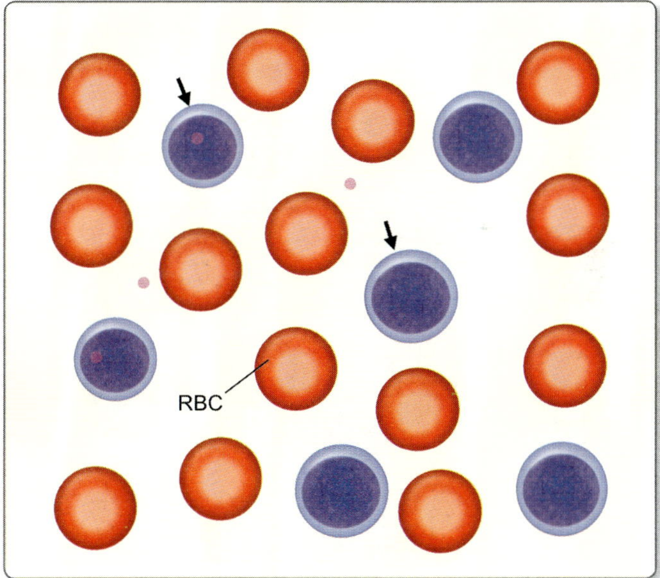

Fig. 12.21: Diagrammatic peripheral blood smear in acute lymphoblastic leukemia showing lymphoblasts (arrows)

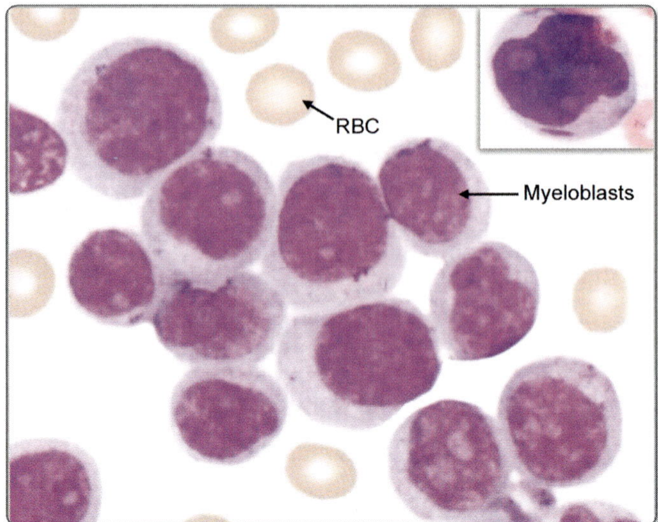

Fig. 12.22: Peripheral smear in AML with myeloblasts. Inset shows myeloblast with Auer rod

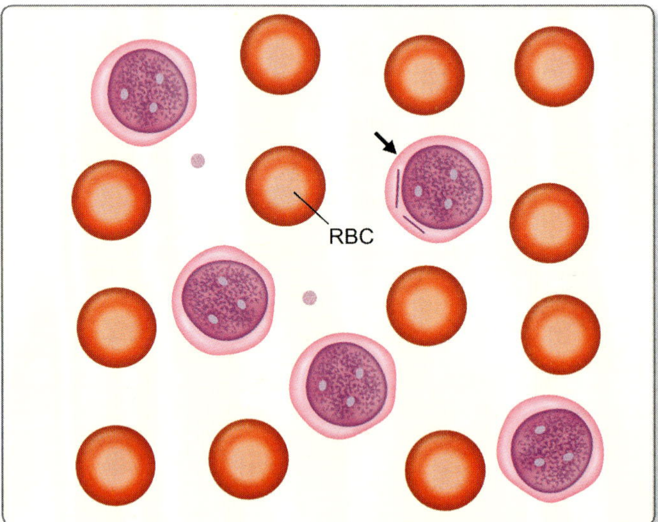

Fig. 12.23: Diagrammatic peripheral blood smear in AML with myeloblasts. One myeloblast with two Auer rods (arrow)

Plate 11

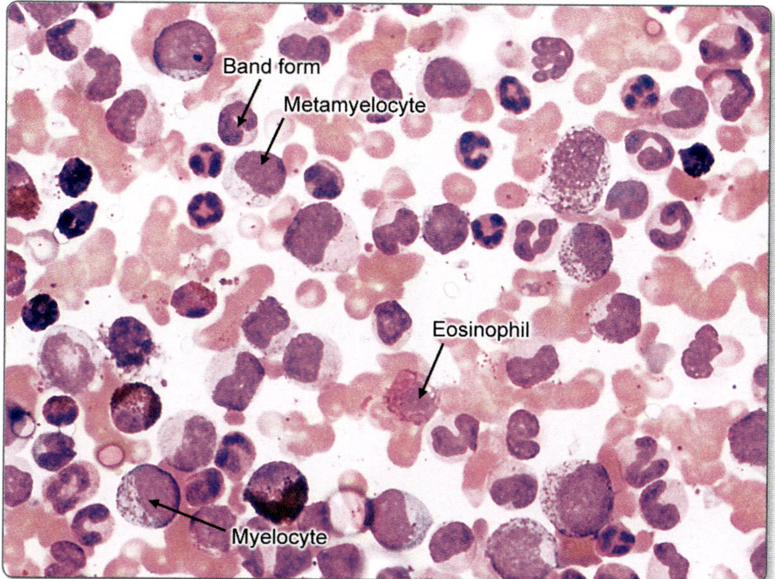

Fig. 12.25: Peripheral blood picture in chronic/stable phase of chronic myeloid leukemia

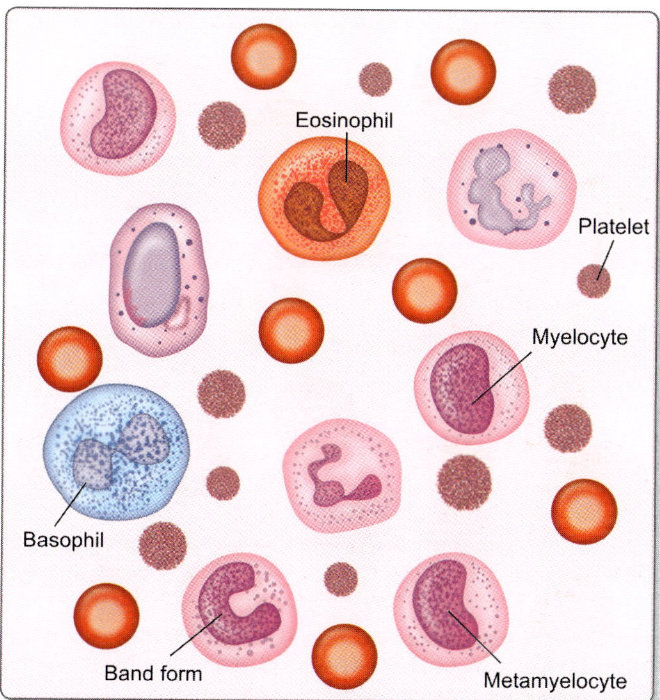

Fig. 12.26: Diagrammatic peripheral blood picture in chronic/stable phase of chronic myeloid leukemia

Plate 12

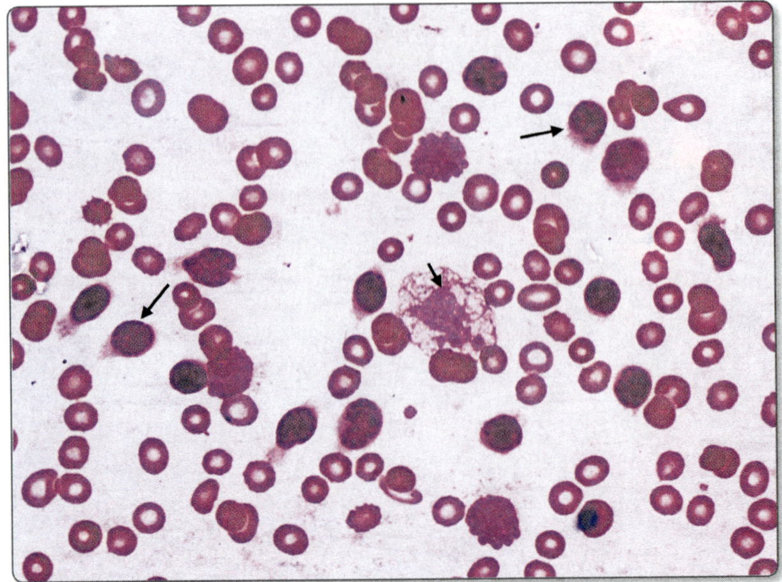

Fig. 12.27: Peripheral blood smears in chronic lymphocytic leukemia showing numerous small lymphocytes (long arrows) and few smudge cells (short arrow)

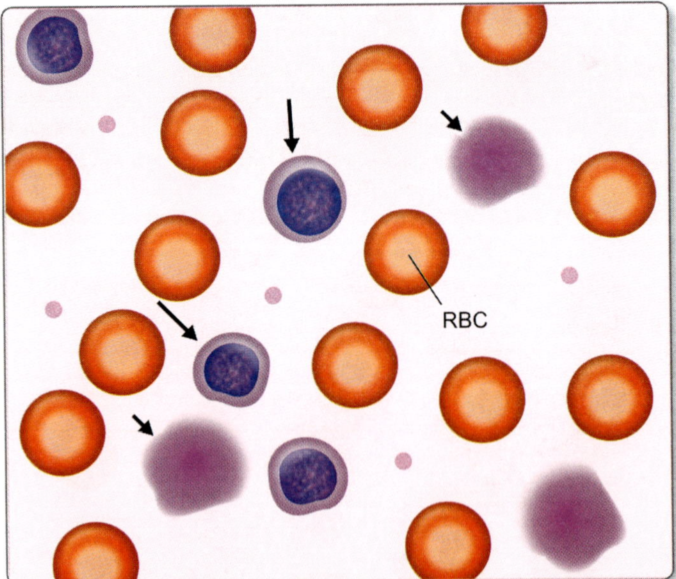

Fig. 12.28: Diagrammatic peripheral blood smears in chronic lymphocytic leukemia showing numerous small lymphocytes (long arrows) and few smudge cells (short arrows)

Plate 13

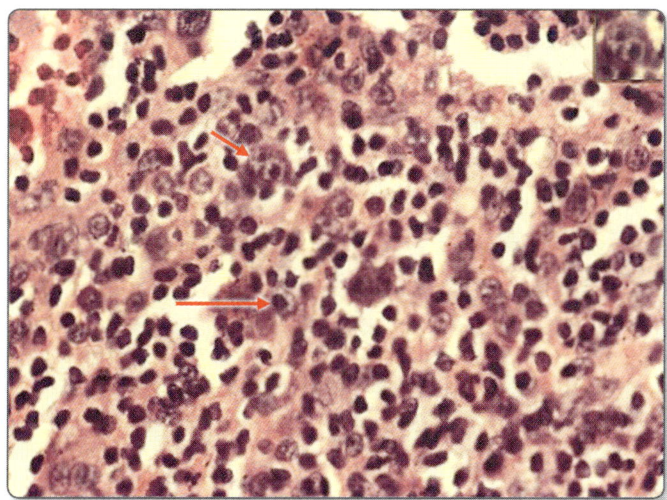

Fig. 13.6: Microscopic appearance of Hodgkin lymphoma showing RS cells (short arrow and inset) and Hodgkin cells (long arrow) within the background of mixed population of reactive cells

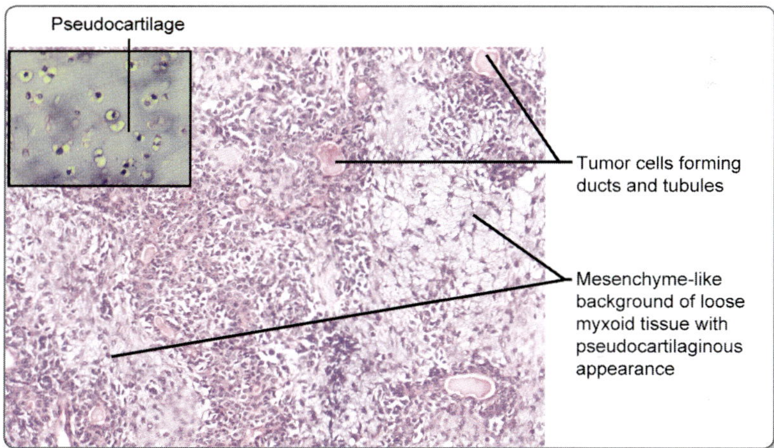

Fig. 15.1: Pleomorphic adenoma showing epithelial cells and myoepithelial cells separated by chondroid matrix Inset shows pseudo-cartilage

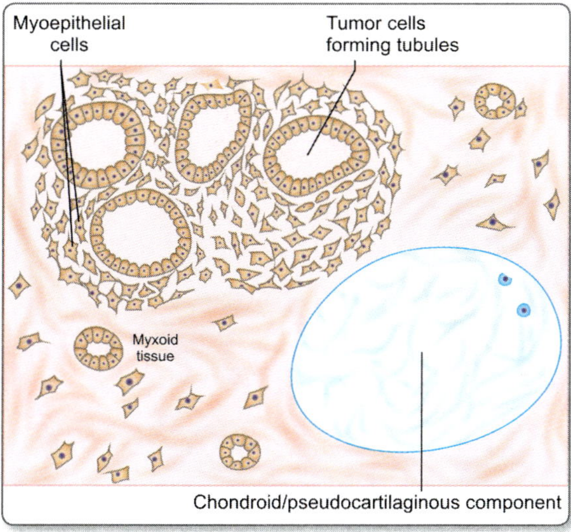

Fig. 15.2: Microscopic features of pleomorphic adenoma of salivary gland (diagrammatic)

Plate 14

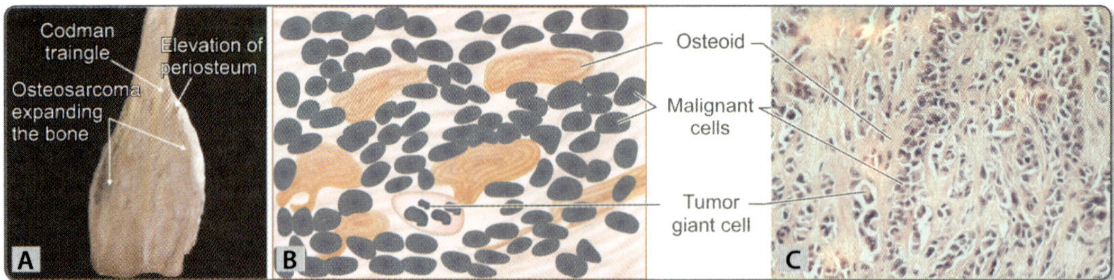

Figs 16.5A to C: A. Gross appearance of osteosarcoma of the lower part of distal femur showing a tan-white tumor filling most of the medullary cavity of the metaphysis and proximal diaphysis. The tumor has infiltrated through the cortex, lifted the periosteum and this region on X-ray appears as Codman triangle; B. Diagrammatic and C. Photomicrograph of microscopy of osteosarcoma composed of pleomorphic tumor cells separated by osteoid

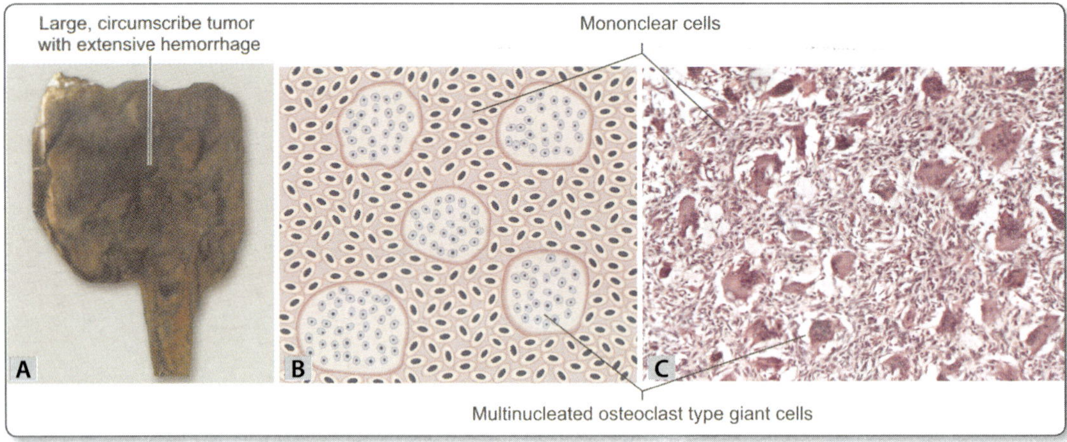

Figs 16.7A to C: Giant-cell tumor of bone. A. Grossly shows a circumscribed tumor with hemorrhage in the upper end of tibia. Microscopically; B. Diagrammatic and C. Photomicrograph, shows numerous multinucleated giant cells. The background shows mononuclear stromal cells

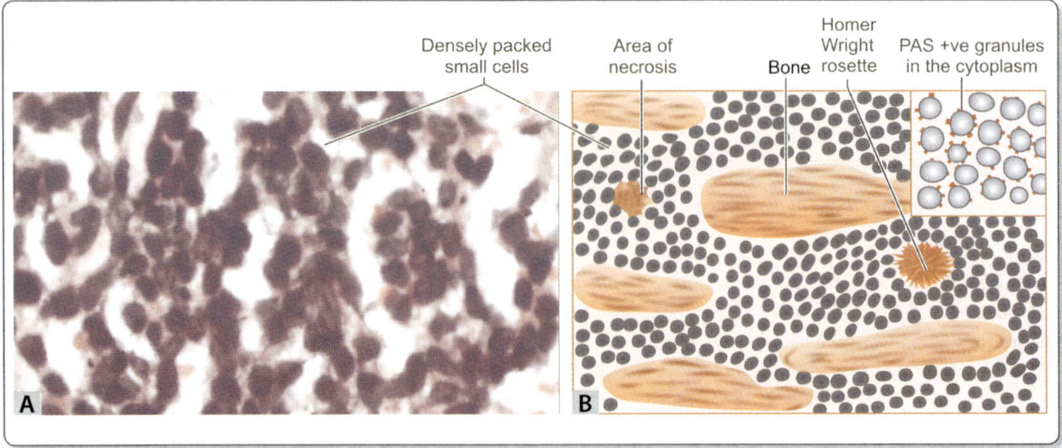

Figs 16.9A and B: A. Photomicrograph; and B. Diagrammatic; Ewing sarcoma composed of sheets of closely packed uniform small round cells with scanty cytoplasm. The inset of B shows PAS positive granules in the cytoplasm

Plate 15

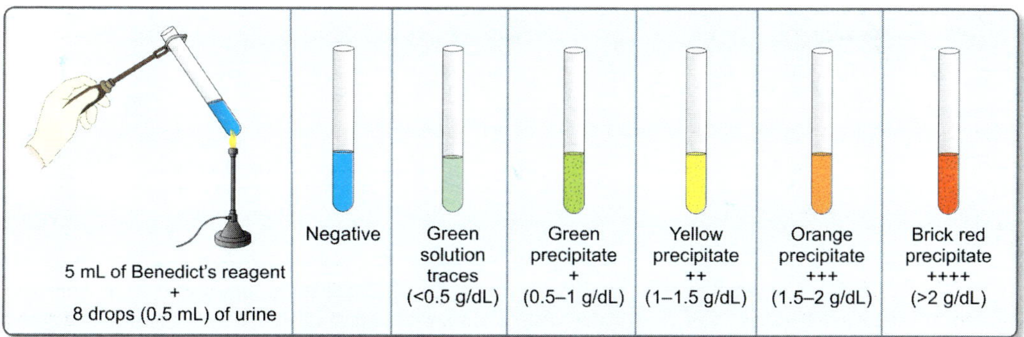

Fig. 18.4: Method and interpretation of Benedict's test

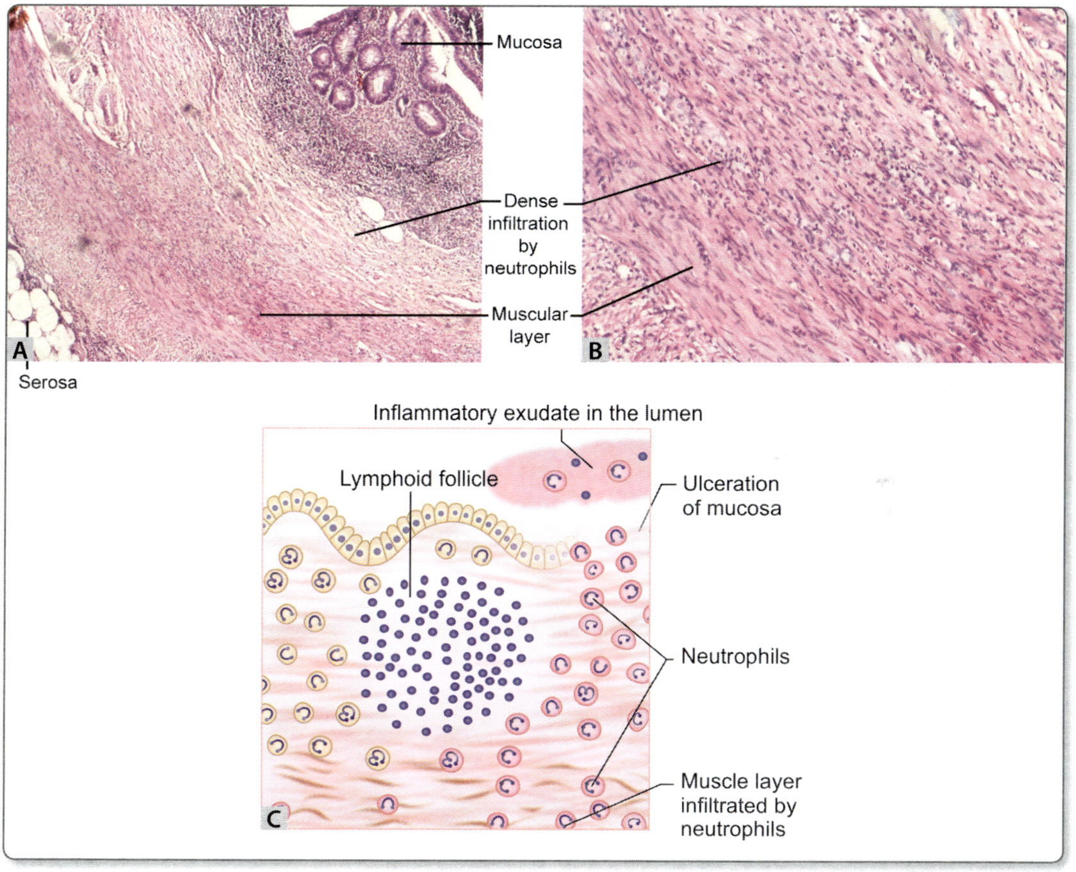

Figs 21.1A to C: A. Photomicrograph (low power) of acute appendicitis showing inflammation of mucosa, submucosa and muscular layer; B. (High power view) shows numerous neutrophils in the muscular layer; C. Diagrammatic appearance of acute appendicitis

Plate 16

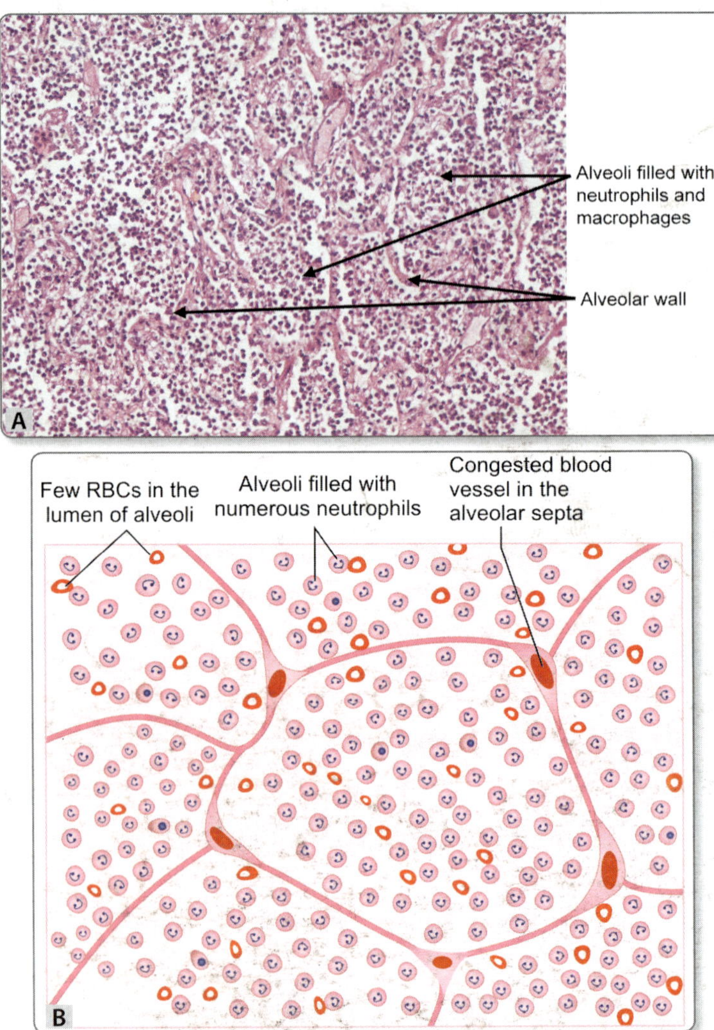

Figs 21.2A and B: Pneumonia A (H & E stain) and B (diagrammatic) shows alveoli filled with neutrophils

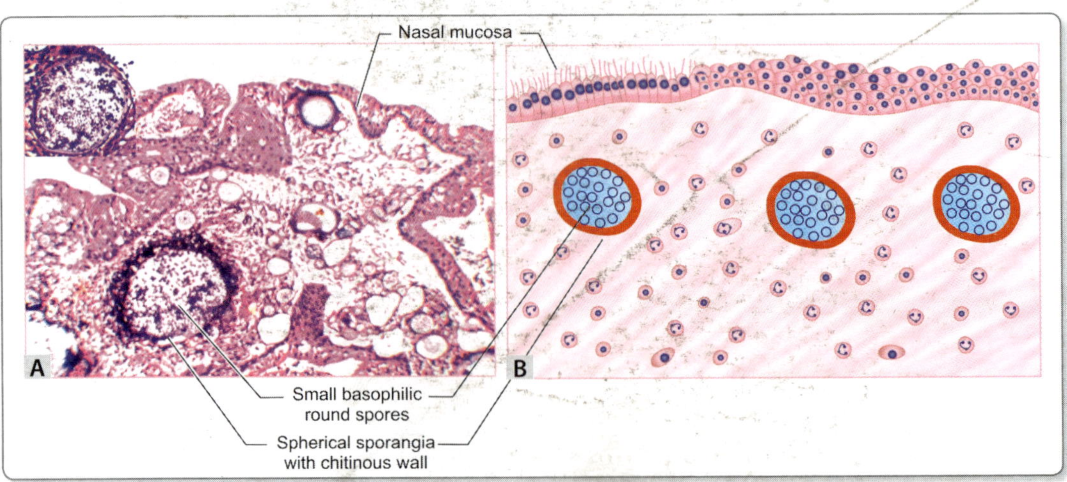

Figs 21.3A and B: Rhinosporidiosis of nasopharynx showing spherical sporangia. A (H & E stain) and B (diagrammatic)

Section 1

Theory

Chapter 1

Introduction

Chapter Outline

- Normal cell structure and functions
- Introduction to pathology

NORMAL CELL STRUCTURE AND FUNCTIONS

- A cell is a fundamental unit of life
- All cells are tridimensional, although when viewed under the light microscope on a glass slide, they appear to be flat
- **Classification of cells**: Except some cells (e.g. RBCs or squamous cells may lose their nucleus in the final stages of their life cycle) all human cells have a distinct nucleus. All nucleated cells are classified as:
    a. **Eukaryotic cells** (from Greek, *karion* = kernel, nucleus): DNA is enclosed by a membrane forming a distinct nuclear structure.
    b. **Prokaryotic cells**: These are primitive cells (e.g. bacteria) in which the DNA is present in the cytoplasm but is not enclosed by a membrane as a distinct nuclear structure.

Components of the Cell (Fig. 1.1)

- All cells share the fundamental structural components. Each cell has three essential components: A) Cell membrane, B) Cytoplasm and C) Nucleus.

A) *Cell Membrane/Unit Membrane*

- It is the outer boundary of the cell
- It facilitates and limits the exchange of substances between the cell and its environment
- Light microscopy: The membrane appears at the periphery as a thin condensation
- Electron microscopy: It is composed of three layers, each about 25 nm thick. The inner and the outer dense (electronopaque) layers are separated by a wider lucent central layer
- Biochemical components: Cell membrane is composed of mixture of phospholipids, glycolipids, cholesterol (adds structural rigidity to the cell membrane), proteins of various sizes and carbohydrates
- Function of cell membrane: Cell membrane plays a critical role in virtually every aspect of cell function.

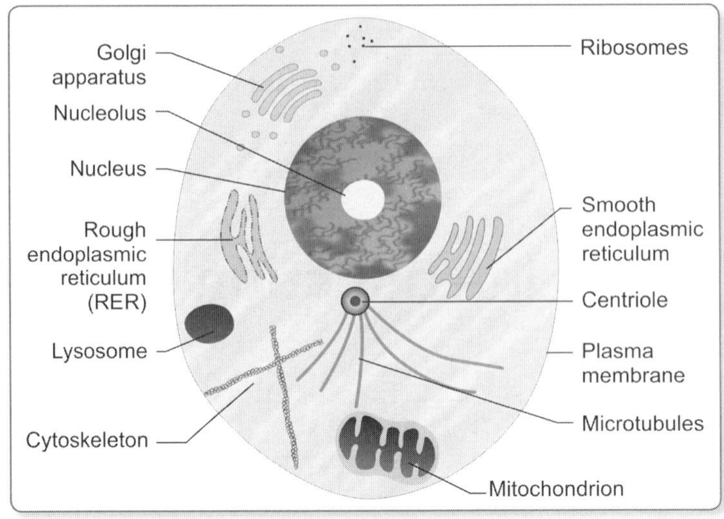

Fig. 1.1: Various constituents of cell.

B) *Cytoplasm*

- Cytoplasm or cytosol is the component of the cell, located between the nucleus and the cell membrane
- Light microscopy: Various products of cell metabolism may be seen in the cytoplasm, and appear as granules or vacuoles.

Cytoplasmic Organelles

Ultrastructurally, the cytoplasm is composed of: 1) organized cell components, or organelles, 2) the cytoskeleton, and 3) a cytoplasmic matrix.

Organized components of the cytoplasm: They mainly consists of: i) membranous systems, ii) ribosomes, iii) mitochondria, iv) lysosomes, and v) centrioles.

i. **Membranous System**: It is composed of: a) the endoplasmic reticulum, and b) the Golgi complex.
   a. **Endoplasmic reticulum**:
      - Appearance: It is a closed system of unit membranes forming tubular canals and flattened sacs or cisternae. It subdivides the cytoplasm into a series of compartments
      - Types: The membranes of the endoplasmic reticulum may be "**rough,**" i.e. **rough endoplasmic reticulum (RER)** [i.e. covered with numerous attached granules composed of ribonucleic acid (RNA) and proteins], or "**smooth**" i.e. **smooth endoplasmic reticulum (SER)** (i.e. free of any particles)
      - Function: Rough endoplasmic reticulum is abundant in metabolically active cells.
   b. **Golgi complex**:
      - Appearance: It consists of a series of parallel, doughnut-shaped flat spaces or cisternae and spherical or egg-shaped vesicles demarcated by smooth membranes
      - Location: In epithelial cells with secretory function, it is usually located between the nucleus and the luminal surface of the cells
      - Function: They synthesize and package cell products for the cells' own use and for export.

ii. **Ribosomes**
   - They are found in all cells
   - Appearance: They are submicroscopic particles composed of RNA and proteins in approximately equal proportions
   - Two types of ribosomes namely free and attached
   - Functions:
     - Free ribosomes produce proteins for the cell's own use
     - Attached ribosomes produce proteins for export.

iii. **Mitochondria**
   - They are present in all eukaryotic cells
   - Appearance:
     - Mitochondria are small, usually elongated structures that vary in size and configuration according to the nutritional status of an organ
     - Each mitochondrion is composed of two membranes. The outer membrane is a continuous, closed-unit membrane. Running parallel to the outer membrane is the inner membrane that forms numerous crests or invaginations.
   - Function: Most important function is the formation of energy-producing adenosine triphosphate (ATP) from phosphorus and adenosine diphosphate (ADP). ATP is exported into the cytoplasm and is an essential source of energy for the cell
   - Mitochondria possess their own DNA that is independent of nuclear DNA.

iv. **Lysosomes**
   - Lysosomes are intracellular organelles that contain degradative enzymes
   - Appearance: Electron microscopically, lysosomes appear as spherical or oval structures of heterogeneous density and variable diameter
   - Function:
     i. Lysosomal enzymes performs the digestion of a wide-range of macromolecules, including proteins, polysaccharides, lipids, and nucleic acids.
     ii. They participate in the removal of phagocytized foreign material.
     iii. Play an important role in certain storage diseases (lysosomal storage disorders).

v. **Centrioles**
   - Appearance: They are short tubular structures, usually located in the vicinity of the concave face of the Golgi complex
   - Function: Play a key role during cell division.

Cytoskeleton

- The skeleton of the cells, and hence, the ability of cells to maintain the particular physical shape, maintain polarity, movement of cells, and organize the relationship of intracellular organelles is provided by a family of fibrillar proteins
- This intracellular scaffolding of fibrillar proteins is called the cytoskeleton
- Types: In eukaryotic cells, there are three major types of cytoskeletal proteins: the actin filaments (microfilaments, tonofilaments), intermediate filaments, and microtubules.

  i. **Actin microfilaments**
     - They interact with many other proteins that regulate their length
     - Electron microscopy: They appear as bundles of longitudinal cytoplasmic filaments crisscrossing the cytoplasm and often converging on specific targets such as desmosomes

  - Functions: Actin microfilaments perform several essential functions within cells as linkage filaments coordinating the activity of divergent cell components.
- **ii. Intermediate filaments**
  - Appearance: They were initially identified in electron microscopy because of their diameter (7 to 11 nm); hence, intermediate filaments (IFs). They are larger than actin microfilaments and smaller than microtubules
  - Functions: Individual types of IFs have characteristic tissue-specific patterns of expression. This can be used for identifying cell of origin of poorly differentiated tumors.
- **iii. Microtubules**
  - They are 25-nm-thick fibrils and appear as hollow, tube-like structures
  - Functions: Microtubules are an integral component of cilia, flagella, and centrioles. Thus, they participate in cellular events requiring motion.

Cytoplasmic matrix

- The space within the cytoplasm, not occupied by the membranous system, the cell skeleton, or by the organelles, is called as the cytoplasmic matrix. It is composed of proteins and free ribosomes.

C) *Nucleus*

- It is present within the cytoplasm
- Nuclear membrane: It is a smaller, approximately spherical dense structure enclosed within the nuclear membrane, or nuclear envelope
- Content: It contains mainly deoxyribonucleic acid (DNA) that governs the genetic and functional aspects of cell activity
- Nucleolus: In normal resting nuclei, the nucleoli are seen as round or oval structures occupying a small area within the nucleus.

INTRODUCTION TO PATHOLOGY

Definition: Pathology is the **scientific study (logos) of disease (pathos)**. It mainly focuses on the study of the structural and functional changes in cells, tissues, and organs in disease.

Learning Pathology

Study of pathology can be divided into general pathology and systemic pathology.

- **General pathology:** It deals with the study of mechanism, basic reactions of cells and tissues to abnormal stimuli and to inherited defects.
- **Systemic pathology:** This deals with the changes in specific diseases/responses of specialized organs and tissues.

Scientific Study of Disease

Disease process is studied under following aspects:

Etiology

The etiology of a disease is its **cause**. The causative factors of a disease can be divided into two major categories: genetic and acquired (e.g. infectious, chemical, hypoxia, nutritional, physical). Most common diseases are multifactorial due to combination of causes.

Pathogenesis

It refers to the **mechanism** by which the causative factor/s produces structural and functional abnormalities. Pathogenesis deals with sequence of events that occur in the cells or tissues from the beginning of any disease process. With the present advances in technology, it is possible to identify the changes occurring at molecular level and this knowledge is helpful for designing new therapeutic approaches.

- **Latent period:** Few causative agents produce signs and symptoms of the disease immediately after exposure. Usually, etiological agents takes **some time to manifest the disease** (e.g. carcinogenesis) and this time period is called as the latent period. It varies depending on the disease.
- **Incubation period:** In disorders caused by infectious (due to bacteria, viruses, etc.) agents, the **period between exposure and the development of disease** is called the incubation period. It usually ranges from days to weeks. Most of the infectious agents have characteristic incubation period.

Morphologic Changes

All diseases start with structural changes in cells. **Rudolf Virchow** (known as the **father of modern pathology**) proposed that injury to the cell is the basis of all diseases. Morphologic changes refer to the **gross and microscopic structural changes** in cells or tissues affected by disease.

Gross

Many diseases have characteristic gross pathology and a fairly confident diagnosis can be given before light microscopy. For example, serous cystadenoma of ovary usually consists of one cystic cavity containing serous fluid; cirrhosis of liver is characterized by total replacement of liver by regenerating nodules.

Microscopy

Light microscopy: Abnormalities in tissue architecture and morphological changes in cells can be studied by light microscopy.

- **Histopathology:** Sections are routinely cut from tissues and processed by pararffin-embedding. The sections are cut from the tissue by a special instrument called microtome and examined under light microscope. In certain situations (e.g. histochemistry, rapid diagnosis), sections are cut from tissue that has been hardened rapidly by freezing (frozen section). The sections are stained routinely by hematoxylin and eosin.
  - **Pathognomonic abnormalities:** If the **structural changes are characteristic of a single disease or diagnostic of an etiologic process** it is called as **pathognomonic.** Pathognomonic features are those features which are restricted to a single disease, or disease category. The diagnosis should not be made without them. For example, **Aschoff bodies** are pathognomonic of **rheumatic heart disease** and **Reed Sternberg cells** are pathognomonic of **Hodgkin lymphoma.**
- **Cytology:** The cells from cysts, body cavities, or scraped from body surfaces or aspirated by fine needle from solid lesions can also be studied under light microscope. This study of cells is known as cytology and is used widely, especially in diagnosis and screening of cancer.
- **Histochemistry (special stains):** Histochemistry (refer Table 2.7) is the study of the chemistry of tissues, where tissue/cells are treated with specific reagent so that the features of individual cells/structure can be visualized, e.g. **Prussian blue reaction for hemosiderin.**
- **Immunohistochemistry and immunofluorescence:** Immunohistochemistry and immunofluorescence utilize antibodies (immunoglobulins with antigen specificity) to visualize substances in tissue sections or cell preparations. Former uses **monoclonal antibodies** linked chemically to enzymes and later **fluorescent dyes.**

Electron microscopy: Electron microscopy (EM) is useful to the study changes at ultrastructural level, and to the demonstration of viruses in tissue samples in certain diseases. The most common diagnostic use of EM is for the interpretation of biopsy specimen from kidney.

Molecular Pathology

Most of the diseases can be diagnosed by the morphological changes in tissues. But, with the present advances in diagnostic pathology, the diseases can be analyzed by the molecular and immunological approaches. Molecular pathology has revealed the biochemical basis of many diseases, mainly congenital disorders and cancer. These techniques can detect changes in a single nucleotide of DNA. *In situ* hybridization can detect the presence of specific genes or their messenger RNA in tissue sections or cell preparations. Minute quantities of nucleic acids can be amplified by the use of the polymerase chain reaction. DNA microarrays can be used to determine patterns of gene expression (mRNA).

Functional Derangements and Clinical Manifestations

- **Functional derangements:** The effects of genetic, biochemical, and structural changes in cells and tissues are **functional abnormalities**. For example, excessive secretion of a cell product (e.g. nasal mucus in the common cold); insufficient secretion of a cell product (e.g. insulin lack in diabetes mellitus).
- **Clinical manifestations:** The functional derangements produce two clinical manifestations of disease, namely symptoms and signs. Diseases characterized by **multiple abnormalities** (symptom complex) are called syndromes.
- **Prognosis:** The prognosis forecasts (predicts) the known or likely **course (outcome) of the disease**, and therefore, the fate of the patient.
- **Complications:** It is a **negative pathologic process** or event occurring **during the disease** which is not an essential part of the disease. It usually aggravates the illness. For example, perforation and hemorrhage are complications which may develop in typhoid ulcer of intestine.

Chapter 2

Cell Injury

Chapter Outline

- Types of cellular responses to injury
- Cellular adaptations
- Cell injury
- Necrosis
- Apoptosis
- Pathologic calcification
- Hyaline change
- Pigments

TYPES OF CELLULAR RESPONSES TO INJURY

Depending on the nature of stimulus/injury, cellular responses can be mainly divided into four types (Fig. 2.1).

1. Cellular adaptations
2. Cell injury
   - Reversible cell injury
   - Irreversible cell injury
3. Intracellular accumulations
4. Pathologic calcification.

CELLULAR ADAPTATIONS

When the cell is exposed to pathological stimuli, the cells can achieve a **new, steady altered state that allows them to survive** and continue to function in an abnormal environment. These are reversible changes and constitute **cellular adaptations**.

Types of adaptations (Fig. 2.2)**:** Hypertrophy, hyperplasia, atrophy and metaplasia.

Hypertrophy

Q. Write short note on hypertrophy.

Definition: Increase in the size of the tissue or organ due to increase in the size of cells.

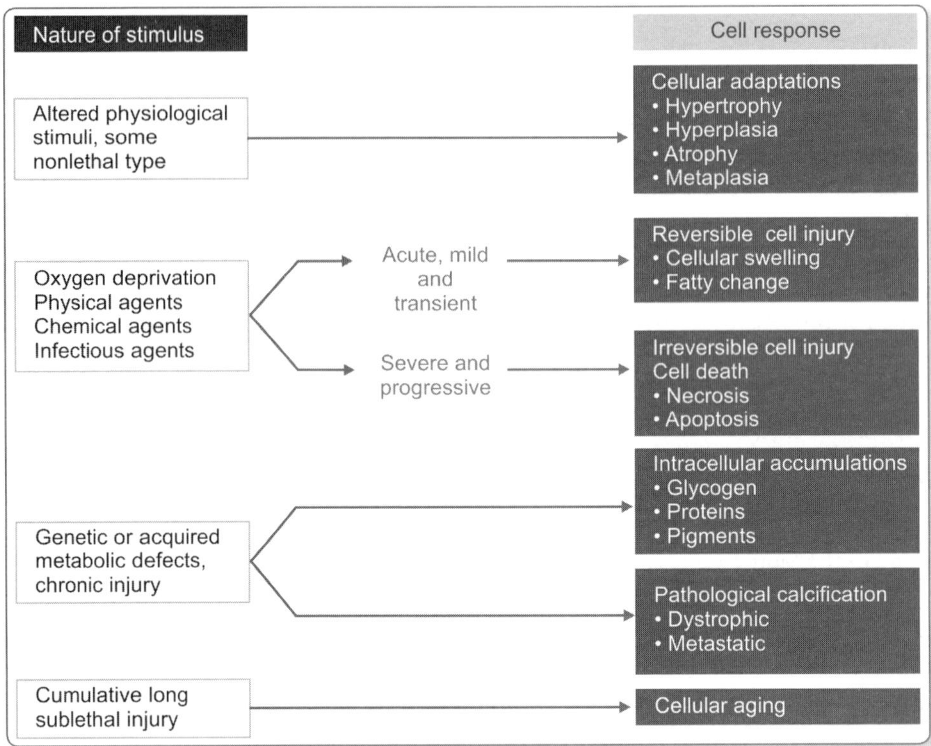

Fig. 2.1: Types of cellular responses to stimuli/injury

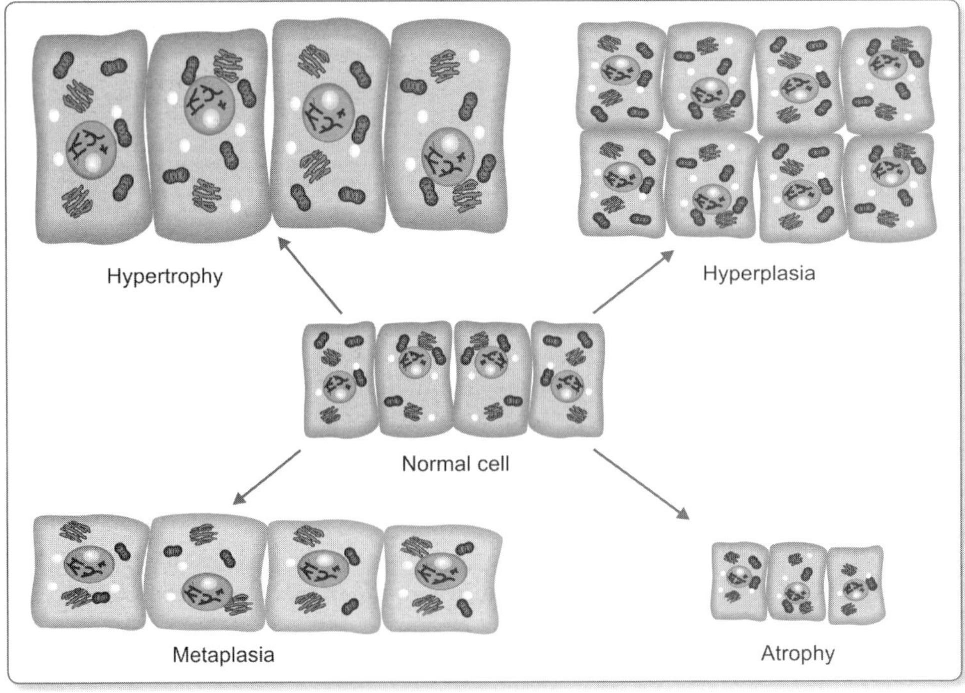

Fig. 2.2: Different types of cellular adaptations

Causes

Increased functional demand/workload.

- **Physiological:**
  - **Hypertrophy of skeletal muscle,** e.g. the bulging muscles of body builders and athletes.
  - **Hypertrophy of smooth muscle,** e.g. growth of the uterus during pregnancy from estrogenic stimulation.
- **Pathological:**
  - **Hypertrophy of cardiac muscle,** e.g. left ventricular hypertrophy (Fig. 2.3) due to hypertension or damaged valves (aortic stenosis, mitral incompetence).
  - **Hypertrophy of smooth muscle,** e.g. hypertrophy of urinary bladder muscle in response to urethral obstruction (e.g. prostate hyperplasia, Fig. 2.4), hypertrophy of muscular layer of stomach due to pyloric stenosis.

Mechanisms of Cellular Hypertrophy

Hypertrophy is due to increased synthesis of cellular proteins. Steps involved in biochemical mechanisms of myocardial (cardiac muscle) hypertrophy are:

1. Activation of the Signal Transduction Pathways

Various mechanisms involved are:

Physiologic Hypertrophy

- **Mechanical stretch:** Increased work load on the myocardium produces mechanical stretch and is the major trigger for physiological hypertrophy.

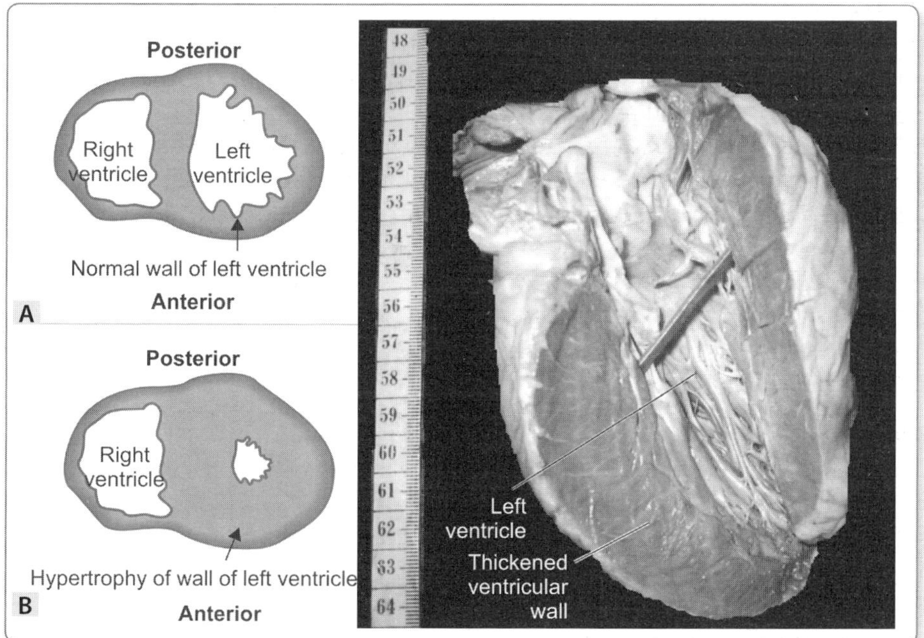

Figs 2.3A to C: A. Transverse section of normal heart; B. Transverse section of heart with thickening of wall of the left ventricle due to hypertrophy; C. Longitudinal section of heart with left ventricular hypertrophy

Pathologic Hypertrophy

Growth factors and hypertrophy agonists are involved in pathologic hypertrophy.

- **Growth factors:** These include (TGF-β), insulin-like growth factor-1 (IGF-1), and fibroblast growth factor (FGF)
- **Hypertrophy agonists:** These include α-adrenergic agonists, endothelin-I, angiotensin II, nitric oxide (NO), and bradykinin.

Mechanical sensors also stimulate production of growth factors and agonists. They cause increased synthesis of muscle proteins.

2. Activation of Transcription Factors

Mechanical stretch, growth factors and hypertrophy agonists activate the signal transduction pathways and transcription factors (e.g. Myc, Fos, Jun).

Morphology

- **Gross:** Involved **organ is enlarged**
- **Microscopy: Increase** in **size of the cells** as well as the **nuclei**.

Hyperplasia

Q. Define hyperplasia and give examples.

Q. Write short note on hyperplasia.

Q. Write short note on pathological hyperplasia.

Definition: Increase in the number of cells in an organ or tissue, resulting in **increased size/ mass of the organ or tissue**.

Causes

- **Physiological hyperplasia:** Hormonal stimulation, or as compensatory process
  - **Hyperplasia due to hormones,** e.g. hyperplasia of glandular epithelium of the **female breast at puberty, pregnancy and lactation**, hyperplasia of the uterus during pregnancy from estrogenic stimulation
  - **Compensatory hyperplasia,** e.g. in liver following partial hepatectomy.
- **Pathological hyperplasia,** Due to **excess** endocrine stimulation or chronic injury/irritation.
  - **Excessive hormonal stimulation,** e.g. endometrial hyperplasia (due to estrogen) and benign prostatic hyperplasia {due to androgens (Figs 2.4A and B)}
  - **Chronic injury/irritation,** Long-standing inflammation or chronic injury may lead to hyperplasia, especially in skin or oral mucosa.

Pathological hyperplasia can progress to cancer, e.g. **endometrial hyperplasia can develop into endometrial cancer**.

Mechanism

- Hyperplasia is characterized by cell proliferation mostly of mature cell mediated **through stimulation by growth factor or hormones**
- **In some instances,** the new cells may be derived from tissue **stem cells**.

Morphology

- **Gross: Size** of the affected organ is **increased**
- **Microscopy:** Increased number of cells with increased number of mitotic figures.

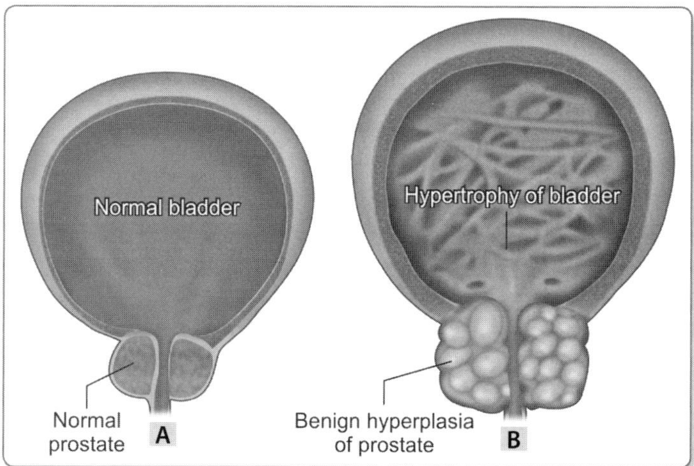

Figs 2.4A and B: Cut section of prostate along with urinary bladder. A. Normal prostate; B. Enlarged prostate due to nodular hyperplasia. The urinary outflow obstruction results in hypertrophy of bladder muscle

Atrophy

Q. Write short note on atrophy.

Definition: Atrophy is the **reduced size of an organ or tissue** resulting from a decrease in cell size and number.

Causes

Physiological atrophy: Common during normal fetal development, and in adult life.

- During fetal development, e.g. atrophy of embryonic structures such as thyroglossal duct
- During adult life, e.g. involution of thymus, atrophy of brain and heart due to aging (senile atrophy).

Pathological atrophy: Local or generalized.

1. **Local**
   - **Disuse atrophy (decreased workload),** e.g. atrophy of limb muscles immobilized in a plaster cast (as treatment for fracture) or after prolonged bed rest
   - **Denervation (loss of innervation) atrophy,** e.g. atrophy of muscle due to damage to the nerves (e.g. poliomyelitis)
   - **Ischemic (diminished blood supply) atrophy,** e.g. brain atrophy produced by ischemia due to atherosclerosis of the carotid artery
   - **Pressure atrophy,** e.g. atrophy of renal parenchyma in hydronephrosis due to increased pressure.
2. **Generalized**
   - **Starvation (inadequate nutrition) atrophy,** e.g. protein-calorie malnutrition.

Mechanisms

Atrophic cells have diminished function. There is **decreased protein synthesis and increased protein degradation** in cells.

Morphology

- **Gross:** The **organ is small and often shrunken**
- **Microscopy:** The **cells are smaller in size** due to reduction in cell organelles.

Metaplasia

Q. Define metaplasia and give examples.

Q. Write short note on metaplasia.

Definition: Metaplasia is a reversible change in which **one adult cell type is replaced by another adult cell type**.

Causes

- Metaplasia is usually **fully reversible adaptive response** to **chronic persistent injury**. If the noxious stimulus is removed (e.g. cessation of smoking), the metaplastic epithelium may return to normal.
- Metaplasia is mainly **seen in association with tissue damage, repair, and regeneration**.
- The **replacing cell type** is usually **more suited to a change in environment**.

Types of Metaplasia

Epithelial Metaplasia

Most common type

Squamous metaplasia: Original epithelium is replaced by squamous epithelium.

- **Respiratory tract:** e.g. chronic irritation due to tobacco smoke, the normal ciliated columnar epithelial cells of the trachea and bronchi undergo squamous metaplasia (Fig. 2.5).
- **Cervix:** Squamous metaplasia in cervix is associated with chronic infection.

Columnar metaplasia: Original epithelium is replaced by columnar epithelium.

- **Squamous to columnar: In Barrett esophagus, the squamous epithelium of the esophagus is replaced by columnar cells.**
- **Intestinal metaplasia:** The gastric glands are replaced by cells resembling those of the small intestine.

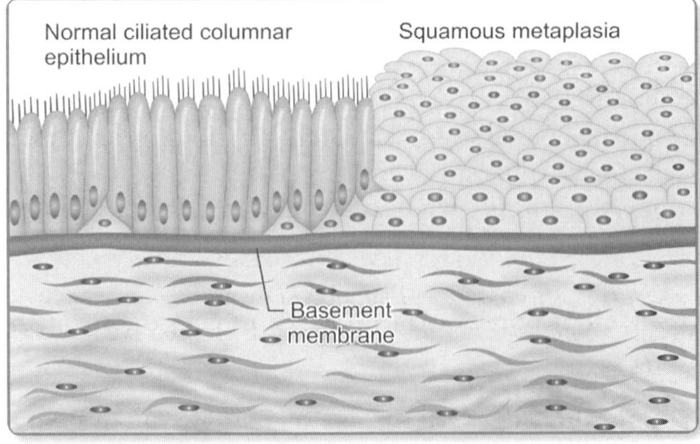

Fig. 2.5: Squamous metaplasia in which columnar epithelium (left) is replaced by squamous epithelium (right)

Connective Tissue Metaplasia

- **Osseous metaplasia:** Formation of new bone at sites of tissue injury is known as osseous metaplasia. Bone formation in muscle, known as **myositis ossificans**, occasionally occurs after intramuscular hemorrhage.

Mechanism

Develops due to the **reprogramming of precursor cells** (i.e. stem cells or undifferentiated mesenchymal cells) that are present in normal tissues.

CELL INJURY

Causes of Cell Injury

Q. Write short note on causes of cell injury.

A. **Hypoxia:** It refers to **inadequate oxygenation of tissue**. It is the **most common cause of cell injury**.

   Causes of hypoxia:
   - **Decreased blood flow** is called **ischemia**. It may be due to thrombosis, embolism, atherosclerosis or external compression of vessel
   - Inadequate oxygenation of the blood (hypoxemia)
     - Due to pulmonary disease
     - Decreased perfusion of tissues, e.g. cardiac failure, hypotension shock
     - Decreased oxygen-carrying capacity of the blood, e.g. anemia
     - Severe blood loss.

   Mechanism of injury: Hypoxia causes cell injury by reducing aerobic oxidative respiration and decreasing the synthesis of adenosine triphosphate (ATP).

   Outcome: Depending on the severity of the hypoxia, cells may adapt, undergo injury, or die.

B. **Physical Agents:**
   - Mechanical trauma, e.g. blunt/penetrating/crush injuries, gunshot wounds
   - Thermal injury: Extremes of temperature (burns and deep cold)
   - Radiation (ionizing radiation and non-ionizing radiation)
   - Electric shock
   - Pressure changes: Sudden changes in atmospheric pressure.

C. **Chemical Agents:**
   - Heavy metals and poisons, e.g. arsenic, mercuric salts or cyanide
   - Simple chemicals, e.g. hypertonic concentrations of glucose or salt
   - Strong acids and alkalies
   - Oxygen at high concentrations is toxic
   - Environmental and air pollutants, e.g. insecticides, and herbicides
   - Industrial and occupational hazards (carbon monoxide and asbestos)
   - Social/lifestyle choices: Addiction to drugs and alcohol, cigarette smoking
   - Therapeutic drugs.

D. **Infectious Agents:** Viruses, bacteria, fungi, rickettsiae and parasites. The mechanism by which these infectious agents cause injury varies.

E. **Immunologic Reactions**
   - **Autoimmunity:** Immune reactions to endogenous self-antigens are responsible for autoimmune diseases.
   - **Hypersensitivity reactions and other immune reactions:** Heightened immune reactions to many external agents (e.g. microbes and environmental agents).

F. **Genetic Derangements:** Genetic defects may cause cell injury because of
   - Deficiency of functional proteins (e.g. enzyme defects in inborn errors of metabolism)
   - Accumulation of damaged DNA or misfolded proteins
   - Variations in the genetic makeup.

G. **Nutritional Imbalances:**
   - **Nutritional deficiencies:**
     - Protein-calorie deficiencies
     - Deficiencies of specific vitamins.
   - **Nutritional excesses:**
     - Excess of cholesterol predisposes to atherosclerosis
     - Obesity is associated with increased incidence of several important diseases, such as diabetes and cancer
     - Hypervitaminosis.

H. **Idiopathic:** Cause is not known.

General Principles of Cell Injury

1. **Cellular response to injury:** It **depends on:** a) type of injury, b) duration of injury and c) severity of injury.
2. **Consequences of injury:** It **depends on:** a) type of cell involved, b) adaptability of cell, c) status of cell and 4) genetic makeup of the cell.
3. **Targets and biochemical mechanism of cell injury:** These include a) mitochondrial damage/dysfunction, b) disturbance of calcium homeostasis, c) damage to cellular membranes and d) damage to DNA and misfolding of proteins.

Mechanisms of Cell Injury

Injurious stimuli that cause cell injury lead to complex cellular, biochemical and molecular changes. Certain mechanism is common for most forms of cell injury and cell death.

Decreased Production of Adenosine Triphosphate (ATP)

ATP is required for all processes within the cell. Injury like hypoxia, chemicals (e.g. cyanide) can cause **decreased production of ATP.**

- **Effects of decreased ATP (Fig. 2.6):**
  - **Failure of the cell membrane sodium pump**
  - **Increased anaerobic glycolysis**
  - **Failure of the calcium pump**
  - **Failure of protein synthesis in the ribosomes.**

Mitochondrial Damage (Fig. 2.7)

- Mitochondria are sensitive to almost all types of injurious stimuli (e.g. hypoxia, toxins).

Consequences of Mitochondrial Damage

1. **Depletion of ATP:** Its effects are mentioned above.
2. **Formation of reactive oxygen species (ROS):** Its effects are mentioned on page 18 (refer Fig. 2.10).

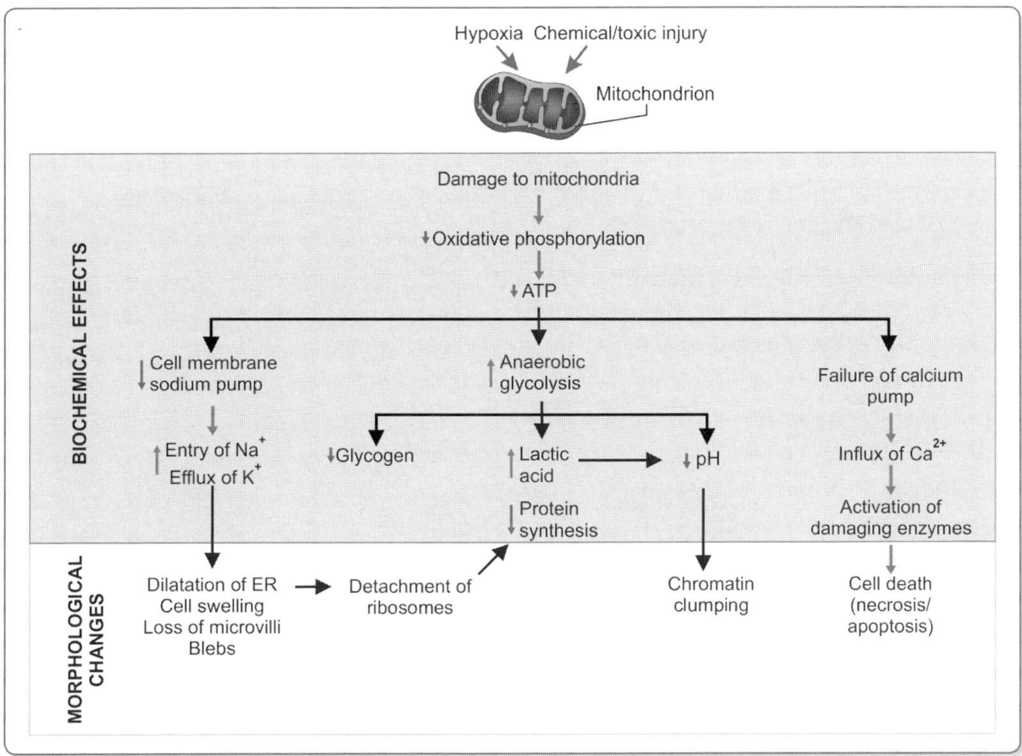

Fig. 2.6: Biochemical and morphological changes due to decreased ATP production

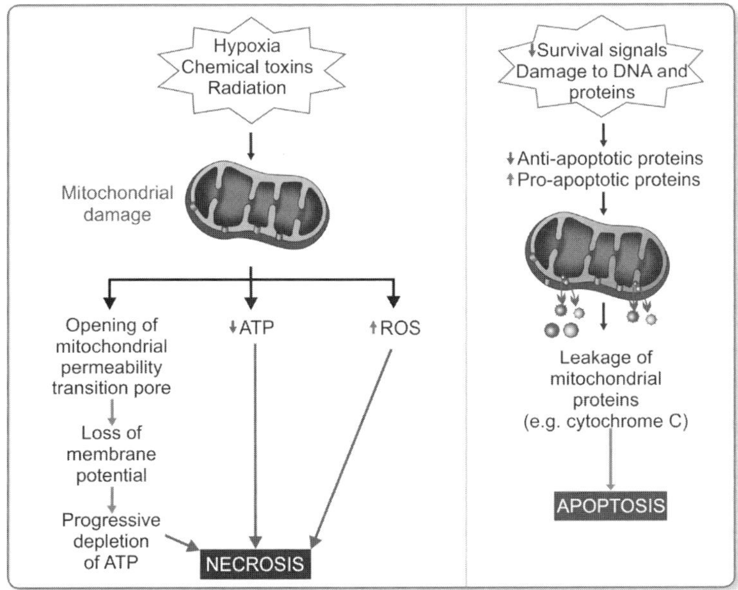

Fig. 2.7: Effects of mitochondrial damage

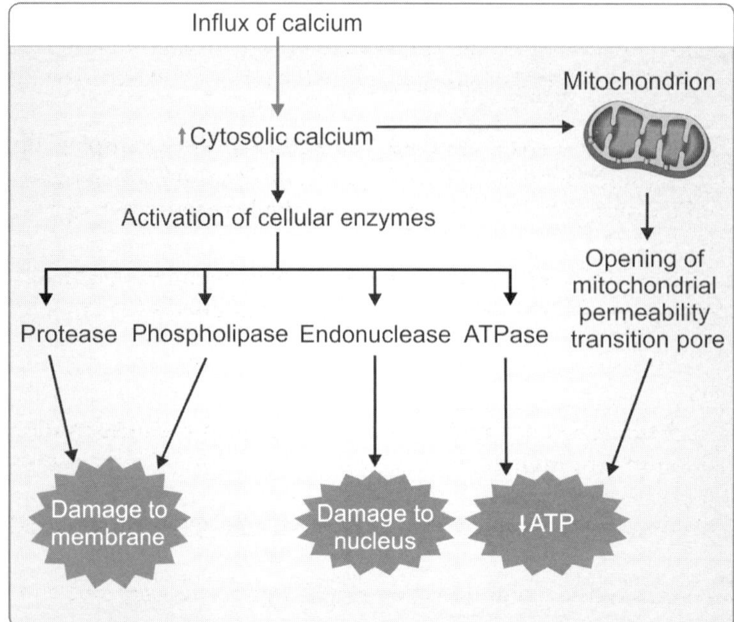

Fig. 2.8: Effects of increased cytosolic calcium in cell injury

Fig. 2.9: Formation of free radical

3. **Formation of mitochondrial permeability transition pore:** It occurs in the mitochondrial membrane. This leads to the **loss of mitochondrial membrane potential, pH changes** and **progressive depletion of ATP** and ultimately **necrosis** of the cell.
4. **Leakage of mitochondrial proteins into cytoplasm:** The mitochondrial membranes contain many proteins **such as cytochrome C and proapoptotic proteins (e.g. Bax and Bak)**. Increased permeability of the mitochondrial membrane may result in leakage of these proteins into the cytosol and induce **apoptosis**.

Influx of Calcium and Loss of Calcium Homeostasis (Fig. 2.8)

Normally, concentration of cytosolic calcium is very low and most of it is sequestered in mitochondria and the endoplasmic reticulum (ER). Ischemia and certain toxins cause an increase in cytoslic calcium. Initially, it is due to the release from intracellular stores and later due to influx across the cell membrane. Increased intracellular calcium stimulates **activation of several damaging enzymes** (e.g. phospholipases, endonucleases, and protease) as well as caspases. The **net result is apoptosis**.

Accumulation of Oxygen-derived Free Radicals (Oxidative Stress)

Free radicals are **unstable chemical compounds** with a **single unpaired electron in an outer orbit (Fig. 2.9)**.

Properties of Free Radicals

- Normally, **free radicals** produced in the cells are **unstable** and are **rapidly destroyed**
- When free radicals react with any molecules they convert those molecules into free radicals and thus initiate **autocatalytic reactions**.
- **Excess** of free radicals may be either **due to increased production or ineffective degradation**.

Types of Free Radicals

- **Oxygen derived free radicals:** Reactive oxygen species (ROS) are oxygen-derived free radicals. ROS includes superoxide anion ($O_2^{\bullet}$), hydrogen peroxide (H_2O_2) and hydroxyl ions ($^{\bullet}OH$).
- **Reactive nitrogen species/nitric oxide (NO) derived free radicals:** For example, nitric oxide (NO) is generated by endothelial cells, macrophages, neurons, and other types of cells. NO can act as a free radical and can also be converted to highly reactive peroxynitrite anion ($ONOO^-$), NO_2 and NO_3^-.
- **Free radicals from drug and chemical:** Enzymatic metabolism of exogenous chemicals or drugs can generate free radicals which are not ROS but have similar effects (e.g. CCl_4 can generate CCl_3).

Mechanism of Production of ROS

1. **In all cells (Fig. 2.10):** ROS are produced normally in **small amounts in the mitochondria** during the reduction-oxidation (redox) reactions occurring during mitochondrial respiration and production of energy.
   - During redox reaction **superoxide ($O_2^{\bullet}$)** is produced when oxygen (O_2) is only partially reduced
   - Superoxide **($O_2^{\bullet}$)** is converted to **hydrogen peroxide (H_2O_2)** spontaneously and by the action of the enzyme superoxide dismutase (SOD)
   - Hydrogen peroxide (H_2O_2) in the presence of metals (e.g. Fe^{2+}) is converted by Fenton reaction to a highly reactive free radical called **hydroxyl radial ($^{\bullet}OH$)**

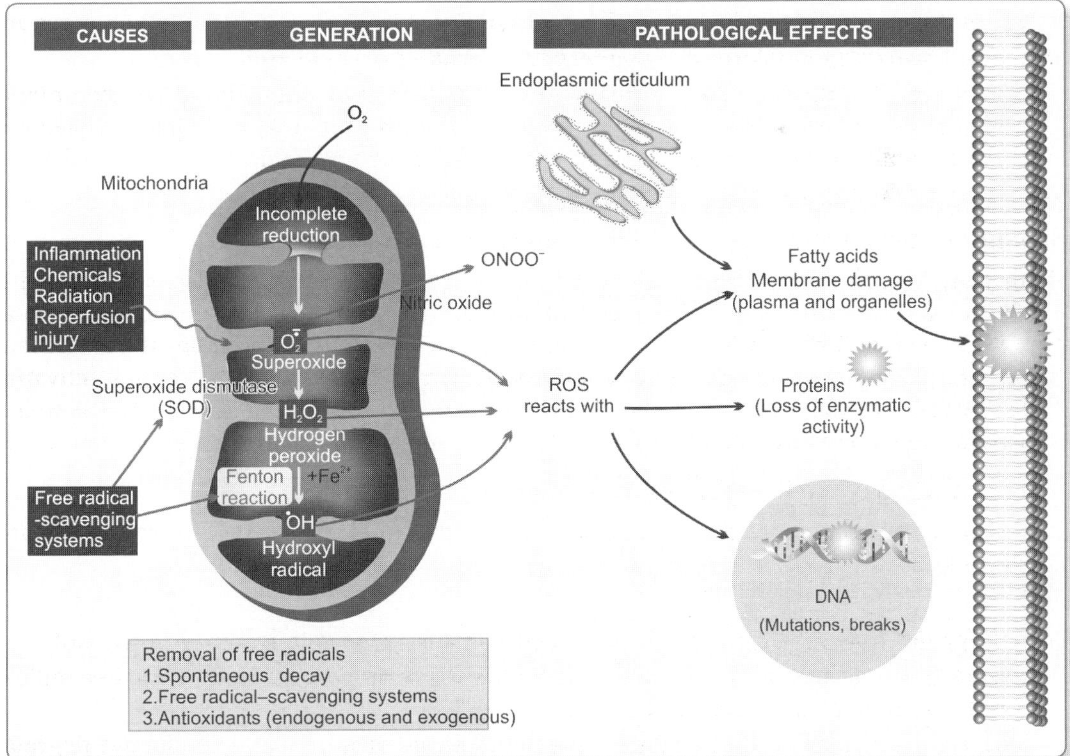

Fig. 2.10: Production of reactive oxygen species in mitochondria of cells and effects in cell injury

- Superoxide ($O_2^{\bar{\bullet}}$) is also converted to peroxynitrite ($ONOO^-$) in the presence of nitric oxide (NO).

2. **In phagocytic leukocytes (Fig. 2.11):** ROS produced to destroy the ingested microbes and other substances produced during inflammation.
   - During phagocytosis **ROS produced in the phagosomes and phagolysosomes** formed in the leukocytes (mainly neutrophils and macrophages) by a process similar to mitochondrial respiration. This process is called as **respiratory burst**
   - Superoxide ($O_2^{\bar{\bullet}}$) is synthesized via NADPH (nicotinamide adenine dinucleotide phosphate/respiratory burst oxidase) oxidase (phagocyte oxidase) present in the phagosome and phagolysosomal membrane of the leukocytes
   - Superoxide ($O_2^{\bar{\bullet}}$) is converted to **hydrogen peroxide (H_2O_2)**
   - Hydrogen peroxide (H_2O_2) in the presence of myeloperoxidase enzyme is converted to **highly reactive compound hypochlorite (HOCl).**

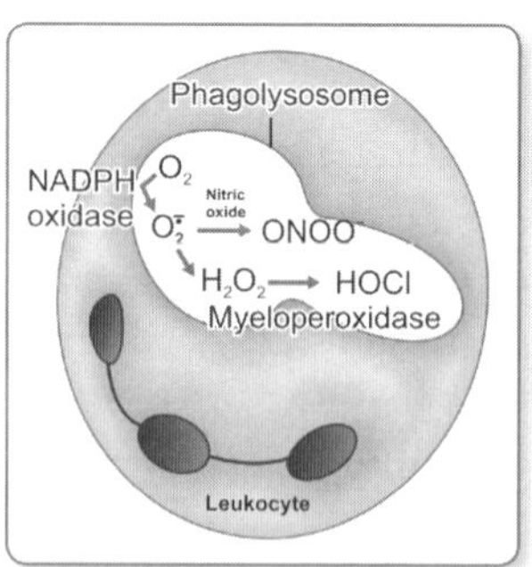

Fig. 2.11: Production of reactive oxygen species in leukocytes

Conditions Associated with Increased Generation of Oxygen-derived Free Radicals

- During inflammation and microbial killing by phagocytes
- Drugs and chemical injury, including chemical carcinogens
- Radiation injury (e.g. ultraviolet light, X-rays)
- Reduction-oxidation reactions
- Ischemia-reperfusion injury induced by restoration of blood flow in ischemic tissue
- Transition metals such as iron and copper donate or accept free electrons during intracellular reactions and catalyze free radical formation, as in the Fenton reaction ($H_2O_2 + Fe^{2+} \rightarrow Fe^{3+} + OH + OH^-$)
- Cellular aging.

Mechanisms of Removal/Neutralization of Free Radicals

Serum, tissue fluids, and host cells have **antioxidant mechanisms,** which protect against potentially harmful oxygen-derived radicals (Table 2.1). These include:

- **Spontaneous decay**
- **Free radical–scavenging systems**
  - Enzyme **catalase** neutralize peroxidase (H_2O_2) free radicals by converting it into water and oxygen
  - Enzyme **superoxide dismutases** (SODs) neutralizes superoxide free radicals by converting it into hydrogen peroxide.
  - Enzyme **glutathione peroxidase** (enhances glutathione) neutralizes peroxidase (H_2O_2), hydroxyl and acetaminophen free radicals.

Table 2.1: Various types of antioxidants

Enzymatic antioxidants	Non-enzymatic antioxidants
• Superoxide dismutase (SOD) • Catalase • Glutathione peroxidase	• Exogenous: Vitamin E, vitamin A, ascorbic acid and sulfhydryl containing compounds (e.g. cysteine and glutathione)
	• Endogenous: Serum proteins such as transferrin, ferritin, albumin and ceruloplasmin

- **Exogenous antioxidants:** For example, vitamins E, vitamin A, ascorbic acid and glutathione
- **Endogenous antioxidants:** Iron and copper are reactive metals, which can catalyze the formation of ROS. Their activities are minimized by binding of these ions to storage and transport proteins (e.g. transferrin, ferritin and ceruloplasmin).

Pathologic Effects of Free Radicals (Fig. 2.12)

Free radicals can cause cell injury in many diseases. Free radicals can activate both **necrosis** and **apoptosis**. Various effects of free radicals are:
- **Lipid peroxidation in membranes** causes extensive membrane damage
- **Cross-linking and oxidative modification of proteins** damages the enzyme activity and causes abnormal folding of proteins
- **Damage to DNA.**

Effects of Cell Injury

Defects in Membrane Permeability and Membrane Damage

- **Reversible injury:** In most forms of cell injury, in the early phase there is selective loss of membrane permeability
- **Irreversible injury:** With the obvious membrane damage, the cell cannot return to normal.

For differences between reversible injury and irreversible injuries see Table 2.3.

Mechanisms of Membrane Damage

- **Indirect damage**
  - **Reactive oxygen species (ROS):** It causes injury to cell membranes by **lipid peroxidation**
  - **Decreased phospholipid synthesis: Hypoxia** through defective mitochondrial function → decreases the production of ATP by **ischemic cells** → leads to decreased phospholipid synthesis in all cellular membranes (including the mitochondria) and energy-dependent enzymatic activities
  - **Increased phospholipid breakdown:** Severe cell injury increases levels of **cytosolic and mitochondrial Ca^{2+}** → results in **calcium-mediated activation** of endogenous **phospholipases** → which degrades membrane phospholipids → leads to the accumulation of **lipid breakdown products** → cause membrane damage
  - **Cytoskeletal damage:** Cytoskeletal filaments connect the plasma membrane to the cell interior. **Increased cytosolic calcium activates proteases** which may **damage the cytoskeletal elements** and **cell membrane**.
- **Direct damage:** The plasma membrane can also be damaged directly by various bacterial toxins, viral proteins, lytic complement components, and a variety of physical and chemical agents.

Consequences of Membrane Damage

Cell injury may damage any membrane, but most important are:
- **Mitochondrial membrane damage:** It results in:
  - Opening of the **mitochondrial permeability transition pore** leading to decreased ATP
  - Release of proteins that trigger apoptotic death.
- **Plasma membrane damage:** It leads to **loss** of:
  - **Osmotic balance** and influx of fluids and ions
  - Cellular contents.
- **Lysosomal membrane damage:** It leads to:
  - **Leakage of lysosomal enzymes** into the cytoplasm
  - **Activation of lysosomal enzymes** → which results in digestion of proteins, RNA, DNA, and glycogen → leads to cell death by necrosis.

Damage to DNA and Proteins

- **Causes of DNA damage:** Exposure to DNA damaging drugs, radiation, or oxidative stress.
- **Repair mechanism:** Cells have mechanisms to repair DNA damage. However, if the damage is too severe to be corrected, the cell initiates a suicide program causing death by apoptosis.

Types of Cell Injury

Two types: **Reversible and irreversible**. Reversible injury may progress to an irreversible stage and result in cell death.

Reversible Cell Injury

If the stimulus is acute and brief or mild, the cell injury produces changes in the cells which are reversible up to a certain point.

Light microscope features of reversible cell injury: Two patterns of reversible cell injury, namely cellular swelling and fatty change.

- **Cellular (hydropic) swelling:** It is due to changes in ion concentrations and fluid homeostasis. There is an increased flow of water into the cells which results in increased water content of injured cells
- **Steatosis (fatty change)** explained below.

Cloudy Swelling (Hydropic Change, Vacuolar Degeneration)

- It was originally applied to the gross appearance of organ involved, but is now applied to the microscopic appearance
- It is closely related to hydropic change, vacuolar degeneration. They represent disturbances in protein and water metabolism. Being a manifestation of a disturbance in protein metabolism, it is also called albuminous degeneration.

Causes: It may be caused by many forms of mild injury but usually due to bacterial toxins, chemical poisons and malnutrition.

Organs involved: Kidney, liver, heart and muscle.

Gross: Organ affected is slightly enlarged due to swelling of its cells. Organ appears pale because of compression of blood vessels by the swollen cells. Cut surface has a cloudy appearance and opaque.

Microscopy: Best example is cloudy swelling highly specialized cells of the convoluted tubule of the kidney. The cell is swollen and projects unevenly into the lumen of the tubule. The cytoplasm appears cytoplasm is discharged into the lumen of the tubule. These granules are proteinaceous in nature.

Steatosis (Fatty Change)

Q. Write short note on fatty liver/steatosis of liver.

Abnormal accumulations of triglycerides within cytosol of the parenchymal cells.

Organs involved: Seen in organs involved in fat metabolism, namely **liver**. It may also occur in heart, muscle, and kidney.

- **Causes**
  - **Disorders with hepatocyte damage:** Alcoholic abuse, protein malnutrition, starvation, anoxia (anemia, cardiac failure), toxins (carbon tetrachloride, chloroform, etc.) and Reye syndrome. **Alcohol is the most common cause** of fatty change in the liver.
  - **Disorders with hyperlipidemia:** Obesity, diabetes mellitus or congenital hyperlipidemia.

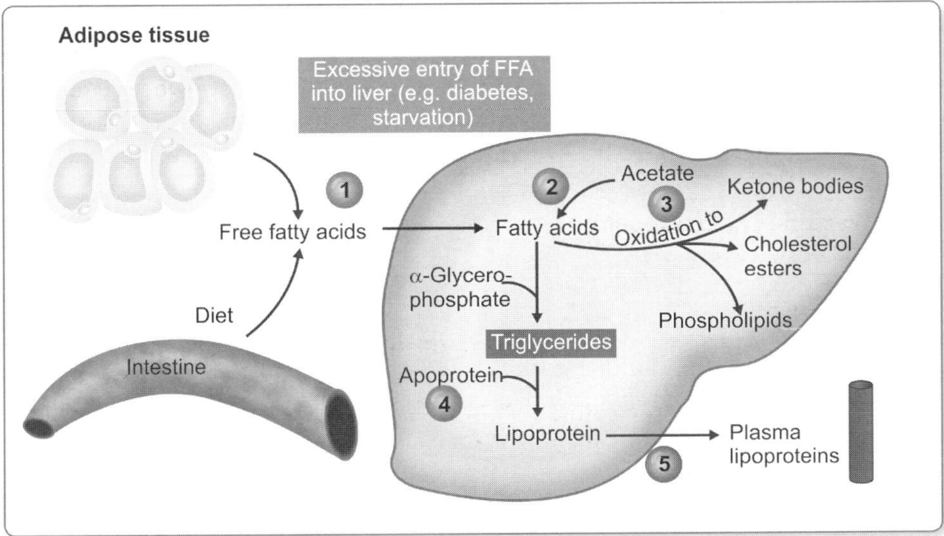

Fig. 2.12: Various mechanisms that can produce accumulation of triglycerides in fatty liver

Pathogenesis of fatty liver

Q. Describe pathogenesis of steatosis/fatty liver.

Various mechanisms are involved in excess accumulation of triglyceride in the liver and one or more mechanism may be responsible.

- **Excessive entry of free fatty acids (FFA) into the liver** (1 in Fig. 2.12): From peripheral stores FFA enters into liver during starvation and diabetes.
- **Defective metabolism of lipids:** This may be due to:
  a. Increased synthesis of fatty acids by liver (2 in Fig. 2.12).
  b. Decreased oxidation of fatty acids into ketone bodies (3 in Fig. 2.12) resulting in increased esterification of fatty acids into triglycerides. **Hypoxia** inhibits fatty acid oxidation.
  c. Decreased synthesis of apoproteins (e.g. in **CCl_4 and protein malnutrition**) causes decreased formation of lipoproteins from triglycerides (4 in Fig. 2.12).
- **Defective excretion of lipoproteins:** Fatty liver may also develop due to defect in excretion lipoproteins from liver into the blood (5 in Fig. 2.12).

Q. Write short note on special stains for fat.

Q. Give gross and microscopic features of fatty liver/steatosis of liver.

- Fatty Liver
  - **Gross (Fig. 2.13 Plate-1):** Liver enlarges and becomes **yellow, soft and greasy to touch**
  - **Microscopy (Fig 2.14 Plate-1):** First fat is seen as small **vacuoles in the cytoplasm** around the nucleus. Later, the vacuoles coalesce, creating cleared spaces that displace the nucleus to the periphery of the cell
  - **Special stains for fat:** Frozen sections stained with Sudan IV or Oil Red-O give an orange-red color to the fat. Osmic acid gives a black color.

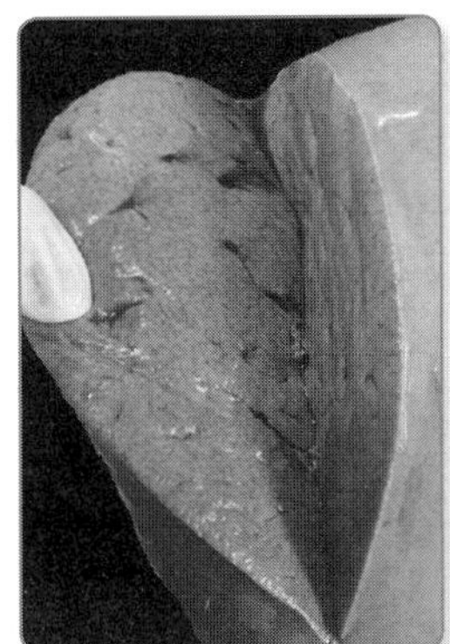

Fig. 2.13: Fatty liver showing a part of liver with yellow color and sharp border

(For color version, see Plate 1)

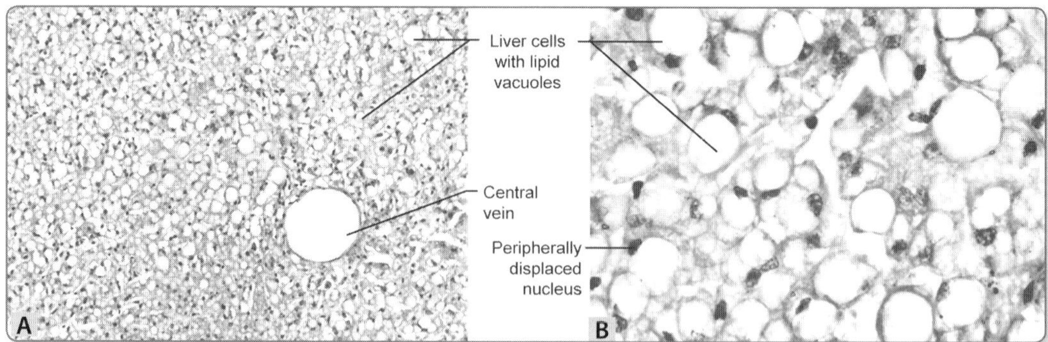

Figs 2.14A and B: A. Fatty liver in which the hepatocytes show accumulation of fat which appear as clear vacuole in the cytoplasm; B. Hepatocytes at higher magnification in which the nucleus is displaced to the periphery by accumulated fat

(For color version, see Plate 1)

Heart

- Lipid in the cardiac muscle can have **two patterns**:
  - **Alternate involvement:** Prolonged moderate hypoxia (e.g. severe anemia), create grossly apparent bands of involved yellow myocardium alternating with bands of darker, red-brown, uninvolved myocardium (**tigered effect, tabby cat appearance**)
  - **Uniform involvement:** More severe hypoxia or some types of myocarditis (e.g. diphtheria infection) show more uniform involvement of myocardial fibers.

Irreversible Cell Injury

If the cell is exposed to continuous injurious stimulus or if the injury is severe, the cells undergo cell death. Two main types of cell death: **Necrosis and apoptosis**.

- **Necrosis:** Always a pathologic process (refer below)
- **Apoptosis:** May be physiological or pathological (refer page 30).

NECROSIS

Q. Define necrosis. Describe the various types of necrosis with suitable examples.

Definition: Morphological changes indicative of cell death in a living tissue following harmful injury. The necrotic cells bring out acute **inflammatory reaction** in the surrounding tissue.

Morphology (Fig. 2.15)

The general changes occurring in necrotic cell are:

- **Cytoplasmic changes:** Increased eosinophilia
- **Nuclear changes:** These may take up one of three patterns
  - **Pyknosis:** Shrinkage of nucleus which appears shrunken and deeply basophilic (similar to ink drop).
  - **Karyolysis:** Progressive fading of basophilic staining of the nuclei and leads to a ghost nuclei.
  - **Karyorrhexis:** Nucleus breaks up into many smaller fragments.

Electron microscopic findings are diagrammatically shown in Figure 2.17.

Necroptosis: Form of cell death which shares features of both necrosis and apoptosis. It is caspase-independent. It resembles morphologically necrosis and mechanistically apoptosis.

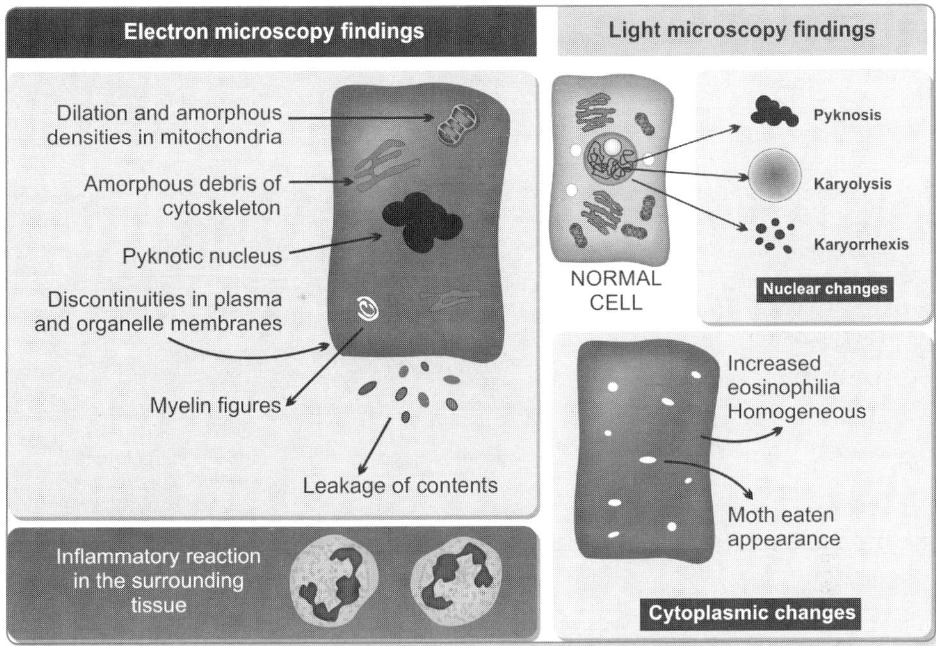

Fig. 2.15: Morphological changes in necrosis

Pyroptosis: A form of programmed cell death associated with the release of fever inducing cytokine IL-1 and has some biochemical similarities with apoptosis.

Patterns/Types of Tissue Necrosis

Coagulative Necrosis

Q. Write short note on types of necrosis.

Q. Write short note on coagulative necrosis.

Common type, outline of dead tissues is preserved (at least for few days). **Infarct** is a localized area of coagulative necrosis.

- **Causes: Ischemia** caused by obstruction in a vessel.
- **Mechanism:** Ischemia denatures and coagulates structural proteins and enzymes.

- **Gross:**
  - **Organs affected:** All organs except the brain. More frequent in **heart, kidney, spleen and limb (dry gangrene).**
  - **Appearance:** Involved region appear **dry, pale, yellow and firm. It is wedge shaped in organs like kidney (Fig. 2.16A) and spleen.**
- **Microscopy** (Figs 2.16B to C): **Indistinct outline of dead tissue.** Nucleus may be either absent or show karyolysis.

Liquefactive Necrosis (Colliquative Necrosis)

Q. Write short note on liquefactive necrosis.

Dead tissue rapidly **undergoes softening** and transforms into a liquid viscous mass.

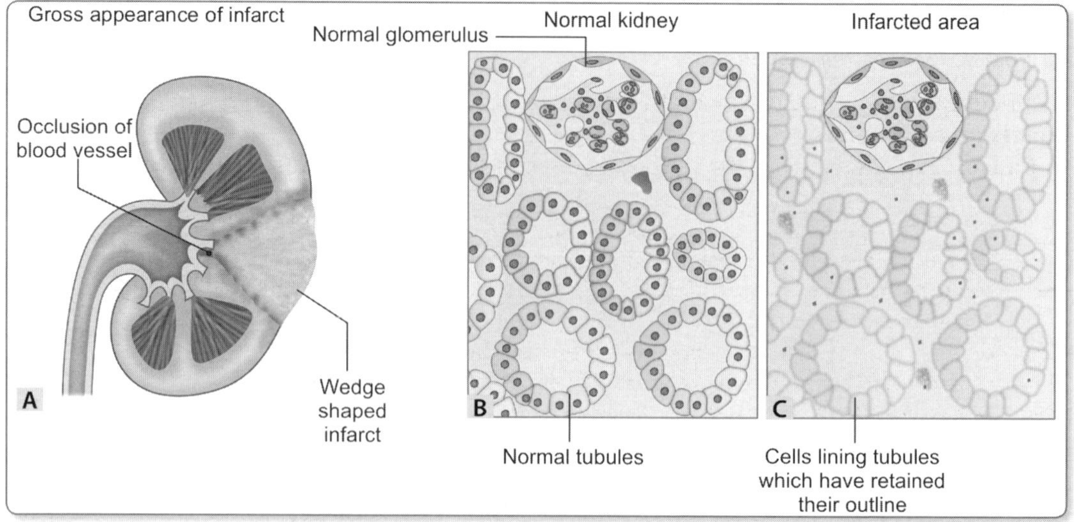

Figs 2.16A to C: A. Gross appearance of infarct of kidney; B. Microscopy of normal kidney parenchyma; C. Infarct of kidney

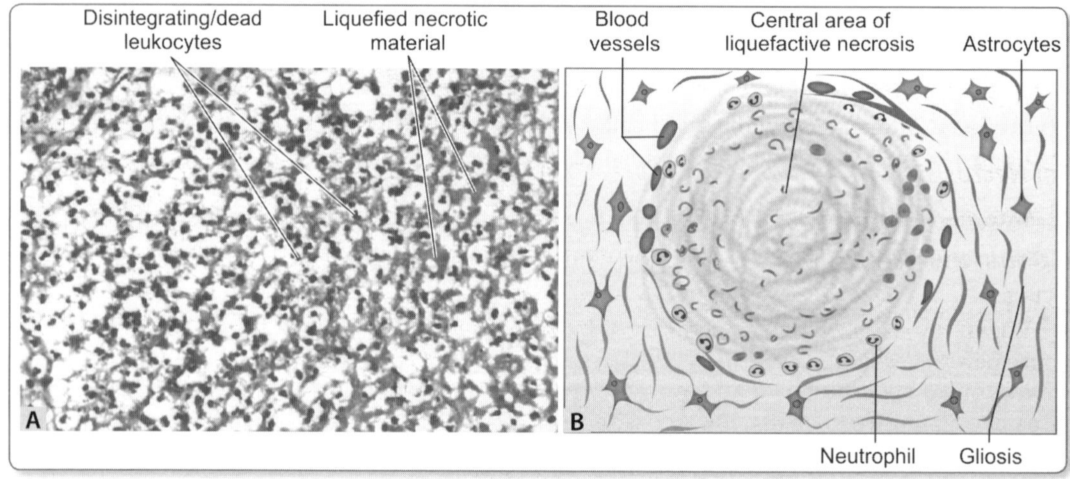

Figs 2.17A and B: Microscopic appearance of an abscess consisting of liquified necrotic cell debris and dead/disintegrating neutrophils. A. H&E and B. diagrammatic appearance of brain abscess

- **Causes:**
  - **Ischemic injury to central nervous system (CNS)**
  - **Suppurative infections:** Infections by bacteria which stimulate the accumulation of leukocytes.
- **Mechanism:** Liquefaction is due to digestive action of the hydrolytic enzymes released from dead cells (autolysis) and leukocytes (heterolysis).

- **Gross:** Organs affected are:
  - **Brain:** Necrotic area is soft and center show liquefaction
  - **Abscess anywhere:** Localized collection of pus
  - It is also seen in wet gangrene and pancreatic necrosis
- **Microscopy (Fig. 2.17): Pus consists of liquefied necrotic cell debris, dead leukocytes and macrophages** (scavenger cells).

Caseous Necrosis

Q. Write short note on caseous necrosis.

Distinctive type of necrosis which shows **combined features of both coagulative and liquefactive necrosis.**

- **Cause:** Characteristic of **tuberculosis** and is due to the hypersensitivity reaction.

- **Gross:**
  - **Organs affected:** Tuberculosis may involve any organ, most common in **lung** and **lymph node**.
  - **Appearance:**
    - Necrotic area appears **yellowish white, soft, granular** and resembles **dry, clumpy cheese**, hence the name caseous (**cheese-like**) necrosis (Figs 2.18).
- **Microscopy:**
  - Focal lesion of tuberculosis is a **granuloma** (Figs 2.19 and 3.11) which may be **caseating (soft granuloma) or noncaseating (hard granuloma)**.
    - Caseous necrosis appears as **eosinophilic, coarsely granular material**. It is surrounded by epithelioid cells; Langhans type giant cells (nuclei arranged in a horse-shoe pattern), lymphocytes and fibroblasts.
    - Caseous necrotic material **may undergo dystrophic calcification.**

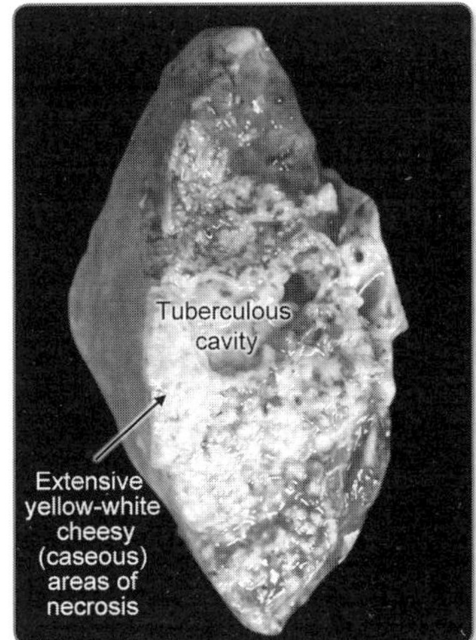

Fig. 2.18: Gross appearance of caseous necrosis. Lung shows cavity with caseous necrosis

(For color version, see Plate 1)

Fat Necrosis

Q. Write short note on fat necrosis.

It refers to **focal areas of fat destruction**, which affects adipose tissue.

Types:

1. **Enzymatic fat necrosis:** Occurs in adipose tissue around acutely inflamed pancreas (in **acute pancreatitis**).

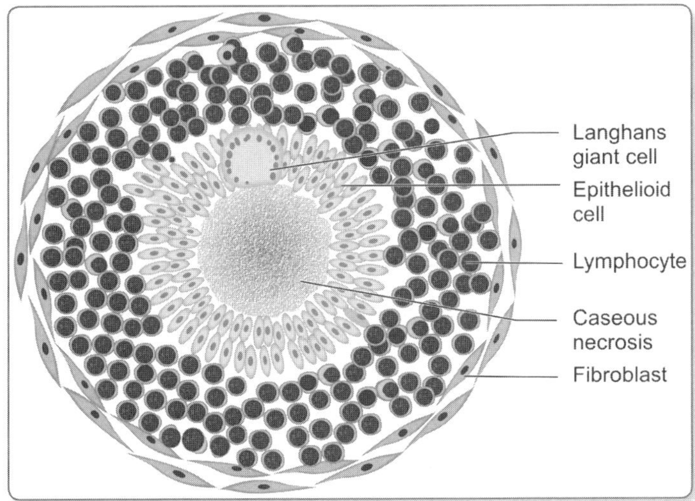

Fig. 2.19: Microscopic (diagrammatic) appearance of a caseous necrosis

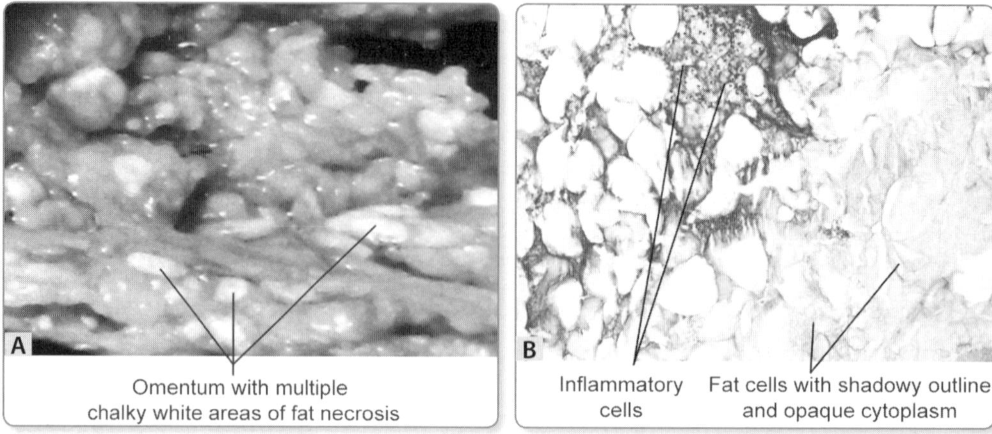

Figs 2.20A and B: A. Omentum shows multiple chalky white areas of fat necrosis caused by acute pancreatitis; B. Fat necrosis shows necrotic fat cells in the right lower part and inflammatory reaction between normal (left upper area) and area of fat necrosis

- **Mechanism:** In pancreatitis, the enzymes (one of them is lipase) leak from acinar cells and causes tissue damage. Lipase destroys fat cells and liberates free fatty acids which combine with calcium and form calcium soaps (fat saponification).

- **Gross:** Appears as **chalky-white areas** (Fig. 2.20A).
- **Microscopy:** The necrotic **fat cells appear pale with shadowy outlines surrounded** by an inflammatory reaction (Fig. 2.20B).

2. **Traumatic fat necrosis:** Occurs in tissues with high fat content (like in **breast and thigh**) following severe trauma.

Fibrinoid Necrosis

Characterized by **deposition of pink-staining (fibrin-like) proteinaceous material** in the tissue matrix with a **staining pattern reminiscent of fibrin**. It obscures the underlying cellular detail.

Gangrene (Gangrenous Necrosis)

Q. Define and classify gangrene. Give examples.

Q. Write short note on gangrene.

It is **massive necrosis with superadded putrefaction**.

Types: Two types, namely **dry and wet gangrene**. A variant of wet gangrene known as **gas gangrene** is **caused by clostridia** (gram-positive anaerobic bacteria).

Dry Gangrene

Q. Write short note on dry gangrene.

- **Causes: Arterial occlusion** (e.g. atherosclerosis).
- **Sites:** It usually involves a **limb**, generally the distal part of lower limb (leg, foot, and toe).

- **Gross:** Affected part is **dry, shrunken** (shriveled) and **dark brown or black** resembling the foot of a **mummy**. The black color is due to the iron sulfide. A **line of demarcation** is seen between gangrenous and adjacent normal area (Fig. 2.21).
- **Microscopy:** The necrosis (coagulative type) shows smudging of soft tissue and overlying skin. The line of demarcation consists of granulation of tissue with inflammatory cells.

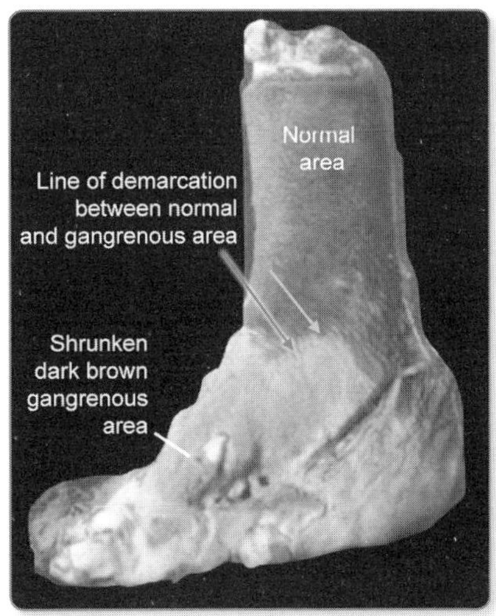

Fig. 2.21: Dry gangrene of left leg shows dry shrunken discolored gangrenous foot separated from adjacent normal area by a line of demarcation

(For color version, see Plate 1)

Wet Gangrene

Q. Write short note on wet gangrene.

- **Causes: Due to the venous blockage** (e.g. strangulated hernia, intussusception or volvulus).
- **Sites:** Occurs in **moist tissues or organs** (e.g. bowel, lung, mouth, etc.).

- **Gross:** The affected part is soft, swollen, putrid and dark. No clear line of demarcation.
- **Microscopy:** Liquefactive type of necrosis.

Differences Between Dry and Wet Gangrene (Table 2.2)

Q. List the differences between dry and wet gangrene.

Table 2.2: Differences between dry and wet gangrene

Characteristics	Dry	Wet
General features		
Common site	Limbs	Bowels
Examples	Senile gangrene	Volvulus, intussusception
Etiological factors		
Cause of ischemia	Arterial obstruction	Commonly venous obstruction
Rate of obstruction	Slow	Abrupt
Gross features		
Appearance of involved part	Shriveled dry (mummification) and black	Swollen, soft and moist
Line of demarcation	Clear cut	Not clear cut
Spread	Slow	Rapid
Prognosis	Fair	Poor due to severe septicemia

Gas gangrene: Special type of wet gangrene caused by infection with a gas forming anaerobic clostridia.

Gummatous Necrosis

The necrotic tissue is firm and rubbery and is usually found in syphilis.

Ultrastructural differences between reversible and irreversible injury are presented in Table 2.3

Q. Describe the ultra-structural changes in reversible cell injury.

Table 2.3: Ultrastructural differences between reversible and irreversible injury

Structure involved	Reversible injury	Irreversible injury
Plasma membrane changes	Blebbing, blunting, loss of microvilli	Discontinuities in plasma and organelle membrane
Mitochondrial changes	Swelling and appearance of small amorphous densities	Marked dilatation with appearance of large amorphous densities (precipitated calcium), aggregates of fluppy material (denatured protein)
Endoplasmic reticulum	Dilatation with detachment of polysomes	Swelling and fragmentation
Myelin figure (large intracellular whorled phospholipid masses)	May be present	Usually present
Nuclear changes	Disaggregation of granular and fibrillar elements	Pyknosis, karyolysis and karyorrhexis

APOPTOSIS

Q. Define apoptosis and give examples.

Q. Write short note on apoptosis.

Apoptosis is a **type of (programmed) cell death**. It is characterized by **activation of cell enzymes that degrade its own nuclear DNA** and **proteins** (nuclear and cytoplasmic).

Causes of Apoptosis

Physiological Situations

- **Removal of excess cells during embryogenesis and developmental processes,** e.g. disappearance of web tissues between fingers and toes
- **Elimination of cells after withdrawal of hormonal stimuli,** e.g. endometrial cell breakdown during the menstrual cycle
- **Elimination of cells after withdrawal of tropic stimuli,** e.g. neutrophils in an acute inflammatory response, lymphocytes after immune response
- **Elimination of potentially harmful cells:** In immunology, the clones of **self-reactive lymphocytes** that recognize normal self antigens are deleted by apoptosis.

Pathological Conditions

Apoptosis eliminates cells that are genetically altered or damaged beyond repair. It is responsible for cell loss in many pathologic states:

- **Elimination of cells with damaged DNA:** DNA may be damaged by many injurious agents like radiation, cytotoxic anticancer drugs and hypoxia
  - Mainly tumor-suppressor gene p53 recognizes cells with damaged DNA and assesses whether it can be repaired. If the damage is too severe to be repaired, p53 triggers apoptosis
  - **Destroying cells with dangerous mutations or with DNA damage** beyond repair by apoptosis prevents the development of cancer
  - In certain cancers, where p53 is mutated or absent, the apoptosis is not induced in cells with damaged DNA.
- **Elimination of cells with excessively accumulated misfolded proteins:** Mutations in the genes encoding proteins or extrinsic factors (damage due to free radicals) may result in accumulation of unfolded or misfolded proteins.

- Excessive intracellular accumulation of these abnormally folded proteins in the ER is known as **ER stress**, which results in apoptotic cell death
- Apoptosis caused by the accumulation of misfolded proteins is found in several degenerative diseases of the central nervous system (Alzheimer, Huntington, and Parkinson diseases) and other organs.

- **Killing of viral infected cells:** In viral infections, the infected cells are lost mainly due to apoptosis induced either by the virus (as in adenovirus and HIV infections) or by host human response by cytotoxic T lymphocytes (as in viral hepatitis)
- **Elimination of neoplastic cells/rejection of transplant:** The T-cell-mediated mechanism is responsible for apoptosis in tumors and cellular rejection of transplants
- **Elimination of parenchymal cells in pathologic atrophy:** Obstruction of duct in the **parenchymal** organs like pancreas, parotid gland and kidney can lead to apoptosis of the parenchymal cells.

Morphology

Electron Microscope

The ultrastructural features of apoptosis (Fig. 2.22) are:

- **Cell shrinkage:** Cytoplasm becomes dense.
- **Nuclear condensation and fragmentation:** Chromatin aggregates peripherally under the nuclear membrane. The nucleus may break up to produce two or more nuclear fragments.
- **Formation of cytoplasmic blebs and apoptotic bodies:** Cell first shows extensive surface blebbing followed by fragmentation into membrane-bound apoptotic bodies. The apoptotic bodies are composed of cytoplasm and tightly packed organelles, with or without nuclear fragments.
- **Phagocytosis of apoptotic cells/bodies:** The apoptotic bodies are rapidly ingested by phagocytes (**usually by macrophages**) and degraded by the lysosomal enzymes of phagocytes.

Light Microscopy

The apoptotic cells appear as round or oval mass having intensely **eosinophilic** cytoplasm. The **nuclei appear as fragments of dense nuclear chromatin** and shows pyknosis. Apoptosis does not elicit an inflammatory reaction in the host.

Mechanisms of Apoptosis

The survival or apoptosis of many cells depends upon balance between two opposite sets of signals, namely: **1) death signal** (pro-apoptotic), and **2) pro-survival** (anti-apoptotic) signals. Unlike necrosis, apoptosis engages the cell's own signaling cascades and results in its own death (suicide). Apoptosis results from **activation of enzymes** called as **caspases**.

Phases of Apoptosis

Divided into: A) initiation phase, and B) execution phase.

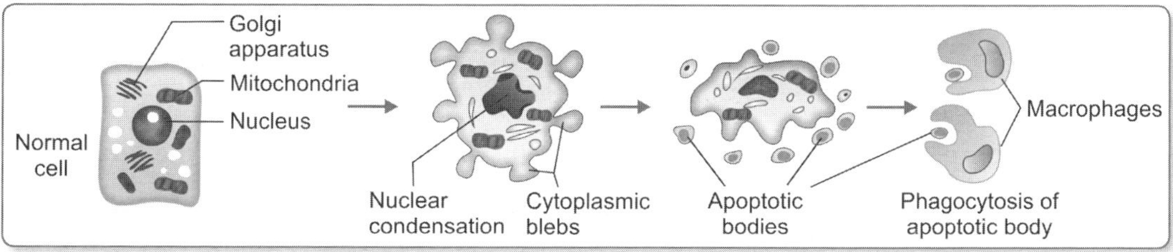

Fig. 2.22: Electron microscopic changes in apoptosis

A. Initiation Phase

Apoptosis is initiated by signals derived from two distinct pathways activated by distinct stimuli, namely: 1) intrinsic or mitochondrial pathway, and 2) extrinsic or death receptor pathway.

1. **Intrinsic (mitochondrial) pathway of apoptosis** (Fig. 2.23): It is activated by intracellular signals.
   - **Role of mitochondria in apoptosis:**
     - **Mitochondrial damage is the major mechanism** in a variety of physiological and pathological apoptosis
     - **Mitochondria contain** proteins capable of inducing apoptosis. These include **cytochrome c and several proapoptotic proteins**
     - Survival or apoptosis of cell is determined by permeability of mitochondria
     - **Mitochondrial permeability is controlled by Bcl-2 family** of more than 20 **proteins.** This family is named after *Bcl-2,* which was identified as an oncogene in a **B-cell** lymphoma. These proteins may be broadly divided into proapoptotic or anti-apoptotic (prosurvival):
       - **Proapoptotic proteins: Bax, Bak,** Bid, Bad, and Bik.
       - **Anti-apoptotic proteins: Bcl-2, Bcl-x_L,** Mcl-1. They prevent leakage of mitochondrial proteins that trigger apoptosis. Growth factors and other survival signals stimulate production of anti-apoptotic proteins.

     If the balance shifts to proapoptotic proteins, the apoptotic cascade is activated.
   - **Causes of mitochondrial injury:** The proapoptotic signals include:
     1. Deprivation/withdrawal of growth factor or survival signals.
     2. DNA damage by radiation, cytotoxic anticancer drugs, hypoxia either directly or through free radical.
     3. Accumulation of excessive amount of misfolded proteins (ER stress).
     4. Increased intracellular free calcium.
   - **Steps in intrinsic (mitochondrial) pathway:** Mitochondrial injury causes increased mitochondrial permeability and **release proapoptotic molecules (death inducers) into the cytoplasm**. The different steps are as follows:
     - The above mentioned causes of mitochondrial injury activate a number of sensors of ***Bcl-2* family** called BH3-proteins. They in turn activate **two critical** proapoptotic ***Bcl-2* family** effector proteins, namely ***Bax*** and ***Bak***
     - **Bax** and **Bak** create channels in the mitochondria that allow release of several **mitochondrial** proteins from the inner mitochondrial membrane to leak out into the cytosol (cytoplasm)
     - One of these proteins is **cytochrome c** which binds to a protein called **Apaf-1 (apoptosis-activating factor-1)** and forms an important caspase cascade activator called **apoptosome**. This complex binds to caspase-9, the critical initiator caspase of the mitochondrial pathway which sets in an auto-amplification process.
     - The cytoplasm of the normal cells contains proteins which block the activation of caspases and function as physiologic **inhibitors of apoptosis (called IAPs)**. Other mitochondrial proteins may enter the cytoplasm and **neutralize** these IAPs and initiate caspase cascade.
     - Sensors of ***Bcl-2* family** namely BH3- proteins also bind to and **block the function of** protective **anti-apoptotic proteins**, namely ***Bcl-2*** and **Bcl-x_L**.

2. **Extrinsic (death receptor–initiated) pathway of apoptosis (Fig. 2.23)**
    - This pathway is **initiated by extracellular signals**
    - **Many cells express "death-receptors" molecules on the surface of plasma membrane that trigger apoptosis**. Death receptors are **members of the TNF (tumor necrosis factor) receptor family** that contain a cytoplasmic domain called the **death domain** because it is essential for delivering apoptotic signals
    - In the extrinsic (death receptor) pathway, **apoptosis is initiated when** the **death receptors** present gets **activated**
    - The **well-known death receptors are the type 1 TNF receptor (TNFR1) and a related protein called Fas (CD95)**. Fas death receptor is expressed on many cell types and the binding ligand for Fas is called Fas ligand (FasL/CD95L)
    - **Functions of extrinsic pathway:** This pathway is **involved in eliminating**:
        - **Self-reactive lymphocytes**, thereby avoiding autoimmunity. FasL is expressed on T-cells that recognize self-antigens and function to eliminate self-reactive lymphocytes.
        - **Virus infected cells** through cytotoxic T lymphocytes
        - **Tumor cells** through cytotoxic T lymphocytes.
    - **Steps in extrinsic pathway:**
        - Extrinsic pathway become activated when CD95/Fas binds to its ligand, CD95L/FasL
        - When FasL binds to Fas receptors, their cytoplasmic death domains binds with an **adapter protein**. This adapter protein also contains a death domain and is called FADD (Fas-associated death domain)

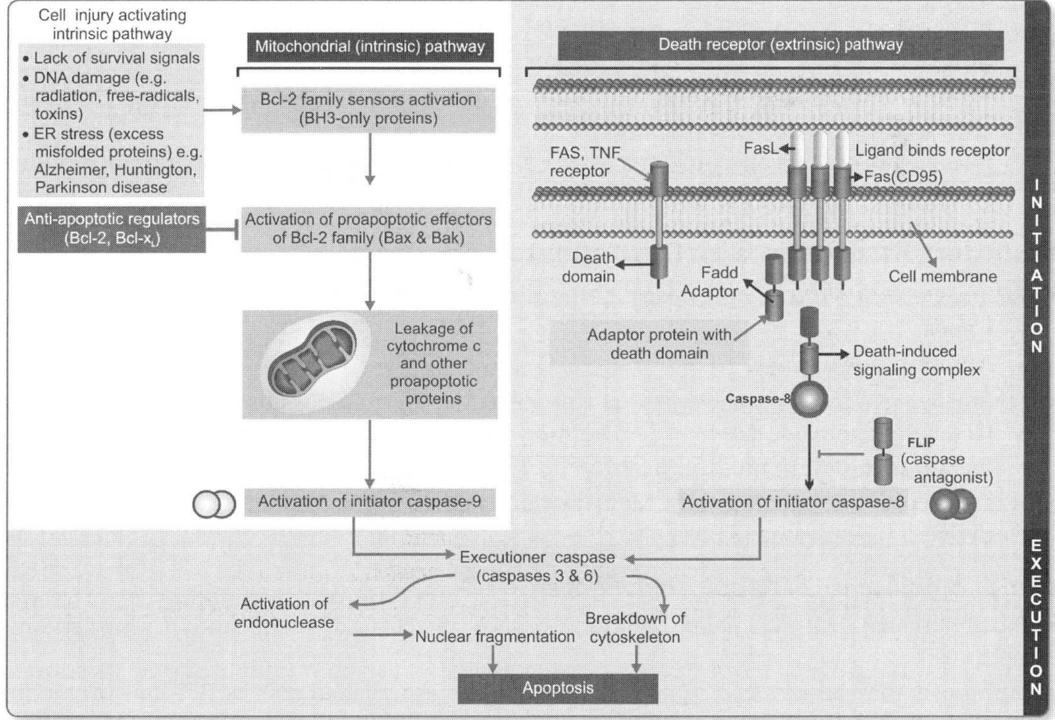

Fig. 2.23: Mechanism of apoptosis

- FADD in turn binds to pro-caspase-8 (an inactive form of caspase-8) via a death domain and generate active caspase-8
- Activated caspase-8 mediate the execution phase of apoptosis.

B. Execution Phase of Apoptosis (Fig. 2.23)

- The above mentioned two initiating pathways produce initiator caspases, namely: 1) the **mitochondrial pathway activates initiator caspase-9**, and 2) the **death receptor pathway activates the initiator caspase-8**
- The initiator caspases activate another series of caspases called **executioner caspases (such as caspase-3 and -6)** that mediates the final phase of apoptosis
- Executioner caspases act on many cellular components and activate DNase, which induces fragmentation of nuclei
- Caspases also degrade components of nuclear matrix and cytoskeleton resulting in fragmentation of involved cells.

Removal of Apoptotic Cells

- **Phagocytosis:** Apoptotic cells and bodies are engulfed and removed by phagocytic cells (mainly macrophages).The phagocytosis is so efficient that these dead cells and apoptotic bodies disappear within minutes. Even when their apoptosis is extensive, their rapid removal prevents release of their cellular contents which may elicit inflammation.
- **Factors favoring phagocytosis:** The apoptotic cells and apoptotic bodies undergo several changes in their membranes and produce signals that favor phagocytosis of these cells/bodies
  - **Expression of phosphatidylserine:** In healthy cells, **phosphatidylserine** is present on the inner leaflet of the plasma membrane. In cells undergoing apoptosis, **phosphatidylserine** turns out and is expressed on the outer layer of the membrane causing easily recognition by receptors present on the macrophage.
  - **Secretion of soluble factors: Apoptotic cells secrete soluble factors** (e.g. **thrombospondin**) that recruit phagocytes.
  - **Natural antibodies and proteins of the complement system** may coat apoptotic bodies which aids in phagocytosis.

Disorders Associated with Dysregulated Apoptosis

- ***Disorders with reduced apoptosis:*** It may allow the survival of abnormal cells.
  - Cancer
  - Autoimmune disease.
- ***Disorders with increased apoptosis:*** This will cause an excessive loss of cells.
  - **Neurodegenerative diseases (Alzheimer, Huntigton, Parkinson disease).**
  - **Ischemic injury:** In myocardial infarction and stroke.
  - **Death of virus-infected cells:** Many viral infections, important being acquired immunodeficiency syndrome (**AIDS**).

Clinical Significance of Apoptosis in Cancers

- Normally, cells with damaged (mutated) DNA are cleared in the body by undergoing apoptosis
- Apoptosis may be reduced in some cancers. Best established role of Bcl-2 in protecting tumor cells from undergoing apoptosis is observed in **follicular lymphoma**. In this type of

non-Hodgkin lymphoma of B cell origin, there **is translocation (14; 18) (q32; q21)** which causes **over expression of anti-apoptotic protein Bcl-2.** This in turn increases the Bcl-2/Bcl-x_L buffer, **protecting abnormal B lymphocytes from undergoing apoptosis** and allows them to survive for long periods.

Differences between apoptosis and necrosis are summarized in Table 2.4.

Q. List the differences between apoptosis and necrosis.

Table 2.4: Differences between apoptosis and necrosis

Features	Apoptosis	Necrosis
Cause	Often physiological, means of eliminating unwanted cells; may also be pathological	Invariably pathological
Biochemical events	Energy-dependent fragmentation of DNA by endogenous endonucleases	Impairment or cessation of ion homeostasis
Lysosomes	Intact	Leak lytic enzymes
Morphology		
Extent	Single or small cluster of cells	Involves group of cells
Cell size	Cell reduced (shrinkage) and fragmentation to form apoptotic bodies with dense chromatin	Cell enlarged (swelling) and lysis
Integrity of cell membrane	Maintained	Disrupted/Lost
Nucleus	Fragmentation into nucleosome-size fragments	Pyknosis, karyorrhexis, karyolysis
Cellular contents	Intact; may be released in apoptotic bodies	Enzymatic digestion; may leak out of cell
Adjacent Inflammatory response	None	Usual
Fate of dead cells	Ingested (phagocytosed) by neighboring cells	Ingested (phagocytosed) by neutrophil polymorphs and macrophages
DNA electrophoresis	DNA laddering is seen	Shows smearing effect
TUNEL staining	Positive	Negative

PATHOLOGIC CALCIFICATION

Q. Write short note on pathologic calcification.

Abnormal **deposition of calcium salts in tissues other than osteoid or enamel**. It is also associated with deposition of small amounts of iron, magnesium and other minerals.

Types of pathologic calcification are: 1) dystrophic, and 2) metastatic.

Dystrophic Calcification

Q. Mention the types of calcification.

Q. Define dystrophic calcification with examples.

Q. Define metastatic calcification with examples.

Deposition of calcium salts in **dying or dead tissues**.

Causes

- **Necrotic tissue:** Calcification in **caseous, enzymatic fat necrosis**, in **dead eggs** of Schistosoma, cysticercosis and hydatid cysts.

- **Degenerating tissue:**
  - **Heart valves:** Occurs in aging or damaged heart valves
  - **Atherosclerosis.**
- **Monckeberg's medial calcific sclerosis:** Calcification in the media of the muscular arteries (Fig. 2.24A) in old people.
- **Psammoma bodies:** Single necrotic cells on which several layers of mineral get deposited progressively to create lamellated shape, called **psammoma bodies** (Fig. 2.24B).

Metastatic Calcification

Deposition of calcium salts in apparently **normal tissues**. It is associated with hypercalcemia **secondary to deranged calcium metabolism**.

Causes

- **Increased secretion of parathyroid hormone** (PTH) with subsequent bone resorption-hyperparathyroidism.
- **Destruction of bone tissue:** Secondary to primary tumors of bone marrow (e.g. multiple myeloma, leukemia and metastatic tumors to bone).
- **Vitamin D-related disorders:** Vitamin D intoxication.
- **Renal failure:** Causes retention of phosphate, leading to secondary hyperparathyroidism.
- **Others:** Sarcoidosis and milk alkali syndrome.

Sites

- **Lungs: Alveolar septa of the lung.**
- **Kidney: Basement membrane of the renal tubules.**
- **Blood vessels:** On the internal elastic lamina of **systemic arteries and pulmonary veins**.
- **Stomach: Interstitial tissues of the gastric mucosa.**

Morphology

Gross: Appear as fine, white granules or clumps, feels gritty and sandlike.
Microscopy: Basophilic, amorphous granular (Fig. 2.24), clumped appearance.

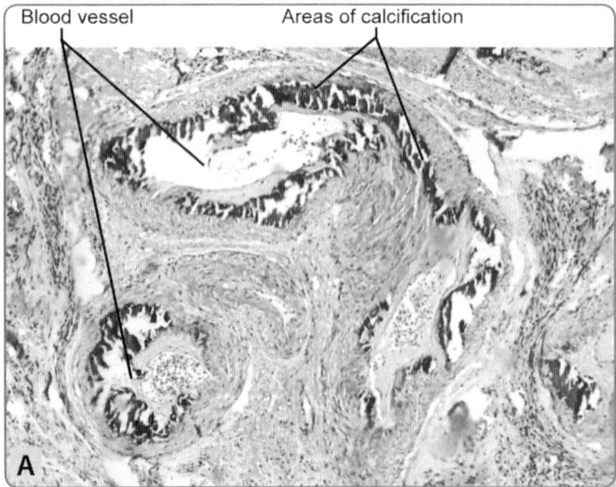

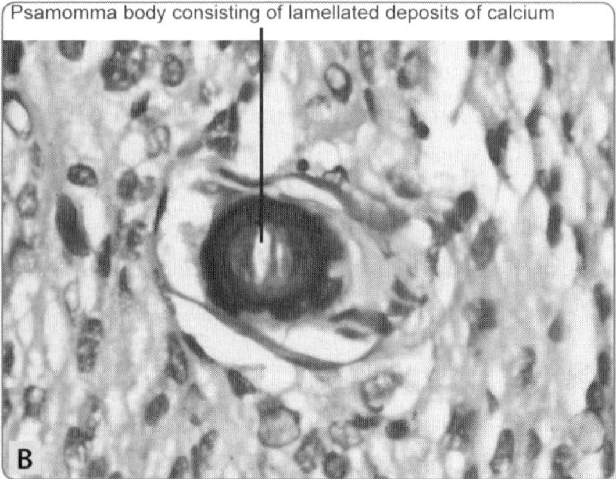

Figs 2.24A and B: A. Monckeberg's medial calcific sclerosis in which the tunica media of arteries in the myometrium of uterus show calcification; B. Photomicrograph of meningioma with psammoma body

HYALINE CHANGE

Q. Write short note on hyaline change.

Hyaline refers to **an alteration within cells or in the extracellular space**, which gives a **homogeneous, glassy, pink appearance** in routine histological sections.

Causes (Table 2.5)

Intracellular Hyaline

- **Mallory body** in the liver is alcoholic hyaline **composed of cytoskeletal filaments.**
- **Russell bodies** are **excessive accumulation of immunoglobulins in the plasma cells.**

Extracellular Hyaline

- Collagenous fibrous tissue in **old scars**
- Hyaline change in **uterine leiomyoma** (Fig. 2.25)
- In **chronic glomerulonephritis,** the **glomeruli** show hyalinization.

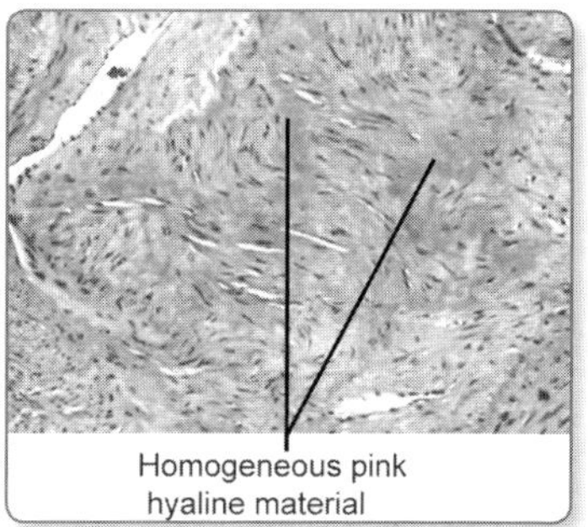

Fig. 2.25: Hyaline change in leiomyoma of uterus

Table 2.5: Examples of hyaline change

Intracellular hyaline	Extracellular hyaline
1. Mallory bodies 2. Russell bodies (e.g. multiple myeloma) 3. Crooke's hyaline 4. Zenker's hyaline change	1. Collagenous fibrous tissue in scar 2. Hyaline change in uterine leiomyoma 3. Hyaline membrane in newborn 4. Hyaline arteriosclerosis 5. Hyalinization of glomeruli in chronic glomerulonephritis 6. Corpora amylacea in prostate, brain, spinal cord in elderly, old infarct of lung

Mucoid Degeneration

- Mucus is the viscid watery secretion produced by mucous glands. It consists of loose combination of proteins and mucopolysaccharides of high molecular weight. Its main constituent is a glycoprotein called mucin
- Mucus is produced by mitochondria and then they move to Golgi apparatus, where they are converted into mucin. When this process is exaggerated with excessive secretion of mucus it is termed mucoid degeneration
- Mucin is normally produced by both epithelial cells of mucus membranes and mucous glands and also by certain connective tissue cells, especially in the fetus (e.g. umbilical cord). Mucoid degeneration may involve both epithelial and connective tissue mucin. Usually, connective tissue mucin is termed as myxoid, i.e. mucus like
- Both epithelial and connective tissue mucin are stained by alcian blue. Epithelial mucin stains positively with periodic acid Schiff (PAS) and connective tissue mucin is PAS negative and stains positively with colloidal iron.

Epithelial mucin: Examples of excessive epithelial mucin secretion are:

- Catarrhal inflammation of the mucus membrane, e.g. inflammation of mucosa of respiratory tract, GI tract
- Obstruction, e.g. mucocele of gall bladder, appendix, oral cavity
- Cystic fibrosis of pancreas
- Mucus secreting tumors (Fig. 2.26A), e.g. of GI tract , ovary.

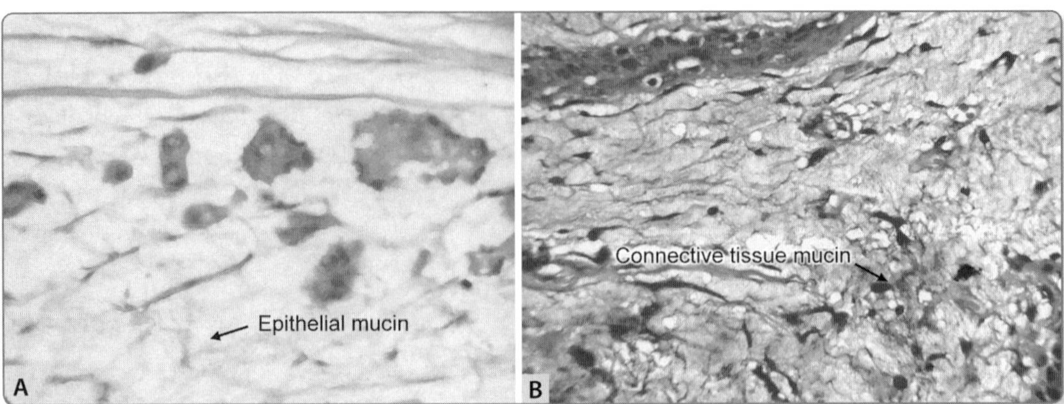

Figs 2.26A and B: A. Epithelial mucin and B. Connective tissue mucin

Connective tissue mucin: Examples—
- Mucoid or myxoid degeneration: Examples of tumors include myxoma, neurofibroma, fibroadenoma (Fig. 2.26B), sarcomas
- Dissecting aneurysm of aorta
- Myxedema: Myxomatous changes in dermis
- Myxoid change in ganglion.

PIGMENTS

Q. Write short note on various pigments.

Pigments are **colored substances**, which are either normal constituents of cells (e.g. melanin), or are abnormal and accumulate in cells. Different types of pigments are listed in Table 2.6.

Table 2.6: Different types of pigments

Endogenous pigments	Exogenous pigments
• Bilirubin • Melanin • Hemosiderin • Hemoglobin derived pigments	• Carbon (anthracotic) • Tattooing • Arsenic • β-carotene

Hemosiderin

It is a hemoglobin-derived, golden yellow-to-brown, granular or crystalline pigment and is one of the major storage forms of iron.

Causes

Local or systemic excess of iron cause hemosiderin to accumulate within cells.
- **Local excesses:**
  - **Bruise**
  - **Brown induration of lung** in chronic venous congestion of lung (refer Fig. 5.1).
- **Systemic excesses: Systemic overload of iron** is known as **hemosiderosis**. The main causes are:
  - **Increased absorption of dietary iron**
  - **Excessive destruction of red cells,** e.g. hemolytic anemias
  - **Repeated blood transfusions.**

Morphology

Site of Accumulation

- **Localized:** Found in the macrophages of the involved area
- **Systemic:** Initially found in **liver, bone marrow, spleen, and lymph nodes**. Later deposited in macrophages of other organs (e.g. skin, pancreas, kidney).

Microscopy: Appears as a coarse, golden, granular pigment within the cytoplasm.

Special stain: Prussian blue histochemical reaction in which hemosiderin converts colorless potassium ferrocyanide to blue-black ferric ferrocyanide.

Other Pigments

- **Hemochromatosis:** Severe accumulation of iron is associated with damage to liver, heart, and pancreas. The triad of cirrhosis of liver, diabetes mellitus (due to pancreatic damage) and brown pigmentation of skin constitute **bronze diabetes**.
- **Hemozoin:** It is a brown-black pigment containing heme in ferric form. This pigment is seen in chronic malaria and in mismatched blood transfusions.
- **Bilirubin** is the normal major pigment found in bile. It is non-iron containing pigment derived from hemoglobin.

Commonly used histochemistry (special stains) in histopathology are listed in Table 2.7.

Table 2.7: Commonly used special stains in histopathology

Stain	Substance	Interpretation
Amyloid		
• Congo red under polarizing microscope	Amyloid	Green-birefringence
Carbohydrates		
• Periodic Acid-Schiff (PAS)	Glycogen, mucin, mucoprotein, glycoprotein, fungi, basement membranes of glomeruli and tubules	Magenta color
• Mucicarmine/Best's carmine	Epithelial mucin	Red color
• Alcian blue	Acid mucin	Blue
Lipids		
• Sudan III	Lipid	Orange
• Oil Red O		Red
• Osmium tetroxide		Brown black
Connective tissue		
• Van Gieson	Extracellular collagen	Red
• Masson's trichrome	Collagen, smooth muscle	Collagen—blue, smooth muscle—red
• Phosphotungstic acid hematoxylin (PTAH)	Cross striation of skeletal muscles, glial filaments, fibrin	Dark blue
• Verhoeff's elastic	Elastic fibers	Black
Microorganisms		
• Gram's stain	Bacteria	Gram +ve= blue Gram –ve= red

Contd...

Contd...

Stain	Substance	Interpretation
• Ziehl-Neelsen (Acid-fast) stain	Tubercle bacilli and other acid-fast organisms	Red
• Fite-Ferraco	Lepra bacilli	Red
• Silver methanamine	Fungi	Black
Pigments and minerals		
• Prussian blue stain (Perl's stain)	Hemosiderin	Blue
• Masson Fontana	Melanin	Black
• Von Kossa	Calcium	Orange red
• Alizarin Red S		Black
• Rubeanic acid	Copper	Greenish-black

Chapter 3

Inflammation

Chapter Outline

- Acute inflammation
- Causes of (stimuli for) acute inflammation
- Sequence of events in acute inflammation
- Reactions of blood vessels (vascular changes)
- Leukocytic/cellular events
- Chemical mediators of inflammation
- Cell-derived mediators
- Plasma-derived mediators
- Outcomes of acute inflammation
- Morphological types/patterns of acute inflammation
- Systemic effects of inflammation
- Chronic inflammation
- Granulomatous inflammation
- Giant cell

ACUTE INFLAMMATION

Q. Define inflammation.

Q. Mention the types of inflammation. List the differences between acute and chronic inflammation.

Definition: Inflammation is a complex **local response of the living vascularized tissues to injury (infections and damaged tissues)** and mainly consists of responses of blood vessels and leukocytes. **It brings cells and molecules of host defense from the circulation to the sites of injury, in order to eliminate the offending agents/cause.**

Protective vs harmful:

- **Protective response**: Inflammation is fundamentally a protective/defensive response. It helps in removal/destruction of the initial cause of cell injury (e.g. microbes, toxins) and the consequences of such injury (e.g. necrotic cells).
- **Harmful consequences of inflammation:** Inflammatory reactions to infections often cause local tissue damage and its associated signs and symptoms (e.g., pain and functional disturbances). Usually, these harmful consequences are self-limited and resolve as the inflammation subsides. However, this normally protective inflammatory reaction may be the cause of the disease and may bring about damage to the tissues. In many diseases, inflammatory reaction may be misdirected (e.g. against own/self tissues in autoimmune diseases), or occurs against normally harmless environmental substances (e.g. in allergies), or is inadequately controlled (e.g. rheumatoid arthritis, atherosclerosis, hypersensitivity reactions).

Type of inflammation: Inflammation may be divided into **acute or chronic**. Differences between acute and chronic inflammation are listed in Table 3.1.

Table 3.1: Differences between acute and chronic inflammation

	Acute inflammation	Chronic inflammation
Onset	Rapid in onset (usually in minutes or hours)	May follow acute inflammation or be slow in onset (days)
Duration	Short duration. Lasts for hours or a few days	Longer duration; may be months
Predominant cells	Neutrophils (also called polymorphonuclear leukocytes)	Lymphocytes, monocytes/macrophages and sometimes plasma cells
Characteristics	Exudation of fluid and plasma proteins (edema) and the emigration of leukocytes	Inflammatory cells associated with the proliferation of blood vessels, tissue destruction and fibroblast proliferation
Injury/damage to tissue and fibrosis	Usually mild and self-limited and can progress to a chronic phase	Usually severe and progressive with fibrosis and scar formation
Signs: Local and systemic	Prominent	Less prominent

Cardinal Signs of Inflammation

Q. Mention the cardinal signs of inflammation and its mechanism.

- The four cardinal signs of inflammation as mentioned by **Celsus** are listed in Table 3.2.
- A fifth clinical sign, **loss of function** (functio laesa), was later added by Rudolf Virchow.

Table 3.2: Cardinal signs of inflammation

Cardinal sign	Mechanism
Rubor (redness)	Increased blood flow and stasis
Calor (heat)	Increased blood flow
Tumor (edema/ swelling)	Increased vascular permeability causing escape of a protein-rich fluid from blood vessels
Dolor (pain)	Chemical mediators: Prostaglandins and kinins

CAUSES OF (STIMULI FOR) ACUTE INFLAMMATION

Q. Mention the various causes of acute inflammation.

- **Infections** (bacterial, viral, fungal, and parasitic) and **microbial toxins**
- **Tissue necrosis:**
  - **Ischemia,** e.g. myocardial infarction
  - **Physical Agents**
    - Mechanical trauma, e.g. blunt/penetrating/crush injuries
    - Thermal injury, e.g. burns or frostbite
    - Radiation
    - Electric shock
    - Sudden changes in atmospheric pressure
  - **Chemical injury,** e.g. strong acids and alkalies, insecticides, and herbicides
- **Foreign bodies,** e.g. sutures, talc
- **Immune reactions:**
  - **Hypersensitivity reactions**
  - **Autoimmune diseases.**

SEQUENCE OF EVENTS IN ACUTE INFLAMMATION

Q. Explain the sequential vascular changes/reactions of blood vessels/hemodynamic changes in acute inflammation.

Acute inflammation has two major components, namely **1) reactions of blood vessels (vascular changes),** and **2) reactions of leukocytes (cellular events)** characterized by leukocyte recruitment to sites of inflammation and their activation to eliminate the causative agent.

REACTIONS OF BLOOD VESSELS (VASCULAR CHANGES)

Purpose: To deliver the circulating cells (leukocytes), fluids and plasma proteins from the circulation to sites of infection or tissue injury.

The reactions of blood vessels in acute inflammation (Figs 3.1 and 3.2) consist of **changes in the vascular flow and caliber** and **increased vascular permeability**.

Changes in Vascular Flow and Caliber

- **Vasodilatation:** It is the earliest feature of acute inflammation; sometimes it follows a transient constriction of arterioles. Vasodilation first affects the arterioles followed by opening of new capillary beds in the area.
  - **Effect:** Result is increased blood flow → local heat and redness.
  - **Chemical mediators involved:** Histamine, prostaglandins, platelet activating factor, kinins and nitric oxide (NO).
- **Increased permeability of the microvasculature:** It leads to escape of protein-rich fluid from the circulation into the extravascular tissues.
  - **Chemical mediators involved:** Histamine, leukotrienes, platelet activating factor, kinins.

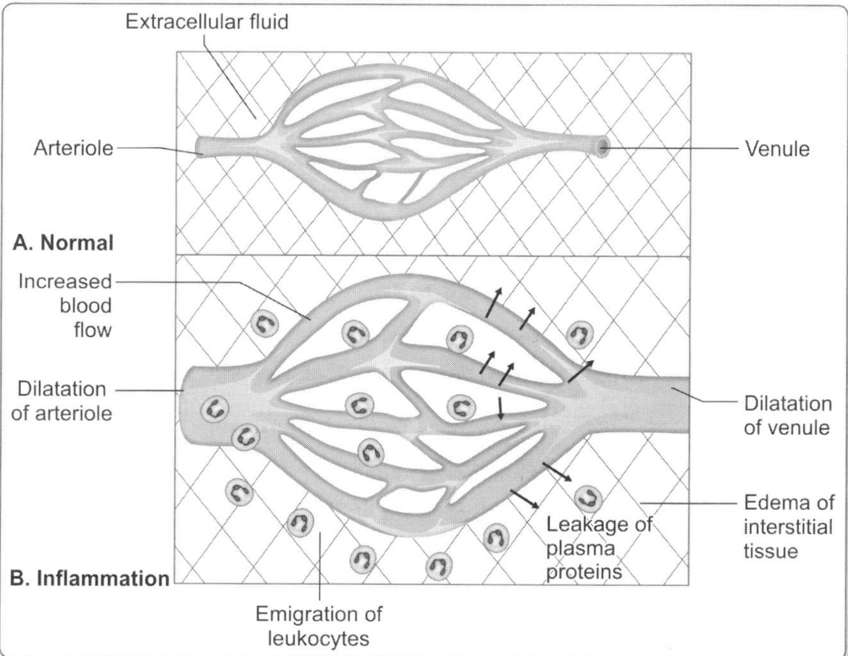

Fig. 3.1: Local features of acute inflammation, compared to normal are vasodilatation, increased blood flow, leakage of plasma fluid and proteins, and emigration of leukocyte

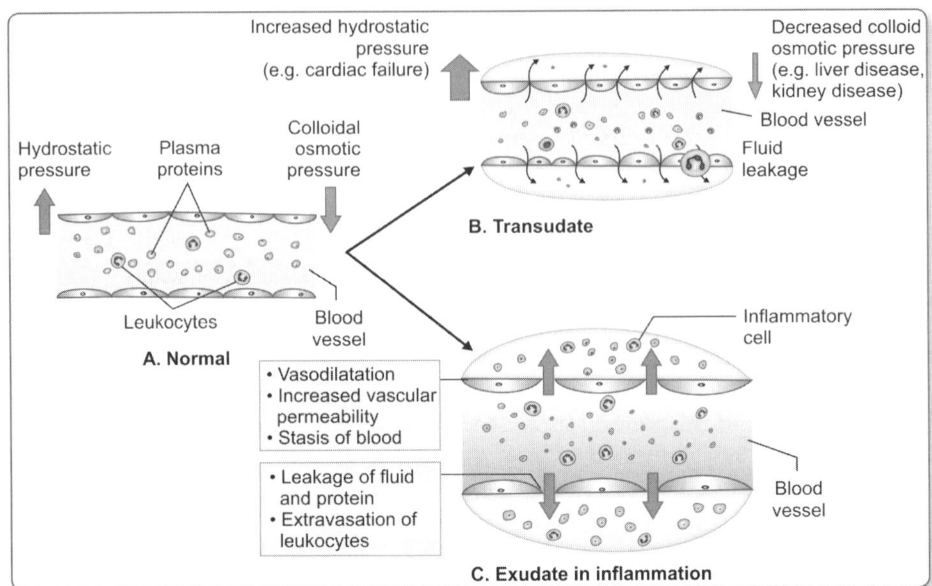

Figs 3.2A to C: A. Normal fluid exchange between blood and extracellular fluid; B. Formation of transudate; C. Formation of exudate in inflammation

- **Slowing of blood flow:** Vasodilatation and loss of fluid leads to concentration of RBCs in small vessels and increased viscosity of the blood. These changes result in ***engorgement of small vessels with slowly moving red cells, a condition termed stasis***.
- **Stasis:** It is responsible for vascular congestion and localized redness of the involved tissue.
- **Leukocyte events:** As stasis develops, **blood leukocytes (mainly neutrophils), accumulate along the vascular endothelium** (leukocyte events are described later on pages 46-50).

Increased Vascular Permeability (Vascular Leakage)

Exudation: It is defined as the process of escape of fluid, proteins and circulating blood cells from the vessels into the interstitial tissue or body cavities.

Escape of a protein-rich fluid **causes edema** and is one of the cardinal signs of inflammation. Differences between transudate and exudate are listed in Table 3.3.

Mechanism of Increased Vascular Permeability

Q. Describe the mechanism of increased vascular permeability.

Several mechanisms can cause increased vascular permeability of postcapillary venules:

1. **Contraction of endothelial cells:** It produces increased interendothelial spaces and results in edema.
   - Most common mechanism of vascular leakage
   - Occurs immediately after injury and is usually short-lived (15–30 minutes) and hence called as **immediate transient response**. In some mild injury (e.g. after burns, irradiation or ultraviolet radiation, certain bacterial toxins), vascular leakage develops after a delay of 2 to 12 hours and it lasts for many hours or even days. This delayed prolonged leakage may be due to contraction of endothelial cells or mild endothelial damage (e.g. sunburn)
   - **Chemical mediators involved:** Histamine, bradykinin, leukotrienes, the neuropeptide substance P.

Q. Mention the differences between transudate and exudate.

Table 3.3: Difference between transudate and exudate

Characteristics	Transudate	Exudate
Cause	Non-inflammatory process	Inflammation process
Mechanism	Ultrafiltrate of plasma, due to increased hydrostatic pressure with normal vascular permeability	Increased vascular permeability
Appearance	Clear, serous	Cloudy/purulent/hemorrhagic/ chylous
Color	Straw yellow	Yellow to red
Specific gravity	< 1.018	> 1.018
Protein	Low, < 2 g/dL, mainly albumin	High, > 2 g/dL
Clot	Absent	Clots spontaneously because of high fibrinogen
Cell count	Low	High
Type of cells	Few lymphocytes and mesothelial cells	Neutrophils in acute and lymphocytes in chronic inflammation
Bacteria	Absent	Usually present
Lactate dehydrogenase (LDH)	Low	High
Examples	Seen in congestive cardiac failure	Pus
Character of edema	Pitting type	No pitting

2. **Direct endothelial injury:** It causes necrosis and detachment of endothelial cells, e.g. burns, or infection by microbes. In most cases, leakage starts immediately after injury and is sustained for several hours until the damaged vessels are thrombosed or repaired. Hence, it is called as immediate sustained response.
3. **Leukocyte-mediated vascular injury:** The leukocyte (mainly neutrophils) which adheres to the endothelium during inflammation may themselves injure the endothelial cells.
4. **Increased transcytosis:** Process of transport of fluids and proteins through the endothelial cell (channels called vesiculovacuolar organelle) is known as transcytosis. However, their role in the vascular permeability of acute inflammation is uncertain.
5. **Leakage from new blood vessels:** During repair new blood vessels are formed (angiogenesis). These vessels are leaky till the endothelial cells mature.

Responses of Lymphatic Vessels and Lymph Nodes

- Apart from blood vessels, lymphatic vessels also participate in acute inflammation. Lymphatic vessels normally drain the small quantity of extravascular fluid that has escaped out of capillaries. Increased vascular permeability in inflammation produces accumulation of fluid in the extravascular space (i.e. edema). In inflammation, there is increased flow of lymph that helps to drain this edema fluid. In addition to fluid, leukocytes, cell debris, and microbes, may also flow into lymph way along with lymph.
- Secondary inflammation may occur in the draining lymphatics (**lymphangitis** characterized by the presence of red streaks along the course of the lymphatic channels draining a skin wound) and also in the draining lymph nodes (**lymphadenitis**). Inflamed draining lymph nodes are often painful and enlarged. These lymph nodes are termed as reactive, or inflammatory, lymphadenitis.

LEUKOCYTIC/CELLULAR EVENTS

Q. Describe leukocyte/cellular events in acute inflammation.

This process **delivers leukocytes** capable of phagocytosis (neutrophils and macrophages) **to the site of injury**. The events can be divided into: **leukocyte recruitment and phagocytosis and clearance of the injurious agent.**

A. Leukocyte Recruitment/Extravasation

Normally, leukocytes move rapidly in the blood, and during inflammation, they slow down and escape to the site of injury/causative agent in the extravascular space. Leukocyte extravasation is the **process of migration of leukocytes from the lumen of the vessel to the site of injury** in the extravascular tissues. It is a multistep process that is mediated and controlled by adhesion molecules and cytokines called chemokines.

Steps in Leukocyte Recruitment/Extravasation (Fig. 3.3)

In the Vascular Lumen:

1. **Margination:** When the blood flow slows down (stasis), **leukocytes** (mainly neutrophils) **move towards the peripheral column** and accumulate along on the endothelial surface of vessels. This process of redistribution of leukocyte is termed margination.
2. **Rolling:** Marginated leukocytes attach weakly to the endothelium, detach and bind again with a mild jumping movement. It causes rolling of leukocyte along the endothelial surface.
   - **Molecules involved:** Selectin family of adhesive molecules and its complementary ligands (Table 3.4).

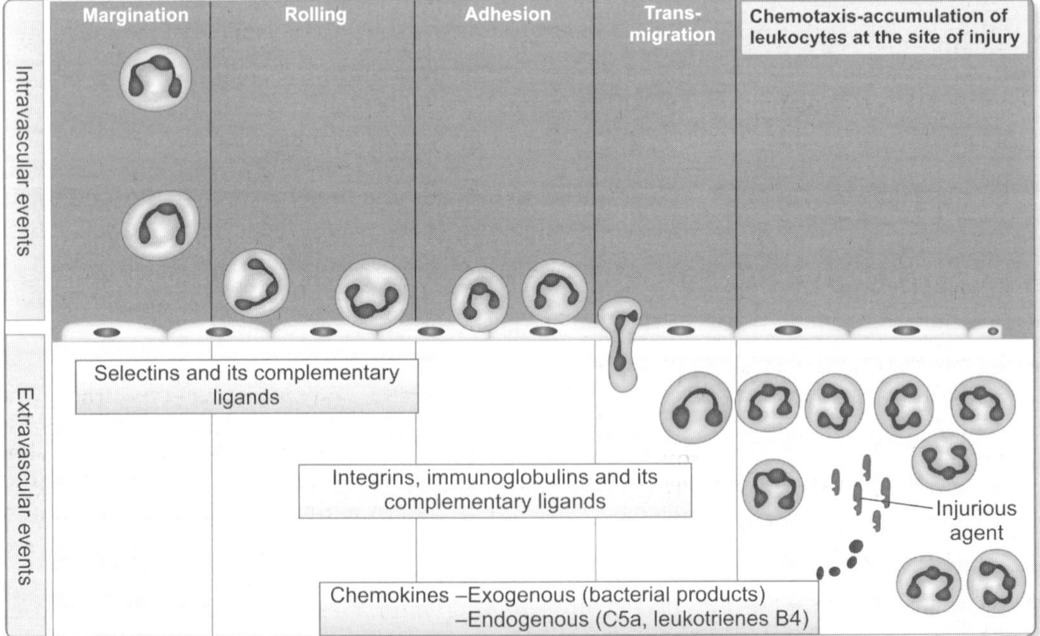

Fig. 3.3: Various steps of leukocyte migration through blood vessels. The leukocytes first roll, and then firmly adhere to endothelium, followed by transmigration across the endothelium. Leukocytes pierce the basement membrane, and migrate toward chemoattractants from the source of injury. Selectins are involved in rolling; integrins in adhesion; and CD31 (PECAM-1) in transmigration

Table 3.4: Selectins and complimentary selectin ligands involved in rolling

Type of selectin	Distribution	Ligand and their expression
L-selectin (CD62L)	Neutrophils, monocytes	Sialyl-Lewis X/PNAd on GlyCAM-1, CD34, MAdCAM-1, others; expressed on endothelium (HEV)
E-selectin (CD62E)	Endothelium activated by cytokines (TNF, IL-1)	Sialyl-Lewis X (e.g., CLA) on glycoproteins; expressed on neutrophils, monocytes
P-selectin (CD62P)	Endothelium activated by cytokines (TNF, IL-1), histamine, or thrombin	Sialyl-Lewis X on PSGL-1 and other glycoproteins; expressed on neutrophils, monocytes

CLA= Cutaneous lymphocyte antigen-1; GlyCAM-1= glycan-bearing cell adhesion molecule-1; HEV= high endothelial venule; IL-1= interleukin-1; MAdCAM-1= mucosal adhesion cell adhesion molecule-1; PSGL-1= P-selectin glycoprotein ligand-1; TNF= tumor necrosis factor.

Table 3.5: Integrins and complimentary ligands involved in endothelial-leukocyte adhesion

Type of integrin	Distribution	Ligands and their expression
LFA-1 (CD11aCD18)	Neutrophils, monocytes	ICAM-1 (CD54), ICAM-2 (CD102); expressed on endothelium (upregulated on activated endothelium)
MAC-1 (CD11bCD18)	Monocytes	
VLA-4 (CD49aCD29)	Monocytes	VCAM-1 (CD106); expressed on endothelium (upregulated on activated endothelium)

ICAM= intercellular adhesion molecule; VCAM= vascular cell adhesion molecule.

- **Chemical mediators involved: Cytokines such as: 1) tumor necrosis factor (TNF), 2) interleukin-1 (IL-1)** and chemokines (chemoattractant cytokines).

3. **Adhesion of leukocyte to endothelium:** Endothelium gets activated and leukocytes bind more firmly.
   - **Molecules involved:** The adhesion/attachment of leukocytes to endothelial cells is mediated by complementary adhesion molecules on these two cell types. The expression of adhesive molecules is enhanced by cytokines (Table 3.5).
   - **Chemical mediators involved:**
     - Endothelial cells are activated by cytokines namely: TNF and IL-1 and increase the expression of two ligands for integrins on leukocyte (Table 3.5).
     - Chemokines are chemoattractant cytokines that cause leukocyte activation and **conversion of low-affinity** integrins **on leukocyte to high-affinity state** resulting in firm adhesion of the leukocytes to the endothelium.

Leukocyte Migration through Vessel Wall:

1. **Leukocyte migration through endothelium: Migration of the leukocytes through the endothelium is called transmigration or diapedesis.** Leukocytes migrate through the vessel wall by squeezing through the intercellular junctions between the endothelial cells.
   - **Molecules involved:** CD31 (platelet endothelial cell adhesion molecule [PECAM-1]) expressed on leukocytes and endothelial cells and ICAM-1. It occurs mainly in postcapillary venules.
2. **Migration across the basement membrane:** Leukocytes penetrate the basement membrane of the vessel by secreting collagenases.

Outside the Vessel Wall

After penetration of the basement membrane of vessel, leukocytes move in the tissues toward the site of injury by a process called chemotaxis. It can be simply defined as locomotion of leukocyte along a chemical gradient.

Q. Define and write short note on chemotaxis.

1. **Chemotaxis of leukocytes**

   Definition: Chemotaxis is defined as process of **migration of leukocytes toward the inflammatory stimulus** in the **direction of the gradient** of locally produced chemoattractants.

   Chemoattractants:
   - **Exogenous:** Bacterial products (e.g. N-formylmethionine terminal amino acid)
   - **Endogenous:**
     - Cytokines, mainly chemokine family (e.g. **IL-8**)
     - Complement components: **C5a, C3a**
     - Arachidonic acid metabolites of lipoxygenase pathway: **Leukotriene B_4 (LTB_4)**.
2. **Accumulation of leukocytes at the sites of infection and injury:** Achieved by binding of leukocytes to the extracellular matrix proteins through **integrins and CD44**.
   - **Type of leukocytes infiltrates:**
     - **Neutrophils:** Predominantly during the first 6 to 24 hours.
     - **Monocytes:** Neutrophils are replaced by monocytes in 24 to 48 hours.

B. Phagocytosis and Clearance of the Offending Agent

Develops in two sequential events:

Recognition of microbes, necrotic cells and foreign substances: Leukocytes recognize microbes, necrotic cells and foreign substances by cell surface receptors known as "**pattern recognition receptors**".

Activation of leukocytes: Recognition of microbes or dead cells by the receptors initiates several responses in leukocytes together known as **leukocyte activation**. The most important functional responses of leukocyte activation is phagocytosis and intracellular killing.

Phagocytosis

Q. Write short note on phagocytosis.

Many leukocytes **recognize, internalize, and digest** foreign materials, microorganisms, or cellular debris by a process termed phagocytosis. It consists of three steps (Fig. 3.4):
- Recognition and attachment
- Engulfment
- Killing or degradation of the ingested material.

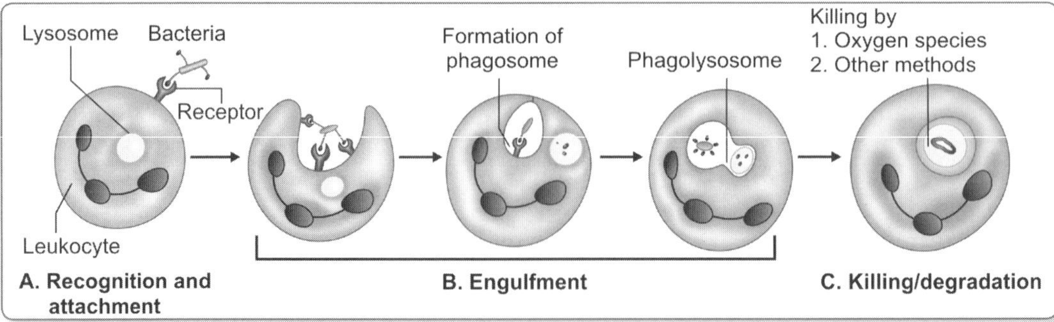

Fig. 3.4: Different steps in phagocytosis. A. Recognition and attachment, which involves binding to receptors on the leukocyte membrane to injurious agent (e.g. bacteria); B. Engulfment, formation of phagosome and fusion of lysosomes with phagocytic vacuoles to form phagolysosome; C. Killing/degradation of ingested particles within the phagolysosomes by lysosomal enzymes and by reactive oxygen and nitrogen species

Table 3.6: Different opsonins and their corresponding receptors on leukocyte

Opsonin	Receptor on leukocyte
IgG antibodies	Fc receptor (FcγRI)
Complement components C3	Type 1 and 3 complement receptor (CR1 and CR3)
Collectins	C1q

Recognition and Attachment

- Receptors on the surface of phagocytic cells recognize components of microbes and necrotic cells. Leukocytes express several receptors that recognize external stimuli. These include 1) receptors for microbial products (e.g. Toll-like receptors—TLRs), 2) G protein-coupled receptors (recognize N-formyl methionie residues), 3) receptors for cytokines (for INF-γ) and 4) receptors for opsonins (described below).
- **Receptors for opsonins (phagocytic receptor):** The phagocytosis is enhanced when leukocyte receptors recognize microbes coated by specific host proteins known as **opsonins.** The major opsonins are IgG antibodies, the C3b breakdown product of complement, and certain plasma lectins called collectins (Table 3.6).

Engulfment

Next step in phagocytosis is engulfment and formation of a phagocytic vacuole. Phagocytosis is dependent on polymerization of actin filaments.

- **Phagosome:** Extensions of the **cytoplasm of leukocyte form pseudopods surrounding the particle to be ingested** and forms a vesicle or vacuole called a phagosome.
- **Phagolysosome:** The membrane of **phagosome fuses** with membrane of **lysosome to form a phagolysosome**. Lysosomal **granules are discharged** into this phagolysosome.

Killing and Degradation

Killing and degradation of ingested microbial agents/particles occurs within neutrophils and macrophages. Most important microbicidal agents are: 1) reactive oxygen species and 2) lysosomal enzymes.

Reactive Oxygen Species (ROS)

Types of ROS are:

- Superoxide anion ($O_2^{\bar{\bullet}}$, one electron)—**weak**
- Hydrogen peroxide (H_2O_2, two electrons)—**weak**
- Hydroxyl ions (•OH), three electrons—**highly reactive.**

Mechanism of production (refer pages 18 to 21)**:** In the phagocytic vacuole of leukocyte, rapid activation of NADPH oxidase (also called **phagocyte oxidase**), oxidizes NADPH (reduced nicotinamide-adenine dinucleotide phosphate) to NADP. During the process oxygen is reduced to superoxide anion ($O_2^{\bar{\bullet}}$).

- $O_2^{\bar{\bullet}}$ is converted into hydrogen peroxide (H_2O_2) by spontaneous dismutation
  $O_2^{\bar{\bullet}} + 2H \rightarrow H_2O_2$
- Amount of H_2O_2 is insufficient to kill most of the microbes by itself but the enzyme **myeloperoxidase** (MPO) present in the azurophilic granules of neutrophils can convert it into a powerful ROS. MPO in the presence of a halide such as Cl^-, converts H_2O_2 to hypochlorous radical (HOCl•), which is a potent oxidant and antimicrobial agent.

Hypochlorite (HOCl•) destroys microbes either by **halogenation** or by proteins and lipid peroxidation.

- H_2O_2 is also converted to hydroxyl radical (•OH) which is also powerful destructive agent.

Reactive nitrogen species: NO, which is generated from arginine by the action of nitric oxide synthase (NOS), can kill microbes similar to ROS.

•NO reacts with superoxide ($O_2^{\bar{\bullet}}$) and produces highly reactive free radical peroxynitrite (ONOO•).

Lysosomal Enzymes

Acid hydrolases of lysosomes degrade the dead microorganisms. Elastase can kill bacteria.

- **Constituents of leukocyte granules:** The microbicidal substances within leukocyte cytoplasmic granules include:
  - Bactericidal permeability—increasing protein
  - Lysozyme and lactoferrin
  - **Major basic protein (MBP) present in eosinophils is cytotoxic to many parasites**
  - Defensins are toxic to microbes
  - Cathelicidins: These are anti-microbial proteins in the neutrophils and other cells. They are very effective against *Mycobacterium tuberculosis*.

CHEMICAL MEDIATORS OF INFLAMMATION

Q. Write short note on role of different mediators in different reactions of inflammation.

Definition: Substances that initiate and regulate inflammatory reactions are called as **mediators of inflammation**. Numerous chemical mediators are responsible for inflammatory reactions.

Q. List chemical mediators of inflammation. Role of chemical mediators in inflammation. Name the cell derived mediators of inflammation. Name the plasma derived mediators of inflammation.

General Features of Mediators

- **Source of mediators:** Mediators are derived either from cells or from plasma proteins (Table 3.7).
  - **Cell-derived mediators:**
    - Present either as **preformed molecules** (e.g. histamine in mast cell granules) or are **synthesized de novo** (e.g. prostaglandins, cytokines) in response to a stimulus.
    - Produced usually by platelets, neutrophils, monocytes/macrophages, and mast cells.
  - **Plasma-derived mediators:** Produced mainly in the **liver** and present in the circulation as **inactive precursors, which require activation** (e.g. complement proteins, kinins).
- **Tightly regulated actions.**
- **Inter-related:** One mediator can stimulate the release of other mediators. The secondary mediators may have the similar, different or even opposite actions.
- Most act by **binding to specific receptor** on target cells.
- **Diverse targets:** Target cell type varies depending on the type of mediator. They can act on one or few or many diverse targets, or may have different effects on different types of cells.
- **Short-lived:** Most of these mediators have a short-lifespan.

Main mediators involved in the inflammatory reaction are listed in Table 3.7.

Table 3.7: Main chemical mediators of acute inflammation

Cell-derived	Plasma protein-derived
• **Vasoactive amines** – Histamine – Serotonin	• **Complement components** – C3a – C5a – C3b – C5b-9 (MAC)
• **Arachidonic acid (AA) metabolites** – Prostaglandins – Leukotrienes	• **Kinins** – Bradykinin – Kallikrein
• **Platelet-activating factor (PAF)**	• **Coagulation/fibrinolytic system**
• **Reactive oxygen species (ROS)**	
• **Nitric oxide (NO)**	
• **Cytokines (TNF, IL-1) and Chemokines**	

Abbreviation: IL-1, interleukin-1; TNF, tumor necrosis factor; MAC, membrane attack complex.

CELL-DERIVED MEDIATORS

Vasoactive Amines: Histamine and Serotonin

Histamine and serotonin are the first mediators to be released during inflammation, which are stored as preformed molecules in cells.

1. **Histamine:** It is a preformed vasoactive mediator. Responsible for immediate transient response.
   Source: Mast cells (richest source), **blood basophils and platelets**.
   Stimuli:
   - **Physical injury** (e.g. trauma, cold, heat)
   - **Immune reactions** in which antibodies bind to mast cells (e.g. **allergic reactions**)
   - **Other chemical mediators:** C3a and C5a, leukocyte-derived histamine-releasing proteins, neuropeptides (e.g. substance P), cytokines (IL-1, IL-8).

   Actions: 1) **Dilation of arterioles** and 2) **increase of the vascular permeability**.
2. **Serotonin (5-hydroxytryptamine):** It is a preformed vasoactive mediator.
   Source: Platelets, some **neurons** and **enterochromaffin cells** in the gastrointestinal tract.
   Stimulus: Platelet aggregation and antigen-antibody complexes.
   Actions: Similar to those of histamine.

Arachidonic Acid (AA) Metabolites (Prostaglandins, Leukotrienes, and Lipoxins)

Arachidonic Acid (AA)

- **Source:** Derived from cell membrane phospholipids mainly by the enzyme phospholipase A_2.
- **Stimuli:** Mechanical, chemical, and physical stimuli or other mediators (e.g. C5a).
- **AA metabolism: Occurs along two major enzymatic pathways (Fig. 3.5)**. These are **cyclooxygenase pathway** (produce prostaglandins) and **lipoxygenase pathway** (produces leukotrienes and lipoxins).

A. **Products of cyclooxygenase pathway:**
   - **Products:** Most important in inflammation are PGE_2, PGD_2, PGI_2 (prostacyclin), and TxA_2 (thromboxane A_2).

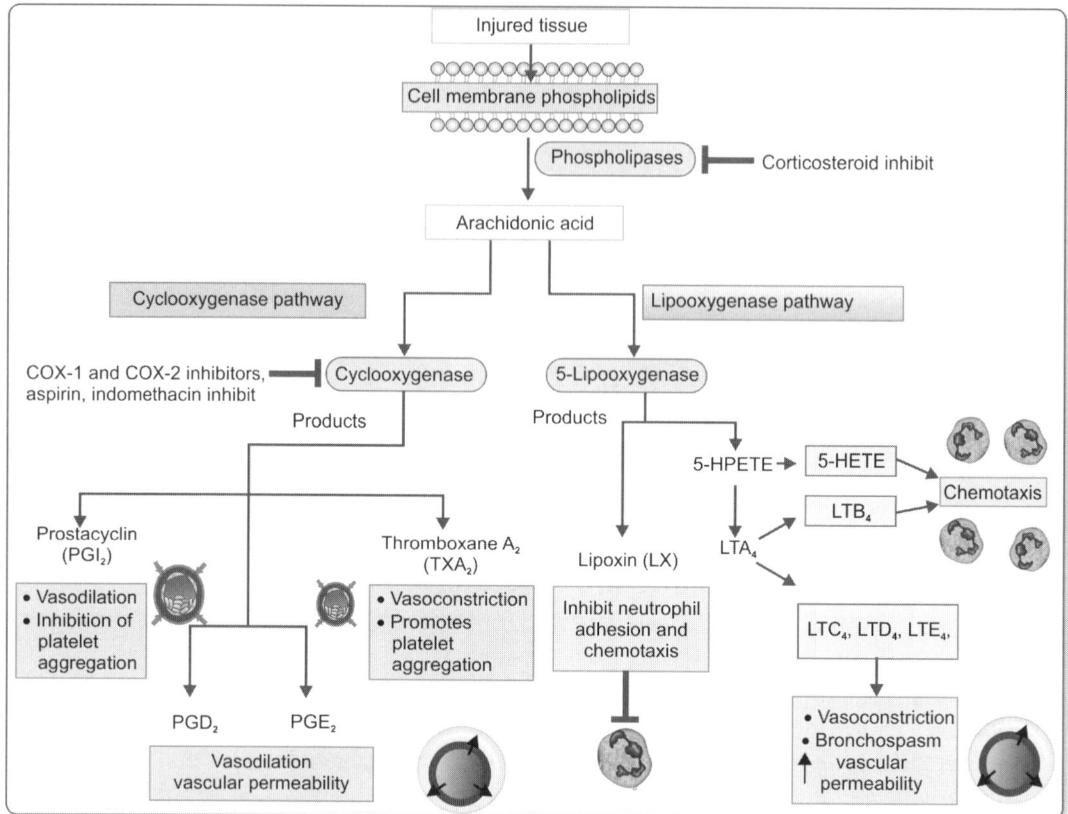

Fig. 3.5: Arachidonic acid metabolites involved in inflammation. The cyclooxygenase pathway generates prostaglandins (PGIs) and thromboxane (TXA_2). The lipoxygenase pathway forms lipoxins (LXs) and leukotrienes (LTEs).
Abbreviation: COX, cyclooxygenase; HETE, hydroxyeicosatetraenoic acid; HPETE, hydroperoxyeicosatetraenoic acid.

- **Mechanism:** They are produced from AA by the actions of two **cyclooxygenases,** COX-1 and COX-2.
- **Local effects:**
  - **TxA_2: Vasoconstriction** and promotes **platelet-aggregation**
  - **Prostacyclin (PGI_2): Vasodilator** and **inhibits platelet aggregation**
  - **PGD_2 and PGE_2: Vasodilation and increased permeability**. PGD_2 is also a chemoattractant for neutrophils.
- **Systemic effects:**
  - Prostaglandins are responsible for **pain and fever** in inflammation.
  - PGE_2 causes cytokine-induced **fever** during infections.

B. Products of lipoxygenase pathway: 1) Leukotrienes and 2) lipoxins.

1. Leukotrienes: Products and their actions:

- **5-hydroxyeicosatetraenoic acid (5-HETE):** Chemotactic for neutrophils, and is the precursor of the leukotrienes.
- **LTB_4**
  - **Chemotactic agent**
  - Neutrophil activation causing adhesion to endothelium, generation of ROS, and release of lysosomal enzymes.

   - **Leukotrienes C_4, D_4, and E_4(LTC_4, LTD_4, LTE_4)**
     - Vasoconstriction
     - Bronchospasm (in asthma)
     - **Increased vascular permeability**.
2. **Lipoxins (LXs):**
   - **Actions: Inhibit inflammation**
     - **Inhibit neutrophil chemotaxis** and recruitment.
     - **Inhibit leukocyte adhesion** to endothelium.

Main actions of arachidonic acid metabolites (eicosanoids) involved in inflammation are presented in Table 3.8.

Table 3.8: Main actions of arachidonic acid metabolites (eicosanoids) in inflammation

Action	Arachidonic acid metabolites (Eicosanoid)
Vasodilation	PGI_2 (prostacyclin I_2), PGE_2, PGD_2
Increased vascular permeability	Leukotrienes C_4, D_4, E_4
Chemotaxis, leukocyte adhesion	Leukotriene B_4, HETE (hydroxyeicosatetraenoic acid)

Platelet-activating Factor (PAF)

Action: Multiple inflammatory effects:
- **Vascular reactions: Vasodilation** and **increased vascular permeability.**
- **Cellular reactions: Increased leukocyte adhesion** to endothelium, **chemotaxis**.
- **Others:** Increases the synthesis of other mediators, mainly eicosanoids.

Reactive Oxygen Species (ROS)

ROS are chemically reactive oxygen-derived free radical. Normally, they are rapidly inactivated. But increased production can cause cell injury.

Cell of origin: Leukocytes (neutrophils and macrophages).

Mechanism of production: Leukocytes during phagocytosis (after exposure to microbes, chemokines, and immune complexes) generate oxygen-derived free radicals (refer chapter 2).

Types: Superoxide anion ($O_2^{\bullet-}$), hydrogen peroxide (H_2O_2), and hydroxyl radical ($^{\bullet}OH$).

$O_2^{\bullet-}$ can combine with NO to form reactive nitrogen species (peroxynitrite $ONOO^-$).

Actions:
- **Physiologic function:** ROS in leukocytes **destroys** phagocytosed **microbes and necrotic cells**.
- **Pathological actions:**
  - Endothelial cell damage, which causes increased vascular permeability
  - Injury to other cells: e.g. tumor cells, parenchymal cells and red blood cells
  - Inactivation of antiproteases, such as α_1-antitrypsin, e.g. destruction of elastic tissues in emphysema of lung.

Nitric Oxide (NO)

NO is a soluble, free radical gas which causes vasodilation (was known as endothelium-derived relaxing factor).

Source: Many cells, such as endothelial cells, macrophages and neurons in the brain.

Synthesis: Synthesized from L-arginine, molecular oxygen, and NADPH by the enzyme nitric oxide synthase (NOS).

Types: Three isoforms of NOS: Type I neuronal (nNOS), type II inducible (iNOS) and type III endothelial (eNOS).

Action: It acts in a paracrine manner on target cells:

- **Vasodilatation** by relaxing vascular smooth muscle cells.
- **Controls inflammatory responses** by inhibiting leukocyte recruitment and adhesion.
- **Reduced platelet adhesion, aggregation and degranulation.**
- **Microbicidal activity.**

Cytokines and Chemokines

These are polypeptides which function as mediators in **immune responses** and in **inflammation (acute and chronic)**.

Source: Cytokines are secreted by many types of cell (activated lymphocytes and macrophages, endothelial, epithelial, and connective tissue cells).

Tumor Necrosis Factor and Interleukin-1

These are the two **major cytokines** involved in inflammation:

Source: Activated macrophages.

Stimuli: Endotoxin and other microbial products, **immune complexes**, **physical injury**, and many **inflammatory stimuli.**

Actions in inflammation (Fig. 3.6):

- **Local effects:**
  - **Endothelial activation:** Endothelial activation and increased expression of **endothelial adhesion molecules**.
  - **Activation of leukocytes and other cells:** TNF increases the responses of neutrophils to other stimuli (e.g. bacterial endotoxin).
  - **During repair:** Proliferation of fibroblasts and increased synthesis of collagen.
- **Systemic effects:**
  - Fever
  - Leukocytosis
  - Systemic acute-phase reactions
  - Suppresses appetite: TNF contributes to cachexia seen in some chronic infections.

Chemokines

Chemotactic cytokines or chemokines are small proteins, which selectively attracts various leukocytes to the site of inflammation.

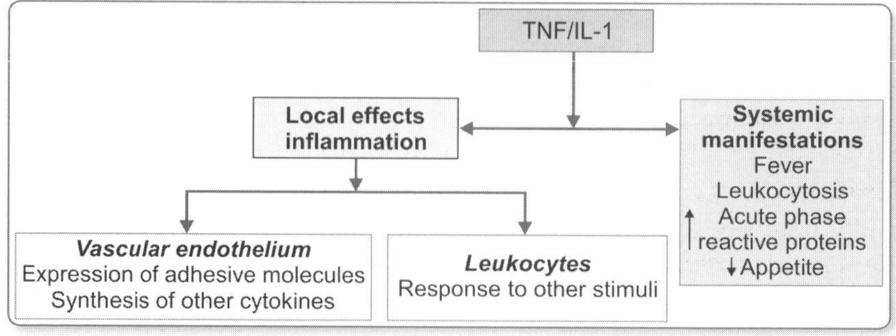

Fig. 3.6: Important local and systemic effects of tumor necrosis factor (TNF) and interleukin-1 (IL-1)

Classification: Chemokines are classified four major groups namely: 1) C-X-C chemokines, 2) C-C chemokines, 3) C chemokines and 4) C-X-3C chemokines.

Action: Chemotaxis of **monocytes, eosinophils, basophils, and lymphocytes** except neutrophils. They activate **leukocyte and promote their recruitment to the sites of inflammation**.

Other Cytokines in Acute Inflammation

- IL-6, produced by macrophages and other cells is involved in local and systemic reactions.
- IL-17 produced by T lymphocytes promotes neutrophil recruitment.

Lysosomal Constituents of Leukocytes

Neutrophils

Types of granules:

1. **Smaller specific (or secondary) granules:** They contain lysozyme, collagenase, gelatinase, lactoferrin, plasminogen activator, histaminase, and alkaline phosphatase.
2. **Larger azurophil (or primary) granules:** They **contain myeloperoxidase**, bactericidal factors (lysozyme, defensins), acid hydrolases, and a variety of neutral proteases (elastase, cathepsin G, nonspecific collagenases, proteinase).

Monocytes and Macrophages

They also contain acid hydrolases, collagenase, elastase, phospholipase, and plasminogen activator. These are active mainly in chronic inflammation.

Neuropeptides

- These are small peptides, such as substance P and neurokinin A.
- **Source:** Secreted by sensory nerves and various leukocytes.
- **Action:** Vasodilation and increased vascular permeability.

PLASMA-DERIVED MEDIATORS

Chemical mediators derived from plasma proteins belong to three interrelated systems:

1. Complement
2. Kinin
3. Clotting systems.

Complement System

Q. What are the three methods of complement activation and its effector function in acute inflammation?

The complement system is a group of plasma proteins synthesize in the liver, and are numbered C1 to C9.

Pathways of complement system activation (Fig. 3.7): The decisive step in complement activation is the proteolysis of the third component, C3.

Cleavage of C3 can occur by any one of three pathways:

1. **Classical pathway:** It is activated by **antigen-antibody** (Ag-Ab) complexes.
2. **Alternative pathway:** It is triggered by microbial surface molecules (e.g. endotoxin, or LPS), complex polysaccharides, cobra venom, and other substances, **in the absence of antibody**.
3. **Lectin pathway:** It directly activates C1 when plasma mannose-binding lectin binds to mannose on microbes.

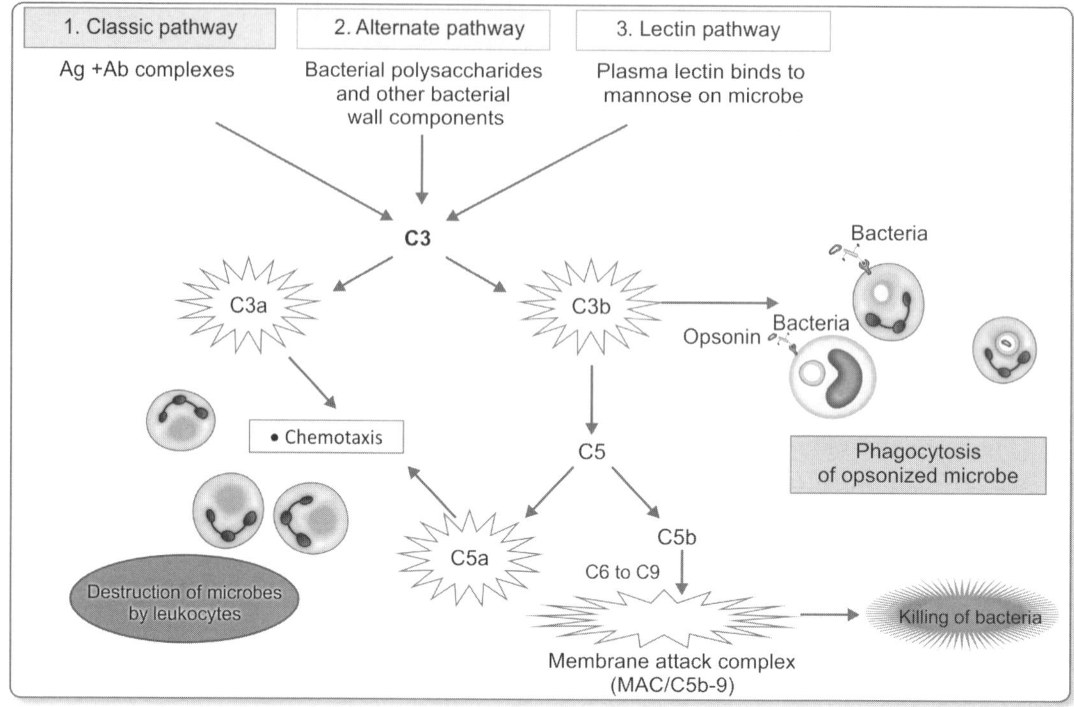

Fig. 3.7: Different pathways of activation and functions of the complement system. All pathways of activation lead to cleavage of C3

Functions of Complement

Anti-infective Functions

1. **Leukocyte activation, adhesion and chemotaxis:** C5a causes **leukocyte activation, adhesion** and C3a and C5a are **powerful chemotactic** agents for neutrophils, monocytes, eosinophils, and basophils.
2. **Opsonization and promote phagocytosis:** C3b and its cleavage product iC3b (inactive C3b) act as opsonins and promote phagocytosis by neutrophils and macrophages through surface receptors for these complement fragments.
3. **Cell and bacterial lysis:** The deposition of the MAC (C5b-C9) on cells creates pores, which allow water and ions to enter into the cells and results in death (lysis) of the cells and bacteria.
4. **Increased vascular permeability:** C3a, C5a complement components stimulate histamine release from mast cells and thus increase vascular permeability and cause vasodilation. They are called anaphylatoxins, because their actions are similar to mast cell mediators involved in anaphylaxis.
5. **Activation of AA:** C5a activates the lipoxygenase pathway of AA metabolism in neutrophils and monocytes, thereby causing release of more chemical mediators.

Interplay between innate and adaptive immune system

- Defense against microbes through innate and adaptive immunity

Other Functions:
- Clearance of:
  - Immune complexes (Clq, C3)
  - Apoptotic cells (Clq, C3).

Coagulation and Kinin Systems

Inflammation and clotting system are intertwined with each other.

Activated Hageman factor (factor XIIa) activate the four systems involved in the inflammatory response (Fig. 3.8).

1. **Activation of fibrinolytic system:** Factor XIIa stimulates fibrinolytic system by converting plasminogen to plasmin. The role of fibrinolytic system in inflammation are:
   a. **Activation of complement system.**
   b. **Fibrin split products:** Plasmin degrades fibrin to form fibrin split products, which may **increase vascular permeability**.
2. **Activation of the Kinin system**
3. **Activation of the alternative complement pathway:** Factor XIIa can activate alternate complement pathway.
4. **Activation of the coagulation system:** Factor XIIa activates coagulation system and form thrombin, which has inflammatory properties.

Kinins System

Kinins are vasoactive peptides derived from plasma proteins.

- **Mechanism of production:** Factor XIIa converts prekallikrein to kallikrein, which in turn cleaves high-molecular-weight kininogen to produce bradykinin.

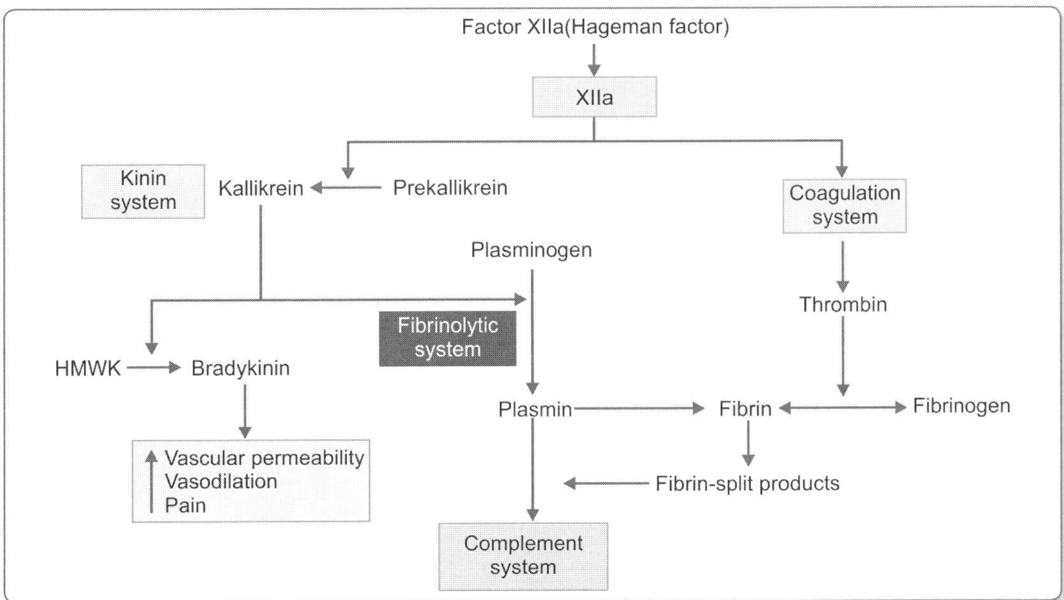

Fig. 3.8: Interrelationships between the four plasma derived chemical mediator systems. Activation of factor XII (Hageman factor) is a key event leading to conversion of plasminogen to plasmin, resulting in generation of fibrin split products and active complement products. Activation of kallikrein produces kinins and activation of the coagulation system results in fibrin formation.

Abbreviation: HMWK, high molecular weight kininogen.

Table 3.9: Important mediators involved in acute inflammation

Action of the mediator	Name of the mediator	Source of the mediator
Vasodilation	Prostaglandins	Mast cells, all leukocytes
	Nitric oxide	Endothelium, macrophages
	Histamine	Mast cells, basophils, platelets
Increased vascular permeability	Histamine	
	Serotonin	Platelets
	C3a and C5a (liberate vasoactive amines from mast cells, other cells)	Plasma (produced in liver)
	Bradykinin	
	Leukotrienes C_4, D_4, E_4	Mast cells, all leukocytes
	Platelet-activating factor (PAF)	All leukocytes, endothelial cell
	Neuropeptides (substance P)	Leukocytes, nerve fibers
Chemotaxis and leukocyte activation	Cytokines (TNF, IL-1, IL-6)	Macrophages, lymphocytes, endothelial cells, mast cells
	Chemokines	Leukocytes, activated macrophages
	C3a, C5a	Plasma (produced in the liver)
	Leukotriene B_4	Mast cells, leukocytes
	Bacterial products (e.g. *N*-formyl methyl peptides)	Bacteria
Fever	IL-1 TNF	Macrophages, endothelial cells, mast cells
	Prostaglandins	Mast cells, leukocytes
Pain	Prostaglandins	
	Bradykinin	Plasma protein
Tissue damage	Lysosomal enzymes	Leukocytes
	Reactive oxygen species	
	Nitric oxide	Endothelium, macrophage

Abbreviations: IL-1, interleukin-1; IL-6, interleukin-6; TNF, tumor necrosis factor.

- **Actions of bradykinin:**
  - **Increases vascular permeability**
  - **Pain** when injected into the skin.
- **Actions of kallikrein:**
  - Potent activator of Hageman factor
  - Chemotactic activity: Directly converts C5 to the chemoattractant product C5a.

Most important mediators involved in acute inflammation are summarized in Table 3.9.

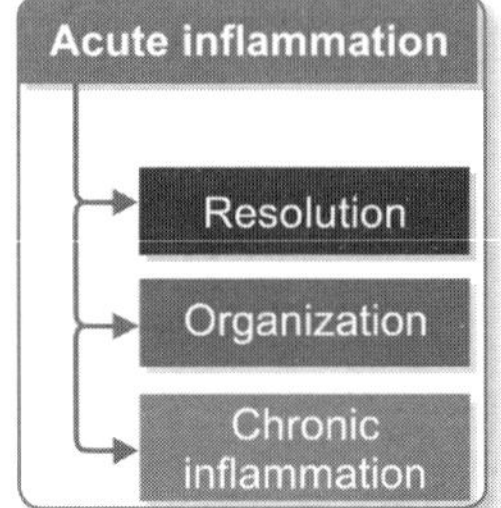

Fig. 3.9: Outcomes of acute inflammation: 1. resolution, 2. organization (healing by fibrosis and scarring), or 3. chronic inflammation

OUTCOMES OF ACUTE INFLAMMATION (FIG. 3.9)

Q. Write short note on outcomes (fate) of acute inflammation.

- **Resolution: Complete return** of tissue architecture **to normal** following acute inflammation. It occurs:

- When the injury is limited or short-lived
- With no or minimal tissue damage
- When injured tissue is capable of regeneration.

- **Organization/healing by fibrosis:** Process of **replacement of dead tissue by living tissue,** which matures to form scar tissue is known as **organization**. It occurs:
  - When there is plenty of fibrin exudation in tissue or serous cavities (pleura, peritoneum) which cannot be removed or cleared.
  - In presence of significant tissue destruction.
  - With inflammation in tissues incapable of regeneration.

  This process involves growing of connective tissue into the area of tissue damage or exudate, and is converted into a mass of fibrous tissue (scar).
  - **Abscess:** Localized collection of pus is called abscess. If the area of acute inflammation is walled off by inflammatory cells and fibrosis, neutrophil products destroy the tissue and form an abscess.
- **Progression to chronic inflammation:** Chronic inflammation may follow acute inflammation, or it may be chronic from the beginning itself. Acute progress to chronic when the acute inflammatory response cannot be resolved. This may be due to:
  - Persistence of the injurious agent or
  - Abnormality in the process of healing.

    Examples:
    - **Bacterial infection of the lung** may begin as acute inflammation (pneumonia). But when it fails to resolve, it can cause extensive tissue destruction and form a cavity with chronic inflammation known as lung abscess.
    - **Acute osteomyelitis** if not treated properly **may progress to chronic osteomyelitis**.
    - Chronic inflammation with a persisting stimulus results in peptic ulcer of the duodenum or stomach, which may persist for months or years.

MORPHOLOGICAL TYPES/PATTERNS OF ACUTE INFLAMMATION

Q. Write short note on morphological types/patterns of acute inflammatory reaction with suitable examples.

Gross and microscopic appearances can often provide clues about the cause:

Serous Inflammation

- Characterized by marked outpouring of a thin serous fluid.
- Serous exudate or effusion is yellow, straw-like in color and microscopically shows either few or no cells.
- **Example:**
  - Skin blister formed in burn or viral infection.
  - Inflammation of synovium (synovitis).
  - Pleural effusion as a complication of lobar pneumonia.

Fibrinous Inflammation

- **Marked increase in vascular permeability** leads to escape of large molecules like fibrinogen from the lumen of the vessel into the extravascular space and forms fibrin. The **exudate rich in fibrin** is called fibrinous exudate.
- A fibrinous exudate is mostly observed with inflammation in the lining of body cavities, such as the meninges, pericardium and pleura. When a fibrinous exudate develops on a

serosal surface, such as the pleura or pericardium, it is known as fibrinous pleuritis or fibrinous pericarditis.
- Microscopically, fibrin appears as an eosinophilic or pink meshwork of threads or pink amorphous coagulum.
- For example fibrinous pericarditis (Fig. 3.10) is seen in rheumatic fever and classically known as "**bread and butter**" pericarditis.

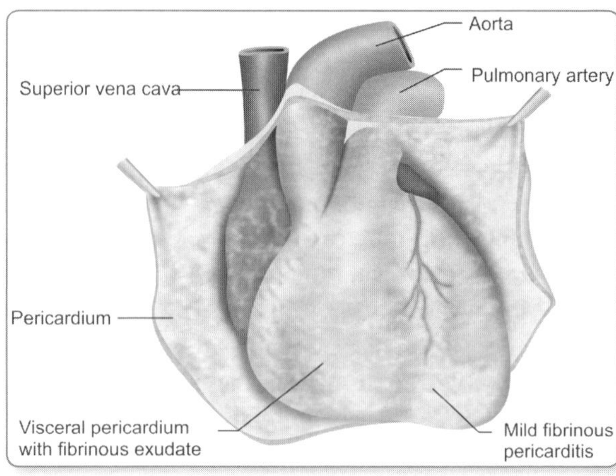

Fig. 3.10: Fibrinous pericarditis developing in rheumatic fever

Suppurative or Purulent Inflammation: Abscess

- It is characterized by the production of large amounts of pus or purulent exudate.
- Microscopically, shows neutrophils, liquefactive necrosis, and edema fluid. Bacteria (e.g. staphylococci) which produce localized suppuration and are called as **pyogenic** (pus-producing) bacteria. For example acute appendicitis.
- **Abscesses**: It is the **localized collections of purulent inflammatory exudates in a tissue**, an organ, or a confined space. Abscesses have a central necrotic focus (consisting of necrotic leukocytes and necrotic parenchymal cells) surrounded by a zone of preserved neutrophils. If pus accumulates in hollow organs or pleural cavity, it is known as empyema e.g. Boil caused by *Staphylococcus aureus*.

Hemorrhagic Inflammation

- When inflammation is associated with severe vascular injury or deficiency of coagulation factors, it causes hemorrhagic inflammation e.g. acute pancreatitis due to proteolytic destruction of vascular walls.

Catarrhal Inflammation

- Acute inflammation of a mucous membrane is accompanied by excessive secretion of mucus and the appearance is described as catarrhal, e.g. common cold.

Membranous Inflammation

- In this type, epithelium is covered by membrane consisting of fibrin, desquamated epithelial cells and inflammatory cells, e.g. pharyngitis or laryngitis due to *Corynebacterium diphtheria*.

Pseudomembranous Inflammation

- Superficial mucosal ulceration covered by sloughed mucosa, fibrin, mucus and inflammatory cells.
- For example pseudomembranous colitis due to *Clostridium difficile* colonization of the bowel, usually following broad-spectrum antibiotic treatment.

Necrotizing (Gangrenous) Inflammation

- The combination of necrosis and bacterial putrefaction is **gangrene** (refer Fig. 2.21) e.g. gangrenous appendicitis.

Ulcer

An ulcer is defined as a local defect, or excavation, of the surface of an organ or tissue. Common sites:

1. Mucosa of the mouth, stomach (e.g. peptic ulcer of the stomach or duodenum intestines, or genitourinary tract.
2. Skin and subcutaneous tissue of the lower extremities (e.g. varicose ulcers).

SYSTEMIC EFFECTS OF INFLAMMATION

Q. Write short note on systemic effects of inflammation.

Systemic changes in acute inflammation are collectively known as **acute-phase response, or the systemic inflammatory response syndrome (SIRS)**.

Causes: Due to **cytokines** produced by leukocytes, in response to infections or immune reactions. Most important cytokines are **TNF, IL-1**, and **IL-6**.

The clinical and pathologic changes of acute-phase response are:

1. **Fever:**
   - **Pyrogens:** These are molecules that cause fever. It may be **exogenous** (bacterial products, like **LPS**), which stimulate leukocytes to release **endogenous** pyrogens **(cytokines such as IL-1 and TNF)**. The cytokines increase the enzymes cyclooxygenases resulting in conversion of AA into **prostaglandins**.
   - Pyrogens and prostaglandins may act on hypothalamic thermoregulatory center causing fever.
2. **Raised plasma levels of acute-phase proteins:** These are plasma proteins synthesized in the liver and may be markedly raised in response to inflammatory stimuli.
   - **Types of acute-phase proteins: 1) C-reactive protein (CRP), 2) fibrinogen, 3) serum amyloid A (SAA) protein**. Their synthesis by hepatocytes is increased by cytokines, especially IL-6 (for CRP and fibrinogen) and IL-1 or TNF (for SAA).
   - **Actions/functions:**
     - Many acute-phase proteins (CRP and SAA) bind to microbial cell walls and **may act as opsonins**.
     - Fibrinogen binds to red cells to form stacks (**rouleaux**) and responsible for **raised erythrocyte sedimentation rate** (ESR).
     - During acute inflammation, acute-phase proteins have beneficial effects but prolonged production (especially SAA) like in chronic inflammation causes **secondary amyloidosis**.
3. **Changes in the leukocytes:**

   A. **Leukocytosis:** Total leukocyte count more than 11,000/μL are termed as leukocytosis. Common in inflammatory reactions, especially those caused by bacterial infections.
   - **Count: May be increased up to 15,000 or 20,000 cells/μL**. Sometimes, it may be extremely high reaching 40,000 to 100,000/μL associated with more immature neutrophils in the blood (shift to the left) and are called as **leukemoid reactions**, similar to the white cell counts found in leukemia. It is important to distinguish it from leukemia which is a malignant disease.
   - **Cause:** It is due to increased release of leukocytes from the bone marrow caused by cytokines, including Colony stimulating factors (CSFs), TNF and IL-1.

- **Bacterial infections** cause an increase in the blood neutrophil count known as **neutrophilia**.

B. **Lymphocytosis:** It is seen in **viral infections** (e.g. Infectious mononucleosis, mumps, and German measles).

C. **Eosinophilia:** It is seen in **bronchial asthma, allergy, and parasitic infestations.**

D. **Leukopenia:** Decreased number of circulating white cells is associated with few infections like **typhoid fever and some viruses, rickettsia, and certain protozoa.**

4. **Other features of the acute-phase response:** It includes:
   - Increased pulse and blood pressure.
   - Anorexia and malaise, probably due to cytokines acting on brain cells.
   - In severe bacterial infections (sepsis), cytokines (mainly TNF and IL-1) may be produced in large quantities and can result in disseminated intravascular coagulation and cardiovascular failure.

CHRONIC INFLAMMATION

Definition: Chronic inflammation is defined as **inflammation of prolonged duration** (weeks or months) in which inflammation, tissue damage, and healing occurs at same time, in varying combinations.

Chronic inflammation may:

1. **Follow an acute inflammation,** which does not resolve (e.g. chronic osteomyelitis) or
2. **Begin as insidious, low-grade, chronic**, response without any acute inflammatory reaction.

Causes of Chronic Inflammation

Q. What are the causes of chronic inflammation?

1. **Persistent infections:** Microbes that are difficult to eradicate elicit delayed-type of hypersensitivity and produce chronic inflammation, e.g. mycobacteria, and certain viruses, fungi, and parasites. Some agents may cause a **distinct pattern of chronic inflammation** known as **granulomatous reaction**.
2. **Immune-mediated inflammatory diseases**
   - **Autoimmune diseases**: e.g. rheumatoid arthritis.
   - **Allergic reactions**: e.g. bronchial asthma.
   - **Unregulated immune response**: e.g. inflammatory bowel disease.
3. **Prolonged exposure to toxic injurious agents**
   - **Exogenous: Silica** is a nondegradable inanimate exogenous material. If persons are exposed to silica particles for long time, it causes an inflammatory lung disease called **silicosis.**
   - **Endogenous**: **Atherosclerosis** is a disease of arterial intima, probably represents a chronic inflammatory process partly due to endogenous toxic plasma **lipid components**.

Morphologic Features

Chronic inflammation is characterized by:

- **Mononuclear cells infiltrate**: Macrophages, lymphocytes, and plasma cells.
- **Tissue destruction:** Due to the persistence of causative agent or by the inflammatory cells.
- **Healing by fibrosis.**

Chronic Inflammatory Cells and Mediators

Q. Write short note on cells of chronic inflammation.

Macrophages

Macrophage is the predominant cell in chronic inflammation.

Macrophage Events in Inflammation

Q. Mention the role of macrophages in chronic inflammation.

- **Monocytes** also emigrate into extravascular tissues early in acute inflammation, and **within 48 hours**, they are the **predominant cell type**.
- **On reaching extravascular tissue**, the monocyte is **transformed into** a larger phagocytic cell known as tissue **macrophage**.

Macrophage Activation

Tissue macrophages are activated by **two major pathways:**

- **Classical macrophage activation**:
  - **Mediators of activation**: It is brought out mainly by
    - **Microbial products : e.g. endotoxin**
    - **T cell-derived signals:** Mainly **cytokines (e.g. IFN-γ)**
    - **Foreign substances: e.g. crystals and particulate matter**
  - **Products of activated macrophages**
    - **Lysosomal enzymes**
    - **Nitric oxide**
    - **Reactive oxygen species (ROS)**
  - **Function:** Phagocytosis and killing/elimination of ingested microbes.
- **Alternate macrophage activation**:
  - **Mediators of activation:** It is brought out mainly by **cytokines** IL-4 and IL-13 produced by T-cells and other cells.
  - **Function:** Initiation of the tissue repair, (they are not bactericidal).

Functions of Macrophages in Inflammation

- **Phagocytosis:** Ingestion and elimination of microbes and necrotic tissue.
- **Initiation of the tissue repair.**
- **Secretion of mediators of inflammation**: These include cytokines (TNF, IL-1, chemokines etc.) and arachidonic acid metabolites.
- **Display signal to T-cells and respond signals from T-cells**: This is responsible for the feedback loop for defense against many microbes by cell-mediated immune response.

Lymphocytes

- **B and T-lymphocyte:** They are found in both antibody-mediated and cell-mediated immune reactions.
- **B lymphocytes:** They may develop into plasma cells and produce antibodies either against foreign or self-antigens in the inflammatory site.
- **T lymphocytes:** Important being **$CD4^+$ helper T** cells which has **3 subtypes** namely:
  - **T_H1:** Produce INF-ϒ and activates macrophage in the classical pathway.

- **T_H2:** Produce IL-4, IL-5 and IL-13 which recruit and activate eosinophils and activate macrophages through alternate pathway. Involved in defense against helminthic infestation and allergic reaction.
- **T_H17:** Produce IL-17 and other cytokines which recruit neutrophils and monocytes.

Other Cells

- **Plasma cells:** They are derived from activated B lymphocytes and produce antibodies either against foreign or self-antigens.
- **Eosinophils:** They are seen in immune reactions mediated by IgE and in parasitic infections. A **chemokine**, which **attracts eosinophil recruitment is eotaxin**. Eosinophils granules contain **major basic protein** which is toxic to parasites and also destroy the epithelial cells.
- **Mast cells:** They are distributed in connective tissues and participate in both acute and chronic inflammatory reactions. They are seen in allergic reactions to foods, insect venom, or drugs.

GRANULOMATOUS INFLAMMATION

Q. Define and classify granuloma.

Definition: A **granuloma** (Fig 3.11) is defined as a **distinctive type of chronic inflammation** characterized by **microscopic aggregation of activated macrophages** (that are transformed into epithelium-like/epithelioid cells) with scattered lymphocytes. Older granulomas in addition show rim of fibroblasts and connective tissue as the outermost layer.

- **Epithelioid cells**: These are **modified macrophages** which resemble epithelial cells.
  - They have a **pale pink granular cytoplasm** with indistinct cell borders, often appearing to merge into one another.
  - The **nucleus is oval or elongate**, and may show folding of the nuclear membrane. The nucleus is less dense than that of a lymphocyte.
- **Giant cells**: **Epithelioid cells** frequently **fuse to form giant cells** and are found in the periphery or sometimes in the center of granulomas. These giant cells may attain diameters of 40 to 50 μm and have many small nuclei. Nuclei may be as many as 20 or more which are and may be arranged either peripherally (Langhans-type giant cell) or haphazardly (foreign body–type giant cell).

Cause of Granuloma Formation (Table 3.10)

Q. Give examples of chronic granulomatous inflammation.

1. **Persistent T-cell response against certain microbes**: e.g. *Mycobacterium tuberculosis.* Granuloma in tuberculosis (Fig. 3.11) is referred to as a tubercle and usually shows central caseous necrosis. **Caseous necrosis is seen in tuberculosis and is rare in other granulomatous diseases**. Sometimes, it may be necessary to perform additional tests/ investigations to identify the etiologic agent.
   - Special stains, e.g. acid-fast stains for tubercle bacilli
   - Culture methods, e.g. in tuberculosis and fungal diseases
   - Molecular techniques (e.g. the polymerase chain reaction in tuberculosis)
   - Serologic studies (e.g. in syphilis).

Table 3.10: Examples of granulomatous inflammation

Disease	Cause	Tissue reaction
Tuberculosis	*Mycobacterium tuberculosis*	Caseating granuloma (tubercle): central necrosis with amorphous granular debris surrounded by epithelioid cells, rimmed by lymphocytes, histiocytes and fibroblasts. Occasional Langhans giant cells, presence of acid-fast bacilli
Leprosy	*Mycobacterium leprae*	Acid-fast bacilli in macrophages; noncaseating granulomas
Syphilis	*Treponema pallidum*	Gumma: microscopic to grossly visible lesion. Consists of histiocytes; plasma cell infiltrate; central necrotic cells without loss of cellular outline (coagulative necrosis)
Cat-scratch disease	Gram-negative *Bacillus*	Rounded or stellate granuloma containing central granular debris and neutrophils; giant cells rare
Sarcoidosis	Unknown etiology	Noncaseating granulomas with plenty of activated macrophages
Crohn disease (inflammatory bowel disease)	Immune reaction against intestinal bacteria, self-antigens	Dense chronic inflammatory infiltrate with occasional noncaseating granulomas in the wall of the intestine

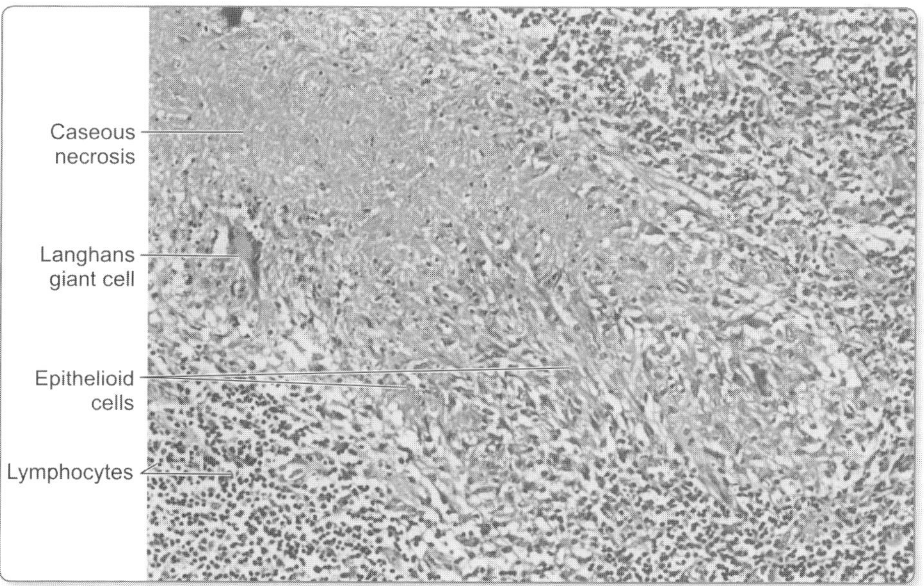

Fig. 3.11: Tuberculous granuloma showing an area of caseous necrosis surrounded by epithelioid cells, Langhans-type giant cell, and lymphocytes

2. **Immune-mediated inflammatory reaction**: e.g. Crohn's disease.
3. **Foreign body granuloma:** These are produced by relatively inert foreign bodies. Examples, foreign body granulomas form around materials such as talc (associated with intravenous drug abuse), sutures, or other fibers. Epithelioid cells and giant cells are apposed to the surface of the foreign body. Sometimes etiology is not known.

GIANT CELL

Q. Write short note on giant cells.

Definition: Cell with more than one nucleus is called as giant cell or multinucleated cell.

Types of giant cells (Fig. 3.12): Various types of giant cells and its associated conditions are given in Table 3.11.

Table 3.11: Types of giant cells

Physiological
Osteoclast *Syncytiotrophoblast* *Megakaryocyte*
Pathological
Damaged muscle fibers • Regenerating sarcolemmal cells in damaged skeletal muscles
Tumor giant cells: They have hyperchromatic nuclei of varying size and shape • Giant cell tumors: Bone (osteoclastoma) • Reed Sternberg cells: Hodgkin lymphoma • Giant cell variants of many malignant tumors, e.g. carcinoma of lung
Giant cells resulting from fusion of cells • Viral infection – Epithelial giant cells e.g. herpes virus infection – Connective tissue e.g. Warthin-Finkeldey giant cells in measles
Fused macrophages • Foreign body giant cells: These have multiple uniform nuclei scattered throughout the cytoplasm. – Reaction to exogenous insoluble material : e.g. suture material, talc, etc. – Reaction to insoluble endogenous material: e.g. keratin (dermoid cyst of ovary, epidermal cyst), cholesterol, urate crystals (in gout) • Touton giant cells: These cells have vacuolated cytoplasm due to lipid, e.g. in xanthoma • Reaction to certain organisms: e.g. tuberculosis (Langhans giant cells in which nuclei are arranged in a horseshoe pattern), fungal infections, syphilis • Fusion of cardiac histiocytes: Aschoff giant cells in rheumatic heart disease.

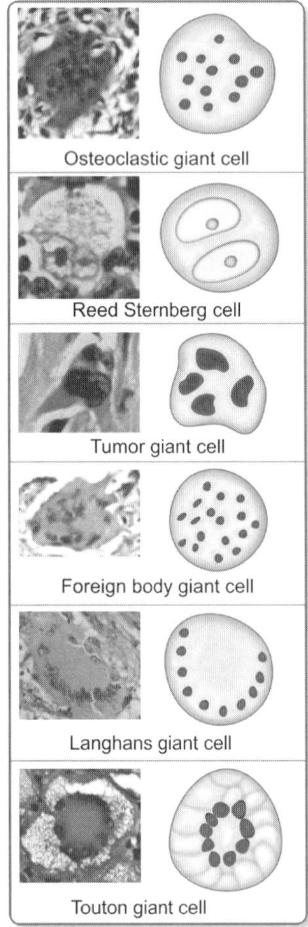

Fig. 3.12: Various types of giant cells

Chapter 4

Repair

Chapter Outline

- Introduction
- Healing
- Cell cycle and cell proliferation
- Healing by repair, scar formation and fibrosis
- Cutaneous wound healing
- Factors that influence wound healing
- Complications of wound healing
- Healing of a fracture

INTRODUCTION

Q. Define the term healing, regeneration and repair.

Injury to cells and tissues **results in loss of cells and tissues.** It sets in inflammation (restrict the tissue damage) and initiate replacement of lost tissue by living tissue.

HEALING

Definition: Healing is a process of replacement of dead tissue by living tissue.

It can be broadly divided into regeneration and repair.

1. **Regeneration**:

Definition: Regeneration is a process in which **lost tissue is replaced by tissue of similar type**. It results in the complete restoration of lost or damaged tissue by proliferation of residual uninjured cells and replacement from stem cells.

2. **Repair**:

Definition: Repair is defined as a process in which **lost/damaged tissue is replaced by fibrous tissue or scar**.

Repair is often used for parenchymal and connective tissues and *healing* for surface epithelia. However, these terms are used interchangeably.

Factors Deciding the Pattern of Healing

The proportion of regeneration and repair process in healing depends on:

Proliferative Capacity of the Tissue

According to proliferative capacity of the cells, the tissues of the body can be divided into three groups:

1. **Labile (continuously dividing) tissues**: The cells of labile tissues proliferate throughout life, replacing the lost cells from stem cells. Examples:
   - Hematopoietic cells of the bone marrow
   - Surface epithelia of the skin, oral cavity, vagina, and cervix
   - Columnar epithelium of the GI tract and uterus.
2. **Stable (quiescent) tissues**: Cells of stable tissue normally do not proliferate; but can **proliferate in response to injury or loss of tissue.** Examples:
   - **Parenchymal cells** of **liver**, kidneys, and pancreas
   - **Mesenchymal cells:** Fibroblasts, vascular endothelial cells, smooth muscle cells, chondrocytes, and osteocytes.
3. **Permanent (nondividing) tissues**: Cells of these tissues **cannot proliferate after birth**. In these tissues, repair is by scar formation. Example:
   - **Neurons: Damaged neurons** are **replaced by** the proliferation of the **glial cells**
   - **Skeletal muscle** cells
   - **Cardiac muscle** cells.

Extent of Tissue Injury

- **Mild and short duration**: The damaged tissue is healed by regeneration without significant scarring.
- **Severe and chronic**: Healing occurs by fibrous tissue forming scar.
  - Severe tissue injury damages both parenchymal cells and the extracellular matrix (ECM) framework
  - Chronic inflammation.

CELL CYCLE AND CELL PROLIFERATION

- Inflammation is the primary response of living tissue to injury.
- With inflammation, there will be damage or loss of tissue, which has to be replaced by living tissue. This replacement is done by transient increase in cellularity due to proliferation of cells by either regeneration and/or by repair.
- Proliferation of cells is characterized by DNA replication and mitosis. The sequence of events that control DNA replication and mitosis is known as the **cell cycle**.

Definition of cell cycle: Cell proliferation is a regulated process, which involves activators and inhibitors, as well as checkpoints.

Phases of Cell Cycle (Fig. 4.1)

- G_1 (presynthetic)
- S (DNA synthesis)
- G_2 (premitotic)
- M (mitotic) phase.

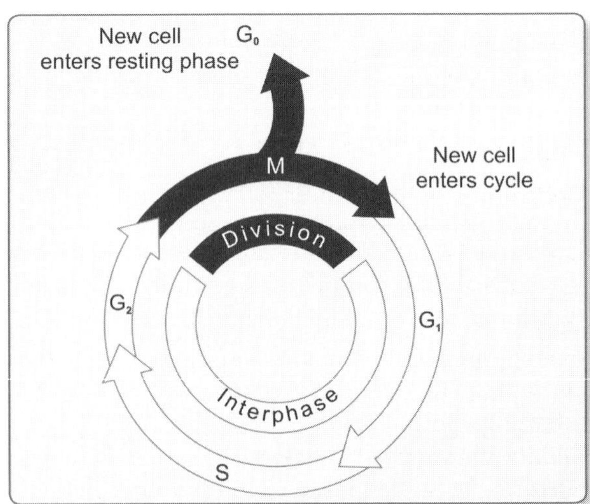

Fig. 4.1: Cell cycle showing different phases (G_0, G_1, G_2, S, and M). Cells from labile tissues (e.g. epidermis) may remain in cycle continuously; stable cells (e.g. liver cells) are quiescent but can enter the cell cycle; permanent cells (e.g. neurons) have lost the capacity to proliferate and cell cycle arrests in the G_1 phase or exit the cycle and are in G_0 phase

Checkpoints: They checks whether there is any damage to DNA and chromosomes in the replicating cells. These checkpoints make sure that only normal cells complete replication. There are two checkpoints:

1. G_1/S checkpoint monitors the integrity of DNA before replication.
2. G_2/M checkpoint checks DNA after replication and monitors whether the cell can safely enter mitosis.

HEALING BY REPAIR, SCAR FORMATION AND FIBROSIS

Healing may be either by **regeneration or repair or combination of both.** With mild and transient injury, there is regeneration. If the tissue injury or damage persists, inflammation becomes chronic, resulting in excessive deposition of connective tissue known as **fibrosis** (repair).

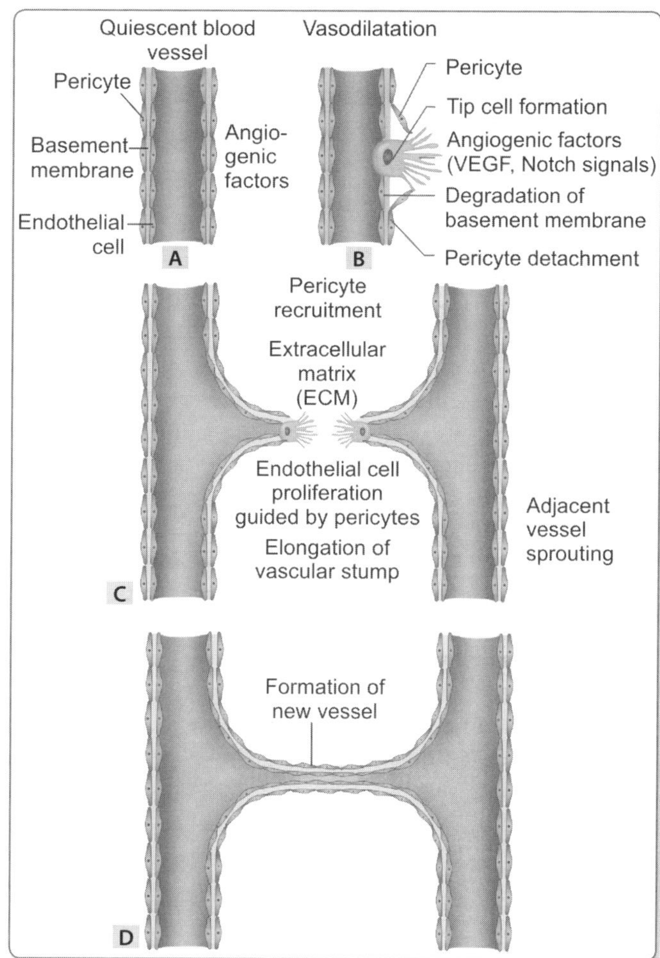

Figs 4.2A to D: Mechanism of angiogenesis. A. Normal blood vessel; B. **Vasodilatation**: First, pericytes separate followed by mobilization and proliferation of endothelial cells from the existing vessel to form capillary sprouts towards the site of injury (angiogenic stimuli); C. Endothelial cells proliferate, loosely following each other, and are presumably guided by pericytes. Maturation of vessel (stabilization) involves the recruitment of pericytes and smooth muscle cells to form the periendothelial layer; D. Finally, blood-vessel sprouts will fuse with other sprouts to build new circulatory systems

Steps in Healing by Repair (Scar Formation)

Inflammation

Whenever there is tissue injury, inflammatory reaction begins, which tries to limit the damage and remove the injured tissue. At the same time, it also promotes the deposition of ECM components at the site of injury and stimulates angiogenesis.

Angiogenesis

Definition: Angiogenesis is the process of formation of new blood vessels from existing vessels. It supplies nutrients and oxygen needed to support the repair process. These vessels are leaky because of incomplete interendothelial junctions and VEGF (the growth factor responsible for angiogensesis).

Steps in angiogenesis (Figs 4.2A to D):

- **Vasodilatation** in response to nitric oxide and **increased permeability of the pre-existing vessel due** to VEGF.

- **Separation of pericytes** from the outer surface of blood vessel and breakdown of the basement membrane. This allows formation of a vessel sprout.
- **Migration and proliferation of endothelial cells** toward the site of injury.
- **Maturation of endothelial cells** into capillary sprouts/tubes.
- **Formation of mature vessel:** It involves recruitment of pericytes and smooth muscle cells to form the periendothelial layer.
- **Suppression of endothelial proliferation** and migration, and deposition of basement membrane.

Formation of Granulation Tissue

Q. Write short note on granulation tissue.

The first 24 to 72 hours of the repair process begins with proliferation of fibroblasts and vascular endothelial cells. It forms a **specialized type of tissue** known as **granulation tissue**, which is a **hallmark/characteristic of tissue repair**. The term granulation tissue is derived from its pink, soft, granular appearance on the surface of healing wounds.

- **Microscopy** (Figs 4.3A and B): Its characteristic features are:
  - Presence of **new small blood vessels** (angiogenesis): The new blood vessels are **leaky**, which allow the passage of plasma proteins and fluid into the extravascular space, which is responsible for edema often seen in granulation tissue.
  - **Proliferation of fibroblasts.**
- **Amount** of granulation tissue formed depends on the:
  - **Size of the tissue deficit** created by the wound
  - **Intensity of inflammation**.

Scar Formation

- The leukocytes, edema, and angiogenesis disappear, accomplished by the **increased accumulation of collagen.** The **granulation tissue scaffolding is converted into a pale, avascular scar.**
- **Components of scar:** It is composed of spindle-shaped fibroblasts, dense collagen, fragments of elastic tissue, and other ECM components.
- **By the end of the first month,** the scar consists of acellular connective tissue without inflammatory infiltrate.

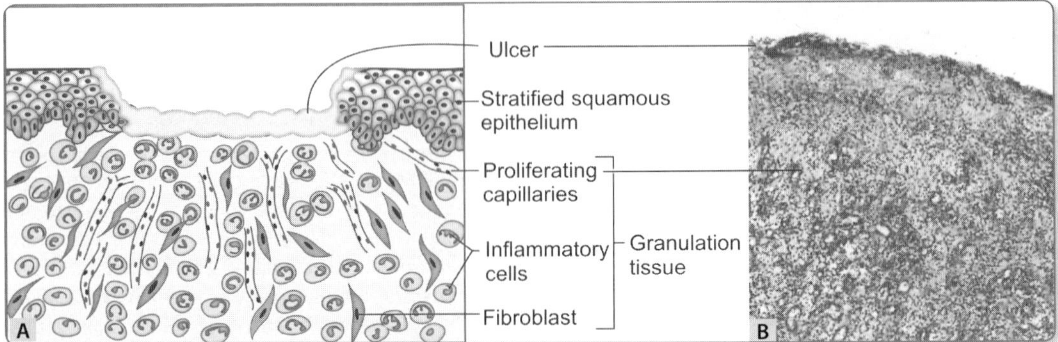

Figs 4.3A and B: Granulation tissue consisting of numerous blood vessels, fibroblasts and edema. A. Diagrammatic; B. Hematoxylin and eosin

(For color version, see Plate 2)

Connective Tissue Remodeling

- Remodeling of the connective tissue framework is an important feature. It is the long-lasting phase of tissue repair.
- Remodeling indicates that the equilibrium/balance between ECM synthesis (collagen deposition) and degradation has been restored.

CUTANEOUS WOUND HEALING

Q. Describe the healing of a clean surgical wound/ healing by first intention.

Healing by Primary Union or by First Intention

Definition: Healing of a **clean, uninfected surgical incision** in the skin joined with surgical sutures is known as healing by **primary union or by first intention**.

Surgical incision causes **death of a minimum number** of epithelial and connective tissue **cells.** The **disruption of epithelial basement membrane** continuity is also **minimal**. Re-epithelialization occurs by regeneration and there is a **relatively thin scar**. This is simplest type of cutaneous wound healing.

Stages in the Healing by First Intention (Figs 4.4A to D)

- **First 24 hours:**
  - **Formation of blood clot**: It is formed in the space between sutured margins. Blood clot contains not only trapped red cells but also fibrin, fibronectin and complement components. Clot stops bleeding and acts as a scaffold for migrating and proliferating cells. **Dehydration at the external surface of the clot** leads to formation of a **scab** over the wound.
  - **Neutrophil infiltration**: Within 24 hours of wound, **neutrophils** appear at the margins of the incision. Neutrophils use the scaffold produced by the fibrin clot for its migration. They **release proteolytic enzymes which clean out debris**.
  - **Epithelial changes:** At the cut edges of the wound, the **basal cells of the epidermis** begin to show **mitotic activity**. Epithelial cells from both the edges of wound proliferate and migration across the wound along the dermis.
- **Two days:**
  - **Neutrophils are replaced by macrophages**.
  - The **epithelial cells fuse in the midline below the surface scab** and epithelial continuity is re-established in the form of a thin continuous surface layer.
- **Three to seven days**:
  - **Granulation tissue** begins to invade incision space. It progressively grows into the **incision space/wound and fills the wound area** by 5 to 7 days. Collagen is progressively laid down.
  - **Surface epidermis** achieves its **normal thickness** and differentiation. It matures with surface keratinization.
  - Acute **inflammatory response** begins to **subside**.
- **Ten to fourteen days**:
  - Leukocytic infiltration, edema, and angiogenesis disappear during the second week.
  - **Increased accumulation of collagen** and **regression of vascular channels**. The **granulation tissue scaffolding is converted into a pale, avascular scar.** Wound normally gains about 10% strength of normal skin. Further fibroblast proliferation occurs with collagen deposition.

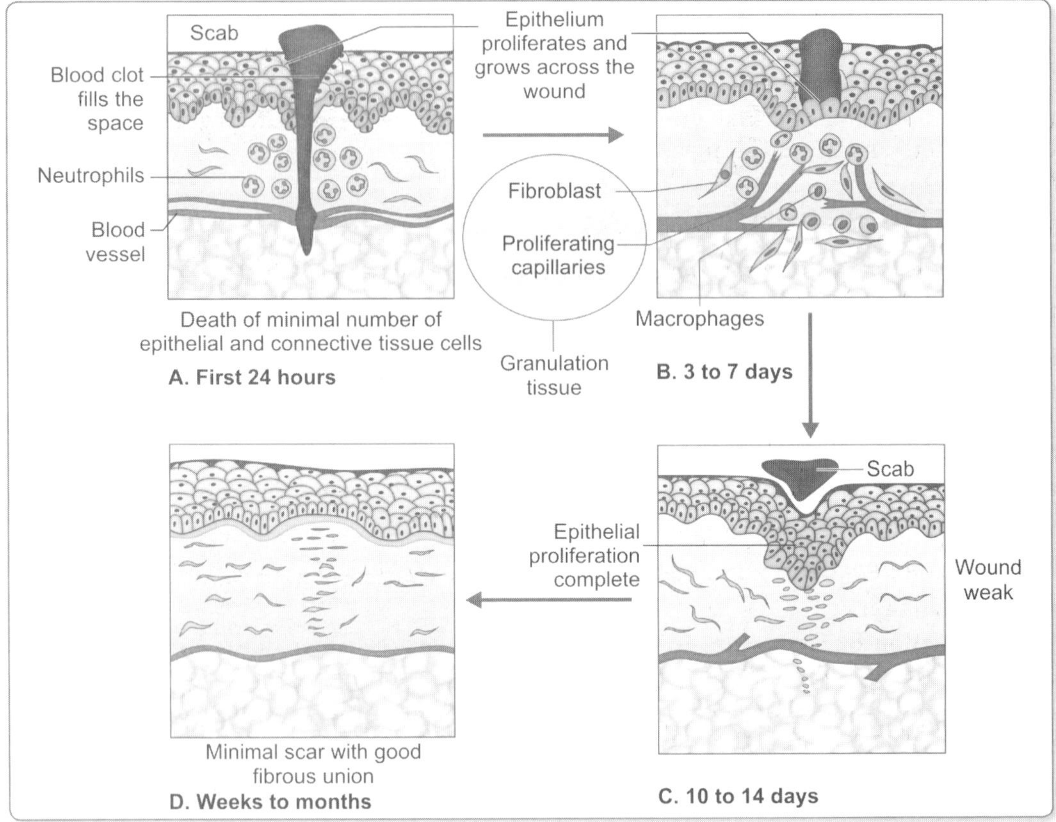

Figs 4.4A to D: Healing by primary intention. A. A wound with closely apposed edges and minimal tissue loss. The blood clots and fills the gap between the edges of the wound; B. Epithelium at the edges proliferates. Minimal amount of granulation tissue is formed; C. The epithelial proliferation is complete and the wound is weak; D. Fibrosis with a small scar

- **Weeks to months**:
  - The **scar** appears as **acellular** connective tissue covered by intact epidermis and without inflammatory infiltrate.
  - Collagen deposition along the line of stress and **wound gradually achieves maximal 80% of tensile strength** of normal skin.

Healing by Secondary Union or by Second Intention

Q. Describe the mode of healing of wound by second intention.

Definition: When injury produces **large defects** on the skin surface with **extensive loss of cells and tissue**, the healing process is more complicated. Healing in such cutaneous wound is referred to as healing by **secondary union or by second intention.**

Features of Healing by Secondary Intention (Figs 4.5A to D)

Q. Mention the differences between healing by first intention and second intention.

- Larger wounds show **more exudate and necrotic tissue**. The **clot or scab** formed at the surface of wound is **large**. Full epithelialization of the wound surface is slow because of the larger gap.

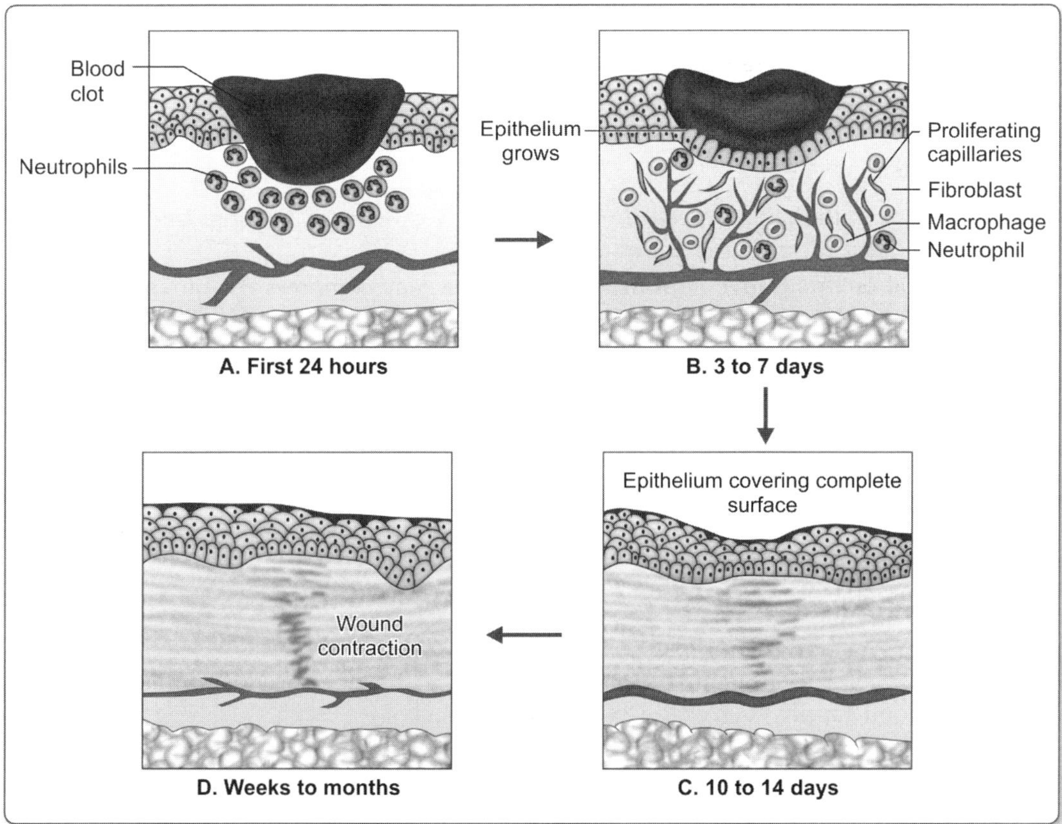

Figs 4.5A to D: Healing by secondary intention. A. There is significant loss of tissue and the edges are far apart. Acute inflammation develops both at the edges and base; B. The cell proliferation starts from the edges and large amount of granulation tissue is formed; C. The wound is covered on the entire surface by the epithelium. The collagen fibers are deposited; D. Granulation tissue is replaced by a large scar. There is significant wound contraction

- **Severe inflammatory reaction** because of larger defect and greater necrotic tissue.
- The **larger defect requires more** amount of (abundant) **granulation tissue**.
- Extensive deposition of collagen with substantial scar formation.
- **Wound contraction:** Wound contraction generally occurs in large surface wounds and is an important feature in healing by secondary union.

Myofibroblasts of granulation tissue **have ultrastructural features of smooth muscle cells**. They contract in the wound tissue and are responsible for wound contraction.

Wound Strength

Major portion of the connective tissue in repair is fibrillar collagens (mostly type I collagen) and are responsible for the development of strength in healing wounds.

Time for a skin wound to achieve its maximal strength

- **At the end of the first week:** When sutures are removed from an incisional surgical wound, **wound strength** is about **10%** that of normal unwounded skin.
- **Four weeks**: Wound strength quickly increases over the next 4 weeks, and then slows down.
- **Three months:** Wound strength **reaches a 70% to 80% of the tensile strength** of unwounded skin.

FACTORS THAT INFLUENCE WOUND HEALING

Q. List the factors that influence wound healing.

Q. List factors which delay healing.

Local Factors

1. **Infection:** It is the single most important cause for delay in healing. Infection causes persistent tissue injury and inflammation.
2. **Mechanical factors: Movement of wounded area** may compress the blood vessels and separate the edges of the wound and can result in delayed healing.
3. **Foreign bodies:** Unnecessary sutures or foreign bodies (fragments of steel, glass), or even bone can delay healing.
4. **Size and type of wound**: Small surgical incisional or other injuries heal quickly with less scar formation than large excisional wounds or wounds caused by blunt trauma.
5. **Location of injury:** Wound over the skin covering bone with little intervening tissue prevents wound contraction (e.g. skin over the anterior tibia). The edges of skin lesions (e.g. burns) in such locations cannot be apposed.

Q. List factors which promote healing.

6. **Blood supply:**
   - Wounds in areas with **good blood supply,** such as the face, heal **faster** than those with **poor blood supply**, such as the foot.
   - **Varicose veins** of the legs decrease the venous drainage and **can cause nonhealing ulceration**.
   - **Bed sores (decubitus ulcers**) result due to prolonged, localized pressure, which diminishes both arterial and venous blood flow.
7. Ionizing radiation decreases repair process.
8. Complications may delay wound healing.

Systemic Factors

1. **Nutritional deficiencies:** Delays wound healing and these include:
   - Protein deficiency (e.g. malnutrition)
   - Vitamin C deficiency: Inhibits collagen synthesis and retard healing
   - Trace elements: Copper and zinc deficiency.
2. **Age:** Wound healing is rapid in young compared to aged individuals.
3. **Metabolic status**: **Diabetes mellitus** is associated with delayed healing due to micro-angiopathy.
4. **Circulatory status**: **Inadequate blood supply** (due to arteriosclerosis) or venous abnormalities (e.g. varicose veins) that retard venous drainage, delay healing.
5. **Hormones: Glucocorticoids have anti-inflammatory effects** and also inhibit collagen synthesis, thereby **impair wound healing**.
6. **Hematological abnormalities:** Quantitative or qualitative defects in neutrophils and bleeding disorders may slow the healing process.

COMPLICATIONS OF WOUND HEALING

Q. Mention the complications of wound healing.

Inadequate Granulation Tissue Formation

Inadequate formation of granulation tissue or a deficient scar formation can cause **wound dehiscence** and **ulceration**.

1. **Dehiscence** (the wound splitting) or rupture of a wound is most common life-threatening complication after abdominal surgery. It is due to increased abdominal pressure/ mechanical stress on the abdominal wound from vomiting, coughing, or ileus.
2. **Ulceration:**
   - Wounds can ulcerate due to inadequate angiogenesis during healing. For example, wounds in the leg of patients with atherosclerotic peripheral vascular disease or varicose veins usually ulcerate.
   - Nonhealing wounds also develop in regions devoid of sensation. These **neuropathic or trophic ulcers** may be seen in diabetic peripheral neuropathy, nerve damage from leprosy.
3. **Incisional hernia** resulting from weak scars of the abdominal wall due to a defect caused by prior surgery. They are due to insufficient deposition of extracellular matrix or inadequate cross-linking in the collagen matrix.

Excessive Scar Formation

Excessive formation of the components of the repair process can result in:

1. **Hypertrophic scar:** The accumulation of excessive amounts of extracellular matrix, mostly collagen may give rise to a raised scar at the site of wound known as a hypertrophic scar. They usually develop after thermal or traumatic injury, which involves the deep layers of the dermis.
2. **Keloid:** If the scar tissue grows/progress beyond the boundaries of the original wound and does not regress, it is called a keloid. Thus, keloid is an exuberant scar that recurs with still larger keloid after surgical excision.
3. **Exuberant granulation:**
   a. **Pyogenic granuloma or granuloma pyogenicum (Fig. 4.6)**:
      i. This consists of the localized formation of excessive amounts of granulation tissue.
      ii. Such exuberant granulation tissue projects above the level of the surrounding skin and prevents re-epithelialization. This mass formed is often named as **proud flesh.**

   b. **Desmoids or aggressive fibromatoses**:
      i. Incisional scars or traumatic injuries may be followed by excessive proliferation of fibroblasts and other connective tissue elements.
      ii. They are known as desmoids, or aggressive fibromatoses, which may recur after excision.

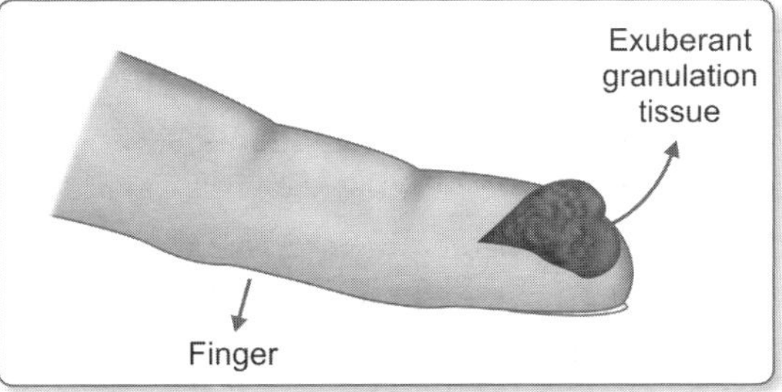

Fig. 4.6: Exuberant granulation tissue at the tip of the finger

Excessive Contraction

- A decrease in the size of a wound due to myofibroblasts is known as **contraction**.
- An exaggeration of this contraction is termed **contracture** and results in deformities of the wound and the surrounding tissues.
- Consequences of contractures:
  - **Compromise movements:** for example, contractures that follow severe burns can compromise the movement of the involved region (Fig. 4.7) and joint movements.
  - **Obstruction:** for example, in GI tract contracture (stricture) can cause intestinal obstruction.

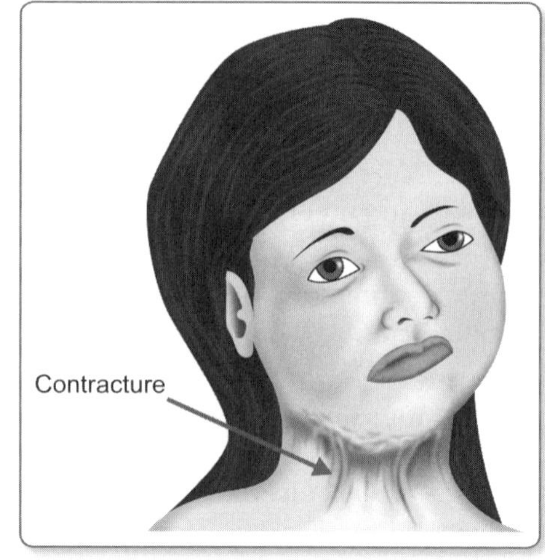

Fig. 4.7: Wound contracture—Severe contracture of a wound on the right side of neck, following burns

Others

1. **Infection** of wound by microbes.
2. **Epidermal cysts** can develop due to persistence of epithelial cells at the site of wound healing.
3. **Pigmentation** may develop due to either colored particle left in the wound or due to hemosiderin pigment.
4. **Neoplasia:** For example squamous cell carcinoma may develop in Marjolin's ulcer, which is the scar that follows burns in skin.

Fibrosis

- Normal wound healing is associated with deposition of collagen.
- The excessive deposition of collagen and other ECM components in a tissue is termed as fibrosis. It is usually observed in chronic inflammation.
- **TGF-β is an important fibrogenic agent**.
- Examples of **disorders with fibrosis**: Cirrhosis of liver, pneumoconioses, chronic pancreatitis and glomerulonephritis.

HEALING OF A FRACTURE

Q. Describe the healing of fractures in long bones.

Phases of Fracture Healing (Figs 4.8A to E)

Bone can repair by reactivating processes that normally takes place during embryogenesis. There are three major phases of fracture healing.

Inflammatory Phase

- **Fracture and hemorrhage:**
  - Soon **after fracture**, **blood vessels** (in the periosteum, cortex and medullary cavity) **rupture** leads to extensive hemorrhage (hematoma), at the fracture site and surrounding tissue.
  - **Necrosis of bone** also occurs at the fracture site.

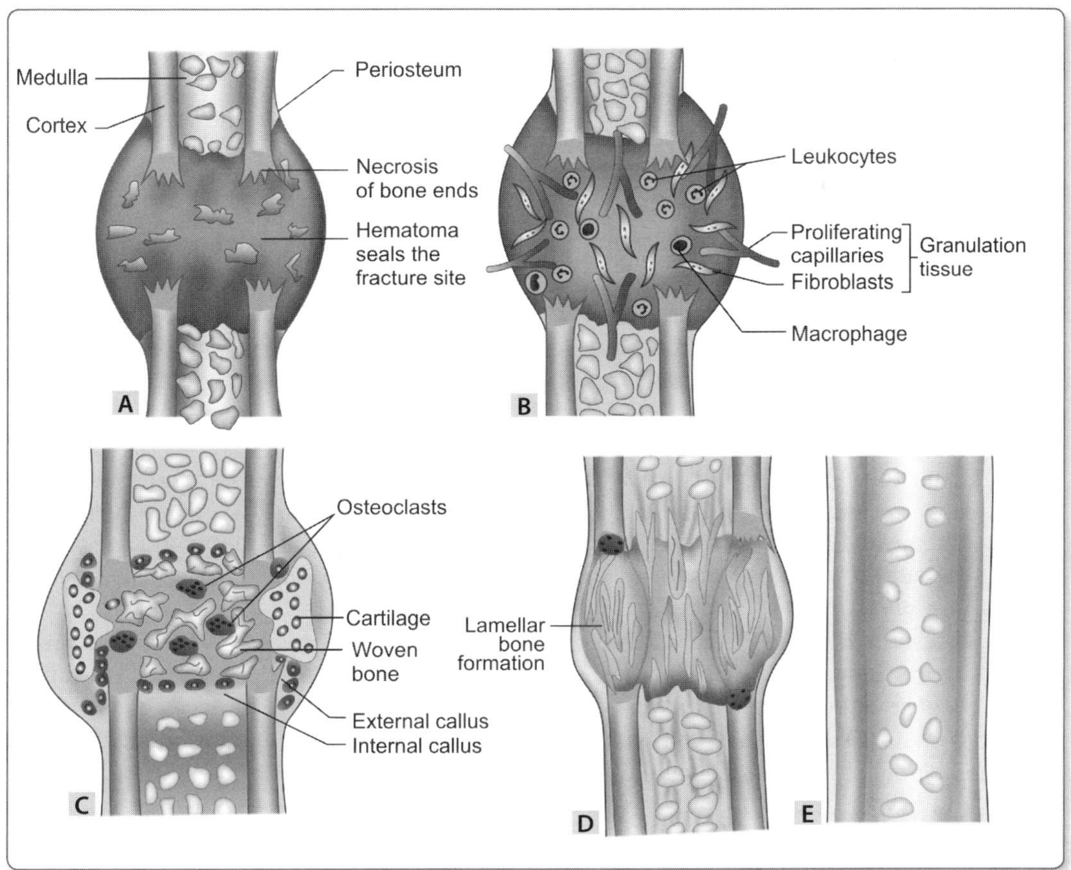

Figs 4.8A to E: Healing of a fracture. A. Immediately after a fracture, blood clot/hematoma forms at the site of fracture; B. During the inflammatory phase of fracture healing, the inflammatory cells (neutrophils and macrophages) migrate to the area of fracture and neovascularization develops; C. The reparative phase of fracture healing is characterized by the formation of a callus near the fracture site; D. In the remodeling phase, the reactive bone (lamellar or woven) develops; E. Healing is complete and bone attains its original contour

- **Inflammatory cells:**
  - **Fibrin mesh work** in the clotted blood **helps**
    - **To seal the fracture site**
    - **Influx of inflammatory cells (neutrophils and macrophages) to the area**
    - **Ingrowth of fibroblasts and new capillary vessels (neovascularization) to the site, producing granulation tissue between the fracture fragments.**
  - **Activation of osteoprogenitor cells**: The **inflammatory cells and platelets release cytokines** (PDGF, TGF-β, FGF and interleukins) → **activate the osteoprogenitor cells** in:
    - **Periosteum**
    - **Medullary cavity**
    - **Surrounding soft tissues.**
- **Formation of granulation tissue:** It consists of proliferating capillaries and fibroblasts and are formed at the site of fractures

- **Soft-tissue callus or procallus formation:**
  - **Osteoprogenitor cells → activate both osteoblastic and osteoclastic activities** at the fracture site.
  - **Osteoblasts** derived from activated osteoprogenitor cells **migrate into the granulation tissue** and **differentiate into osteoid synthesizing units**. They **deposit** large quantities of **osteoid collagen in a haphazard pattern** producing **woven bone** (unmineralized bone is called osteoid).
  - **Granulation tissue containing** (mineralized or unmineralized) **bone or cartilage** is termed a **callus.**
  - At this stage, **callus** is predominantly **uncalcified** and is called **soft-tissue callus or procallus**, which **provides a type of temporary connection between the ends of the fractured bones**. However, procallus does not have any structural rigidity for any weight bearing. The callus depending on its site and appearance can be divided into external and internal callus.
    - **External callus:** It is formed from the osteoprogenitor cells of periosteum and surrounding soft tissue and is found on the surface of the bone. It bridges the fracture site outside the bone and continues to grow inwards toward the fracture site. In this region, the osteoprogenitor cells may also differentiate into chondroblasts, which form fibrocartilage and hyaline cartilage around the fracture site.
    - **Internal callus:** It is derived from osteoprogenitor cells of medullary cavity and grows outward toward the fracture site. This bridges the fracture in the region of medullary cavity but in contrast to external callus does not contain cartilage.
  - The **repair tissue** attains **maximal thickness at the end of the second or third week** and consists of hyaline cartilage and woven bone.

Reparative Phase

- **Lamellar bone formation:** As the healing advances, the hyaline cartilage and woven bone of the original fracture **callus are replaced by lamellar bone.** This is stronger and consists of **parallel collagen fibers**.
- **Endochondral ossification:** The replacement process is known as **endochondral ossification** with respect to the hyaline cartilage and **bony substitution** with respect to the woven bone.
- **Bony callus:** At this stage, the **callus is mineralized** (calcified) and is known as **bony (osseous) callus**. As the mineralization proceeds, the stiffness and strength of the callus increases. By the second or third week, controlled weight bearing can be tolerated.

Remodeling Phase

- Several weeks after a callus has sealed the bone ends, the remodeling phase begins.
- **Resorption of excess portions of bony callus**: During healing, **excess of bony callus is formed around the fracture site**. As the callus is subjected to weight-bearing forces, the portions of bony callus that are not physically stressed by this weight are **slowly resorbed by osteoclasts**. Thus, the osteoclasts act to remodel bone and decrease the size of callus.
- The remodeling phase **substitutes the trabecular bone with compact bone**.
- Remodeling phase continues till the original bone shape (contour), outline and strength of the fractured bone is re-established.

The **whole process of healing** of a bone fracture usually takes **about 6 to 8 weeks**.

Major Causes of Delayed Fracture Healing (Table 4.1)

Table 4.1: Major causes of delayed fracture healing

Local factors	General factors
• Excessive movement of fractured bone during healing process • Infection of the fractured site • Severe local soft tissue injury • Wide separation of fracture ends • Extensive necrosis of the fractured bone • Poor or impaired blood supply (e.g. tibia, head of femur)	• Old age • Poor general health • Drugs, e.g. corticosteroids

Complications of Healing

Q. Mention the complications of healing of fracture bone.

- **Delayed union and nonunion** of fracture.
- **Pseudoarthrosis:** In case of nonunion, too much movement along the fracture gap can cause cystic degeneration in the callus, creating a false joint or pseudoarthrosis.
- **Large callus with deformity**.

Chapter 5

Immunity

Chapter Outline

- Immunity
- Cells of the immune system
- Cytokines
- Hypersensitivity: Immunologically mediated tissue injury
- Type I (Immediate) hypersensitivity
- Antibody-mediated (type II) hypersensitivity
- Immune complex-mediated (type III) hypersensitivity
- T cell-mediated (type IV) hypersensitivity
- Autoimmune diseases
- Systemic lupus erythematosus (SLE)
- Major histocompatibility complex (MHC) molecules
- Acquired immunodeficiency syndrome (AIDS)
- Amyloidosis

The normal immune system is essential for protection against infection. Immune system is like a double-edged sword. Though it is protective in most of the situations, sometimes an hyperactive immune system may cause fatal diseases.

IMMUNITY

Definition: Immunity is **resistance** (defense mechanism) exhibited **by host against invasion by any foreign antigen**, including microorganisms.
Types: There are two types namely innate and adaptive immunity.

Innate (Natural/Native) Immunity

General Features

- **First line of defense present by birth**.
- Provides **immediate initial protection** against an invading pathogen and **can eliminate damaged cells.**
- **Does not depend on the prior contact** with foreign antigen or microbes.
- **Lacks specificity**, but **highly effective**. No memory, and no self/non-self recognition.
- **Triggers the adaptive immune response**.

- **No memory** is seen.
- It functions in stages: 1) recognition of microbes and damaged cells, 2) activation of various mechanisms, and 3) elimination of the unwanted substances.

Major Components

1. **Physical/anatomical barriers:** It includes epithelium lining skin, gastrointestinal and respiratory tracts act as **mechanical barriers**, produce anti-microbial molecules, such as defensins.
2. **Cells:**
   a. **Phagocytic-cells:** It consists of mainly **monocytes (macrophages in tissue) and neutrophils** in the blood. Phagocytic cells use several receptors to sense microbes and are called as "microbial sensors" (pattern recognition receptors).
      i) **Pathogen-associated molecular patterns (PAMPs):** Microbes have few highly conserved common molecular structures shared by entire classes of pathogens. These structures are called **pathogen-associated molecular patterns** (PAMPs) and are essential for the infectivity of these pathogens.
      ii) **Pattern-recognition receptors (PRRs):** Phagocytic cells involved in innate immunity recognizes PAMP using a group of cellular receptors (microbial sensors) called pattern recognition receptors. Examples for PAMPs:
         - **Toll-like receptors (TLRs)**. These are transmembrane receptors and about 10 types of human TLRs have been identified. Each receptors recognize a unique set of microbial patterns.
         - **Receptors for mannose residues.**
         - **NOD (nucleotide-oligomerization domain protein)-like receptors** (NLRs) **and the inflammasome:** They are located in the cytoplasm and serve as intracellular sensors for microbial products. Many NLRs signal via a cytosolic multiprotein complex called the inflammasome, which activates an enzyme (caspase-1). This cleaves a precursor form of the cytokine interleukin-1 (IL-1) to generate the biologically active form. IL-1 is a mediator of inflammation that recruits leukocytes and produces fever.
         - **Receptors for opsonins.**

   b. **Dendritic cells:** These cells **function as antigen presenting cells** to T cells. They produce type I interferons (IFN) (e.g. IFN-α), which inhibit viral infection and replication.
   c. **Natural killer (NK) cells:** They provide defense against many viral infections and other intracellular pathogens.
3. **Soluble molecules in the blood and tissues:**
   - **Complement system**
   - Proteins that coat microbes and aid in phagocytosis. e.g., mannose-binding lectin and C-reactive protein.

Functions of Innate Immune Response

- **Inflammation** and destruction of invading microbe
- **Antiviral defense** is mediated by **dendritic cells and NK cells**.
- Provides the danger signals that stimulate the subsequent more powerful adaptive immune response.

Adaptive Immunity

If the innate immune system fails to provide effective protection against invading microbes, the adaptive immune system is activated.

General Features

- **Second line of defense** acquired during life
- **Capable of recognizing both microbial and nonmicrobial substances**
- **Takes more time to develop** and is **more powerful than innate immunity**
- **Long-lasting protection**
- Prior exposure to antigen is present
- Three **characteristic features** are: 1) **specificity**, 2) **diversity** and 3) **memory**.

Components

Q. Write short note on cellular immunity.

Q. Write short note on humoral immunity.

1. **Humoral immunity**: B lymphocytes and their soluble protein products called antibodies (also called **immunoglobulins**, Ig) and helper T cells.
2. **Cellular immunity:** T lymphocytes and their soluble products called cytokines.

Functions of Adaptive Immune Response

- **Antibodies:** Protection against extracellular microbes in the blood, mucosal secretions and tissues.
- **T lymphocytes**:
  - Defense against viruses, fungi and intracellular bacteria either by direct killing of infected cells by cytotoxic T lymphocytes or by activation of phagocytes to kill the ingested microbes.
  - Important immunoregulatory role, orchestrating and regulating the responses of other components of the immune system.

Different types of adaptive immunity and their differences are shown in Table 5.1.

Table 5.1: Differences between two types of adaptive immunity

Type	Mediator	Protection against
Humoral immunity	B lymphocytes, which secrete antibodies	Extracellular microbes and their toxins
Cell-mediated (or cellular) immunity	T (thymus-derived) lymphocytes	Intracellular microbes

Both B and T lymphocytes express highly specific receptors for a wide variety of substances, called **antigens**.

CELLS OF THE IMMUNE SYSTEM

Cells of immune responses (lymphocytes and other cells) migrate among lymphoid and other tissues and the vascular and lymphatic circulations.

Naïve Lymphocytes

These are mature lymphocytes which have not encountered the antigen (immunologically inexperienced). After the lymphocytes are activated by recognition of antigens, they differentiate into:

- **Effector cells:** They perform the function of eliminating microbes.
- **Memory cells:** They live in a state of heightened awareness and are better able to combat the microbe in case it infects again.

T Lymphocytes

- **Development:** T (thymus derived) lymphocytes develop from precursors in the thymus.
- **Distribution:** Mature T cells are found in:
  - Peripheral blood where it constitute 60% to 70% of lymphocytes
  - T-cell zones of peripheral lymphoid organs namely paracortical region of lymph node and periarteriolar sheaths of spleen.
- **T-cell Receptor:** T cell recognizes a specific cell-bound antigen by means of an antigen-specific T-cell receptor (TCR).
- **Markers:** Leukocyte cell surface molecules are named systematically by assigning them a 'cluster of differentiation' (CD) antigen number that helps in their identification.
  - **Primarily T-cell associated** CD molecules: **CD1, CD3, CD4, CD5, and CD8.**
  - **CD3** is involved in signal transduction and is also known as **pan T-cell marker**.
- **Subsets of T lymphocytes:** Naïve T cells can differentiate into two subtypes namely **CD4 and CD8.** Both subtypes serve as "coreceptors" in T-cell activation. They are called as coreceptors because they work with the antigen receptor in responses to antigen.

B Lymphocytes

- **Development:** B (bone marrow derived) lymphocytes develop from precursors in the bone marrow.
- **Distribution:**
  - **Peripheral blood:** Mature B cells constitute 10% to 20% of the circulating peripheral lymphocyte population
  - **Peripheral lymphoid tissues:** Lymph nodes (cortex), spleen (white pulp), and mucosa-associated lymphoid tissues (pharyngeal tonsils and Peyer's patches of GIT).
- **B-cell Receptor (BCR):** B cells have receptors composed of IgM and IgD on their surface and has unique antigen specificity.
- **Functions of B cells:** B cells recognize antigen via these BCRs.
  - **Production of antibodies:** The primary function of B cells is to **produce antibodies and are the only cells in the body capable of producing antibody molecules (mediators of humoral immunity).** After stimulation by antigen and other signals, B cells develop into **plasma cells**. These cells secrete antibodies which are the mediators of humoral immunity.
  - **Antigen presenting cell:** B cells also serve as APCs and are very efficient at antigen processing.
- **Markers:** B cell markers include: CD10 (CALLA), CD19, CD20, CD21 (EBV receptor), CD23, CD79a.

Dendritic Cells

As the name suggests these cells have numerous fine cytoplasmic processes that resemble dendrites. These are important antigen presenting cells (APC) in the body.

Macrophages

- Macrophages are a part of the mononuclear phagocyte system.
- **Role in adaptive immune responses:**
  - **Processing of antigen:** Macrophages process the antigens present in the phagocytosed microbes and protein antigens. After processing, the antigen is presented to T cells and thus, they function as APCs in T-cell activation.
- **Effector cell in immunity:**
  - **Cell-mediated immunity:** Macrophages are main effector cells in certain types of cell-mediated immunity, the reaction that serves to eliminate intracellular microbes.
  - **Humoral immunity:** Macrophages also participate in the effector phase of humoral immunity.
  - **Phagocytosis:** Macrophages efficiently phagocytose and destroy microbes which are opsonized (coated) by IgG or C3b through their respective receptors.

Natural Killer Cells

- Non-phagocytic **large** (little larger than small lymphocytes), **granular** (numerous cytoplasmic **azurophilic granules**) **lymphocytes**.
- Comprise about **5%** to 15% **of** human **peripheral lymphoid cells**.
- **Function:** NK cells provide **defense against many viral infections** and other **intracellular pathogens** and also **has antitumor activity**, causing lysis of cells with which they react.

CYTOKINES

- Immune responses involve multiple interactions among many cells. These include lymphocytes, dendritic cells, macrophages, other inflammatory cells (e.g. neutrophils), and endothelial cells.
- Some of these interactions are cell-to-cell contact. However, many interactions and effector functions of leukocytes are mediated by **short-acting soluble proteins** called **cytokines**. These cytokines represent the **messenger molecules of the immune system** and mediate communications between leukocytes are called **interleukins**.

Classification

Most of the cytokines have a many effects and can be classified depending on their functions.

Cytokines of Innate Immunity

- These cytokines are produced rapidly in response to microbes and other stimuli
- Mainly secreted by macrophages, dendritic cells, and NK cells
- Mediate inflammation and anti-viral defense
- These cytokines include TNF, IL-1, IL-12, type I IFNs, IFN-γ, and chemokines.

Cytokines of Adaptive Immune Responses

- These cytokines are produced mainly by CD4+ T lymphocytes in response to antigen and other signals
- They promote lymphocyte proliferation and differentiation and activate effector cells
- This category include IL-2, IL-4, IL-5, IL-17, and IFN-γ.

Colony-stimulating Factors

- These cytokines stimulate hematopoiesis and are assayed by their ability to stimulate formation of blood cell colonies from bone marrow progenitors.
- They increase leukocyte numbers during immune and inflammatory responses.

HYPERSENSITIVITY: IMMUNOLOGICALLY MEDIATED TISSUE INJURY

Immune response is usually a protective process but sometimes it may be injurious. Hypersensitivity means that the body responds to a particular antigens in an exaggerated fashion, where it does not happen in normal circumstances. **Injurious immune reactions are called *hypersensitivity*.**

Definition: Hypersensitivity reaction is a **pathological, excessive, and injurious immune response to antigen leading to tissue injury, disease** or sometimes death **in a sensitized individual.** The resulting diseases are named as hypersensitivity diseases.

General Features of Hypersensitivity Disorders

Individuals who have been previously exposed to an antigen manifest detectable reactions to that antigen, i.e. individual is said to be sensitized to that antigen. Hypersensitivity indicates an excessive or harmful reaction to antigen.

- **Priming or sensitization:** It occurs in **individuals who had previous contact with the antigen** (allergen).
- **Nature of antigens:** It may be **exogenous or endogenous** origin.
  - **Exogenous environmental antigens: Examples for environmental antigens (microbial and nonmicrobial)** include antigens in dust, pollens, foods, drugs, microbes, chemicals, and few blood products.
  - **Endogenous self antigens:** Self or autologous antigens → cause **autoimmune diseases.**
- **Genetic susceptibility:** Hypersensitivity diseases **(both allergic and autoimmune)** are usually associated with the inheritance of particular susceptibility genes (e.g. HLA genes).
- **Imbalance between control and effector mechanisms:** It produces damage to host tissues.
- **In hypersensitivity reactions, the mechanisms of tissue injury are the same as the effector mechanisms of defense against infectious pathogens.** Hypersensitivity reactions are poorly controlled, excessive, or misdirected (e.g. against normally harmless environmental and self antigens).

Classification of Hypersensitivity Reactions (Table 5.2)

Hypersensitivity diseases are classified on the basis of the immunologic mechanism that mediates the disease. This classification helps in distinguishing the manner in which the immune response causes tissue injury and disease, and also the pathological and clinical manifestations. However, multiple mechanisms may be operative in any one hypersensitivity disease.

Table 5.2: Classification of hypersensitivity reaction according to the effector immune mechanism

Types	Effectors
1. Immediate hypersensitivity reaction (type I hypersensitivity) 2. Antibody-mediated disorders (type II hypersensitivity) 3. Immune complex-mediated disorders (type III hypersensitivity)	Antibody molecules
4. Cell-mediated immune disorders (type IV hypersensitivity)	Antigen-specific effector T cells

TYPE I (IMMEDIATE) HYPERSENSITIVITY

Q. Write short note on type I hypersensitivity reactions.

Usually known as **allergic or atopic disorders** and the environmental antigens that elicit these reactions are known as **allergens**.

Definition: Type I hypersensitivity reaction is a type of immunological tissue reaction, which **occurs rapidly (within 5–10 minute) after the interaction of antigen** (allergen) **with a IgE antibody on the surface of the mast cells in a previously sensitized person**.

Characteristics

- **Immediate** reaction occurring within minutes (5–10 minutes).
- **Antibodies:** Mediated by IgE antibody.
- **Develops after the interaction of an antigen with IgE bodies** bound to **mast cells.**
- **Genetic susceptibility:** Occurs in genetically susceptible individuals **previously sensitized** to the antigen.
- **Antigens (allergens):** Many allergens (e.g. house dust mites, pollens, animal danders or moulds) in the environment are **harmless for majority of individuals**. Allergens elicit significant IgE reactions only in **genetically predisposed individuals**, who are said to be **atopic**.

Sequence of Events (Figs 5.1A and B)

A. During Initial Exposure to Antigen (Sensitization)

In a genetically susceptible individual, the following events occur:

1. **Exposure to sensitizing antigen:** Individuals are exposed to environmental allergens and may be introduced by: **1) inhalation, 2) ingestion, or 3) injection**.

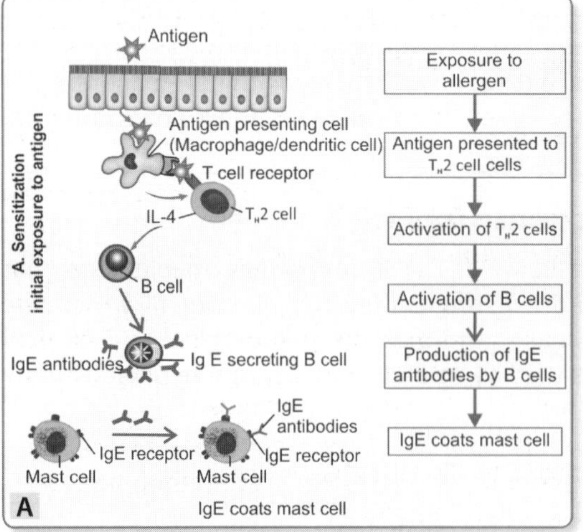

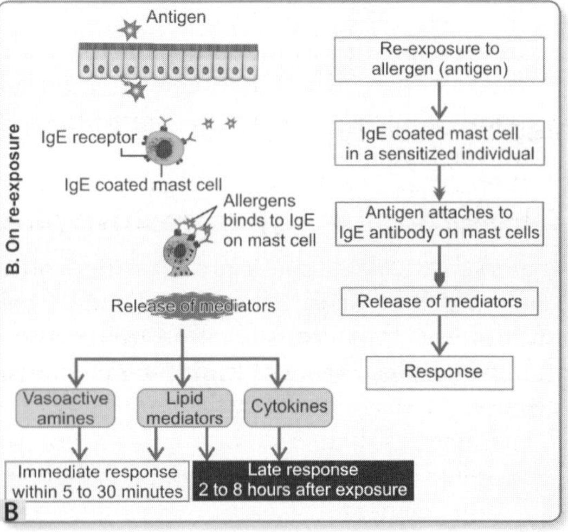

Figs 5.1A and B: Sequence of events in type I hypersensitivity. A. It is initiated by the exposure to an allergen, which stimulates T_H2 responses and IgE production, in genetically susceptible individuals. IgE binds to mast cells; B. On re- exposure to the allergen, antigen binds to IgE on the mast cells and activates it to secrete the mediators. These mediators produce the manifestations of type I hypersensitivity

2. **Presentation of the antigen:** The **sensitizing antigen (allergen)** is **presented to T cells**. However, T cells do not recognize antigens by themselves but recognize when presented **by APC** (antigen presenting cell), which capture the antigen.
3. **Activation of T_H2 cells:** In genetically susceptible individual, antigens (allergens) activates **T_H2 subset of CD4+ helper T cells → secrets cytokines (e.g. IL-4, IL-5 and IL-13).**
4. **Production of IgE antibody:** IL-4 secreted by T_H2 cells stimulates B cells to secrete cytotropic IgE antibodies.
5. **Sensitization of mast cells by IgE antibody:**
   - Mast cells possess Fc-epsilon (FcεRI) receptor, which have high affinity for IgE antibodies.
   - IgE antibodies produced by B cells, attach to the FcεRI on the mast cells. These **IgE antibody bearing mast cells are sensitized to react if antigens binds to these antibodies.**
   - **Eosinophils** also express FcεRI and are involved in IgE mediated defense against helminth infections.

B. During Subsequent Exposure to Antigen

In sensitized individual (the mast cell has attached IgE antibodies), during subsequent re-exposure to the specific allergen, following events occur:

- **Mast cell activation:** The **antigen (allergen) binds** to the more than one **IgE antibody molecules on mast cells** → generate signals → **causes mast cell degranulation** → **secretion of preformed (primary) mediators** that are stored in the granules.
- **Two phases:** IgE triggered reactions can be divided into two phases:
  1. **Immediate response:**
     - Develops **within 5 to 30 minutes** after exposure to an allergen and **subside in 60 minutes**.
     - Characterized by **vasodilation**, **vascular leakage**, and **smooth muscle spasm or glandular secretions**.
  2. **Late-phase reaction:**
     - Develops in **2 to 8 hours after** the exposure to antigen which may **last for several days**.
     - Characterized by **infiltration of tissues with eosinophils, neutrophils, basophils, monocytes, and T_H2 cells**. It also shows mucosal **epithelial cell damage**.

Mediators of Type I Hypersensitivity (Fig. 5.2)

1. **Preformed mediators (primary mediators):** They are stored in mast cell granules. Their biological effects start immediately following their release. These include:
   - **Vasoactive amines:** Most important being **histamine**, which causes
     - **Vasodilatation**
     - **Increased vascular permeability**
     - **Smooth muscle contraction**
     - **Increased secretion of mucus** by nasal, bronchial, and gastric glands.
   - **Enzymes:** It include neutral proteases (chymase, tryptase) and several acid hydrolases. These enzymes **cause tissue damage** and generate kinins and activates components of complement (e.g. C3a) by acting on their precursor proteins.
   - **Proteoglycans:** It include heparin (anticoagulant), and chondroitin sulfate.
   - Neutrophil and eosinophil chemotactic factors (NCF and ECF).

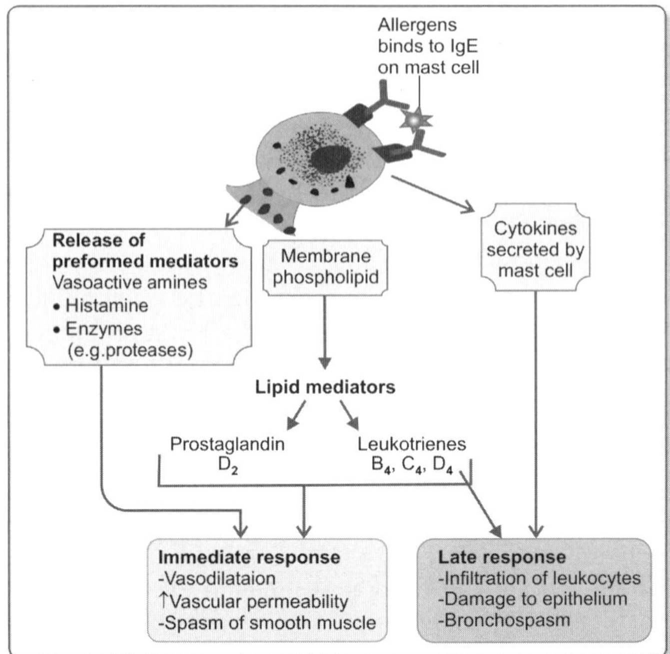

Fig. 5.2: Mast cell mediators involved in type I hypersensitivity

2. **Secondary (newly synthesized) mediators:**
   A. **Lipid mediators:** They are synthesized and secreted by mast cells, includes leukotrienes and prostaglandins.
      - **Leukotrienes C_4 and D_4** (previously known as the slow-reacting substances of anaphylaxis-SRS-As): These are the most powerful (several thousand times than histamine) and cause **increased vascular permeability** and **bronchial smooth muscle contraction**.
      - **Leukotriene B_4:** It is **chemotactic** for neutrophils, eosinophils, and monocytes.
      - **Prostaglandin D_2:** It causes bronchospasm and increased mucus secretion.

   B. **Cytokines:** Mast cells can produce many cytokines, which may be involved in immediate hypersensitivity reactions.

Clinical Manifestations

Systemic Anaphylaxis

- **Acute, potentially fatal form** and known as anaphylaxis (ana = without, phylaxis = protection).
- Usually **follows injection of an antigen into a sensitized individual**.
- **May cause shock and death**.
- **Causes:** It develops.
  - After **administration of foreign proteins** (e.g. antisera), **drugs** (e.g. penicillin), hormones, and enzymes
  - Following exposure to **food allergens** (e.g. peanuts, shellfish) or **insect toxins** (e.g. bee venom)
- **Dose:** Systemic anaphylaxis may be triggered by extremely small doses of antigen.

- **Clinical features:**
  - Itching, hives, and skin erythema appear within minutes after exposure
  - Followed by difficulty in breathing and respiratory distress due to contraction of respiratory bronchioles
  - Laryngeal edema results in hoarseness and laryngeal obstruction, which further aggravates respiratory difficulty
  - Vomiting, abdominal cramps, diarrhea may follow
  - May lead to shock and death within the hour.

Local Reactions

- Recurrent and non-fatal.
  - Site of local reaction depends on the portal of entry of the allergen.
- **Causes:** Develop against common environmental allergens, such as pollen, animal dander, house dust, and foods.

Atopy

- **Susceptibility to type I hypersensitivity reactions is genetically determined. Atopy** refers to a familial predisposition to produce an **exaggerated localized immediate hypersensitivity** (IgE mediated) **reactions to inhaled and ingested environmental** substances (allergens) that are otherwise harmless.
- Atopic individuals tend to **have higher serum IgE levels**, and **more IL-4–producing T_H2 cells**.
- A positive family history of allergy is found in 50% of atopic individuals.

Examples of type I hypersensitivity reactions are listed in Table 5.3.

Table 5.3: Examples of type I hypersensitivity reactions

Localized type I hypersensitivity	Systemic type I hypersensitivity
• Bronchial asthma (extrinsic) • Hay fever/allergic rhinitis • Allergic conjunctivitis • Urticaria • Atopic dermatitis/eczema • Angioedema • Allergic gastroenteritis (food allergy)	Anaphylaxis due to: • Antibiotics: Most commonly penicillin • Bee stings • Insect bite • Foreign proteins (e.g. antisera) • Foods (peanuts, fish and shellfish) • Food additives

ANTIBODY-MEDIATED (TYPE II) HYPERSENSITIVITY

Q. Write short note on type II hypersensitivity reactions.

Definition: Type II hypersensitivity disorders are **caused by antibodies (IgG/IgM)**, which react with **target antigens on the surface of cells or fixed in the extracellular matrix. These antibodies cause disease by destroying the involved cells, triggering inflammation, or interfering with normal functions.**

Characteristics

Antibodies: IgG (usually) and IgM (rarely) type of antibodies mediate type II reactions.

Antigen: It may be endogenous or exogenous

- **Endogenous antigens:** It may be normal molecules intrinsic to the cell membrane or extracellular matrix (e.g. autoimmune diseases).

- **Exogenous antigens:** These antigens may get adsorbed on a cell surface or extracellular matrix → may cause altered surface antigen (e.g. drug metabolite).

Mechanisms of Injury

Mechanism of tissue injury can be broadly divided into: **1) complement dependent and 2) antibody-dependent**.

A. Complement Dependent Reactions

1. **Opsonization and phagocytosis (Fig. 5.3):** Complement injure the target cells by promoting their phagocytosis.
   - **Production of antibodies: Antigen may be intrinsic to target cells** (e.g. RBC or platelets) **or exogenous antigen adsorbed to its cell surface.** B **cells produce IgG antibodies** (e.g. autoantibodies) against target antigens.
   - **Activation of complement:** Antigen-antibody complexes are formed on the surfaces of the target cells → may activate the complement system by the classical pathway.
   - **Opsonization: Complement components such as C3b**, which **acts as opsonins** and get deposited on the surfaces of the target cells.
   - **Phagocytosis:** Opsonized cells are recognized by phagocytes through Fc and C3b receptors on its surface → results in **phagocytosis of the opsonized cells → destruction of cells by phagocytes** (e.g. macrophages in spleen).

     Examples:
     - **Autoimmune hemolytic anemia: Target antigen is RBC membrane protein (Rh or I antigen).**
     - **Autoimmune thrombocytopenia purpura: Target antigen is GpIIb/IIIa** of platelets
     - **Drug-induced hemolytic anemia.**
2. **Lysis of target cells through membrane attack complex (Fig. 5.4):** Complement causes lysis of target cells by generating membrane attack complex (C5-9)
   - **Complement activation on cells** also **generates membrane attack complex** (MAC).
   - MAC disrupts membrane integrity and causes **lysis of the cells.**
   - **Example: Transfusion reactions** in which the cells from an incompatible donor react with and are opsonized by preformed antibody in the recipient. Hemolytic disease of newborn.

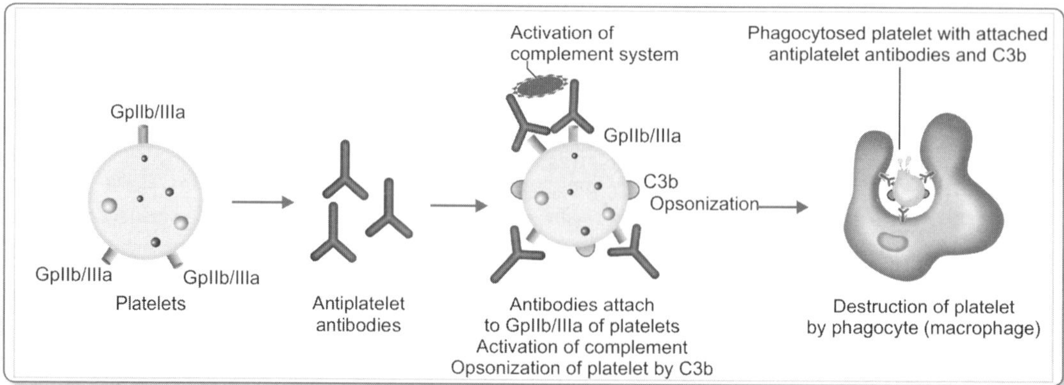

Fig. 5.3: Type II hypersensitivity reaction. Complement dependent opsonization and phagocytosis. The antibody binds to antigens on the target cell. Activation of complements produces opsonin C3b. Opsonization of target cells by antibodies and complement leads to ingestion by phagocytes (phagocytosis of target cell) via either Fc or C3b receptors

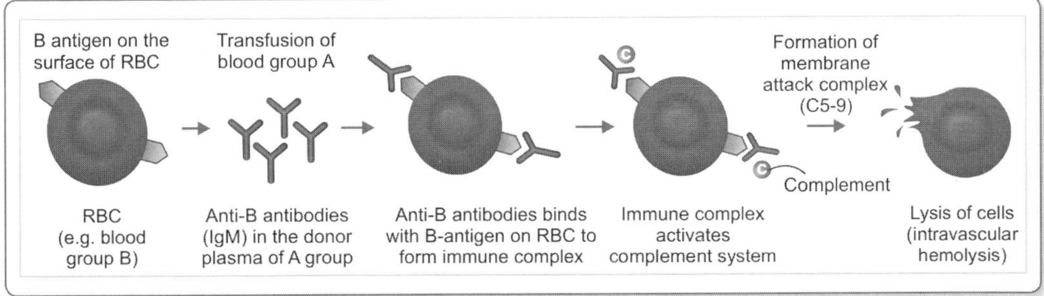

Fig. 5.4: Type II hypersensitivity reaction-lysis through MAC. Binding of IgG or IgM antibody to an antigen promotes complement fixation. Activation of complement leads to formation of membrane attack complex (MAC) which causes cell lysis. Example transfusion of A group blood to individual with B group

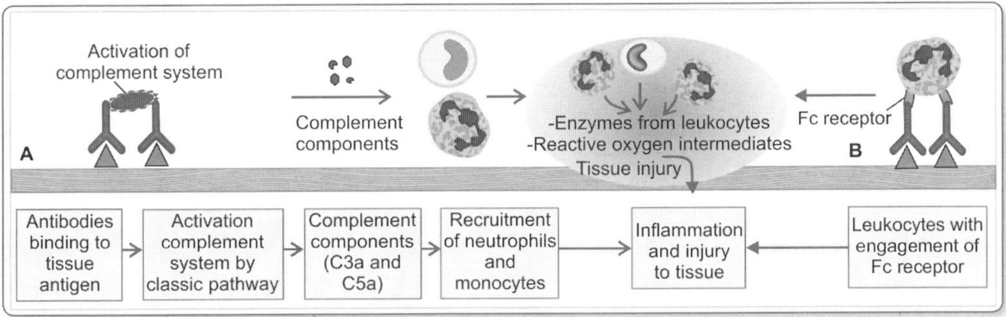

Fig. 5.5: Type II-hypersensitivity reaction-complement and Fc receptor mediated inflammation: A. Antibody binds to a surface antigen, activates the complement system and leads to the recruitment of tissue-damaging inflammatory cells. Several complement-derived peptides (e.g. C5a) are potent chemotactic factors; B. Inflammation may also be induced by antibody binding to Fc receptors of leukocytes

3. **Tissue injury by complement and Fc receptor mediated inflammation (Fig. 5.5)**: Complement induces inflammation and causes injury to target cells.
   - **Antibodies against matrix components in fixed tissue antigens**, such as basement membranes and extracellular matrix may **activate complement system by classical pathway**.
   - Complement components may **cause injury due to inflammation**. This may be due to 1) chemotactic agents (mainly C5a) produced at the site of deposition of antibody and 2) anaphylatoxins (C3a and C5a), which increase vascular permeability.
   - Activated **inflammatory cells** (leukocyte) **release lysosomal enzymes and reactive oxygen species** which **damage tissues**.
   - Inflammation may also be induced by antibody binding to Fc receptors of leukocytes

     Example: Goodpasture syndrome in which anti-glomerular basement membrane antibody binds to a glomerular basement membrane antigen and activates the complement system. The recruitment of inflammatory cells damages the basement membrane.

B. Antibody-dependent (Complement Independent) Cellular Dysfunction

It is characterized by deposition of antibodies against target cell surface receptors, which may impair or dysregulate function of the target cell without causing cell injury or inflammation. Examples:

- **Antibody-mediated stimulation of cell function: In Graves' disease**, antibodies against the thyroid-stimulating hormone receptor on thyroid epithelial cells stimulate the cells. This results in hyperthyroidism (Fig. 5.6).
- **Antibody-mediated inhibition of cell function:** In **myasthenia gravis** (Fig. 5.7), antibodies directed against acetylcholine receptors in the motor end plates of skeletal muscles block neuromuscular transmission. This causes muscle weakness.

Mechanism of type II hypersensitivity reactions are summarized in Figure 5.8.

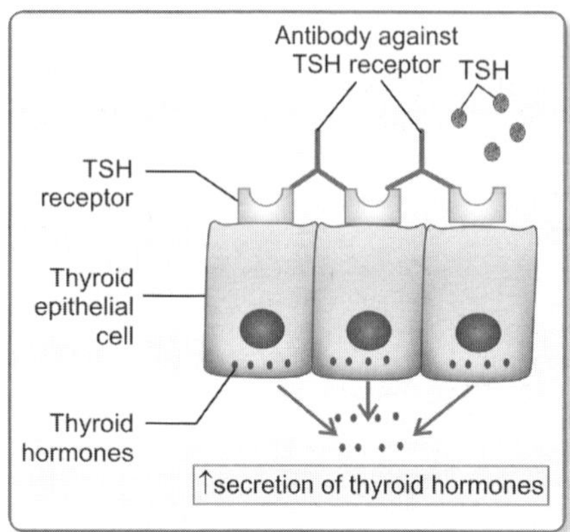

Fig. 5.6: Type II hypersensitivity reaction- antibody mediated stimulation of cell function. Autoantibodies bind against the thyroid-stimulating hormone (TSH) receptor and activate thyroid cells to produce excessive production of hormones and causing hyperthyroidism in Graves' disease

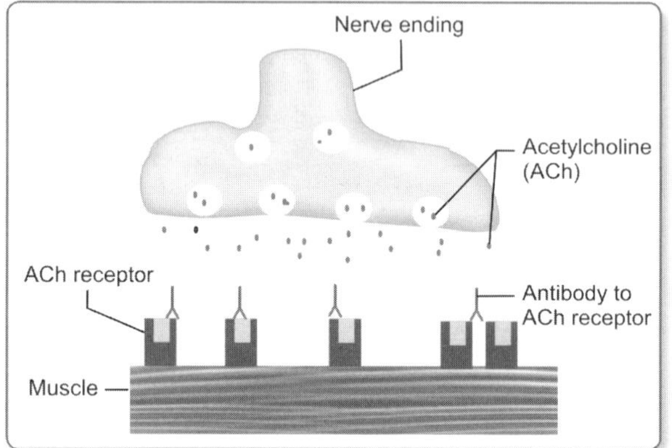

Fig. 5.7: Type II hypersensitivity reaction- antibody mediated inhibition of cell function. Anti-receptor antibodies may inhibit/disturb the normal function of receptors. Example, autoantibodies to the acetylcholine (ACh) receptor on skeletal muscle cells in myasthenia gravis, produce disease by blocking neuromuscular transmission and causing progressive muscle weakness

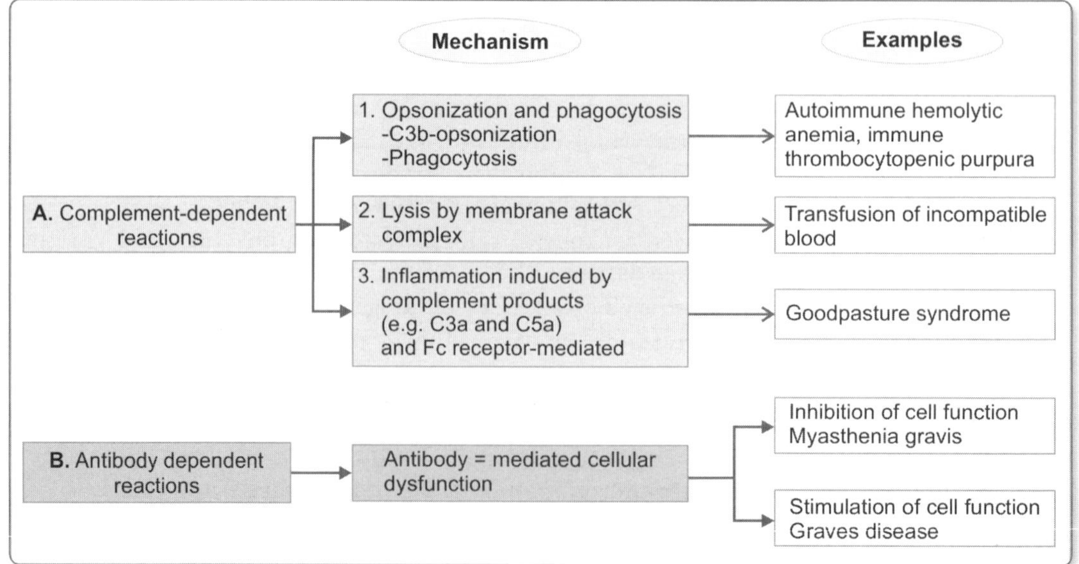

Fig. 5.8: Summary of mechanism of type II hypersensitivity reactions

Examples of type II hypersensitivity diseases are presented in Table 5.4

Table 5.4: Examples of type II hypersensitivity (antibody-mediated) diseases

Disease	Target antigen	Mechanisms of disease
A. Complement dependent reactions		
1. Opsonization and phagocytosis (IgG-mediated)		
Autoimmune hemolytic anemia	Cell-surface antigens (Rh blood group antigens, I antigen)	Opsonization and phagocytosis of RBCs
Autoimmune thrombocytopenic purpura	Platelet membrane glycoprotein IIb:IIIa integrin	Opsonization and phagocytosis of platelets
2. Complement mediated lysis by membrane attack complex (IgM-mediated)		
Transfusion reactions	The cells from an incompatible donor react with and are opsonized by preformed antibody in the recipient	Complement activation and lysis by membrane attack complex
3. Complement and Fc receptor mediated inflammation (IgG-mediated)		
Goodpasture syndrome	Antibody against matrix antigens (basement membrane noncollagenous protein of kidney glomeruli and lung alveoli)	Complement and Fc receptor-mediated inflammation
B. Antibody-mediated (complement independent) cellular dysfunction		
Graves' disease (hyperthyroidism)	Antibody against receptors: thyroid-stimulating hormone (TSH) receptor (agonistic antibodies)	Antibody-mediated stimulation of TSH receptors
Myasthenia gravis	Antibody against receptors: acetylcholine receptor (antagonistic antibodies)	Antibody inhibits acetylcholine binding, to receptors

IMMUNE COMPLEX–MEDIATED (TYPE III) HYPERSENSITIVITY

Q. Write short note on type III hypersensitivity reactions.

Definition: Type III hypersensitivity reactions are **characterized by formation of immune** (antigen and antibody) **complexes in the circulation** and may **get deposited in blood vessels, leading to complement activation and acute inflammation**. The inflammatory cells recruited (neutrophils and monocytes) **release lysosomal enzymes → generate toxic free radicals → cause tissue damage**.

Characteristics

Antibodies: Complement-fixing antibodies namely IgG, IgM, and occasionally IgA.

Antigen:

- **Exogenous:** Various **foreign proteins**, e.g. foreign serum protein injected (e.g. diphtheria antitoxin, horse antithymocyte globulin) or produced by an infectious microbe.
- **Endogenous: Antibody against self-components** (autoimmunity), e.g. nucleoproteins.

Sites of Antigen-antibody Formation

- **Circulating** immune complexes: They are **formed within the circulation**.
- **In situ immune complex:** Less frequently, the immune complexes may be formed at sites where antigen has been "planted" previously producing in situ immune complexes.

Sites of Immune Complex Deposition

- **Systemic:** Circulating immune complexes may be **deposited in many organs**.

- **Localized:** Immune complexes may be **deposited or formed in particular organs/tissues: kidney** (glomerulonephritis), **joints** (arthritis), **small blood vessels of the skin.**

Cause of Tissue Damage

- **Activation of complement**
- **Inflammation at the sites of deposition**

Examples of immune complex disorders are listed in Table 5.5.

Table 5.5: Examples of immune complex-mediated diseases

Disease	Antigen	Manifestations
Exogenous antigen		
Poststreptococcal glomerulonephritis	Streptococcal cell wall antigen(s)	Glomerulonephritis
Serum sickness	Various proteins, e.g. foreign serum protein (horse antithymocyte globulin)	Arthritis, vasculitis, nephritis
Arthus reaction	Various foreign proteins	Cutaneous vasculitis
Endogenous antigen		
Systemic lupus erythematosus (SLE)	Nuclear antigens	Glomerulonephritis, skin lesions, arthritis, others

Systemic Immune Complex Disease—Acute Serum Sickness

Q. Write short note on serum sickness.

This was a frequent sequela to the administration of large amounts of foreign serum (e.g. serum from immunized horses used for protection against diphtheria). Nowadays it is infrequent.

Pathogenesis (Fig. 5.9)

Divided into three phases:

1. **Formation of immune complexes:**
   - **Introduction of protein antigen:** It initiates an immune response.
   - **Formation of antibody:** It usually forms a week (7 to 12 days) after the injection of the foreign protein and are secreted into the blood.
   - **Formation of immune complexes:** They are formed in the circulation when antibodies react with the antigen.
2. **Deposition of immune complexes:**
   - **Immune complexes** of **medium size** and with **slight antigen excess** are the **most pathogenic**.
   - **Sites of deposition:**
     - **Blood vessels:** It causes vasculitis.
     - **Renal glomeruli:** It causes glomerulonephritis.
     - **Joints:** It causes arthritis.
3. **Inflammatory reaction and tissue injury:** Mechanism of tissue injury include:
   - **Inflammatory reaction: Immune complexes** in the tissues **activates complement**, the products (e.g chemotactic C5a) of which causes chemotactic **recruitment of acute inflammatory cells** (neutrophils and monocytes) to the site.
   - **Tissue damage:** Activated inflammatory cells (leukocyte) **release lysosomal enzymes, arachidonic acid products and reactive oxygen species** → which produce **tissue damage**.

Clinical features: Fever, urticaria, joint pains (arthralgias), lymph node enlargement, and proteinuria appear during this phase.

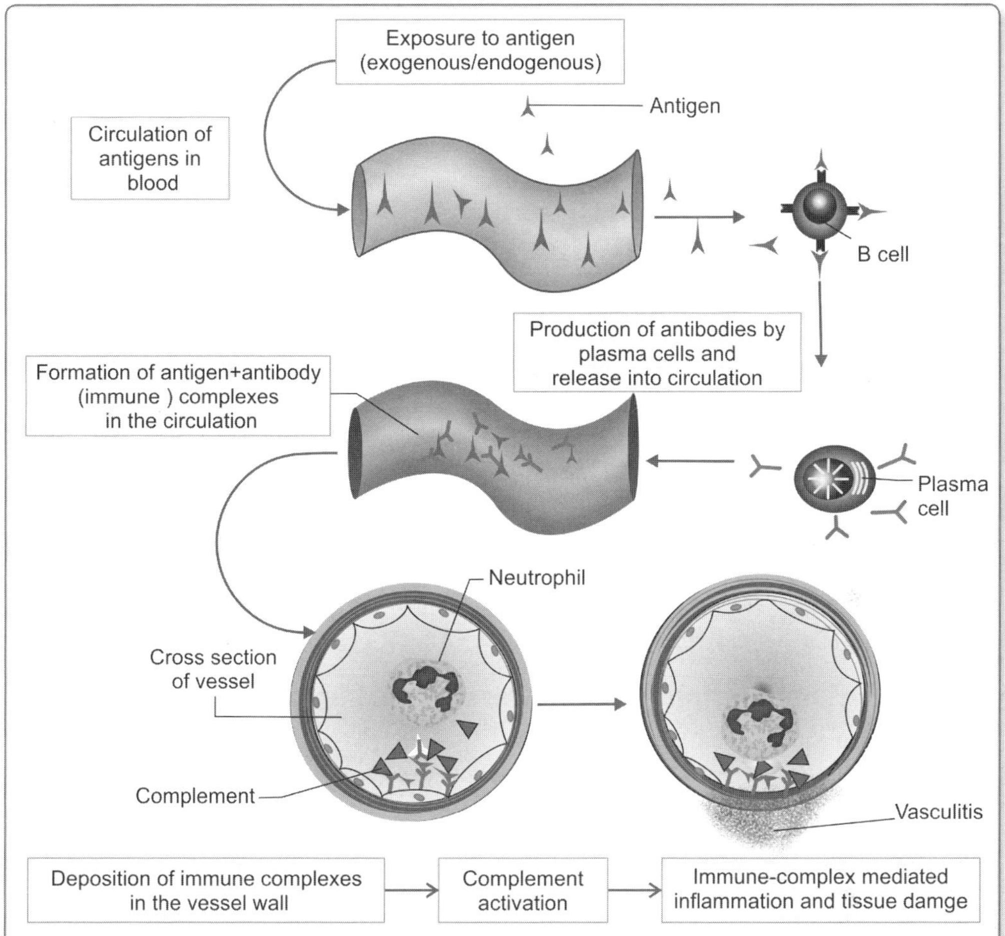

Fig. 5.9: Pathogenesis of systemic immune complex–mediated disease (type-III hypersensitivity). Immune complexes are deposited in tissue activate complement system and recruit tissue-damaging inflammatory cells. The pathogenic ability of immune complexes to mediate tissue injury depends on size, solubility, net charge, and ability to fix complement

Morphology

- **Acute necrotizing vasculitis:** It is the **main feature** and is characterized by **necrosis of the vessel wall and intense neutrophilic infiltration**.
- **Fibrinoid necrosis:** It consists of necrotic tissue, immune complexes deposits, complement, and plasma protein. It produces a **smudgy eosinophilic appearance** at the site of deposit and obscures the cellular detail.

Local Immune Complex Disease—Arthus Reaction

Q. Write short note on Arthus reaction.

Q. Differences between serum sickness and Arthus reaction.

- Arthus reaction is a **local area of tissue necrosis usually in the skin**, resulting from acute immune complex vasculitis.

- Arthus reaction can be experimentally produced by intracutaneous injection of an antigen to a previously immunized animal (with circulating antibodies against the antigen). As the antigen diffuses into the vascular wall, it locally binds to the antibody, and form large immune complexes at the site of injection.
- **Immune complexes deposited in the vessel walls, cause fibrinoid necrosis, and thrombosis leading to ischemic injury**.

T CELL-MEDIATED (TYPE IV) HYPERSENSITIVITY

Q. Write short note on type IV hypersensitivity reactions/delayed hypersensitivity reactions.

- Type IV hypersensitivity reaction is **mediated by T lymphocytes** including **CD4+ and CD8+ T cells**.
- It develops in response to antigenic exposure in a previously sensitized individual.
- Reaction is delayed by 48 to 72 hours after exposure to antigen. Hence also called as delayed-type hypersensitivity (DTH).
- This hypersensitivity reaction is involved in several **autoimmune diseases** (e.g. rheumatoid arthritis, Hashimoto thyroiditis), pathological **reactions to environmental chemicals** (e.g. poison ivy, nickel) and **persistent microbes (e.g. tuberculosis, leprosy)**.

Types: Two types namely: 1) **Cytokine mediated** inflammation in which **CD4+ T cells produce cytokines** and 2) **Direct cell toxicity** mediated by **CD8+ T cells**.

Cytokine Mediated Inflammation Elicited By CD4+ T Cells (Fig. 5.10)

A. **First exposure to antigen:**
   - **Type of antigen:** Antigen may be either **exogenous** environmental antigens or **endogenous** (**self-antigens** causing autoimmune disease).
   - **Processing of antigen:** Upon exposure to an **antigen**, it should be **processed by the antigen presenting cells (APC**- dendritic cells or macrophages) before **presenting it to T cells**, because T cells cannot directly recognize the antigen.
   - **Recognition of antigen by naïve CD4+ T cells** in **association with II MHC molecules** on APC.

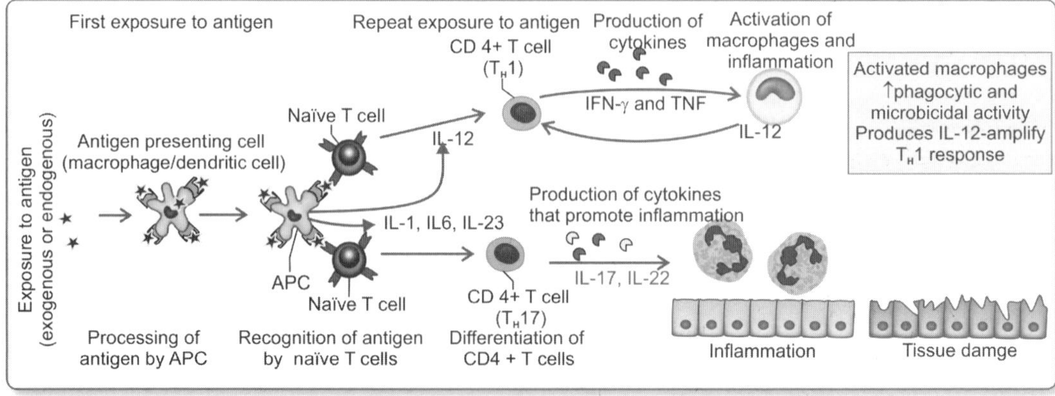

Fig. 5.10: Mechanisms of CD4+ T cell–mediated (type IV) hypersensitivity reactions. In delayed-type hypersensitivity reactions, antigens are phagocytized, processed by APC (antigen presenting cells, e.g. dendritic cell, macrophage). They are presented to naïve T cells. Depending on the cytokines produces by APC naïve cells T may differentiate into CD4+ T_H1 or CD4+ T_H17. CD4+ T_H1 cells secret cytokines that activate macrophage leading to tissue injury. CD4+ T_H17 cells produce cytokines that produce inflammation by recruiting neutrophils. Both mechanisms produce tissue damage

- **Differentiation of CD4+ T cells:**
  - If the APCs secrete **IL-12**, the **naïve CD4+ T cells differentiate into effector cells of T_H1 type**.
  - If the APCs secrete **IL-1, Il-6, or IL-23** (instead of IL-12), the **naïve CD4+ T cells differentiate** into **effector cell of T_H17 type**.

B. **On repeat exposure to an antigen: Previously activated T cells recognize the antigen** presented by APCs. Depending on the cytokines produced, one of two effector cells, i.e. either **T_H1 or T_H17** cells respond.

- **T_H1 cells → production of cytokines** (e.g. **IFN-γ and TNF**). IFN-γ (**most powerful macrophage activating cytokine) → activates macrophages.**
  - **Activated macrophages** have **increased phagocytic and microbicidal power**. They **secrete IL-12** which **amplify the T_H1 response.**
- **T_H17 cells:** They are **activated by** some **microbial antigens** as well as **self-antigens** in autoimmune diseases. They **produce IL-17, IL-22, chemokines, and other cytokines.** These cytokines **promote inflammation** by recruiting more **neutrophils and monocytes** to the site of reaction.

Tuberculin Reaction (Montoux Test)

- Tuberculin reaction is a classical example for delayed-type hypersensitivity.
- It is produced by the **intracutaneous injection of purified protein derivative** (PPD, also called tuberculin), a protein-containing antigen of the tubercle bacillus.
- **In a previously sensitized individual, the injection site becomes red and indurated** in 8 to 12 hours, reaches a peak (usually 1 to 2 cm in diameter) in 24 to 72 hours, and thereafter slowly subsides.
- Microscopically, the injected site shows perivascular accumulation "cuffing" of CD4+ T cells and macrophages.

Contact Dermatitis

Contact with various environmental antigens (e.g. poison ivy, metals such as nikel and chromium, chemicals like hair dyes, cosmetics, soaps) may evoke inflammation with blisters in the skin at the site of contact known as contact dermatitis.

Direct Cell Toxicity Mediated By CD8+ T Cells

It is a type of T-cell mediated tissue injury due to CD8+ T lymphocytes (also called as cytotoxic T lymphocytes- CTLs), which kill antigen-bearing target cells. Example—killing of virus infected cells (e.g. in viral hepatitis) and some tumor cells.

Examples of T cell-mediated (type IV) hypersensitivity are shown in Table 5.6.

Table 5.6: Examples of T cell-mediated (type IV) hypersensitivity

Disease	Antigen	Manifestations
Type 1 diabetes mellitus	Antigens of pancreatic islet β cells (insulin, glutamic acid decarboxylase, others)	Insulitis (chronic inflammation in islets), destruction of β cells; diabetes mellitus
Rheumatoid arthritis	Collagen; citrullinated self-protein	Chronic arthritis, inflammatory destruction of articular cartilage and bone
Inflammatory bowel disease	Enteric bacteria, self-antigen	Chronic inflammation of intestine, ulceration
Hashimoto thyroiditis	Thyroglobulin and other thyroid proteins	Hypothyroidism
Contact sensitivity (dermatitis)	Environmental chemicals (e.g. poison ivy)	Inflammation of skin and blisters

Salient features and differences between hypersensitivity reactions are presented in Table 5.7.

Table 5.7: Salient features and differences between hypersensitivity reactions

Features	Type I	Type II	Type III	Type IV
Antigens	Exogenous allergens include: pollens, moulds, mites, drugs, food etc.	Cell surface or tissue bound	Soluble exogenous (viruses, bacteria, fungi, parasites) or endogenous autoantigens	Cell/tissue bound
Antibody involved	IgE	IgG and IgM	IgG, IgM, IgA	None
Mediators	From mast cells	Complement and lymphokines	Complement	T lymphocytes Activated macrophages
Time taken for reaction to develop	5–10 min	6–36 hours	4–12 hours	48–72 hours
Immunopathology	Edema, vasodilatation, mast cell degranulation, eosinophils	Antibody-mediated damage to target cells/ tissue	Acute inflammatory reaction, neutrophils, vasculitis	Perivascular inflammation, mononuclear cells, fibrin, granulomas caseation and necrosis in TB
Examples of diseases and conditions produced	• Asthma (extrinsic) • Urticaria/edema • Allergic rhinitis • Food allergies • Anaphylaxis	• Autoimmune hemolytic anemia • Transfusion reactions • Hemolytic disease of newborn • Goodpasture's syndrome • Acute rheumatic fever • Pernicious anemia • Myasthenia gravis	• Autoimmune e.g. SLE • Glomerulonephritis • Rheumatoid arthritis • Farmer's lung disease • Hypersensitivity pneumonitis • Arthus reaction (localized)	• Pulmonary TB • Contact dermatitis • Tuberculin test • Leprosy • Graft-versus-host

AUTOIMMUNE DISEASES

Definition: Autoimmunity is defined as **immune reactions** in which **body produces autoantibodies** and **immunologically competent T- lymphocytes against self-antigens.**

Autoimmunity is an important cause of certain diseases in humans (Table 5.8).

- **Organ-specific disease:** It may be restricted to a single organ or tissue (e.g. type 1 diabetes).
- **Systemic or generalized disease:** e.g. systemic lupus erythematosus (SLE).
- **Involving more than one organ:** e.g. Goodpasture's syndrome, in which lung and kidney are involved.

Normal individuals are unresponsive (tolerant) to their own (self) antigens and autoimmune disorders results from the loss of self-tolerance.

Immunological Tolerance

Immunological tolerance is the phenomenon in which there is **no immune response to specific (usually self) antigens.** It is the result of exposure of lymphocytes to that specific antigen.

Self-tolerance: It is absence of immune response to an individual's own antigens.

Q. List autoimmune diseases.

Table 5.8: Examples of autoimmune diseases

Diseases mediated by antibodies	Diseases mediated by T cells
Organ-specific	**Organ-specific**
Autoimmune hemolytic anemia	Type 1 diabetes mellitus
Autoimmune thrombocytopenia	Hashimoto thyroiditis
Goodpasture syndrome	Crohn's disease
Myasthenia gravis	Multiple sclerosis
Graves' disease	
Systemic	**Systemic**
Systemic lupus erythematosus (SLE)	Rheumatoid arthritis

Autoimmunity develops from a combination of the inheritance of susceptibility genes, which may contribute to the breakdown of self-tolerance, and environmental triggers (e.g. infections and tissue damage), which promote the activation of self-reactive lymphocytes.

General Features of Autoimmune Diseases

- Autoimmune diseases are usually chronic, sometimes with relapses and remissions.
- Damage caused is often progressive.
- Clinical and pathological features of an autoimmune disease depend on the nature of the underlying immune response.

SYSTEMIC LUPUS ERYTHEMATOSUS (SLE)

SLE is a **chronic autoimmune disease** having following characteristics:

1. **Protean manifestation and variable behavior**.
2. **Remission and relapses**.
3. **Multisystemic involvement:** Mainly affects **skin, kidneys, joints, serous membranes and heart**.
4. **Broad spectrum of autoantibodies**, most important is antinuclear antibodies (ANAs).

Etiology

SLE is an **autoimmune disease** in which fundamental defect is **failure of self-tolerance**. It leads to production of **many autoantibodies** that **damages the tissue either directly or indirectly by depositing immune complex deposits**. A combination of genetic and environmental factors plays a role in the pathogenesis of SLE.

Genetic Factors

Evidence to support genetic predisposition are:

1. **Familial association:**
   - **Family members** of SLE patients have an **increased risk** of SLE. About 20% of unaffected first-degree relatives may show autoantibodies.
   - **High rate** of concordance (>25%) in **monozygotic twins** when compared with dizygotic twins (1%–3%).
2. **HLA association:** Risk is more with HLA-DR2 or HLA-DR3.

3. **Other genetic factors:**
   - Genetic deficiencies of early complement components (such as C2, C4, or C1q): It may result in: 1) impaired removal of circulating immune complexes by the mononuclear phagocyte system, 2) defective phagocytic clearance of apoptotic cells and 3) failure of B cell tolerance. If apoptotic cells are not cleared, their nuclear components may elicit immune responses.
   - Polymorphism in the inhibitory Fc receptor → inadequate control of B cell activation.

Immunological Abnormalities

Several immunological abnormalities of both innate and **adaptive immune** system have been observed in SLE.

1. **Type I interferons:**
   - These are antiviral cytokines normally produced by B cells during innate immune responses to nucleic acid of viruses.
   - **INF-α** is a type I interferon produced by plasmacytoid dendritic cells and **large amounts is produced** in SLE. It may indirectly produce autoantibodies.
2. **TLR signals:**
   - TLRs present in B lymphocytes normally sense microbial products, including nucleic acids.
   - In SLE, nuclear DNA and RNA within the **immune complexes may activate B lymphocytes by engaging with TLRs**. These **activated B cells** specific for nuclear antigens may **produce antinuclear autoantibodies**.
3. **Failure of B cell tolerance:** Occurs due to **defects in both central** (i.e. bone marrow) and **peripheral tolerance → higher autoreactive B cells**.

Environmental Factors

1. **Ultraviolet (UV) radiation:** Exposure to sunlight exacerbates the lesions of the disease.
   - **Mechanism:** UV irradiation → causes **apoptosis** of host cells → **increases burden of nuclear antigens** and **promote inflammation**.
2. **Cigarette smoking:** It is associated with development of SLE.
3. **Sex hormones:** SLE is 10 times greater during the reproductive period (17–55 years) **in women** than in men. SLE shows exacerbation during normal menses and pregnancy.
4. **Drugs:** Examples include **hydralazine, procainamide, isoniazid, and D-penicillamine** can produce SLE-like disease and disease remits after withdrawal of the drug.

Pathogenesis of SLE (Fig. 5.11)

Different steps are:

1. **Increased apoptosis triggered by environmental agents:** UV irradiation and other environmental agents may cause death of cells by **apoptosis**.
2. **Inadequate clearance of apoptotic bodies:** It results in accumulation of large amount of nuclear antigens. It is partly due to defect in complement proteins.
3. **Susceptibility genes with failure of self-tolerance:** Genetic abnormality in B and T lymphocytes is responsible for failure of self-tolerance.
4. **Stimulation of self-reactive B cells:** It produces antibodies against the self-nuclear antigens.
5. **Formation of antigen-antibody (immune) complexes** in the circulation.

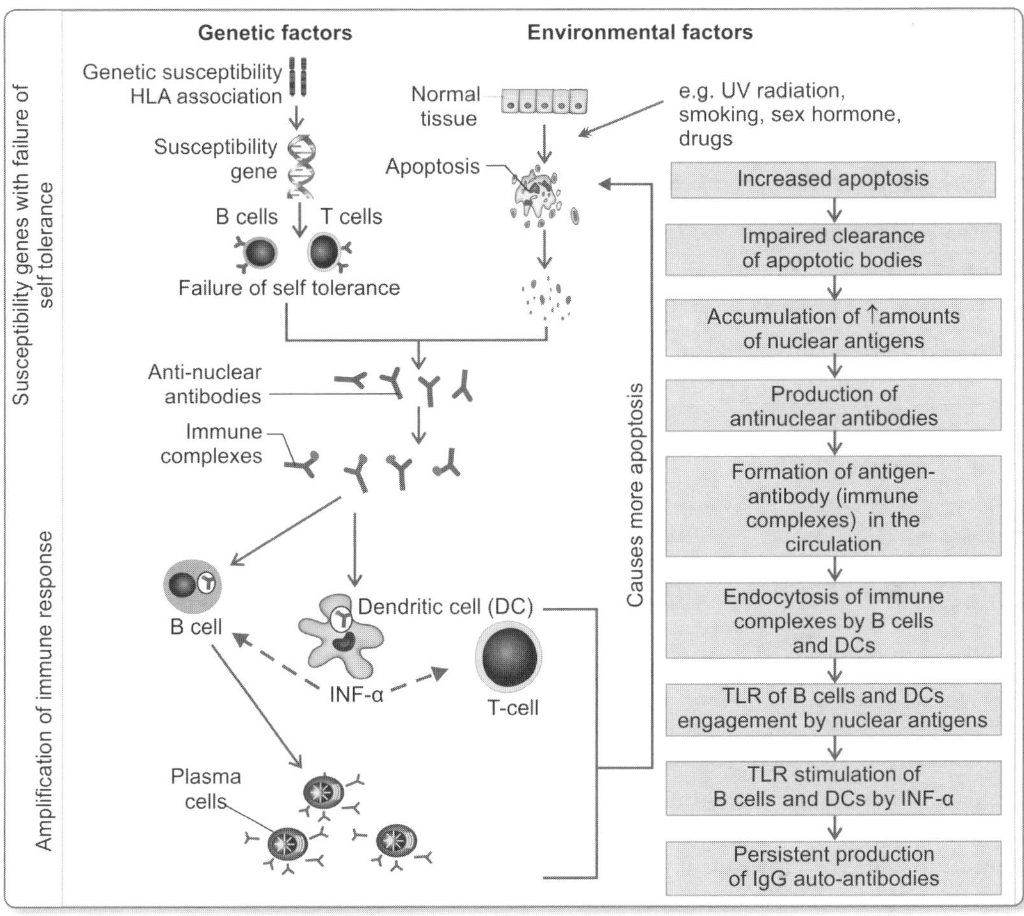

Fig. 5.11: Pathogenesis of systemic lupus erythematosus
Abbreviation: TLRs, Toll-like receptors; DCs, Dendritic cells

6. **Endocytosis of immune complexes:** The antibodies portion of immune complexes bind to Fc receptors on B cells and dendritic cells (DCs), and the immune complexes may be internalized by endocytosis.
7. **TLR engagement by nuclear antigens:** Nucleic acid components of immune complexes bind to TLRs (Toll-like receptors) of B cells and DCs.
8. **TLR stimulation of B cells and DCs:** Binding to TLR
   - Stimulate B cells to produce autoantibodies
   - Activate dendritic cells (mainly plasmacytoid DCs) to produce INF-α → stimulate B and T cells to further amplify immune response → cause more apoptosis.
9. **Persistent production of autoantibodies:** Thus, a cycle of antigen release and immune activation → results in the persistent production of IgG autoantibodies.

Autoantibodies in SLE

SLE is characterized by the production of **several diverse autoantibodies**. Some antibodies are against different nuclear and cytoplasmic components of the cell that are not organ specific. Other antibodies are directed against specific cell surface antigens of blood cells.

Antinuclear antibodies (ANAs): They are directed against various nuclear antigens including DNA, RNA, and proteins (all together called generic ANAs) and can be grouped into different categories (Table 5.8).

Q. List autoimmune diseases.

Table 5.9: Important antinuclear antibodies and their clinical utility

Type of antinuclear antibodies	Antigen recognized	Clinical utility
Anti-dsDNA*	DNA (double-stranded-ds)	High titers of IgG antibodies are SLE-specific (but not to single-stranded DNA)
Anti-Sm*	Nonhistone proteins bound to RNA	Specific for SLE; do not usually correlate with disease activity or clinical manifestations
Antihistone antibodies	Histones associated with DNA	More frequent in drug-induced lupus than in SLE
Antibodies to DNA	Multiple nuclear	Best screening test; if repeated test are negative SLE unlikely
Anti-Ro (SS-A)	RNP (ribonucleoprotein)	Not specific for SLE; predictive value indicates increased risk for neonatal lupus, and sicca syndrome

*Antibodies specific to SLE. Females with child-bearing potential and SLE should be screened for aPL and anti-Ro.

Mechanisms of Tissue Injury

Autoantibodies mediate tissue injury.

- **Type III hypersensitivity:** It occurs with deposition of **immune complexes**. It is the most **common cause of tissue injury and visceral lesions**.
- **Type II hypersensitivity: Autoantibodies against cell surface antigens** specific for **RBCs, white cells, and platelets** → opsonize these cells → promote their phagocytosis and lysis → **cytopenias**.

LE Bodies or Hematoxylin Bodies

Q. Write short note on LE cell.

LE Bodies

- ANAs cannot penetrate intact cells, but if nuclei of the cell are exposed, they can bind to them.
- In tissues, nuclei of damaged cells react with ANAs, lose their chromatin pattern, and appear homogeneous, to produce **LE bodies or hematoxylin bodies**.

LE Cell (Figs 5.12A and B)

- It is related to LE bodies and can be demonstrated in vitro.
- The blood sample is agitated to damage the nucleated cells and it releases the nuclei.
- The nuclei of damaged cells react with ANAs to form a homogenous denatured nuclear material.

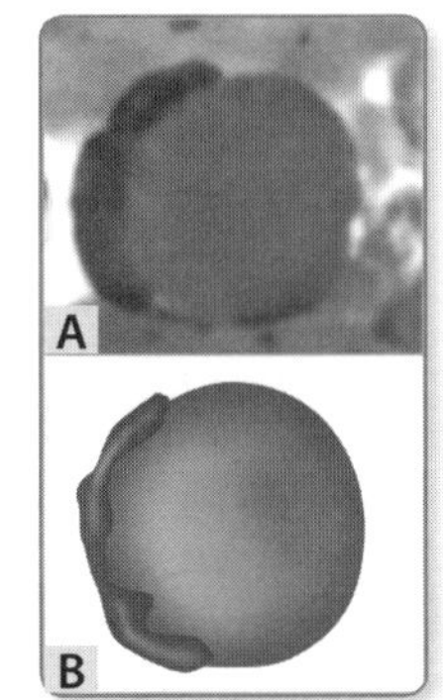

Figs 5.12A and B: Appearance of LE cell (A, Leishman stain and B, diagrammatic)

- The LE cell is any phagocytic leukocyte (blood neutrophil or macrophage) that has engulfed this denatured nucleus of an injured cell.
- The demonstration of LE cells in vitro was used as a test for SLE.
- With the advent of new techniques for detection of ANAs, this test is of only historical interest.
- Sometimes, LE cells can be found in body fluid, such as pericardial or pleural effusions.

Morphology

SLE is a systemic autoimmune disease and morphologic changes in SLE are **extremely variable.**

The most **characteristic lesions** of SLE are **due to deposition of immune complexes** in **blood vessels, kidneys, connective tissue, and skin.**

Kidney

Kidney may be **involved in about 50%** of SLE patients and is one of the most important organs involved. However, it involves tubules and interstitium.

Pathogenesis of glomerulonephritis: Immune complexes composed of **DNA and anti-DNA antibodies** gets deposited in the glomeruli → inflammation → proliferation of cells (endothelial, mesangial and/or epithelial).

Morphologic classification of lupus nephritis: Six patterns are recognized but none of these is specific for SLE.

1. **Minimal mesangial** lupus nephritis (class I)
2. **Mesangial proliferative** lupus nephritis (class II)
3. **Focal proliferative** lupus nephritis (class III)
4. **Diffuse proliferative** lupus nephritis (class IV)
5. **Membranous** lupus nephritis (class V)
6. **Advanced sclerosing** lupus nephritis (class VI)

Clinical Features

- SLE is a **multisystem** disease with **variable clinical presentation**.
- **Age:** It usually occurs in young woman between **20 to 30 years**, but may manifest at any age.
- **Sex:** It predominantly affects **women**, with female-to-male ratio of 9: 1.
- **Onset:** Acute or insidious with fever.
- **Typical presentation: Butterfly rash over the face, fever, pain** without deformity in one or more **peripheral joints, pleuritic chest pain, and photosensitivity**. SLE patients are **susceptible to infections**, because of immune dysfunction and treatment with immunosuppressive drugs.

MAJOR HISTOCOMPATIBILITY COMPLEX (MHC) MOLECULES

- All human cells have a series of molecules on their surfaces that are recognized by other individuals as foreign antigens. **Major histocompatibility complex** (MHC) **molecules** were discovered as **products of genes that evoke rejection of transplanted organs** and responsible for tissue compatibility between individuals.
- The **human major histocompatibility complex** (MHC) are commonly called the **human leukocyte antigen (HLA) complex** is the name of the **loci of genes** densely packed (clustered) on a **small segment on chromosome 6** (6p21.3). They were named HLA because in humans MHC-encoded proteins were initially detected on leukocytes by the binding of antibodies.
- **Physiologic function of MHC molecules**: To **display peptide fragments of proteins for recognition by antigen-specific T cells.**

- The MHC molecules are products of MHC gene. The best known of these genes are the HLA class I and class II genes. Their products are important for immunologic specificity and transplantation histocompatibility, and they play a major role in susceptibility to a number of autoimmune diseases.
- **Polymorphism of MHC gene:**
  - **MHC gene is highly polymorphic**. Polymorphism means that there are many alleles of each MHC gene resulting in extreme (high degree) variation in the MHC in human population (genetic diversity). Each person inherits one set of these alleles that is different from the alleles in most other persons. The possibility of two different individuals having the same combination of MHC molecules is very remote. Therefore, grafts exchanged between individuals are recognized as foreign and attacked by the immune system. **Polymorphism is an important barrier in organ transplantation.**
  - **HLA haplotype:** It is the combination of HLA alleles in each individual. Each individual inherits one set of HLA genes from each parent and thus typically expresses two different molecules for every locus.
- **Importance of MHC:** 1) In organ/tissue transplantation and 2) HLA is linked to many autoimmune diseases.

Classification

MHC gene product is classified based on their structure, cellular distribution, and function into **three groups** (Fig. 5.13). MHC class I and class II gene products are critical for immunologic specificity and transplantation histocompatibility, and they play a major role in susceptibility to a number of autoimmune diseases.

Class I MHC Molecules

- They are the products of MHC class I genes and are **expressed on all nucleated cells and platelets** (except erythrocytes and trophoblasts).
- They are **encoded by three closely linked loci, designated *HLA-A*, *HLA-B*, and *HLA-C*.**
- **Highly polymorphic** in the population and most highly polymorphic segment known within the human genome.
- **Functions:** Products of MHC class I gene are integral participants in the **immune response to intracellular infections, tumors, and allografts**. Class I MHC molecules display peptides that are derived from proteins, such as viral and tumor antigens, that are located in the cytoplasm. These peptides are usually produced in the cell.

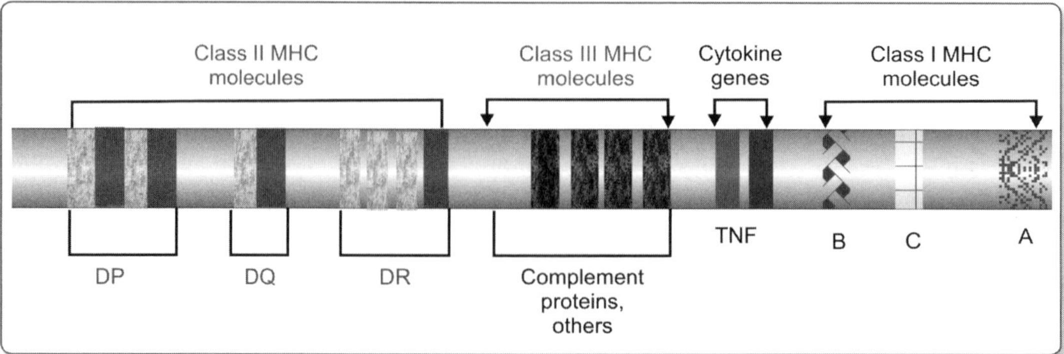

Fig. 5.13: Major histocompatibility complex [human leukocyte antigen (HLA) complex] showing location of genes

- **The class I–associated peptides are recognized by CD8+ T lymphocytes.** Class I molecules **interact with CD8+ T lymphocytes during antigen presentation** and are **involved in cytotoxic reactions.** CD8+ T lymphocytes recognize antigens only in the context of self-class I molecules, they are referred to as class I MHC-restricted.

Class II MHC Molecules

- They are encoded in a region called ***HLA-D***, which has three sub-regions: ***HLA-DP, HLA-DQ*, and *HLA-DR***.
- Class II antigens (HLA-D and -DR, D-related) **are expressed only on professional antigen-presenting cells (B lymphocytes, monocytes/macrophages, Langerhans' cells, dendritic cells) and activated T cells.**
- **Function: Class II MHC molecules present antigens that are internalized into vesicles, and are usually derived from extracellular microbes and soluble proteins. HLA-D locus** contains genes that **encode many proteins involved in antigen processing and presentation.** The **class II–peptide complex is recognized by CD4+ T cells** (function as helper cells) and these CD4 molecule acts as the co-receptor. Because **CD4+ T cells can recognize antigens only in the context of self–class II molecules** → they are referred to as **class II MHC–restricted.**

Class III MHC Molecules

- Their gene **encode** components of the **complement system, cytokines, tumor necrosis factor (TNF), lymphotoxin**, and some proteins without apparent role in the immune system.

ACQUIRED IMMUNODEFICIENCY SYNDROME (AIDS)

AIDS is caused by the retrovirus **human immunodeficiency virus** (HIV).

Characteristic Features

- **Infection and depletion of CD4+ T lymphocytes.**
- **Severe immunosuppression → leads to opportunistic infections, secondary neoplasms, and neurologic manifestations.**

Route of Transmission

Transmission of HIV occurs when there is an exchange of blood or body fluids containing the virus or virus-infected cells. The three major routes of transmission are:

1. **Sexual transmission:** It is the **main route of infection** in more than 75% of cases of HIV.
    - **Homosexual or bisexual men** or **heterosexual contacts:** It may be male-to-male, or male-to-female or female-to-male transmission.
    - **HIV is present in genital fluids,** such as vaginal secretions and cervical cells (in women), and semen (in men).
    - Risk of sexual transmission of HIV is increased when there is coexisting sexually transmitted diseases, especially those associated with genital ulceration (e.g. syphilis, chancroid, and herpes).
    - **Viral transmission** can occur in two ways:
        - **Direct inoculation of virus or infected cells into the blood vessels** at the site of breach caused by trauma, and
        - **By uptake into the mucosal dendritic cells** (DCs).

2. **Parenteral transmission:** Three groups of individuals are at risk
   - **Intravenous drug abusers:** Transmission occurs by **sharing of needles, and syringes contaminated** with HIV-containing blood.
   - **Hemophiliacs:** Mainly those who received large amount of factor VIII and factor IX concentrates before 1985. Now increasing use of recombinant clotting factors have eliminated this mode of transmission.
   - **Transfusion of blood or blood components:** Recipients of blood transfusion of **HIV-infected whole blood or components** (e.g. platelets, plasma) was one of the modes of transmission. Screening of donor blood and plasma for antibody to HIV has reduced the risk of this mode of transmission. Because of recently infected individual may be antibody-negative (seronegative), there is a small risk of acquiring AIDS through transfusion of blood. Organs from HIV-infected donors can also transmit AIDS.
3. **Perinatal transmission (mother-to-infant transmission):**
   - **Major mode of transmission of AIDS in children**.
   - Transmission of infection can occur by **three routes**:
     - **In utero:** It is transmitted by transplacental spread.
     - **Perinatal spread:** During normal vaginal delivery or child birth (intrapartum) **through an infected birth canal** and in the immediate period (peripartum).
     - **After birth:** It is transmitted by ingestion of breast milk or from the genital secretions.

Transmission of HIV infection to healthcare workers: There is an extremely small risk of transmission to healthcare professionals, after accidental needle-stick injury or exposure of nonintact skin to infected blood.

Etiology

Properties of HIV

AIDS is caused by HIV, which is a **nontransforming human retrovirus** belonging to the lentivirus family. Retroviruses are **RNA viruses having an enzyme called reverse transcriptase**, which **prepares a DNA copy of the RNA genome of the virus in host cell**.

Genetic forms: HIV occurs in two genetically different but related main forms, **HIV-1 and HIV-2**.
- **HIV-1** is most common in the United States, Europe, and Central Africa.
- **HIV-2 is common** in West Africa and India.

Structure of HIV (Fig. 5.14)

Q. Write short note on structure of HIV.

- HIV-1 is **spherical enveloped** virus which is about 90–120 nm in diameter.
- It consists of electron-dense, cone-shaped core surrounded by nucleocapsid cell which is covered by lipoprotein envelope.

A. **Viral core:** It contains
   1. **Major capsid protein p24:** This viral antigen and the antibodies against this are **used for the diagnosis of HIV infection** in enzyme-linked immunosorbent assay (**ELISA**).
   2. **Nucleocapsid protein p7/p9.**
   3. **Two identical copies of single stranded RNA genome.**
   4. **Three viral enzymes: 1) protease, 2) reverse transcriptase** (RNA-dependent DNA polymerase), and **3) integrase. When the virus infects a cell, viral RNA** is not translated, instead **transcribed by reverse transcriptase into DNA**. The **DNA form of the retroviral genome** is called a **provirus** which can be **integrated into the chromosome of host cell.**

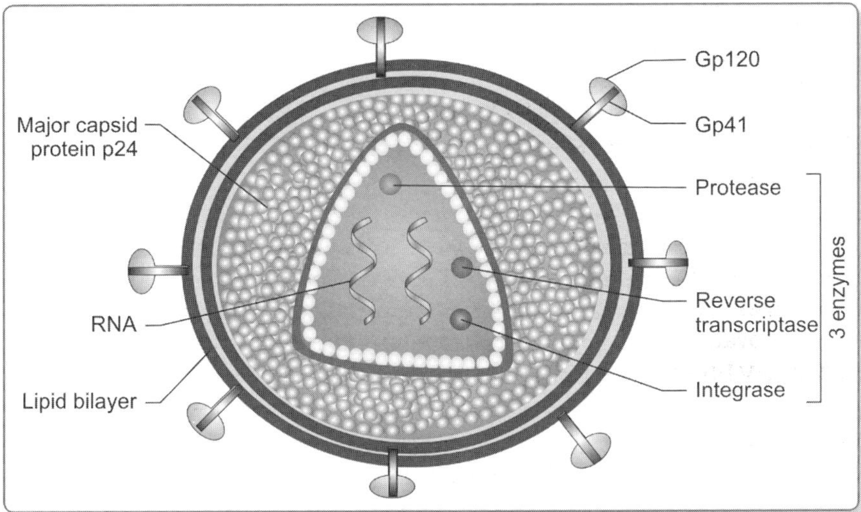

Fig. 5.14: Diagrammatic representation of structure of the human immune deficiency virus (HIV)–1 virion. The viral particle is covered by a lipid bilayer derived from the host cell and studded with viral glycoproteins gp41 and gp120

B. **Nucleocapsid:**

The **viral core is surrounded by a matrix protein p24 and p17**, which **lies underneath the lipid envelope** of the virion.

C. **Lipid envelope:**

The virus contains a lipoprotein envelope, which **consist of lipid derived from the host cell and two viral glycoproteins**. These glycoproteins are: **1) gp120** which project as a knob-like spikes on the surface and **2) gp41** anchoring transmembrane pedicle. **These glycoproteins are essential for HIV infection of cells.**

HIV Genome

It contains two main groups of genes and their products act as antigens.

1. **Standard genes:** HIV-1 RNA genome **contains three standard retroviral genes**, which are **typical of retroviruses**. These include: **gag**, **pol**, and **env** genes. Initially, the protein products of the **gag** and **pol** genes are translated into **large precursor proteins** and are later cleaved by the viral enzyme protease to form → **mature proteins.**
2. **Accessory genes:** HIV contains accessory genes: e.g. tat, rev, vif, nef, and vpr, and vpu. They **regulate the synthesis and assembly of infectious viral particles** and the **pathogenicity of the virus.**

Pathogenesis of HIV Infection and AIDS

Q. Write short note on pathogenesis of HIV infection and AIDS.

Infection is transmitted when the virus enters the blood or tissues of an individual.

Major targets: HIV can infect many tissues, but two major targets of HIV infection are the:

- **Immune system**
- **Central nervous system (CNS).**

Life Cycle of HIV

Q. Write note on life cycle of HIV.

Consists of four main steps namely: 1) infection of cells by HIV, 2) integration of the provirus into the host cell genome, 3) activation of viral replication, and 4) production and release of infectious virus (Fig. 5.15).

1. **Infection of Cells by HIV**:
   - **Cell tropism:** HIV has **selective affinity** for host cells with **CD4 molecule receptor**. The cells with such receptors include **CD4+ T cells** and other CD4+ cells such as **monocytes/ macrophages** and **dendritic cells.** The HIV envelope contains two glycoproteins, surface gp120 noncovalently attached to a transmembrane protein, gp41.
   - **Gp120 of HIV binding to CD4 molecule receptor** on the host cell is the first step in HIV infection. Binding alone is not enough for infection and **requires participation of a coreceptor molecule.**
   - **Conformational change:** Binding to CD4 leads to a conformational change **in the HIV, that results in the formation of a new recognition site on gp120 for the coreceptors CCR5 or CXCR4.**
   - **Gp120 binding to chemokine receptor:** New recognition site on gp120 of HIV bind to **chemokine receptors,** i.e. CCR5 and CXCR4.
   - **Penetration of host cell membrane by gp41:** Binding of gp120 to the chemokine coreceptors leads to **conformational changes in gp41.**
   - **Membrane fusion:** The conformational change in gp41 allows **HIV to penetrate the cell membrane of the target cells** (e.g. CD4+ T cells or macrophages), **leading to fusion of the virus with the host cell.**
   - **Entry of viral genome into cytoplasm of host cell:** Once internalized, the virus core containing the HIV genome enters the cytoplasm of the host cell.
2. **Integration of the proviral DNA into the genome of the host cell**
   - After the internalization of the virus core, the **RNA genome of the virus undergoes reverse transcription** → leading to the **synthesis of double-stranded complementary DNA (cDNA/proviral DNA).**
   - **Episomal form: In quiescent T cells, HIV cDNA** may remain as a linear **episomal form in the cytoplasm of infected cell.**
   - **Integration of cDNA: In dividing T cells,** HIV **cDNA enters the nucleus,** and **becomes integrated into the genome** of the host cell using a viral integrase protein.

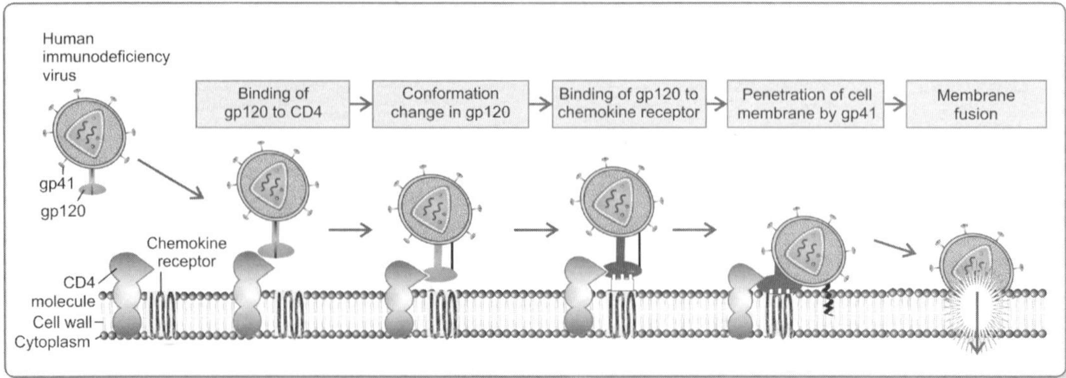

Fig. 5.15: Various molecular steps involved in the life cycle of HIV

3. **Viral replication:** After the integration of proviral DNA it can either be latent or productive infection.
   - **Latent infection:** During this, the **provirus remains silent** for months or years.
   - **Productive infection:** In this the **proviral DNA is transcribed** → leading to **viral replication** → formation of **complete viral particles**.
4. **Production and release of infectious virus:** The complete **virus particle** formed, **buds from the cell membrane** and **release new infectious virus**. This productive infection when extensive, leads to death of infected host cells.

The virus **infection remains latent for long periods in lymphoid tissues. Active viral replication is associated with more infection of cells and progression to AIDS.**

Dissemination: Virus disseminates to other target cells. This occurs either by fusion of an infected cell with an uninfected one or by the budding of virions from the membrane of the infected cell.

Progression of HIV Infection

Acute Infection

HIV infection starts as an acute infection. It is only partially controlled by the host immune response and progresses to chronic infection of peripheral lymphoid tissue.

- **Primary infection: HIV first infects memory CD4+ T cells** (express CCR5), which are present in **the mucosal lymphoid tissue** (largest reservoir of **T cells** and where majority of memory cells are lodged). HIV **causes death of these cells** resulting in **significant depletion of T cells.**
- **Spread to lymphoid tissue: Dendritic cells at the primary site of infection capture the virus** and **migrate to lymphoid tissue** such as lymph nodes and spleen. In the lymphoid tissues, **DCs is passed on to CD4+ T cells by direct cell to cell contact.**
- **Acute HIV syndrome: Virus replicates** and **causes viremia**, accompanied by **acute HIV syndrome** (nonspecific signs and symptoms similar to many viral diseases).
- **Host immune response against HIV:** Virus spreads throughout body and infects helper T cells, macrophages and DCs in the peripheral lymphoid tissues. During this period, the host humoral and cell-mediated immune response develops against viral antigens. These include **anti-HIV antibodies** and **HIV-specific cytotoxic T cells.** Immune responses partially control the infection and viral replication.

Clinical Latency Period

Following acute phase it progress to chronic phase. This phase is **characterized by dissemination of virus, viremia,** and **development of immune response by host.**

- **Minimal/no symptoms:** In this phase, **virus continuously replicates in the lymph nodes and spleen.**
- **Progressive decrease of CD4+ T cells:** There is **continuous destruction of CD4+ T cells in the lymphoid tissue** accompanied by steady **decrease in their number in the peripheral blood.**

Inversion of CD4+/CD8+ ratio: Normal CD4+/CD8+ ratio is 1:2. Loss of CD4+ cells in AIDS patient leads to inversion of ratio of 0.5 or less.

HIV Infection of Non-T Cells: HIV can infect non-T cells such as macrophages and dendritic cells **(mucosal and follicular).**

Abnormalities of B-cell Function

- **Polyclonal activation of B cells → hypergammaglobulinemia → circulating immune complexes.**

- **Impaired humoral immunity → disseminated infections** caused by capsulated bacteria, such as *S. pneumoniae* and *H. influenzae.*

Natural History of HIV Infection

Virus usually enters the body through mucosal epithelia and clinical course can be divided into three main phases:

1. **Early acute phase:** It may present as an acute (refer above), usually **self-limited nonspecific illness. These symptoms include sore throat, myalgias, fever, weight loss, and fatigue. Other features, such as rash, cervical adenopathy**, diarrhea, and vomiting, may also occur.

   Centers for Disease Control (CDC) classification of HIV infection: IT depends on blood CD4+ T-cell count. This divides the patients into three categories with counts being:
   - **Greater than 500 cells/μL**
   - **Between 200 to 500 cells/μL**
   - **Less than 200 cells/μL.**
2. **Middle chronic phase:** It may have **few or no clinical manifestations**, and is called the clinical latency period. The **symptoms may be due to minor opportunistic infections**, such as oral candidiasis (thrush), vaginal candidiasis, herpes zoster, and perhaps mycobacterial tuberculosis.
3. **Final crisis phase:** It is **final phase of HIV with progression to AIDS**. It presents with **fever, weight loss, diarrhea, generalized lymphadenopathy, multiple opportunistic infections, neurologic disease, and secondary neoplasms**. Most of untreated (but not all) patients with HIV infection **progress to AIDS after a chronic phase lasting from 7 to 10 years**.

The opportunistic infections and neoplasms found in patients with HIV infection are presented in Table 5.10.

Q. Write briefly on common neoplasms in HIV patients.

Table 5.10: AIDS-defining opportunistic infections and neoplasms found in patients with HIV infection

Opportunistic Infections	
Protozoal and helminthic infections	**Organ or site involved or type of damage**
Cryptosporidiosis or isosporidiosis	Enteritis
Toxoplasmosis	Pneumonia or CNS infection
Fungal Infections	
Pneumocystosis	Pneumonia or disseminated infection
Candidiasis	Esophageal, tracheal, or pulmonary
Cryptococcosis	Infection of central nervous system
Coccidioidomycosis	Disseminated
Histoplasmosis	Disseminated
Bacterial Infections	
Mycobacteriosis	
• Atypical," e.g. *Mycobacterium avium*-intracellulare	Disseminated or extrapulmonary
• *M. tuberculosis*	Pulmonary or extrapulmonary
Nocardiosis	Pneumonia, meningitis, disseminated
Salmonella infections	Disseminated

Contd...

Contd...

Opportunistic Infections	
Viral Infections	
Cytomegalovirus	Pulmonary, intestinal, retinitis, or CNS infections
Herpes simplex virus	Localized or disseminated
Varicella-zoster virus	Localized or disseminated
Progressive multifocal leukoencephalopathy	Central nervous system
Neoplasms	**Cause**
Kaposi sarcoma (KS)	Kaposi sarcoma herpes virus
Non-Hodgkin B-cell lymphoma—Primary lymphoma of the brain	Epstein Barr Virus (EBV)
Cervical cancer in women	Human papilloma virus (HPV)
Anal carcinoma	HPV

Diagnosis of HIV Infection or AIDS

1. **ELISA:** Detects antibodies against viral proteins. It is the **most sensitive** and best screening test for the diagnosis of AIDS.
2. **Western blot: Most specific** or the **confirmatory test** for HIV.
3. **Direct detection of viral infection:**
   a. **p24 antigen capture assay**
   b. **Reverse transcriptase polymerase chain reaction (RT-PCR)**
   c. **DNA-PCR**
   d. **Culture of virus from the monocytes and CD4+T cells.**

Prognosis: The prognosis of AIDS is poor.

AMYLOIDOSIS

Define amyloidosis.

Definition: Amyloid is a **pathologic fibrillar protein deposited in the extracellular space** in **various tissues and organs** of the body in variety of clinical condition.

General Features

- **Associated with** number of **inherited and inflammatory disorders**.
- **Extracellular deposits** cause structural and functional damage to involved tissue.
- **Basically a disorder of protein misfolding** and is produced by aggregation of misfolded proteins (normal folded proteins are soluble) or protein fragments.
- It also contains abundant charged sugar groups and has staining characteristics that were thought to resemble starch (amylose) and were called as amyloid. But these deposits are not related to starch.
- **Usually a systemic** (sometimes localized) disease.

Forms of Amyloid

All amyloid have same morphological and staining property but amyloidosis is **not a single disease**. It is a **group of diseases** having **in common the deposition of similar-appearing proteins** in which biochemical structure (more than 20 different proteins) and mechanism of formation are different.

Physical Nature of Amyloid

All types of amyloid are **composed of nonbranching fibrils of 7 to 10 nm diameter**.

- **Each fibril consists of β-pleated sheet polypeptide chains** and is wound around one another.
- **Congo red dye** binds to these fibrils and produces **classic apple-green birefringence** (dichromism). Hence, Congo red stain is used to identify amyloid deposits in tissues.

Chemical Nature of Amyloid

Q. Write short note on physical and chemical nature of amyloid.

Fibrillar proteins bind with variety of substances:

- **About 95%** of the amyloid material consists of **fibril proteins**.
- **Remaining 5%** consists of **proteoglycans, glycosaminoglycans, serum amyloid P, etc**.

Biochemical Forms of Amyloid

It consists of three major distinct proteins and more than 20 minor forms.

A. Major forms: These are **AL, AA** and **Aβ amyloid**

1. **AL (amyloid light chain) protein:**
   - Consists of **complete immunoglobulin** (Ig) **light chains** or the **aminoterminal fragments of light chains, or both.**
   - **Produced by plasma cells** and associated with some monoclonal B cell proliferation (e.g. plasma cell tumors).
2. **AA (amyloid-associated) protein:**
   - **Non-immunoglobulin.**
   - **Derived from** a larger precursor in the serum called **SAA (serum amyloid-associated)** protein **synthesized by the liver. Increased synthesis of SAA** protein occurs under the influence of cytokines (e.g. IL-6 and IL-1) **during inflammation**.
   - Associated with **chronic inflammation** (called as secondary amyloidosis).
3. **Aβ amyloid:**
   - **Derived from** transmembrane glycoprotein called **amyloid precursor protein (APP)**.
   - **Found in the cerebral lesions** of **Alzheimer disease**.

B. Minor types:

1. **Transthyretin (TTR):**
   - **It is a normal serum protein** that transports thyroxine and retinol.
   - **Mutations** in gene encoding TTR → **alter its structure** → misfolds.
   - **Found in a familial amyloid polyneuropathies, heart of aged individuals** (senile systemic amyloidosis).
2. **β_2-microglobulin:**
   - It is a **normal serum protein**.
   - Amyloid fibril subunit namely **Aβ_2m is derived from β_2-microglobulin** and is found in amyloidosis of **patients on long-term hemodialysis**.
3. **Other minor types:** Serum amyloid P component, proteoglycans, and highly sulfated glycosaminoglycans.

Pathogenesis of Amyloidosis (Fig. 5.16)

Q. Write short note on pathogenesis of amyloidosis.

Misfolding of Proteins

Amyloidosis is a **disorder due to abnormal folding or misfolding of proteins**.

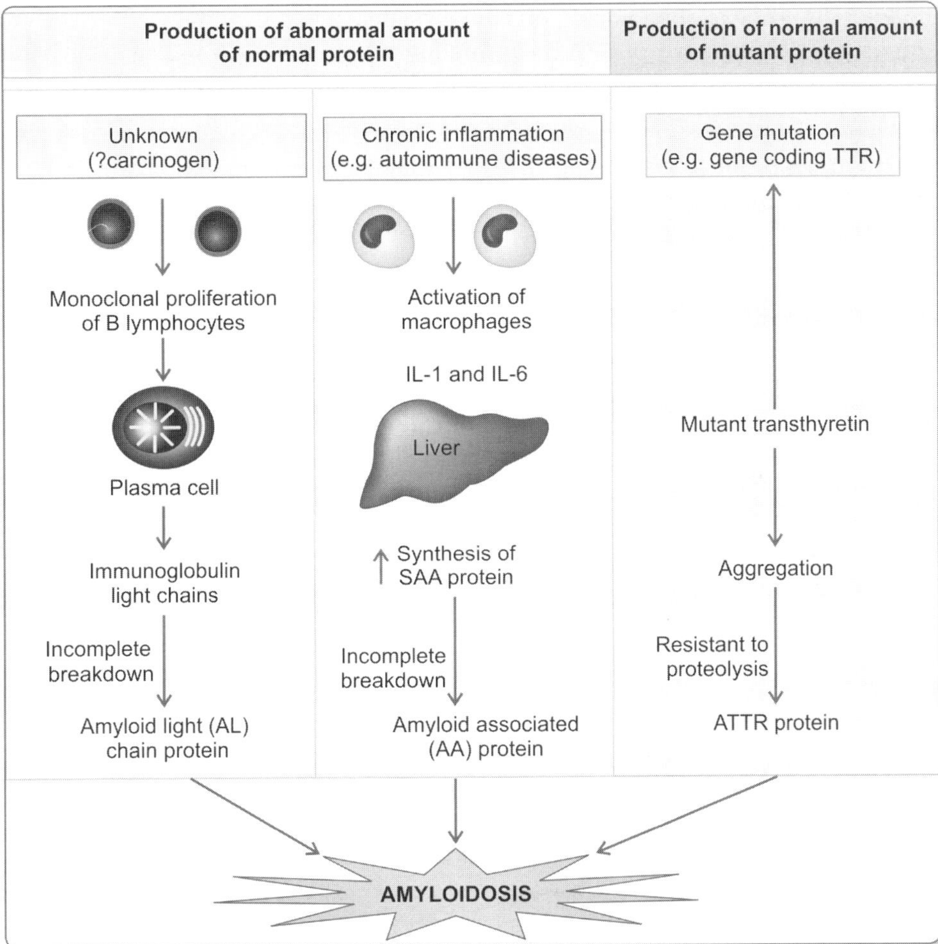

Fig. 5.16: Pathogenesis of amyloidosis. AL protein is seen in association with B lymphocyte and plasma cell proliferation which secrete immunoglobulin light chains that are amyloidogenic. AA protein is seen in variety of diseases associated with the activation of macrophages, which in turn leads to the synthesis and release of SAA. The SAA is converted to AA protein. ATTR protein is due to mutant proteins which aggregate and deposit as amyloid

Abbreviation: SAA, serum amyloid; ATTR, transthyretin.

- **Normally, misfolded proteins are degraded either intracellularly** in proteasomes, or **extracellularly** by macrophages.
- **In amyloidosis**, there is **failure of control mechanism** → production of misfolded proteins, which exceeds the degradation → accumulation outside cells. These misfolded proteins are unstable and self-associated → deposited as fibrils in extracellular tissues.

Categories of Proteins

Misfolded proteins that form amyloid may be the result of:

1. Production of Abnormal Amounts of Normal Protein

- These proteins have an inherent tendency to fold improperly or undergo misfolding → associate and form fibrils. Example: During inflammation, SAA is synthesized by the liver cells under the influence of cytokines such as IL-6 and IL-1 secreted by activate macrophages, and is degraded by monocyte-derived enzymes.

- In individuals prone to amyloidosis, there may be defect in the monocyte-derived enzymes → incomplete breakdown of SAA → formation of insoluble AA molecules. Genetically, defective SAA may also be responsible for resistant degradation by macrophages.

2. Production of Normal Amount of Mutant Protein

This protein that is prone to misfolding and subsequent aggregation to form amyloid.

Example: In familial amyloidosis, mutation of gene encoding TTR → alterations in structure serum protein TTRs → proteins prone to misfolding → aggregate → are resistant to proteolysis.

Pathological Effects

- **Pressure on adjacent normal cells** → leads to **atrophy of cells.**
- **Deposition in the blood vessel wall** causes:
  - Narrowing of the lumen → lead to **ischemic damage**.
  - **Increased permeability** → escape of protein out of vessel.

Classification of Amyloidosis

Q. Classify amyloidosis.

Amyloidosis is classified **depending on biochemical and clinical characteristics** (Table 5.11).

Table 5.11: Classification of amyloidosis

Type	Precursor protein	Fibril protein	Associated disease/s
A. Systemic (generalized) amyloidosis			
1. Immunocyte dyscrasias with amyloidosis (primary amyloidosis)	Immunoglobulin light chains (mainly λ)	AL	Multiple myeloma, other plasma cell dyscrasias
2. Reactive systemic amyloidosis (secondary amyloidosis)	Serum amyloid associated (SAA)	AA	Chronic inflammatory process
3. Hemodialysis-associated amyloidosis	β_2-microglobulin	$A\beta_2m$	Chronic renal failure
B. Hereditary or familial amyloidosis			
1. Familial mediterranean fever	SAA	AA	
2. Familial amyloidotic neuropathies	Transthyretin	ATTR	
3. Systemic senile amyloidosis			
C. Localized amyloidosis			
1. Senile cerebral	Amyloid precursor protein (APP)	Aβ	Alzheimer disease
2. Endocrine			
• Thyroid	Calcitonin	A Cal	Medullary carcinoma
• Islets of Langerhans	Islet amyloid peptide	AIAPP	Type 2 diabetes

A. Systemic (Generalized)

It involves several organ systems.

1. Primary Amyloidosis:

Q. Describe the pathology of primary amyloidosis.

Immunocyte Dyscrasias with Amyloidosis

- Usually **systemic** and is of **AL type**.
- **Many have underlying plasma cell dyscrasia**, e.g. **multiple myeloma.**

- **Multiple myeloma:**
  - **About 5% to 15% of patients** develop amyloidosis.
  - **Tumor synthesize abnormal amounts of a single specific Ig** (monoclonal gammopathy) → appears as an **M (myeloma) protein spike on serum electrophoresis.**
  - Tumor **also synthesizes the light chains (known as Bence-Jones protein) of either the** κ **or the** λ **type** which are found in the serum.
  - **Bence-Jones protein** being of small molecular size **can be excreted in the urine.** The amyloid deposits in these patients contain the same light chain protein.

Primary amyloidosis without plasma cell dyscrasia:
  - Majority of patients with AL amyloid do not have multiple myeloma or any other overt plasma cell neoplasm.
  - But almost all these patients **have monoclonal immunoglobulins or free light chains, or both, in the serum or urine.**
  - **Bone marrow** in most show **increase in the number of plasma cells,** which may secrete the precursors of AL protein. Thus, these may represent plasma cell dyscrasia characterized by production of an abnormal protein, instead of production of tumor masses.

2. Reactive Systemic (Secondary) Amyloidosis

Q. Write short note on reactive systemic amyloidosis.

- **Systemic in distribution** and is of **AA** type.
- Occurs as a **complication of** (secondary to) **chronic inflammatory** or **tissue-destructive process.** Hence, was known as **secondary amyloidosis.**
- **Complicates or occurs in association with diseases,** such as:
  i. **Chronic inflammatory conditions:** e.g. **tuberculosis, bronchiectasis,** and chronic osteomyelitis.
  ii. **Autoimmune states:** e.g. **rheumatoid arthritis**, ankylosing spondylitis, inflammatory bowel disease (Crohn's disease and ulcerative colitis).
  iii. **Heroin abusers:** These patients develop with chronic skin infections or abscesses due to subcutaneous self-administration of narcotics.
  iv. **Nonimmunocyte-derived tumors:** e.g. renal cell carcinoma and Hodgkin lymphoma.

3. Hemodialysis-associated Amyloidosis

Patients with **chronic renal failure on long-term hemodialysis** have high **levels of** β_2-**microglobulin** in the serum because it cannot be filtered through dialysis membranes → gets deposited as amyloid.

B. Hereditary or Familial Amyloidosis

It constitutes a heterogeneous group, are rare and occur in certain geographic areas.

1. Familial Mediterranean Fever

- **Autosomal recessive** disorder.
- Characterized by recurrent attacks of fever accompanied with inflammation of serosal surfaces (peritoneum, pleura, and synovial membrane).
- The gene encodes a protein called **pyrin** (for its relation to fever), regulate inflammatory reactions by producing high levels of proinflammatory cytokines IL-1.
- The amyloid fibril proteins are of AA type probably produced due to recurrent bouts of inflammation.

2. Familial Amyloidotic Neuropathies

It is characterized by **deposition of amyloid in peripheral and autonomic nerves** and the **fibrils are made up of mutant TTRs.**

C. Localized Amyloidosis

- Amyloid deposits are **limited to a single organ** (e.g. **heart**) or tissue.
- Either grossly visible as nodular masses or detected only by microscopic examination.
- **Sites:** Lung, larynx, skin, urinary bladder, and tongue.
- **Microscopy:** Amyloid deposits may be surrounded by lymphocytes and plasma cells.

1. Endocrine Amyloid

- Endocrine tumors such as **medullary carcinoma of the thyroid**, islet tumors of the pancreas, pheochromocytomas, and undifferentiated carcinomas of the stomach.
- **Islets of Langerhans in type II diabetes mellitus.**

2. Amyloid of Aging

- **Senile systemic amyloidosis** characterized by the systemic deposition of amyloid in elderly patients usually between 70 to 80 years. Also called senile cardiac amyloidosis because of the symptoms related to restrictive cardiomyopathy and arrhythmias. **The amyloid is composed of the normal TTR molecule.**

Q. Write short note on special stains for amyloid.

Morphology

Main Organs Involved:

- **Secondary amyloidosis:** Kidneys, liver, spleen, lymph nodes, adrenals, and thyroid.
- **Primary amyloidosis:** Heart, GI tract, respiratory tract, peripheral nerves, skin and tongue.

Gross:

- May or may not be apparent grossly.
- If large amount accumulates → affected organs are **enlarged, firm and have a waxy appearance.**
- **Cut surface:** If the amyloid deposits are large, **painting** the cut surface **with iodine** gives a **yellow color, which is transformed to blue violet after application of sulfuric acid** (which acidifies iodine). This method was used for demonstrating cellulose or starch. This staining property was responsible for the coining of the **term amyloid (starch-like). But it is neither starch nor cellulose.**

Microscopy

Hematoxylin and Eosin Stain

- Amyloid deposits are always **extracellular** (Fig. 5.17A) and begin between the cells. In AL form perivascular and vascular deposits are common.
- Progressive accumulation of **amyloid produces pressure atrophy of adjacent cells.**
- Appears as an **amorphous, eosinophilic, hyaline, glassy, extracellular substance.**
- Many other substances (e.g. collagen, fibrin) also stain eosinophilic with hematoxylin and eosin. Hence, it is necessary to differentiate amyloid from these other hyaline deposits by using special stains.

Staining (Tinctorial) Properties of Amyloid

1. **Congo red stain:** It is the **special stain used for the diagnosis of amyloidosis.** Amyloid **stains pink or red** with the Congo red dye **under ordinary light (Fig. 5.17B).** But **more specific** when viewed **under polarizing microscope;** amyloid gives **apple-green birefringence (Fig. 5.17C).** This reaction is due to the cross-β-pleated configuration of amyloid fibrils. Can be confirmed by electron microscopy.

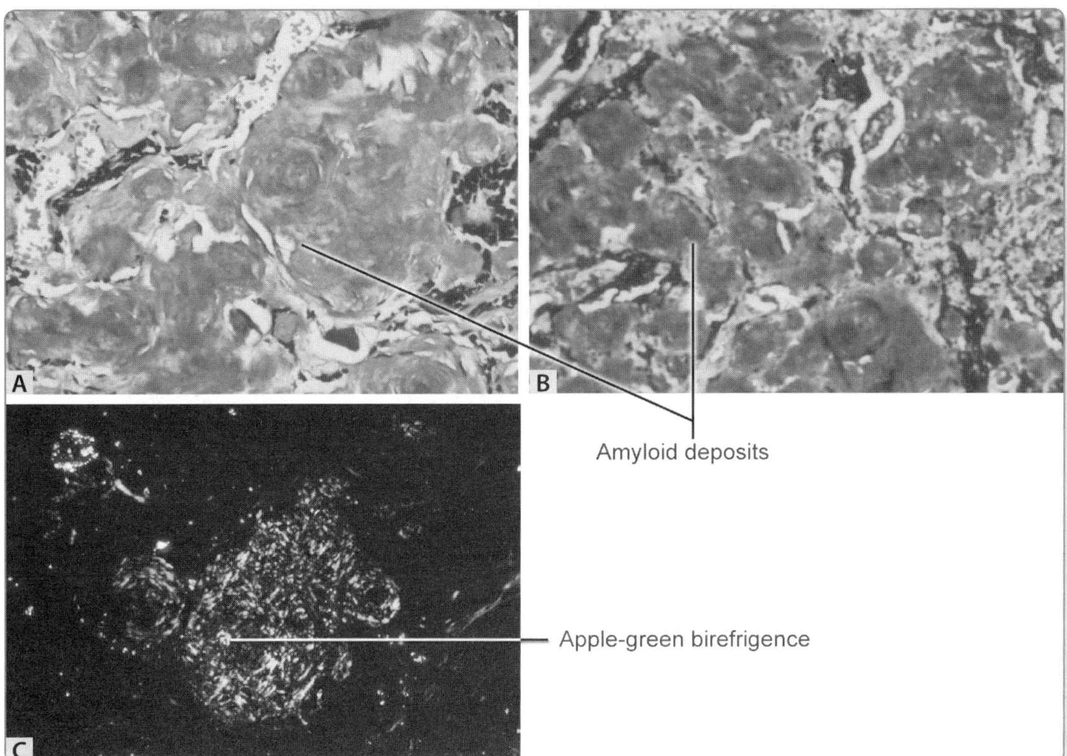

Figs 5.17A to C: Amyloid deposits in medullary carcinoma of thyroid. A. Amyloid appear as extracellular, amorphous, eosinophilic substance under H and E stain. B. Congo red stain gives red color to the amyloid deposits. C. Congo red stain viewed under polarizing microscope gives apple-green birefringence to amyloid deposits

(For color version, see Plate 2)

2. **Van Gieson stains:** It takes up khaki color.
3. **Alcian blue:** It imparts blue color to glycosaminoglycans in amyloid.
4. **Periodic acid Schiff reaction (PAS):** It stains pink.
5. **Methyl violet and cresyl violet:** These metachromatic stains give rose pink color.
6. **Thioflavin T:** It is not specific for amyloid, but amyloid gives fluorescence when viewed in ultraviolet light.
7. **Immunohistochemical staining:** It can distinguish AA, AL, and ATTR types.

Q. Write short note on spleen in amyloidosis.

Morphology of Major Organs Involved

Kidney:

Kidney involvement is the **most common** and the **most serious** form of organ involvement.

- **Gross:** It may be of normal size and color during early stages. In advanced stages, it may be shrunken due to ischemia, which is caused by vascular narrowing induced by the amyloid deposit within arterial and arteriolar walls.

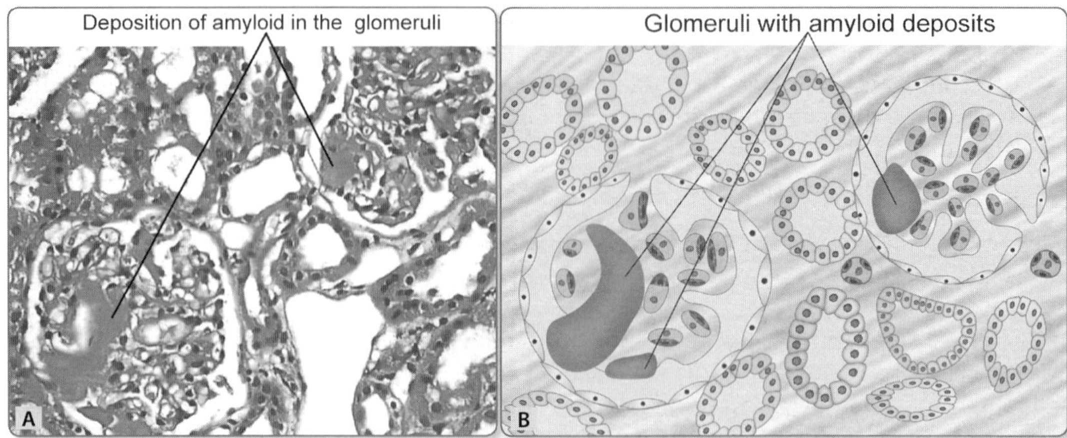

Figs 5.18A and B: Amyloidosis of kidney. A, showing pink, amorphous extracellular amyloid deposits in the glomeruli; B, Diagramatic appearance

- **Microscopy:** Most commonly renal amyloid is of light-chain (AL) or AA type.
  - **Glomeruli:** It is the main site of amyloid deposition (Fig. 5.18).
    - First, focal deposits within **mesangial matrix**, accompanied by diffuse or nodular thickening of the **glomerular basement membranes.**
    - Later, both the mesangial and basement membranes deposits cause **capillary narrowing.** Progressive accumulation of amyloid results in **obliteration of the capillary lumen** and glomerulus shows broad ribbons of amyloid.
  - Amyloid may also be deposited in the **peritubular interstitial tissue**, **arteries**, and **arterioles.**

Q. Describe the gross and microscopic appearance of spleen in amyloid (Sago and Lardaceous spleen).

Spleen:

- **Gross:** It may be normal in size or may cause moderate to marked splenomegaly (200–800 g). It may show one of **two patterns of deposition.**
  - **Sago spleen:** Amyloid **deposits are limited to the splenic follicles**, which **grossly appear like tapioca/sago granule**; hence known as **sago spleen.** Microscopically, the **amyloid is deposited in the wall of arterioles in the white pulp.**
  - **Lardaceous spleen: Amyloid is deposited in the walls of the splenic sinuses** and connective tissue framework in the red pulp. This may result in moderate to marked enlargement of spleen. Fusion of the early deposits gives rise to large, maplike areas of reddish color on cut surface. This resembles pig fat (lardaceous) and hence called as **lardaceous spleen.** Microscopically, it shows amyloid deposits in the wall of the sinuses.
- **Light microscopy:** These deposits appear homogenous pink, which when stained with Congo red and viewed under polarizing microscope, give rise to characteristic green birefringence.

Clinical Features

- Amyloidosis may not produce any clinical manifestations, or it may produce symptoms related to the sites or organs affected. Clinical manifestations **initially may be nonspecific** (e.g. weakness, weight loss). Specific symptoms appear later and are related to renal, cardiac, and gastrointestinal involvement.
- **Renal involvement:** It gives rise to **proteinuria** sometime massive enough to cause nephrotic syndrome. In advanced cases, the obliteration of glomeruli causes renal failure and uremia.

- **Cardiac amyloidosis:** It may present as **congestive heart failure**, conduction disturbances and arrhythmias.
- **Gastrointestinal amyloidosis:** It may be asymptomatic, or present as **malabsorption, diarrhea, and digestive disturbances**. Amyloidosis of the tongue may hamper speech and swallowing.

Diagnosis

It depends on the **histologic demonstration of amyloid deposits** in tissues.

- **Biopsy:** The most common sites are the **kidney, rectum or gingival tissues** in systemic amyloidosis.
- **Examination of abdominal fat aspirates** stained with Congo red is quite specific, but has low sensitivity.
- In immunocyte-associated amyloidosis, **serum and urine protein electrophoresis and immunoelectrophoresis** should be done. Bone marrow aspirates may show monoclonal plasmacytosis, even in the absence of multiple myeloma.
- **Scintigraphy with radiolabeled serum amyloid P** (SAP) component is a **rapid and specific test**.

Chapter 6

Infections

Chapter Outline

- Granulomatous diseases
- Tuberculosis
- Leprosy
- Syphilis
- Typhoid fever
- Viral hepatitis
- Chronic hepatitis
- Actinomycosis

GRANULOMATOUS DISEASES

Mycobacterium is bacteria, which appear as slender aerobic rods that grow in straight or branching chains. Mycobacteria have a waxy cell wall composed of mycolic acid, which is responsible for their **acid fast nature**. Mycobacteria are weakly Gram-positive.

TUBERCULOSIS

Tuberculosis (also called Koch's disease) is a **communicable, chronic granulomatous disease** caused by ***Mycobacterium tuberculosis***.

- Most cases of tuberculosis are caused by ***Mycobacterium tuberculosis hominins*** (human strain). The source of infection is patients with **active open case of tuberculosis**.
- **Oropharyngeal and intestinal tuberculosis** can be caused by drinking milk contaminated with ***M. bovis*** (bovine strain) from infected cows. Routine pasteurization has almost eliminated this source of infection.
- ***M. avium* and intracellular**, which are nonpathogenic to normal individuals but cause infection **in patients with AIDS**.

Characteristics of Mycobacteria

- It is an aerobic, slender, rod-shaped bacteria measuring 2 to 10 μm in length.
- It has a lipid coat which makes it difficult to stain, but **once stained resists decolorization by acids and alcohol**. Hence, it is termed as acid-fast bacilli (AFB), because once stained by carbol fuchsin (present in **Ziehl-Neelsen stain**), it is not decolorized by acid and alcohol.

Epidemiology

- Tuberculosis is common in India. Incidence of tuberculosis is high wherever there is **poverty, overcrowding, and chronic debilitating illness**.
- Diseases are associated with increased risk: diabetes mellitus, Hodgkin lymphoma, malnutrition, immunosuppression, alcoholism, chronic lung disease (e.g. silicosis), and chronic renal failure.
- **HIV is the most important risk factor**.

Infection Versus Disease

Infection with *M. tuberculosis* is to be differentiated from disease.

- **Infection**: Tuberculous infection **indicates the presence of organisms in a person**, which **may or may not cause symptomatic disease**.
- **Disease**: Active tuberculosis refers to subset of **tuberculous infections manifested by destructive, symptomatic disease**.

Mode of Transmission

Inhalation

- It is the **most common mode** of transmission.
  - **Source of organisms** is from an **active open case of tuberculosis** to a susceptible host.
  - Tubercle bacilli will be expelled while coughing, sneezing that creates aerosolized respiratory droplets. When an individual inhales the droplets, it lodges in the lung and causes infection.

Ingestion

- Tuberculosis may be transmitted by drinking nonpasteurized milk from infected cows contaminated with *M. bovis.*
- Site of infection: *Mycobacterium bovis* causes oropharyngeal and intestinal tuberculosis.
- Eradication of tuberculous herds with tuberculosis and **pasteurization** has almost **eliminated this mode of transmission** of tuberculosis. Nowadays the ingestion mode of transmission occurs when a patient with open case of tuberculosis swallows the infected sputum results in tuberculosis of intestine.

Inoculation

- It **is extremely rare mode** of transmission. May develop during postmortem examination, while cuts resulting from handling tuberculous infected organs.

Tuberculin (Mantoux) Test

- Infection by mycobacteria → development of delayed hypersensitivity to *M. tuberculosis* antigens → which is detected by the tuberculin skin test.
- About 2 to 4 weeks after infection, **intracutaneous injection of 0.1 mL of purified protein derivative** (PPD) of *M. tuberculosis* produces a **visible and palpable induration of 10 mm diameter or more** at the site of injection of PPD. The induration peaks in 48 to 72 hours.
- **Significance:**
  - **Positive tuberculin test: It indicates T cell-mediated immunity** to mycobacterial antigens.
  - **False-negative reactions**: It is seen in certain viral infections, sarcoidosis, malnutrition, Hodgkin lymphoma, immunosuppression, and overwhelming active tuberculous disease.

- **False-positive reactions:** It seen in infection by **atypical mycobacteria** or prior **vaccination with BCG** (*Bacillus Calmette-Guerin*).

Pathogenesis

Q. Pathogenesis of tuberculosis.

Immunity and hypersensitivity: Infection with tubercle bacillus results in two simultaneous immunological responses.

- Cell-mediated immunity
- Type IV hypersensitivity reaction.

The effector cells for both cell-mediated immunity and hypersensitivity reaction are **T_H1** cells.

- **Cell-mediated immunity**: Tuberculosis developing first time in an immunocompetent individual depends on the cell-mediated immunity.
- **Type IV hypersensitivity reactions**: Develops to mycobacterial antigens and is **responsible for the tissue destruction such as caseating granulomas and cavitation**. Appearance of type IV hypersensitivity reaction also signals the development of protective immunity.

Mechanism of Granuloma Formation in Tuberculosis (Fig. 6.1)

Tuberculosis is a chronic granulomatous disease, caused by *M. tuberculosis*. Lung being commonly involved in tuberculosis, the pathogenesis is considered with respect to pulmonary tuberculosis.

A. **First 0–3 weeks after exposure: Initial infection** with *Mycobacterium tuberculosis* **in a nonsensitized individual** is called **primary tuberculosis**. The following sequence of events occur:

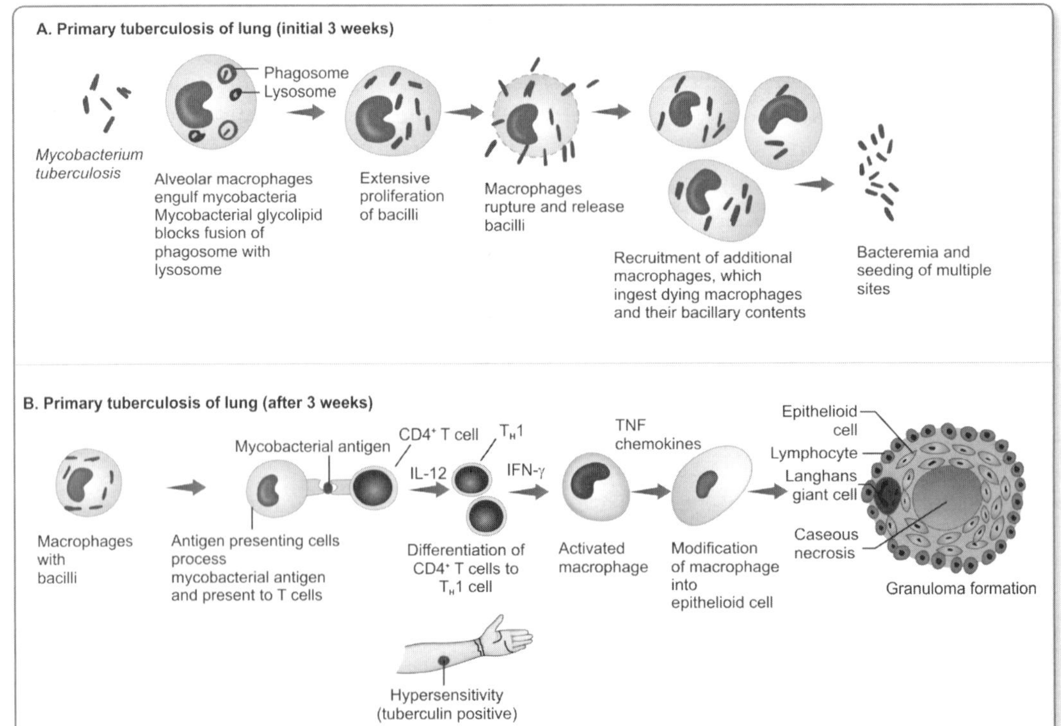

Figs 6.1A and B: Sequence of events in primary tuberculosis of lung

- **Phagocytosis of mycobacteria by macrophages**: **First time**, when the **virulent tubercle bacilli** are deposited in the tissue, they primarily **infect macrophages**. In the lung, they **undergo endocytosis** into the alveolar macrophages through **macrophage receptors** These receptors include:
  - **Mannose receptors** bind lipoarabinomannan (LAM), a glycolipid in the cell wall of tubercle bacilli
  - **Complement receptors** (C3b receptor) which bind mycobacteria opsonized by C3b.
- **Proliferation of mycobacteria within macrophages:**
  - **First 3 weeks**: Tubercle **bacilli proliferate freely** within the phagosome of the macrophage by **blocking fusion of the phagosome and lysosome**. It **may result in bacteremia** and seeding of tubercle bacilli at many sites. This bacteremia may be either asymptomatic or may have a mild flulike illness.
  - **Genetic factor**: **NRAMP1 is a transmembrane protein** (a product of *NRAMP1* gene) **inhibits microbial growth**. In individuals with **polymorphisms in the *NRAMP1*** (**n**atural **r**esistance-**a**ssociated **m**acrophage **p**rotein **1**) **gene**, **tuberculosis may progress due to the absence of an effective immune response**.

B. **After 3 weeks of infection**
- **Cell-mediated immunity:** It develops about 3 weeks after exposure.
- **Presentation of antigen to CD4⁺ T cells:** Antigen-presenting cells (APCs which includes macrophages, dendritic cells) process the mycobacterial antigen and present it to naïve $CD4^+$ T cells. Processed antigen reaches regional lymph nodes.
- **Differentiation of $CD4^+$ T cells into T-helper 1 (T_H1) cell**: It is due to the action of IL-12 secreted by macrophages. **Role of T_H1 cells**:
  - **T_H1 cells** produce **IFN-γ** which has several functions.
    - i. **Activation of macrophages:** These macrophages become bactericidal and secrete TNF → which promotes recruitment of more monocytes → **differentiation into epithelioid (epithelium-like) cells.**
    - ii. **Stimulates formation of the phagolysosome** in infected macrophages → exposes the bacteria to acidic environment.
    - iii. **Stimulates nitric oxide synthase** → to produce nitric oxide → antibactericidal.
    - iv. **Generation of reactive oxygen species** → antibacterial.
  - **T_H1** is also responsible for the **formation of granulomas and caseous necrosis.**
    - i. **Transformation of macrophages into epithelioid cells:** Activated macrophages are transformed into epithelioid cells. Some of these "epithelioid cells" may fuse to form giant cells.
    - ii. **Granuloma formation**: A microscopic aggregates of epithelioid cells, surrounded by a rim of lymphocytes, is referred as a granuloma and this pattern of inflammation, known as **granulomatous inflammation. Hypersensitivity reaction results in tissue destruction → caseation and cavitation.**

Primary Tuberculosis

Q. Write short note on primary tuberculosis.

- **Initial infection** that occurs on first exposure to the organism **in an unsensitized** (previously unexposed) **individual** is known as primary tuberculosis.
- About 5% of newly infected people develop clinically significant disease.
- **Source** of the organism is always **exogenous.**

Q. Write short note on Ghon focus.

Q. Write short note on Ghon complex.

Morphology

Sites of Primary Tuberculosis

Lung, intestine, tonsil and skin (very rare).

Lung: It is the **commonest site** of primary tuberculosis.

- **Ghon lesion**: Following inhalation, tubercle bacilli gets deposited in the distal airspaces.
  - **Site of deposit**: Usually **lower part of the upper lobe or upper part of the lower lobe near the pleural surface** (subpleural).
  - **Ghon focus (Fig. 6.2):** About 2 to 4 weeks after the infection, a circumscribed **gray-white area** of about **1- to 1.5-cm develops in the lung** known as the Ghon focus→ the center of which undergoes caseous necrosis.
  - **Regional lymphadenitis**: Tubercle bacilli (free or within macrophages) are carried along the lymphatics to the regional draining nodes → which often show caseous necrosis.
- **Ghon complex**: It is the combination of subpleural parenchymal lung lesion (**Ghon focus**) and **regional lymph node** involvement.
- **Fate of Ghon complex**:
  - **Healing:** In **majority** (about 95%), cell-mediated immunity controls the infection and primary tuberculosis **heals**. The **hallmark of healing is fibrosis** and Ghon complex undergoes progressive fibrosis, followed by radiologically detectable **calcification** (Ranke complex), and very rarely ossification.
  - **Spread:** During the first few weeks **lymphatic and hematogenous dissemination** occurs to other organs or parts of the body.

Other Sites of Primary Complex

- **Intestine:** Primary focus in the small intestine (usually ileal region) along with mesenteric lymphadenitis.
- **Tonsils:** Primary focus in the pharynx and tonsil with cervical lymph node enlargement.
- **Skin**: Primary focus in the skin along with regional lymph node involvement.

Microscopy (Fig. 6.3)

Granuloma in tuberculosis is called as tubercle. Tubercle may show central area of caseous necrosis (caseating granuloma) or may not show caseation (noncaseating tubercles). Individual tubercles are identified only by microscopic examination. When multiple granulomas coalesce → they may be grossly identified.

Caseating granuloma (Fig. 6.3) consists of:

- **Central area of caseous necrosis**
- **Surrounded by epithelioid cells** (modified macrophages), some of which may fuse to form multinucleate giant cells. The **giant cells may be Langhans** type (nuclei arranged in horseshoe pattern) **or foreign body type** (nuclei in the center).
- The epithelioid cells are **surrounded by rim of lymphocytes.**
- These granulomas are usually enclosed within fibroblasts.

Secondary Tuberculosis

(Synonyms: Post-primary tuberculosis, reactivation tuberculosis)

- **Tuberculosis** developing **in a previously sensitized** individual is known as secondary tuberculosis.
- It may follow shortly or many years after primary tuberculosis, usually when resistance host decreases.

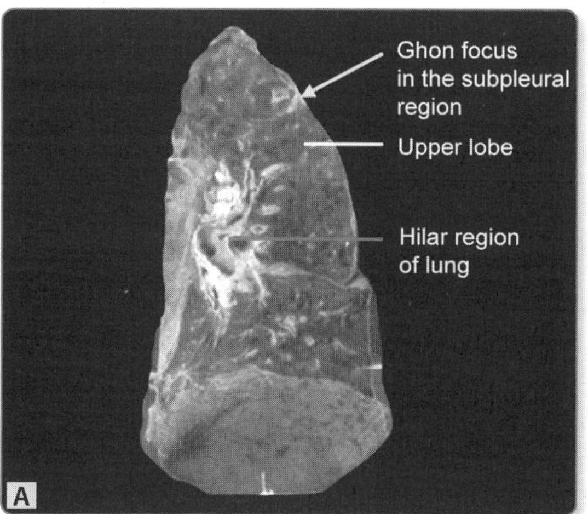

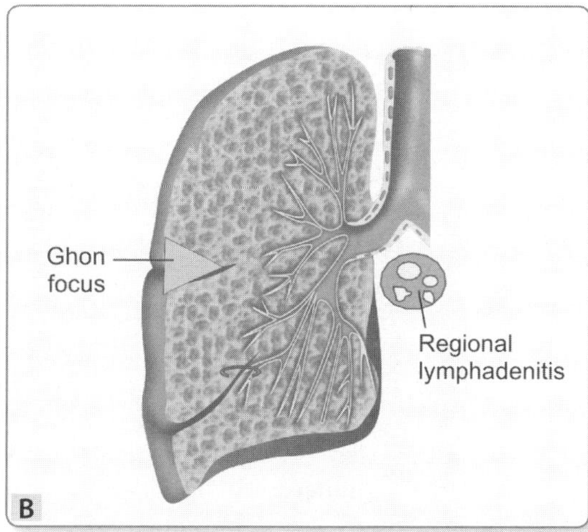

Figs 6.2A and B: Gross appearance of primary pulmonary tuberculosis (B diagrammatic). Ghon complex consists of gray-white parenchymal focus is under the pleura and enlarged hilar lymph nodes with caseation

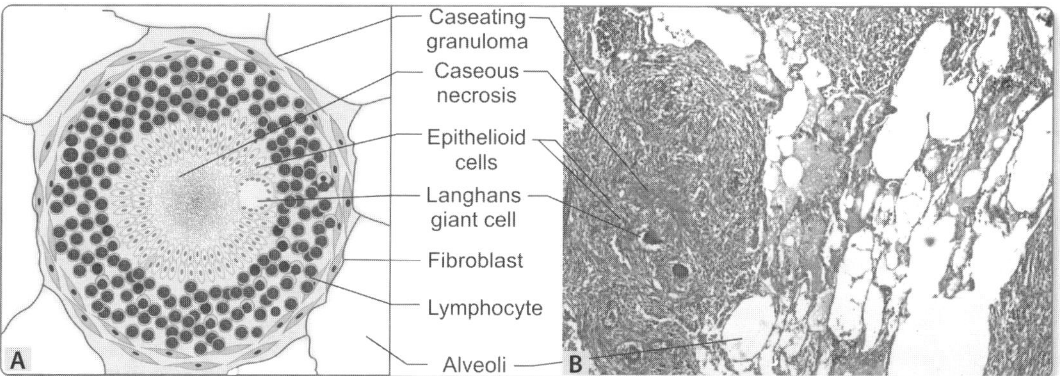

Figs 6.3A and B: Microscopic appearance of tuberculosis of lung. A. (diagrammatic); B. (photomicrograph). Central area of caseation surrounded by epithelioid and multinucleated giant cells

(For color version, see Plate 3)

- **Source of infection**:
  - Most common source is **reactivation of a latent infection**
  - Rarely exogenous reinfection.
- Any location may be involved in secondary tuberculosis, but the lungs are by far the most common site.

Morphology

Gross (Fig. 6.4)

- **Site:** In the lungs, secondary tuberculosis usually involves the **apex of the upper lobes** of one or both lungs, **within 1 to 2 cm of the apical pleura**.
- **Appearance: Initially- small focus** (less than **2 cm in diameter) of consolidation**, sharply circumscribed, firm, and **gray-white to yellow** in color.
- **Regional lymph nodes involvement is less prominently** than in primary tuberculosis.

Microscopy: Active lesions show **caseating granulomas** and **acid-fast stain** often shows **tubercle bacilli**.

Natural history and various stages of tuberculosis are depicted in Figure 6.5.

Tuberculous cavity with caseous material
Lower lobe shows caseous pneumonia
A
B

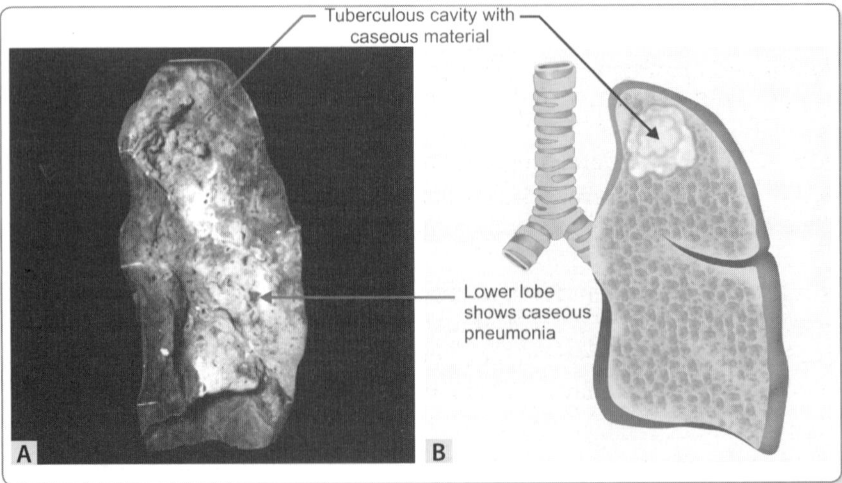

Figs 6.4A and B: Secondary pulmonary tuberculosis. A. (specimen); B. (diagrammatic). The lung shows gray-white areas of caseation with a cavity in the upper lobe

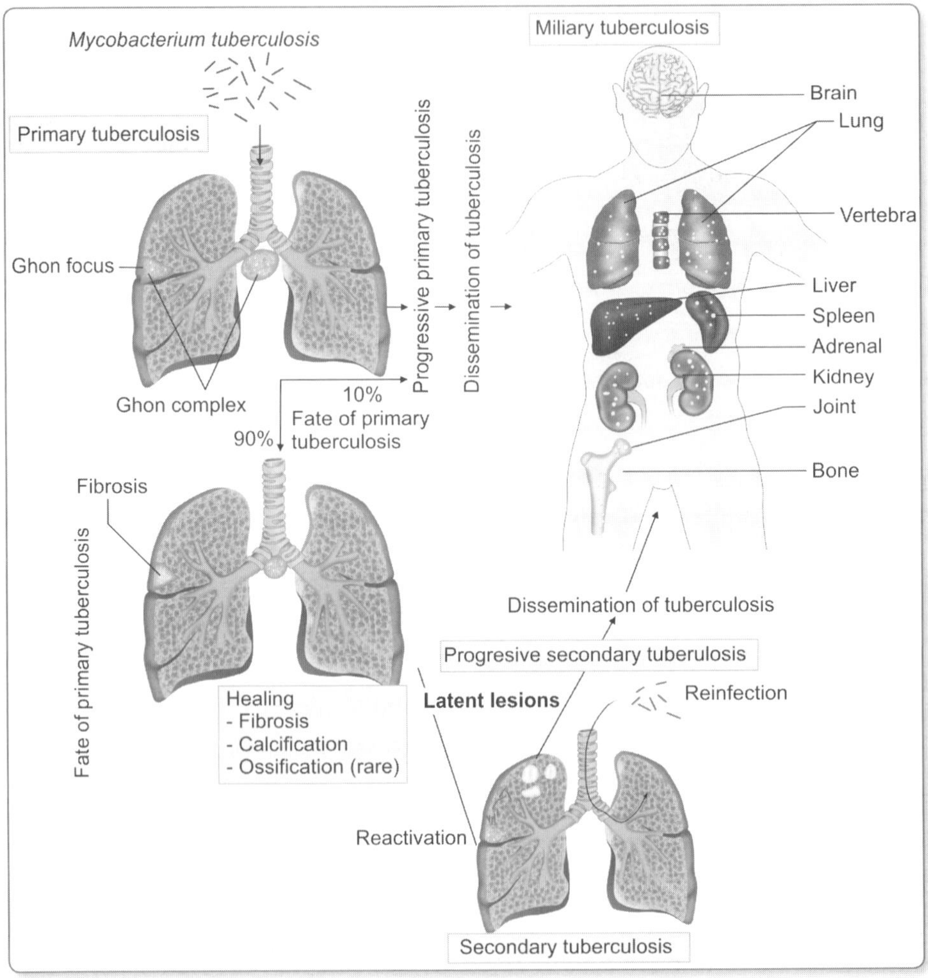

Mycobacterium tuberculosis
Primary tuberculosis
Ghon focus
Ghon complex
10%
Fate of primary tuberculosis
90%
Progressive primary tuberculosis
Dissemination of tuberculosis
Miliary tuberculosis
Brain
Lung
Vertebra
Liver
Spleen
Adrenal
Kidney
Joint
Bone
Fibrosis
Fate of primary tuberculosis
Healing
- Fibrosis
- Calcification
- Ossification (rare)
Dissemination of tuberculosis
Progresive secondary tuberulosis
Latent lesions
Reinfection
Reactivation
Secondary tuberculosis

Fig. 6.5: Natural history and various stages of tuberculosis

Fate of Secondary Tuberculosis (Fig. 6.6)

Healing: In immunocompetent individuals, localized, apical, focus may **heal with fibrosis and calcification** rarely ossification.

Progress: It may occur along several different pathways.

A. **Progressive pulmonary tuberculosis:** It occurs mainly in the elderly and immunosuppressed. Apical lesion may expand into surrounding lung and may erode into bronchi and vessels.
   - **Erosion into bronchi:** It leads to release of the central area of caseous necrosis → resulting in a ragged, irregular **apical cavity** surrounded by fibrous tissue. This produces an **important source of infection**, because when the patient coughs, sputum contains bacteria.
   - **Erosion of blood vessels**: may results in hemoptysis.

   With prompt treatment, it may undergo healing by fibrosis.

B. **Spread of infection**: If the treatment is inadequate or if host defenses are impaired, the infection may spread via: 1) airways, 2) lymphatics or 3) blood vessels.
   1. **Local/direct spread:** Tuberculosis can directly spread to the surrounding tissue. In the lung local spread to the pleura and shift up as first bullet. Result in serous **pleural effusions**, **tuberculous empyema**, or **obliterative fibrous pleuritis**.
   2. **Spread through bronchi/airways:** It may produce tuberculous pneumonia.
      - **Intestinal tuberculosis**: In the past, intestinal tuberculosis resulted by the drinking of contaminated milk and with pasteurization of milk, now it is rare. Nowadays caused by the **swallowing of coughed-up infective material** in patients with open case of advanced pulmonary tuberculosis. **Mainly develops in the ileum.**

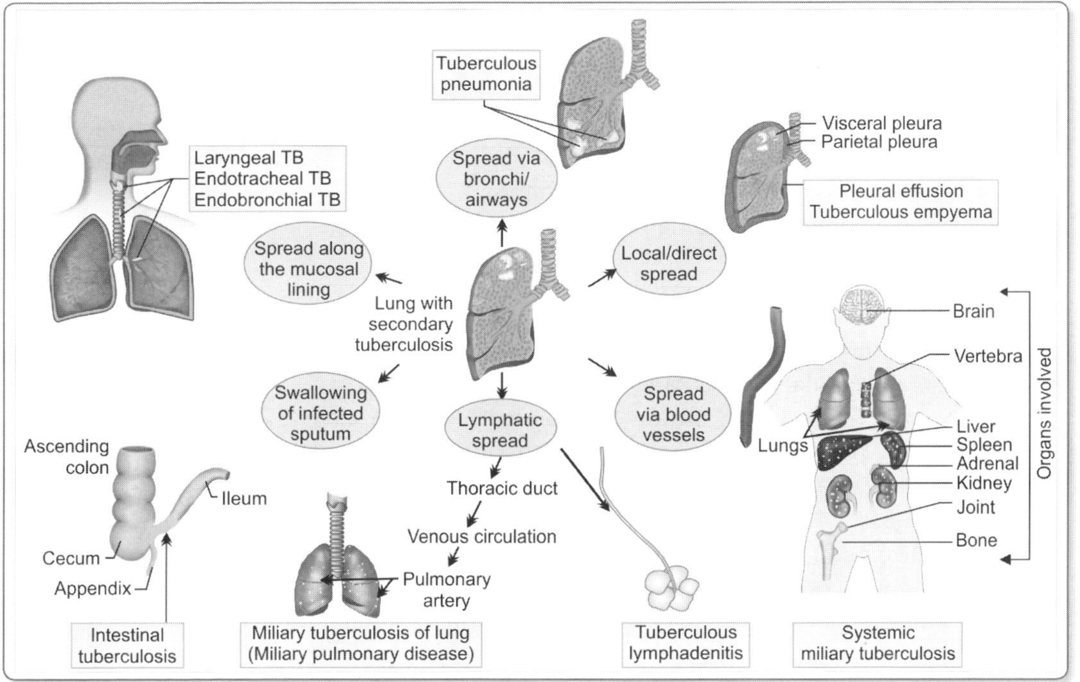

Fig. 6.6: Progress and complications of secondary tuberculosis of lung

3. **Spread along mucosal lining:** Spread through lymphatic channels or along the mucosal lining from mycobacteria present in the expectorated infectious material may lead to **endobronchial**, **endotracheal**, and **laryngeal tuberculosis**.
4. **Lymphatic spread:** Spread through lymphatic channels mainly reach regional lymph nodes. It may also cause disseminated disease.
   - **Miliary pulmonary disease:** It is the disseminated form of tuberculosis. When the dissemination occurs only to the lungs, it is called miliary pulmonary disease.
     - **Mechanism of development**: Tubercle bacilli draining through lymphatics → enter the venous blood → to the right venous side of the heart → through pulmonary artery → to the lung.
     - **Lesions: Multiple**, **small**, **yellow**, **nodular** lesions in the lung parenchyma of both the lungs. Each lesion is either microscopic or small, visible (2-mm) foci of **yellow-white** consolidation → **resemble to millet seeds, hence named "miliary"**.
   - **Lymphadenitis**: It is most frequent presentation of extrapulmonary tuberculosis, and usually occurs in the cervical region ("scrofula").
     - HIV-negative individuals: Unifocal and localized.
     - HIV-positive individuals: Multifocal and systemic disease.
5. **Spread via blood vessels:**
   - **Systemic miliary tuberculosis** occurs when tubercle bacilli disseminate through the systemic arterial system. Miliary tuberculosis most commonly involves liver, bone marrow, spleen, adrenals, meninges, kidneys, fallopian tubes, and epididymis. But no organ is exempt and can involve any organ.
   - **Isolated-organ tuberculosis:** Dissemination of tubercle bacilli through blood may seed any organ or tissue → resulting in isolated organ tuberculosis. Commonly involved organs are:
     - Meninges (tuberculous meningitis)
     - Kidneys (renal tuberculosis)
     - Adrenals
     - Bones (osteomyelitis): When it involves the vertebrae, the disease is referred to as **Pott disease**. Paraspinal "cold" abscesses may track along tissue planes and present as an abdominal or pelvic mass.
     - Fallopian tubes (salpingitis).

Clinical Features

- Localized secondary tuberculosis may remain asymptomatic.
- **Systemic symptoms of pulmonary tuberculosis**:
  - **Nonspecific**: malaise, anorexia, weight loss, and fever.
  - **Low-grade fever:** It is **remittent** (appearing late each afternoon and then subsiding-commonly known as **evening rise of temperature**), and **night sweats**.
  - **Sputum**: It is first mucoid and later purulent.
  - **Hemoptysis:** It is present in 50% of cases of pulmonary tuberculosis.
  - **Pleuritic pain:** It is due to infection to the pleural surfaces.
- **Extrapulmonary manifestations** depend on the organ/system involved.

Main differences between primary and secondary tuberculosis of lung are listed in Table 6.1.

Table 6.1: Main difference between primary and secondary tuberculosis of lung

Characteristics	Primary TB	Secondary TB
Type of infection	Initial infection in an unsensitized individual	Infection in a previously sensitized individual
Source of infection	Exogenous	Usually endogenous activation of latent infection
Site of lung involved	Lower part of upper lobe or upper part of lower lobe and subpleural	Apex and posterior segments of the upper lobe and superior segments of lower lobe
Regional lymph node involvement	Significant and prominent	Not prominent
Sputum for AFB	Rarely positive	Commonly positive
Cavity formation	Rare	Common
Healing	Mainly by calcification	By fibrosis
Extrapulmonary complications	Very common	Lesion usually localized to lung

Diagnosis: Pulmonary Disease

Q. Write short note on diagnosis of tuberculosis.

- Based on the **history, physical and radiographic** findings.
- Identification of **acid-fast tubercle bacilli in the sputum**.
- **Culture of the sputum**: Conventional cultures require up to 10 weeks. Culture is the gold standard.
- **PCR amplification** of *M. tuberculosis:* DNA is the rapid method of diagnosis. PCR can detect as few as 10 organisms in clinical specimens.

Prognosis: Generally good if infections are localized to the lungs. All stages of HIV infection are associated with an increased risk of tuberculosis.

LEPROSY

Leprosy (Hansen disease), is a **chronic**, **granulomatous**, slowly progressive, destructive infection caused by ***Mycobacterium leprae***.

Sites of involvement: Mainly involves the **peripheral nerves, skin and mucous membranes** (nasal) and results in disabling deformities.

Leprosy is one of the oldest human diseases and lepers were isolated from the community in the olden days.

Mycobacterium leprae

- Slender, **weakly acid-fast** intracellular bacillus.
- **Proliferates at low temperature** of the human skin.
- **Cannot be cultured** on artificial media or in cell culture.
- **Experimental animals**: Lepra bacilli grow at sites where the temperature is below that of the internal organs. Examples: **foot pads of mice**, ear lobes of hamsters, rats, and other rodents.
- **Experimentally transmitted to nine branded armadillos** (they have low body temperature ranging from 32° to 34°C).

Mode of transmission: It has comparatively low communicability.

1. **Inoculation/inhalation:** Likely to be transmitted from person to person through aerosols from asymptomatic lesions in the upper respiratory tract. Inhaled *M. leprae*, is taken up by

alveolar macrophages and disseminates through the blood, but replicates only in relatively cool tissues of the skin and extremities.

2. **Intimate contact:** For many years.

Source of infection: *M. leprae* is present in nasal secretions or ulcerated lesions of patients suffering from leprosy.

Incubation period: Generally 5 to 7 years.

Classification

Q. Classify leprosy.

A. **Ridley-Jopling (1966) classification:** It depends on the clinicopathological spectrum of the disease, which is **determined by the immune resistance of the host** (Fig. 6.7). They are classified into five groups with two extremes or polar forms, namely tuberculoid and lepromatous types.
   1. **Tuberculoid leprosy (TT):** It is the polar form that has maximal immune response.
   2. **Borderline tuberculoid (BT):** In this type, the immune response falls between BB and TT.
   3. **Borderline leprosy (BB):** It exactly falls between two polar forms of leprosy.
   4. **Borderline lepromatous (BL):** It has the immune response that falls between BB and LL.
   5. **Lepromatous leprosy (LL):** It is the other polar form with least immune response.

B. **WHO classification:**
   - Paucibacillary: All cases of tuberculoid leprosy and some cases of borderline type.
   - Multibacillary: All cases of lepromatous leprosy and some cases of borderline type.

Pathogenesis

- *M. leprae* does not secrete any toxins, and its virulence depends on properties of its cell wall (similar to that of *M. tuberculosis*) and immunization with BCG may provide some protection against *M. leprae* infection.
- Cell-mediated immunity is reflected by delayed-type hypersensitivity reactions to dermal injections of a bacterial extract called **lepromin**.
- The **T-helper (T_H1) lymphocyte response** to *M. leprae*, determines whether an individual develop tuberculoid or lepromatous type of leprosy.
   a. **Tuberculoid leprosy** patients have a T_H1 response which secretes IL-2 and IFN-γ. The later (IFN-γ) is essential for an effective host macrophage response.
   b. **Lepromatous leprosy** patients have a weak T_H1 response and, in some a relative increase in the T_H2 response → results in a poor cell-mediated immunity → proliferation of lepra bacilli. Sometimes, antibodies may be produced against *M. leprae* antigens, but they are usually not protective. These can form immune complexes with free antigens and lead to erythema nodosum, vasculitis, and glomerulonephritis.

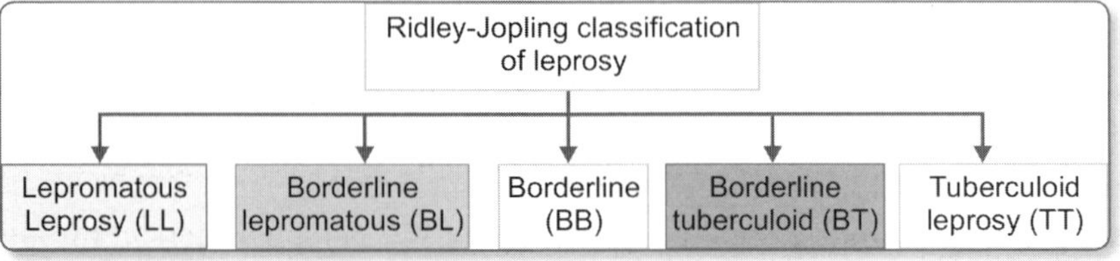

Fig. 6.7: Ridley-Jopling classification of leprosy

Q. Write short note on morphology of tuberculoid leprosy.

Q. Write short note on morphology of lepromatous leprosy.

Morphology

Two extremes or polar forms of the diseases are the tuberculoid and lepromatous types.

1. **Tuberculoid leprosy:** It is the **less severe form** of leprosy. It is **very slow in its course** and most patients die with leprosy.
   - **Lesion in skin**:
     - **Number of lesions**: Single or very few lesions.
     - **Site:** Usually on the **face, extremities, or trunk**
     - **Type**: **Localized, well-demarcated, red or hypopigmented, dry, elevated**, skin **patches** having raised outer edges and depressed pale centers (central healing). As they progress they develop irregular shapes with induration.
   - **Nerve involvement:**
     - **Dominating feature** in tuberculoid leprosy.
     - Nerves are surrounded by granulomatous inflammatory reactions and, may destroy small (e.g. the peripheral twigs) nerves.
     - Nerve involvement → causes **loss of sensation** in the skin → atrophy of skin and muscle. These affected parts are liable to trauma, and lead to the development of chronic skin ulcers.
     - **Consequences:** It may lead to **contractures, paralyses, and autoamputation** of fingers or toes. Involvement of facial nerve can lead to paralysis of the eyelids, with keratitis and corneal ulcerations.
   - **Microscopy (Fig. 6.8):**
     - **Granuloma:** These are well-formed, circumscribed and **non-caseating** (no caseation). Seen in all involved sites and in the dermis of skin. Termed tuberculoid leprosy because the granulomas resemble those found in tuberculosis. Granulomas are composed of epithelioid cells (modified macrophages), Langhans giant cells, and lymphocytes.
     - **Absence of Grenz zone**: Granulomas in the dermis extend to the basal layer of the epidermis (without a clear/Grenz zone).
     - **Fite-Faraco** (modified Z-N stain for demonstration of lepra bacillus) stain generally **does not show lepra bacillus**, hence the name **"paucibacillary"** leprosy.
     - **Perineural (surrounding nerve fibers) inflammation**: By lymphocytes.
     - **Strong T-cell immunity:** It is responsible for granulomas formation, without lepra bacilli.
2. **Lepromatous leprosy**: It is the **more severe form** and is also called **anergic leprosy**, because of the unresponsiveness (anergy) of the host immune system.

   Sites involved:
   - **Lesion in skin**:
     - **Thickening of skin** and **multiple, symmetric, macular, papular, or nodular lesions.** The nodular skin lesions may ulcerate. Most skin lesions are **hypoesthetic or anesthetic.**
     - More severe involvement of the **cooler areas of skin** (e.g. earlobes, wrists, elbows, and knees, and feet), than warmer areas (e.g. axilla and groin).
     - With progression, the nodular lesions in the face and ear lobes may coalesce to produce a lion like appearance known as **leonine facies** (Fig. 6.9). This may be accompanied by loss of eyebrows and eyelashes.
   - **Peripheral nerves:**
     - Particularly the **ulnar and peroneal nerves** are symmetrically invaded with mycobacteria.
     - **Loss of sensation and trophic changes** in the hands and feet may follow the damage to the nerves.
   - **Testes:** Usually severely involved, leading to destruction of the seminiferous tubules → sterility.
   - **Other sites:**
     - Anterior chamber of the eye: **Blindness.**
     - Upper airways: Chronic nasal discharge and voice change.

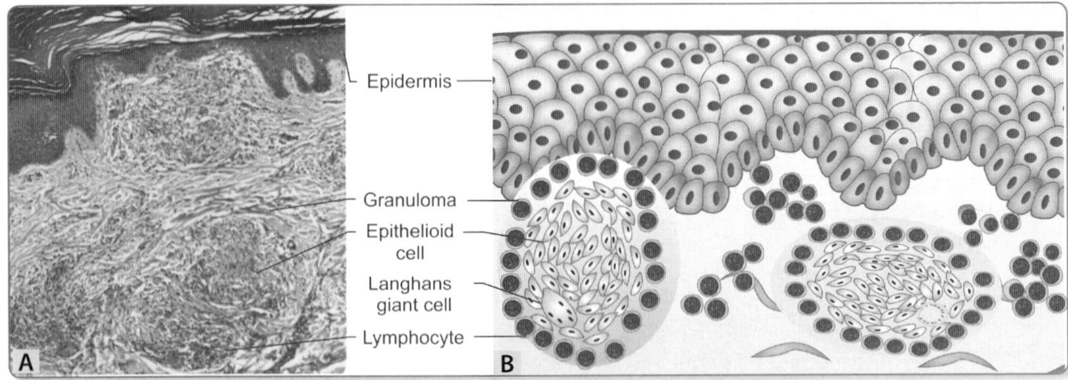

Fig. 6.8: Microscopy of tuberculoid leprosy with circumscribed non-caseating granulomas. A. Photomicrograph; B. Diagrammatic

- **Microscopy of skin lesion (Fig. 6.10):**
  - **Flattened epidermis**: Epidermis is thinned and flattened (loss of rete ridges) over the nodules.
  - **Grenz** (clear) **zone:** It is a characteristic **narrow, uninvolved dermis** (normal collagen) which separates the epidermis from nodular accumulations of macrophages.
  - **Lepra cells:** The nodular lesions contain large aggregates of lipid-laden foamy macrophages (lepra cells, Virchow cells), filled with aggregates ("globi") of acid-fast lepra bacilli (*M. leprae*).
  - **Fite-Faraco (acid-fast) stain:** It shows **numerous lepra bacilli** ("red snappers") within the foamy macrophages. They may be arranged in a parallel fashion like **cigarettes in a pack.**
  - Due to the presence of numerous bacteria, lepromatous leprosy is also referred to as **"multibacillary"**.

Fig. 6.9: Leonine facies of lepromatous leprosy

In advanced cases, *M. leprae* may be present in sputum and blood.

Individual with intermediate forms of disease, called **borderline leprosy**.

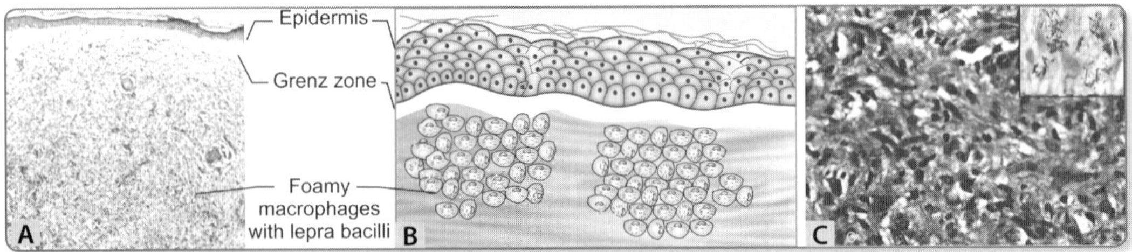

Fig. 6.10: Microscopic appearance of lepromatous leprosy. A. Photomicrograph. B. Diagrammatic. The epidermis is thinned and the dermis shows dense collections of lepra cells. The epidermis is separated from the collections of lepra cells by an uninvolved Grenz zone; C. Photomicrograph. High power view showing foamy macrophages. Inset of C shows acid-fast lepra bacilli within macrophages (Fite-Faraco stain).

Lepromin Test

Q. Write short note on lepromin test.

It is **not a diagnostic test** for leprosy. It is **used for classifying** the leprosy based on the immune response.

- **Procedure:** An antigen extract of *M. leprae* called lepromin is intradermally injected.
- **Reaction:**
  - An **early positive reaction** appears as an indurated area in 24 to 48 hours is called **Fernandez reaction.**
  - A **delayed granulomatous reaction** appearing after 3 to 4 weeks is known as **Mitsuda reaction.**
- **Interpretation:**
  - **Lepromatous leprosy**—shows **negative lepromin test** due to suppression of cell-mediated immunity.
  - **Tuberculoid leprosy**—show **positive lepromin test** because of delayed hypersensitivity reaction.

Differences between lepromatous and tuberculoid leprosy are presented in Table 6.2.

Q. List the differences between lepromatous and tuberculoid leprosy.

Diagnosis of Leprosy

1. **Clinical examination:**
   - **Sensory testing**
   - Examination of peripheral nerve

Table 6.2: Differences between lepromatous and tuberculoid leprosy

Characteristics	Lepromatous leprosy	Tuberculoid leprosy
Clinical features		
Skin lesions	Symmetrical, multiple, ill-defined, macular, nodular	Asymmetrical, hypopigmented, well defined macular
Disfigurement	Leonine facies, loss of eyebrows, pendulous ear lobes, claw-hands, saddle nose	Minimal disfigurement
Nerve involvement	Seen, but with less severe sensory loss than tuberculoid	Common with sensory disturbances
Microscopy of skin lesions		
Type of lesion	Nodular or diffuse collections of Lepra cells within dermis	Noncaseating granulomas composed of epithelioid cells and giant cells
Grenz/clear zone between inflammatory cells and epidermis	Present	Absent
Lepra bacilli	Plenty within the lepra cells as globular masses (globi)	Rare if any
Bacillary index	4 or 5	0
Other features		
Immunity	Suppressed-low resistance	Good immunity-high resistance
Lepromin test	Negative	Positive

2. **Demonstration of acid-fast bacilli**
   - Skin smears prepared by **slit and scrape method**
   - **Nasal swabs stained by Ziehl-Neelsen method**
3. **Skin biopsy**
4. **Nerve biopsy**
5. **Molecular method: PCR.**

SYPHILIS

Introduction: Spirochetes are gram-negative, slender corkscrew-shaped bacteria covered in a membrane called an outer sheath, which may mask its antigens from the host immune response.

Syphilis (lues) is a **chronic, sexually transmitted** disease **caused by spirochete *Treponema pallidum*.**

Etiology

- ***Treponema pallidum (Fig. 6.11)*:**
  - It is a **thin, delicate, corkscrew-shaped spirochete**, measures about 10 μm long with tapering ends and has about 10 regular spirals.
  - Actively motile, showing rotation round the long axis, backward and forward motion.
  - Cannot be grown in artificial media.
  - **Staining:** It does not stain with ordinary bacterial stains and is too slender to be seen in Gram stain. It can be visualized by **silver stains, dark-field examination, and immunofluorescence techniques**.
- **Source of infection:** An open lesion of **primary or secondary syphilis**. Lesions in the mucous membranes or skin of the genital organs, rectum, mouth, fingers, or nipples.
- **Mode of transmission:**
  - **Sexual contact:** It is the usual mode of spread.
  - **Transplacental transmission**: From mother with active disease to the fetus (during pregnancy) → congenital syphilis.
  - **Blood transfusion**
  - **Direct contact**: With the open lesion is rare mode of transmission.

Basic Microscopic Lesion

Irrespective of stage, the basic microscopic lesion of syphilis consists of

- **Mononuclear inflammatory infiltrate**: Predominantly of **plasma cells and lymphocytes**.
- **Obliterative endarteritis:** It is a characteristic obstructive vascular lesion in which mononuclear infiltrates surround small arteries and arterioles (**periarteritis**).

Stages of Syphilis (Fig. 6.12)

T. pallidum passes from the site of inoculation to regional lymph nodes and enters to the systemic circulation, and disseminate throughout the body. Syphilis can be **1) congenital or 2) acquired.** The course of acquired syphilis is divided into three stages:

1. Primary syphilis
2. Secondary syphilis
3. Tertiary syphilis.

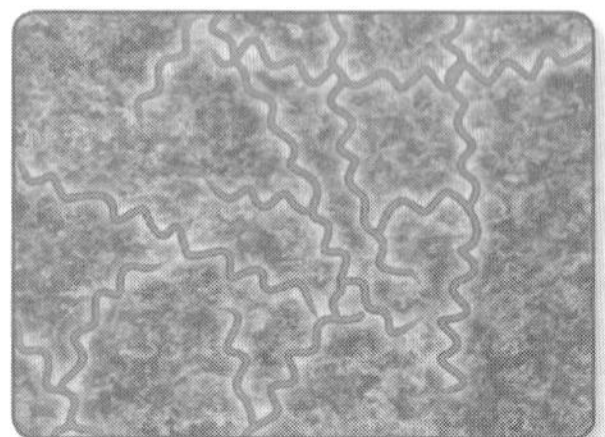

Fig. 6.11: Appearance of *Treponema pallidum* under dark field examination

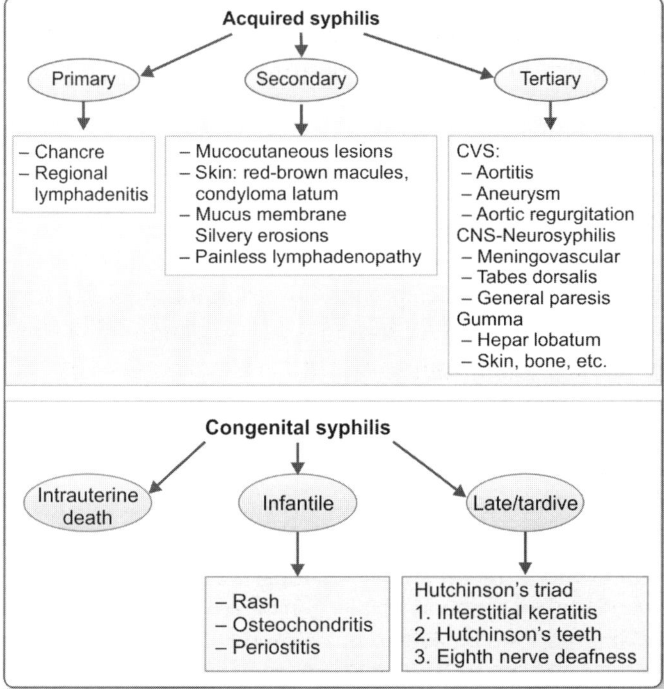

Fig. 6.12: Various manifestations of syphilis

Primary Syphilis

Develops about **3 weeks after contact** with an infected individual and the lesion is primary chancre.

Primary Chancre

It is the classical lesion of primary syphilis.

- **Sites: Penis or scrotum** in men and **cervix, vulva** and **vaginal** wall in women. It may also be seen in the anus or mouth.

Q. Write short note on chancre.

- **Gross features:** It is single, firm, **nontender (painless)**, slightly raised, **red papule** (chancre) up to several centimeters in diameter. It erodes to create a clean-based shallow ulcer. Because of the induration surrounding the ulcer, it is designated as **hard chancre.**
- **Demonstration of treponema**: Plenty of treponemes can be demonstrated in the chancre by 1) silver stains (e.g. Warthin-Starry stain) or 2) immunofluorescence techniques or 3) dark field examination.
- **Microscopy:**
  - **Mononuclear infiltration**: Consisting of **plasma cells,** with scattered macrophages and lymphocytes. These cells are also seen surrounding the blood vessels (periarteritis).
  - **Blood vessels with endarteritis:** It is characterized by endothelial cell proliferation which progresses to intimal fibrosis.

Regional Lymphadenitis

It is due to nonspecific acute or chronic inflammation.

- Treponemes may spread throughout the body by blood and lymphatics even before the appearance of the chancre.
- **Symptoms:** Usually painless and often unnoticed.
- **Fate:** It heals in 3 to 6 weeks with or without therapy.

Secondary Syphilis

It develops 2 to 10 weeks after the primary chancre in approximately 75% of untreated patients. Its manifestations are due to systemic spread and proliferation of the spirochetes within the skin and mucocutaneous tissues.

Q. Write short note on oral lesions of syphilis.

Lesions of Secondary Syphilis

Mucocutaneous Lesions

These are painless, superficial lesions and contain spirochetes and are infectious.

- **Skin lesions**:
  - **Skin rashes:** Consist of **discrete red-brown macules** less than 5 mm in diameter, but it may be scaly/pustular/annular. They are more frequent on the **palms** of the hands, or **soles** of the feet.
  - **Condylomata lata:** These are **broad-based, elevated plaques** with numerous spirochetes. They are seen in moist areas of the skin, such as the **anogenital region (perineum, vulva, and scrotum),** inner thighs, and axillae.
- **Mucosal lesions***:* Usually occurs in the mucous membranes of **oral cavity or vagina as silvery-gray superficial erosions**. These lesions contain numerous *T. pallidum* and are the **highly infectious.**

  Microscopy: Similar to primary chancre, i.e. infiltration by plasma cells and endarteritis obliterans.

Painless Lymphadenopathy

Especially involves **epitrochlear nodes** and shows plenty of spirochetes.

Symptoms: Mild fever, malaise, and weight loss are common in secondary syphilis, which may last for several weeks. The lesions subside even without treatment.

Tertiary Syphilis

- After the lesions of secondary syphilis have subsided patients enters an asymptomatic latent phase of the disease.
- The latent period may last for 5 years or more (even decades), but spirochetes continue to multiply.
- This stage is rare if the patient gets adequate treatment, but can occur in about one-third of untreated patients.
- Focal ischemic necrosis due to obliterative endarteritis is responsible for many of the processes associated with tertiary syphilis.

Manifestations: Three main manifestations of tertiary syphilis are: **cardiovascular syphilis, neurosyphilis, and so-called benign tertiary syphilis.** These may occur alone or in combination.

Cardiovascular Syphilis

Most **frequently involves the aorta** and known as syphilitic aortitis.

i. **Syphilitic aortitis:** Accounts for more than 80% of cases of tertiary disease, and affects the **proximal aorta.**

ii. **Saccular aneurysm and aortic valve insufficiency:**
   - **Occlusion of the vasa vasorum** due to endarteritis leads to **necrosis and scarring of the aortic media,** causing a loss of elasticity, strength and resilience.
   - Gradual weakening and slow progressive **dilation of the aortic root and arch** causes, **aortic valve insufficiency** and **aneurysms of the proximal aorta.** Syphilitic aneurysms are saccular and seen in the ascending aorta, which is unusual site for the more common atherosclerotic aneurysms.
   - On gross examination, the aortic intima appears rough and pitted (**tree-bark appearance**).

iii. **Myocardial ischemia**: Narrowing of the coronary artery ostia (at the origin from aorta) caused by subintimal scarring may lead to myocardial ischemia/infarction.

Neurosyphilis

It may be asymptomatic or symptomatic.

- **Asymptomatic neurosyphilis**: It is detected by CSF examination, which shows pleocytosis (increased numbers of inflammatory cells), elevated protein levels, or decreased glucose. Antibodies can also be detected in the CSF, which is the most specific test for neurosyphilis.
- **Symptomatic disease**: Takes one of several forms
  1. **Chronic meningovascular disease:** Chronic meningitis → involves base of the brain, cerebral convexities and spinal leptomeninges.
  2. **Tabes dorsalis:** It is characterized by **demyelination of posterior column, dorsal root and dorsal root ganglia**.
  3. **General paresis of insane:** Shows generalized brain parenchymal disease with **dementia**; hence called as general paresis of insane.

Benign Tertiary Syphilis

Q. Write short note on gumma

It is characterized by the formation of nodular lesions called **gumma**s in any organ or tissue. Gammas reflect development of delayed hypersensitivity to the spirochete. Gummas are very rare and may be found in patients with AIDS.

Syphilitic gummas:

- May be single or multiple.
- **White-gray and rubbery.**
- Vary in size from microscopic lesions to large tumor-like masses.
- **Site:** They occur in most organs but mainly involve
  1. **Skin, subcutaneous tissue** and the mucous membranes of the upper airway and mouth.
  2. **Bone and joints:** It causes local pain, tenderness, swelling, and sometimes pathologic fractures.
  3. In the **liver,** scarring due to gummas may cause a distinctive hepatic lesion known as **hepar lobatum.**
- **Microscopy:** Center of the gammas show **coagulative necrosis** → surrounded by plump, **palisading macrophages**, fibroblasts and plenty of **plasma cells.** Treponemes are scant in gummas.

Congenital Syphilis

Q. Write short note on congenital syphilis.

Q. Oral lesions of congenital syphilis.

Q. Features of congenital syphilis.

Transplacental Transmission

- *T. pallidum* can cross placenta and spread from infected **mother to the fetus** (during pregnancy).
- Transmission occurs, when **mother is suffering from primary or secondary syphilis** (when the spirochetes are abundant. Because of routine serologic testing for syphilis in done in all pregnancies) congenital syphilis is rare.

Manifestations: can be divided into

1. **Intrauterine death and perinatal death.**
2. **Early (infantile) syphilis**: It occurs in the **first 2 years of life** and often manifested by **nasal discharge** and congestion (**snuffles**).
   - A **desquamating or bullous eruption/rash** can lead to epidermal sloughing of the skin, mainly in the hands, feet, around the mouth and anus.
   - **Skeletal abnormalities:**
     - **Syphilitic osteochondritis:** Inflammation of bone and cartilage is more distinctive in the nose. Destruction of the vomer causes collapse of the nasal bridge → produces characteristic **saddle nose deformity**.
     - **Syphilitic periostitis:** It involves the tibia and causes excessive new bone formation on the anterior surfaces and leads to anterior bowing, or **saber shin**.
   - **Liver: Diffuse fibrosis** in the liver.
   - **Lungs:** Diffuse interstitial fibrosis → lungs appear pale and airless (**pneumonia alba**).
3. **Late (tardive) syphilis**: Manifests **2 years after birth**, and about 50% of untreated children with neonatal syphilis will develop late manifestations.
   - **Manifestations:** Distinctive manifestation is **Hutchinson's triad** are
     - **Interstitial keratitis.**
     - **Hutchinson's teeth**: They are like small screwdrivers or peg-shaped incisors, with notches in the enamel.
     - **Eighth-nerve deafness.**

Laboratory Diagnosis

- **Immunofluorescence of exudate** from the chancre is important for diagnosis in primary syphilis.
- Microscopy and PCR are also useful.
- **Serological tests:**
  - **Nontreponemal antibody tests:** These tests measure antibody to cardiolipin, a phospholipid present in both host tissues and *T. pallidum*.
    - These antibodies are detected by the rapid plasma reagin and **Venereal Disease Research Laboratory (VDRL) tests**.
    - **False-positive VDRL test:** Found in certain acute infections, collagen vascular diseases (e.g. systemic lupus erythematosus), drug addiction, pregnancy, hypergammaglobulinemia of any cause, and lepromatous leprosy.
    - **Antitreponemal antibody tests:** These measure antibodies, which react with *T. pallidum*. These include
      - Fluorescent treponemal antibody absorption test (FTA)
      - Microhemagglutination assay for *T. pallidum* antibodies.

Jarisch-Herxheimer reaction:

- Treatment of syphilitic patients having a high bacterial load, by antibiotics can cause a massive release of endotoxins, and cytokine that may manifest with high fever, rigors, hypotension, and leukopenia.

- This **syndrome** is called the Jarisch-Herxheimer reaction, which **can develop not only in syphilis but also in other spirochetal diseases**, such as Lyme disease.

TYPHOID FEVER

- Typhoid fever (enteric) is an **acute systemic disease** caused by infection with *Salmonella typhi*.
- Paratyphoid fever is a clinically similar but milder disease caused by *Salmonella paratyphi*. **Enteric fever** is the general term, which includes **both typhoid and paratyphoid** fever.

Etiology

Causative agent: Enteric fevers are caused by ***Salmonella typhi*** **and** ***Salmonella paratyphi***. *Salmonella* are gram-negative, motile bacilli (rods). Boiling or chlorination of water and pasteurization of milk destroy the bacilli.

Source of infection: Humans are the only natural reservoir and includes:

1. **Patient suffering from disease:** Infected urine, feces, or other secretions from patients.
2. **Chronic carriers of typhoid fever**: *S. typhi* or *S. paratyphi* **colonizes in the gallbladder** or biliary tree → may be associated with gallstones and the chronic carrier state.

Mode of transmission: From **person-to-person contact.**

- **Ingestion** of **contaminated food** (especially dairy products) and shellfish or **contaminated water**.
- **Direct spread:** Rare by **finger-to-mouth contact** with feces, urine, or other secretions is rare.

Incubation period: Usually 7 to 14 days.

Pathogenesis (Fig. 6.13)

Q. Write short note on pathogenesis of typhoid fever.

- The typhoid bacilli (*Salmonella*) are **ingested through contaminated food or water** → able to **survive in gastric acid of the stomach** → reach mucosa of small intestine.
- **Events during incubation period**:
  - During the initial asymptomatic period (about 2 weeks), the *Salmonella* **attach to the microvilli** and penetrate the **ileal mucosa** of the small intestine → reach lamina propria and submucosa.
  - *Salmonella* are **phagocytosed by the macrophages** (mononuclear phagocytes) present in the lymphoid tissue and **Peyer's patches** in the submucosa of small intestine.
  - *Salmonella* **multiply within the macrophages** and are **carried to** the **mesenteric lymph node** via lymphatics. They multiply in the lymph nodes and **via** the **thoracic duct** enter the **bloodstream** causing **transient bacteremia**.
  - During bacteremia, the bacilli are **seeded in many organs.** They colonize reticulo-endothelial tissues (**liver, gallbladder, spleen, bone marrow**), where bacilli multiply further causing **massive bacteremia** (occurs towards the end of incubation period) → disease clinically manifests.
- **Bile is a good culture medium for the typhoid bacillus**, and bacilli **multiplies in the gall-bladder** → bacilli are continuously shed through the bile into the → intestine.
- In the intestine, the bacilli are localized to the **Peyer's patches and lymphoid follicles** of the terminal ileum. They cause inflammation, plateau-like elevations of Peyer's patches and necrosis, which results in characteristic **oval typhoid ulcers.**

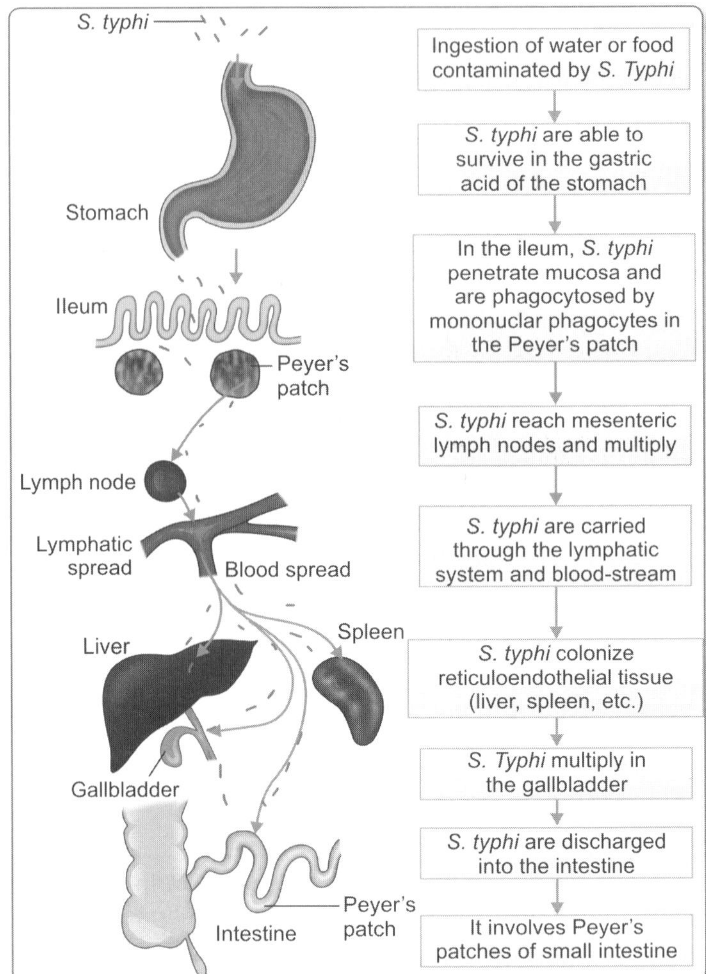

Fig. 6.13: Pathogenesis of typhoid fever

Q. Morphology of intestine in typhoid fever.

Morphology

Lesions may be 1) intestinal and 2) extraintestinal.

Intestinal Lesions

Gross (Fig. 6.14)

- **Site:** Most commonly involved is **terminal ileum**, but may be seen in the jejunum and colon.
- **Appearance**: Peyer's patches in the terminal ileum enlarge into sharply delineated, plateau-like elevations → shedding of mucosa produces → typhoid ulcers. **Characteristics of typhoid ulcer**:
  - **Number: Varies.**
  - **Orientation: Oval ulcers oriented along the long axis of the bowel** (tuberculous ulcers of small intestine are transverse).
  - **Base of the ulcer:** It is **black** due to sloughed mucosa.
  - **Margins: Slightly raised** due to inflammatory edema and cellular proliferation.
  - **No fibrosis:** Hence, narrowing of the intestinal lumen seldom occur in healed typhoid lesions.

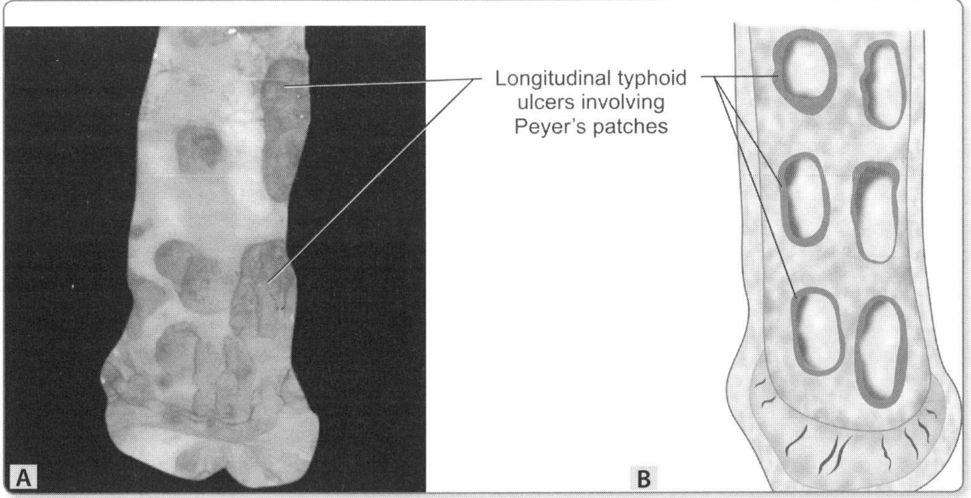

Figs 6.14A and B: Gross appearance of typhoid ulcers in the ileum of small intestine. A. specimen; B. diagrammatic

Microscopy

- **Mucosa: Oval ulcers** over the Peyer's patches.
- **Lamina propria**:
  - **Macrophages** containing bacteria, red blood cells (erythrophagocytosis) and nuclear debris
  - **Lymphocytes and plasma cells**
  - **Neutrophils** within the superficial lamina propria.

Extraintestinal Lesions

- **Typhoid nodules:** Systemic dissemination of the bacilli leads to **formation of focal granulomas** termed **typhoid nodules.** These nodules are composed of **aggregates of macrophages** (typhoid cells) containing ingested bacilli, red blood cells, and lymphocytes. They are **common in the lymph node, liver, bone marrow and spleen**.
- **Mesenteric lymph nodes**: They are enlarged due to accumulation of macrophage, which contains typhoid bacilli.
- **Liver:** It shows small, scattered foci of hepatocyte necrosis replaced **typhoid nodules.**
- **Spleen:** It is enlarged and soft.
- **Abdominal muscles**: Zenker's degeneration.
- **Gallbladder: Typhoid cholecystitis.**

Clinical Features

- Onset is gradual and patients present with anorexia, abdominal pain, bloating, nausea, vomiting, and diarrhea.
- **Fever: Continuous rise in temperature** (step-ladder fever).
- **Rose spots:** These are small erythematous maculopapular lesions on the skin that fade on pressure appear on the chest and abdomen, which occur during second or third week.
- **Spleen:** It is soft and palpable may be accompanied by hepatomegaly.

Complications

- *Intestinal complications:* It can be fatal.
  - **Perforations of ulcer**
  - **Hemorrhage from the ulcer.**
- *Extraintestinal complications*: **Encephalopathy, meningitis, seizures, endocarditis, myocarditis, pneumonia, and cholecystitis. Sickle cell disease → susceptible to *Salmonella* osteomyelitis.**
- *Carrier state*: Persistence of bacilli in the **gallbladder or urinary tract** may result in passage of bacilli in the feces or urine → causes a '**carrier state**' → source of infection to others.

Laboratory Diagnosis

Isolation of Bacilli

- **Blood culture**: It is positive in **first week** of fever in 90% of patients and remains positive in second week till the fever subsides. Blood culture rapidly becomes negative on treatment with antibiotics.
- **Stool cultures:** It is almost as valuable as blood culture and become positive in the **second and third** weeks.
- **Urine culture**: It reveal is the organism in approximately 25% of patients by **third week.**

Other Tests

- **Widal reaction:** Classic Widal test **measures antibodies against O and H antigens** of *S. typhi* but **lacks sensitivity and specificity**. Widal test (immunological reactions) become positive from end of the first week till fourth week. There are many false-positive and occasional false-negative Widal reactions.
- **Other serologic tests**: They are available for the rapid diagnosis of typhoid fever with a higher sensitivity.
- **Total leukocyte count**: It shows **leukopenia with relative lymphocytosis.** Eosinophils are usually absent.

VIRAL HEPATITIS

Definition: Viral hepatitis may be defined as viral **infection of hepatocytes** that produces necrosis and inflammation of the liver.

Cause

Most cases of hepatitis are caused by a group of **five separate, unrelated** viruses that have a particular affinity for the liver known as **hepatotropic virus** (hepatitis viruses A, B, C, D, and E). **All except HBV are RNA viruses.**

Hepatitis A Virus

- **Hepatitis A virus** (HAV): It is a **nonenveloped, 27 nm, RNA virus.**
- **Source of infection**: Only source of infection is **acutely infected person.**

Mode of Transmission

- **Fecal-oral route** by ingestion of contaminated water and foods.

Incubation period: 3 to 6 weeks (mean ~ 4 weeks).

Outcome of HAV Infection

- HAV cause a mild, **benign, self-limited** disease **acute hepatitis**. HAV **does not produce chronic hepatitis or a carrier state** and fulminant hepatitis develops only rarely.

Hepatitis B Virus (HBV)

Structure of HBV

- Hepatitis B virus (HBV): It is a **hepatotropic DNA virus** belonging to the family Hepadnaviridae.
- HBV **virion**: It is spherical and **double-layered**.
- **Dane particle**: It is the complete viral particle/virion.

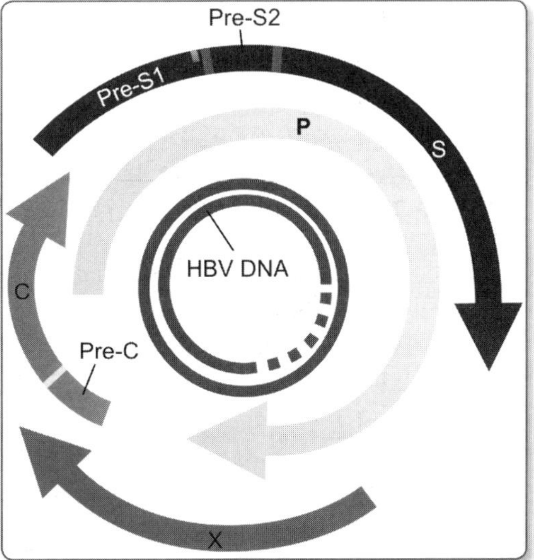

Fig. 6.15: Diagrammatic representation of various genes and respective encoded proteins in HBV. HBV-DNA encodes four proteins namely 1) DNA polymerase required for viral replication (P), 2) surface protein (S), 3) core protein (C) and 4) X protein

Genome of HBV

It consists of partially double-stranded circular DNA and has four genes (Fig. 6.15).

- **HBsAg (S gene): HBsAg, hepatitis B surface antigen** is **secreted into the blood in large amounts**. HBsAg is **immunogenic**.
- **HBcAg (C gene):** The **C** gene produces two antigenically different products:
  - Hepatitis B core antigen (HBcAg):
  - Hepatitis B e antigen (HBeAg):
- **HBV polymerase (P gene):**
- **HBxAg (X gene):**

Source of infection: Human suffering from hepatitis or carrier is the only source of infection.

Mode of Transmission

- **Vertical/congenital transmission**: From mother [who is carrier for HBV (90% HbeAg$^+$, 30% HbeAg$^-$)] to child may occur in utero, **during parturition or soon after birth**.
- **Horizontal transmission**: It is the **dominant mode** of transmission.
  - **Parenteral:**
    - **By percutaneous and mucous membrane:** Exposure to infectious body fluids, through minor cuts/abrasions in the skin or mucous membranes. HBV can survive for long periods on household articles, e.g. toys, toothbrushes and may transmit the infection.
    - **Intravenous route:** Through transfusion of unscreened infected blood or blood products. This mode of spread is rare now, because of routine screening of all blood donors for HBV and HBC. Other modes include intravenous drug abuse with sharing of needles and syringes, tattooists or acupuncturists.
  - **Close personal contact:** Unprotected heterosexual or homosexual intercourse. The virus can be found in semen and saliva.

Incubation period: It ranges from **4 to 26 weeks**.

Q. Write short note on sequelae of hepatitis B virus infection.

Sequelae/Outcome of HBV Infection (Fig. 6.16)

1. **Acute hepatitis** with recovery and clearance of the virus.
2. **Chronic hepatitis.**
3. Progressive chronic disease ending in **cirrhosis.**
4. **Fulminant hepatitis** with massive liver necrosis.
5. Asymptomatic **carrier** state.
6. Hepatocellular carcinoma.

Sequence of Serological Markers for HBV Hepatitis

The natural course of the disease can be followed by serum markers (Fig. 6.17).

Q. Discuss the laboratory diagnosis (serological markers) of hepatitis B virus infection.

HBsAg

- It is the **first virologic marker**

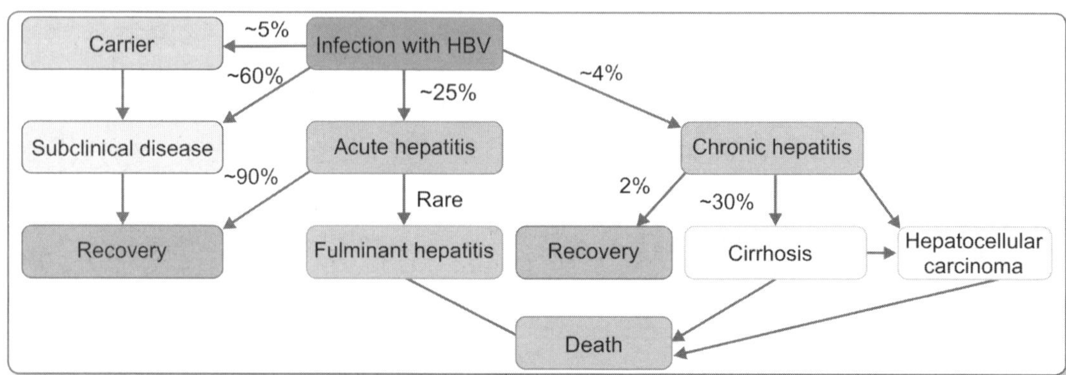

Fig. 6.16: Potential outcomes of hepatitis B infection

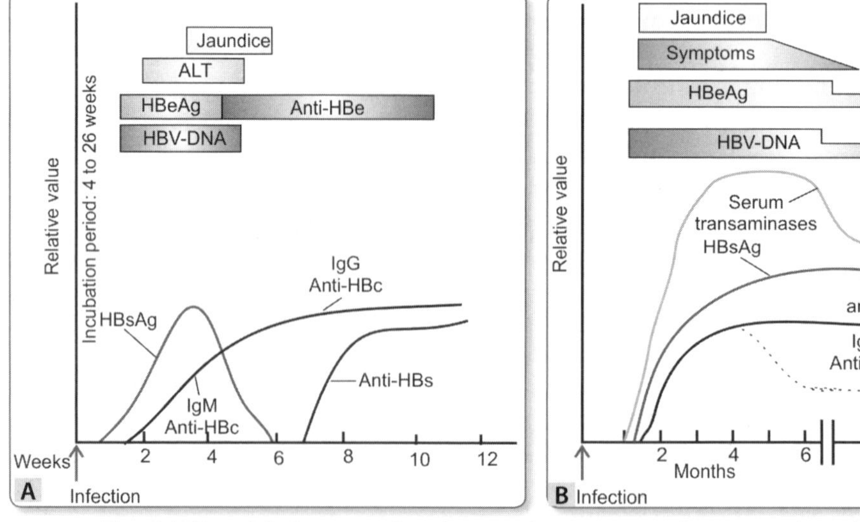

Figs 6.17A and B: Sequence of serologic markers in, A. Acute hepatitis with resolution and in; B. Chronic hepatitis caused by HBV

- **Significance**:
  - **Present in the serum in both acute and chronic hepatitis B; indicates an infectious state. Loss of HBsAg** plus the development of anti-HBs **denotes recovery**.

Anti-HBs

- Anti-HBs is a **protective antibody** and present in the serum in the recovery phase and in immunity (i.e. vaccination) and **may persist for life providing protection.**

HBeAg, HBV-DNA, and DNA Polymerase

- They appear in serum soon after HBsAg,

Anti-HBc

- **HBcAg is not found in the serum**. But its antibody, IgM anti-HBc appears in serum a week or two after the appearance of HBsAg.

Serological findings in HBV are summarized in Table 6.3.

Table 6.3: Summary of serological findings in HBV

Antigens		Antibodies			Interpretation
HBsAg	HBeAg	Anti-HBc	Anti –HBs	Anti-HBe	
+	+	IgM	-	-	**Acute hepatitis B**, highly infectious
+	+	IgG	-	-	**Chronic infection** or carrier state, **high infectivity**
+	-	IgG	-	+/-	**Chronic infection** or carrier state, **low infectivity**
-	-	-	+	-	**Immunity** following HBV vaccine

Prevention

Hepatitis B can be prevented by **vaccination** and by the **screening of donor blood, organs, and tissues**. The **vaccine is purified HbsAg** and induces a protective anti-HBs antibody response.

Hepatitis C Virus

- HCV is a **small, enveloped, single-stranded RNA virus**. It is a member of the *Flaviviridae* family.

Mode of spread: It mainly spreads by the **parenteral route** as a bloodborne infection. It may also spread by **sexual contact.**

Incubation period: 2 to 26 weeks (mean 6 to 12 weeks).

Q. Sequelae of hepatitis C virus infection.

Sequelae/Outcome of HCV Infection

1. **Acute hepatitis**.
2. **Chronic hepatitis:** It **occurs in the majority of individuals infected by HCV.** It can be prevented by screening procedures.
3. **Cirrhosis:** It develops over 5 to 20 years in 20 to 30% of patients.
4. Fulminant hepatic failure is rare.

Hepatitis D Virus

Hepatitis D virus (HDV) is a **defective RNA virus,** which requires HBV for its replication and expression. Because HDV is dependent on HBV, the duration of HDV infection is determined by the duration of HBV infection.

Patterns of HDV Hepatitis

HDV causes **Delta hepatitis** with two clinical patterns.

- **Acute coinfection**: It develops when an individual is **exposed simultaneously** to serum containing **both HDV and HBV**. The HBV infection first becomes established and the HBsAg is necessary for development of complete HDV virions.
- **Superinfection**: It occurs when an **individual is already infected with HBV** is exposed to a **new dose HDV**.

Mode of spread: Parenteral route and sexual contact.

Hepatitis E Virus

- HEV is an unenveloped, RNA virus in the **Hepevirus** genus.
- Hepatitis E occurs primarily in young to middle-aged adults.

Source of infection: HEV is a **zoonotic disease with animal reservoirs**, such as monkeys, cats, pigs, and dogs. Virions are shed in stool during the acute illness.
Mode of transmission: It is an **enterically transmitted, waterborne** infection.
Incubation period: ~6 weeks.

Outcome of HCV Infection

It causes self-limiting acute hepatitis. It does not cause chronic liver disease. But it has a **high mortality rate (about 20%) among pregnant women.**
Salient features of hepatitis viruses are presented in Table 6.4.

Table 6.4: Summary of features of hepatitis viruses

Type	Type of virus	Route of transmission	Mean incubation period	Frequency of chronic liver disease	Diagnosis
A	ssRNA	Fecal-oral	2–4 weeks	Never	IgM anti-HAV
B	Partially dsDNA	Parenteral, sexual contact, perinatal	1–4 months	10%	HBsAg or antibody to HBcAg
C	ssRNA	Parenteral	7–8 weeks	~80%	Anti-HCV, HCV RNA
D	Circular defective ssRNA	Parenteral	Same as HBV	5% (coinfection); ≤70% (superinfection)	Anti-HDV, HDV RNA; Coinfection—IgM anti-HBc and anti-HDV; Superinfection—IgG anti-HBc and anti-HDV
E	ssRNA	Fecal-oral	4–5 weeks	Never	IgM/IgG anti-HEV

Abbreviations: ss, single stranded; ds, double-stranded DNA; HBcAg, hepatitis B core antigen; HBsAg, hepatitis B surface antigen; HBV, hepatitis B virus; HCV, hepatitis C virus; HDAg, hepatitis D antigen; HDV, hepatitis D virus; HEV, hepatitis E virus.

Clinical Features

1. Asymptomatic acute infection with recovery (serologic evidence only).
2. Acute hepatitis (anicteric or icteric).
3. Fulminant hepatitis with massive to submassive hepatic necrosis.
4. Chronic hepatitis (without or with progression to cirrhosis).
5. Chronic carrier state.

Acute Hepatitis

It can be caused by any one of four hepatotropic viruses.

It presents with nonspecific symptoms such as malaise, nausea, poor appetite, and vague abdominal pain. Jaundice and yellow sclera, dark colored urine (conjugated hyperbilirubinemia), light-colored stool, and pruritis (bile salt retention).

Investigations

- **Biochemical**: Raised serum bilirubin and aminotransferase levels.
- **Serology:** Hepatitis viral genome in the liver and serum followed by antibodies to viral antigens.

Morphology of Acute and Chronic Hepatitis

Q. Morphology of liver in viral hepatitis.

- **General morphological features**: Majority of microscopic changes caused by hepatotropic viruses (A, B, C, D and E) are generally similar.

Acute Hepatitis

Microscopy (Fig. 6.18)

1. **Hepatocyte injury:**
   - **Ballooning degeneration:** It is characterized **swelling of hepatocytes**, empty and pale stained cytoplasm, with clumping of cytoplasm around the nucleus.
   - **Hepatocyte necrosis:**
     i. **Dropout necrosis**: Rupture of the cell membrane of ballooned hepatocytes → leads to cell death and focal loss of hepatocytes → necrotic cell **dropout** → collapse of sinusoidal collagen reticulin framework → **aggregates of macrophage** around necrotic hepatocyte.
     ii. **Acidophilic or apoptotic or Councilman body:** It is caused by anti-viral cytotoxic (effector) T cells. Apoptotic hepatocytes shrink → become **intensely eosinophilic** and have with a densely staining **pyknotic or fragmented nuclei**. The remnants of apoptotic hepatocytes may be extruded into the sinusoids → appear as **acidophilic or Councilman bodies.**
     iii. **Bridging necrosis (Fig. 6.19):** It is a confluent (uniting band/zone) necrosis of hepatocytes observed in severe acute hepatitis. This **band/zone of necrosis** may extend from **portal tract to portal tract, central vein to central vein, or portal-to-central regions of adjacent lobules.**
2. **Inflammation:** It involves **all areas** of the lobule and is a **characteristic and prominent feature** of acute hepatitis.
   - **Mononuclear inflammatory cells:** mainly consists of **lymphocytes and macrophages.**
   - **Lobular hepatitis:** It is **inflammation** involving **liver parenchyma away from portal tract.**
   - **Interface hepatitis:** It can **occur in acute and chronic hepatitis.**
3. **Kupffer cells:** They show **hypertrophy and hyperplasia.**
4. **Lobular disarray**: It is due to combination of necrosis of hepatocytes, accompanying regeneration and mononuclear inflammatory infiltrate → disruption of the normal orderly architecture of the liver cell plates.

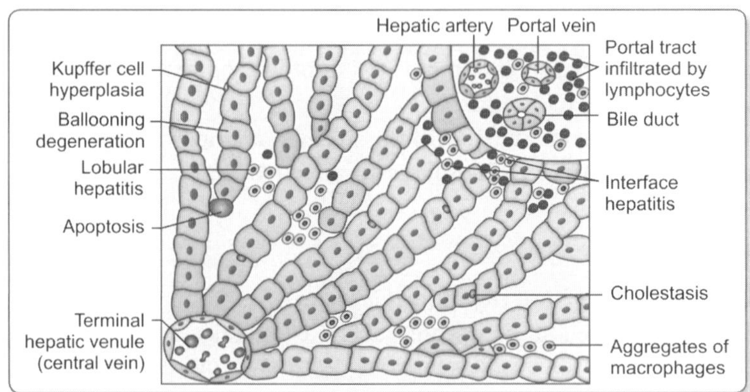

Fig. 6.18: Microscopic features of acute hepatitis

CHRONIC HEPATITIS

Definition: Chronic hepatitis is defined as **symptomatic, biochemical, or serologic evidence of hepatic disease** for **more than 6 months**. Microscopically, there should be inflammation and necrosis in the liver.

Causes

Hepatitis may be caused by viruses (HCV, HBV and HDV+HBV) as well as other etiological agents:

Q. Write short note on chronic hepatitis.

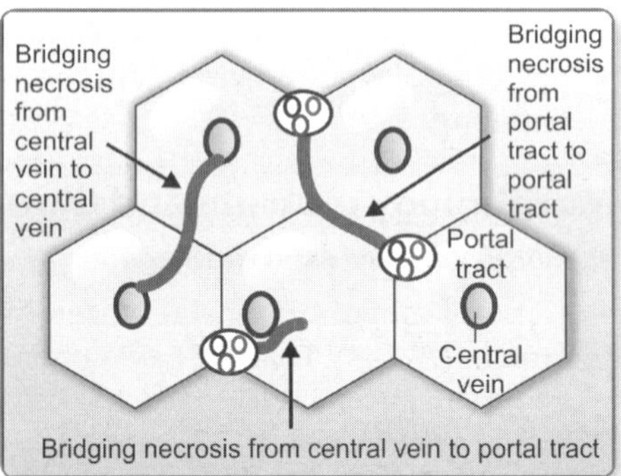

Fig. 6.19: Patterns of bridging necrosis in severe hepatitis

Morphology

Microscopy (Fig. 6.20)

It is characterized by a combination of 1) portal inflammation, 2) interface hepatitis, 3) parenchymal inflammation and necrosis, and 4) fibrosis.

1. **Portal inflammation:** Predominantly consists of **lymphocytes, macrophages, and occasional plasma cells.**
2. **Interface hepatitis (piecemeal necrosis/periportal necrosis):** It is an **important feature** characterized by **spillover of inflammatory cells** (lymphocytes and plasma cells) **from portal tract into the adjacent parenchyma** at the limiting plate → associated with degenerating and apoptosis of periportal hepatocytes.
3. **Parenchymal inflammation and necrosis.**
4. **Fibrosis:** It is the **hallmark of chronic liver damage.** Continued inflammation and associated necrosis → leads to progressive fibrosis at the limiting plate and enlargement of the portal tract.

Consequence

- Continued loss of hepatocytes and fibrosis → results in **cirrhosis**.

Fulminant Hepatic Failure

Definition: Hepatic insufficiency progresses **within 2 to 3 weeks** from **onset of symptoms** to hepatic encephalopathy, in patients who do not have chronic liver disease.

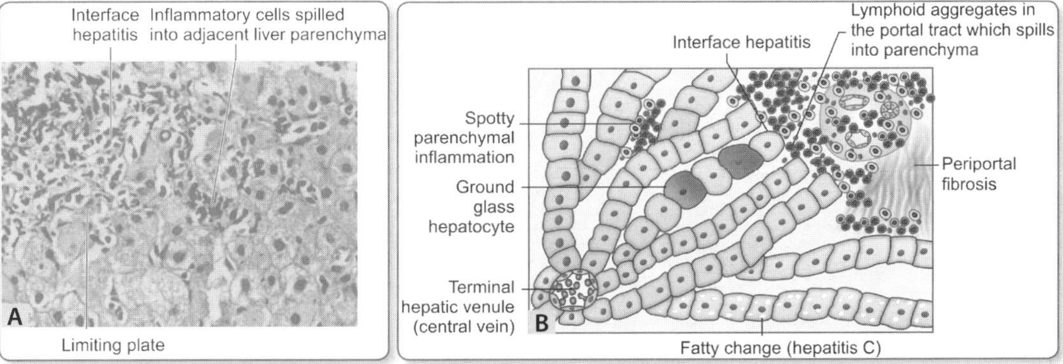

Fig. 6.20: Microscopic features of chronic hepatitis (A, photomicrograph B, diagrammatic)

ACTINOMYCOSIS

- It is a chronic suppurative disease caused by anaerobic bacteria, *Actinomycetes israelii.* It is not a fungus.
- The organisms are commensals in the oral cavity, gastrointestinal (GI) tract and vagina.
- Mode of infection: Infection is always endogenous in origin and not due to personal contact.
- Break in mucocutaneous continuity, diminished immunity due to some underlying disease favors the organism to invade, proliferate and disseminate.

Morphology

Depending on the anatomic location of lesions, actinomycosis is divided into four types:

1. Cervicofacial actinomycosis
   a. It is the most common form (60%) and has best prognosis.
   b. Infections gains through tonsils, carries teeth, periodontal diseases or trauma following extraction of tooth.
   c. In the beginning, a firm swelling develops in the lower jaw (i.e. lumpy jaw). Later, the mass breaks down and form abscess and sinuses. Typically the sinus discharges yellow Sulfur granules. The infection may spread into the adjacent soft tissues and may destroy the bone.
2. Thoracic actinomycosis:
   a. The infection of lung is as a result of aspiration of organism from the oral cavity or extension of infection from abdominal or hepatic lesions.
   b. Initially, lung lesions resemble pneumonia but as the disease progresses it spreads to the whole lung, pleura, ribs and vertebrae.
3. Abdominal actinomycosis:
   a. The common sites are appendix, cecum and liver.
   b. The infection occurs as a result of swallowing of organism from oral cavity or as an extension from thoracic cavity.
4. Pelvic actinomycosis: It develops as a complication of intrauterine contraceptive devices (IUCDs).

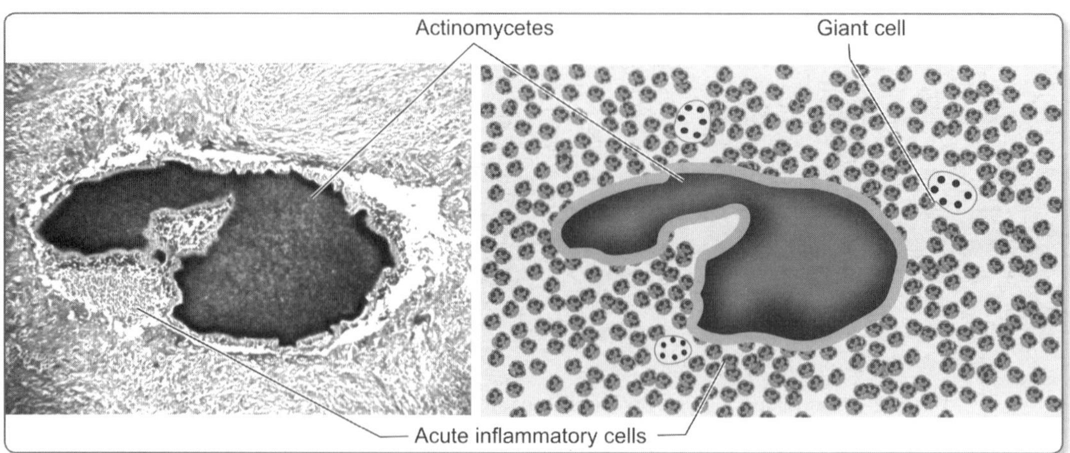

Fig. 6.21: Microscopy of actinomycosis showing central bacterial colony surrounded inflammatory cells. (A-H&E and B-diagrammatic)

Microscopy (Fig. 6.21):

Following features are seen irrespective of the location of actinomycosis:

- **Granulomatous reaction with central suppuration**: There is formation of abscesses in the center of lesions and the periphery of the lesions show chronic inflammatory cells, giants cells and fibroblasts.
- The **central abscess** contains bacterial colony (Sulfur granule) characterized by radiating filaments (was called as ray fungus) surrounded by hyaline, eosinophilic, club-like ends which represent immunoglobulins.
- **Special stains for bacteria**: The organisms are gram positive filaments and nonacid-fast. They stain positively with Gomori's methenamine silver (GMS) stain.

Chapter 7

Hemodynamic Disorders

Chapter Outline

- Hyperemia and congestion
- Edema
- Thrombosis
- Embolism
- Infarction
- Shock

HYPEREMIA AND CONGESTION

Q. Write short note on hyperemia.

Hyperemia and congestion are characterized by **locally increased blood volume.**

Hyperemia

Definition: Hyperemia is an **active process** in which **arteriolar dilation** leads to increased **blood flow to a tissue/organ**.

Causes

- **Physiological:** Response to **increased functional demand** (e.g. heart and skeletal muscle during exercise).
- **Pathological:** Seen in **inflammation** and is responsible for the two cardinal signs of inflammation namely **heat** (calor) and **redness** (rubor/**erythema**).

Congestion

Q. Write short note on chronic passive congestion.

Definition: Congestion is a **passive process** resulting from **reduced venous outflow of blood** from a tissue/organ.

Types and Causes

1. **Systemic:** for example, congestive heart failure, congestion involves liver, spleen, and kidneys.

2. **Local:** examples
   - Congestion of leg veins due to deep venous thrombosis → edema of the lower extremity.
   - Local congestion at various sites due to compression of veins: for example, tight bandage, plasters, tumors, pregnancy, hernia, etc.

Onset

1. **Acute congestion**: It develops during shock, or sudden right-sided heart failure. It may occur in lung and liver.
2. **Chronic passive congestion:** It usually produces edema in the organ/tissue in which the venous outflow is reduced.
   - **Appearance**: Congested tissues have a **dusky reddish-blue color (cyanosis)** due to stasis of RBCs and the accumulation of deoxygenated hemoglobin.

Chronic Venous Congestion of Lung

Q. Write short note on CVC lung/brown induration of lung.

Causes

- **Mitral stenosis**: for example, rheumatic mitral stenosis.
- **Left-sided heart failure**: It develops secondary to coronary artery disease or hypertension.

Mechanism

- Chronic left ventricle failure → reduces the flow of blood out of the lungs → leads to chronic passive pulmonary congestion → **increases pressure in the alveolar capillaries** and they become excessively filled with blood.

Consequences

Q. Write short note on heart failure cells and the special stain used for its demonstration.

Four major consequences are:

- **Microhemorrhages**: The wall of alveolar capillaries may rupture → minute hemorrhages into the alveolar space → release RBCs → hemoglobin breakdown → **liberation of iron containing hemosiderin pigment** (brown color) → alveolar macrophages phagocytose hemosiderin. **Hemosiderin-laden macrophages** are known as **heart failure cells**. When stained by Perl's stain, the hemosiderin in these cells appear blue-black in color.
- **Pulmonary edema**: It is due to forced movement of fluid from congested vessels into the alveolar spaces.
- **Fibrosis:** It develops due to increased fibrous tissue in the interstitium of lung.
- **Pulmonary hypertension**: It is due to transmission of pressure from the alveolar capillaries to the pulmonary arterial system.

Morphology

Gross

- Lung is **heavy**.
- Cut section (c/s) **rusty brown color** (due to hemosiderin pigment), **firm in consistency** (due to fibrosis) → known as **brown induration of lung**.

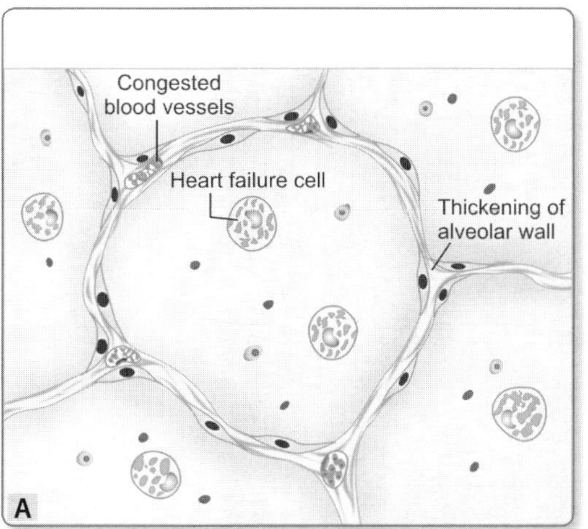

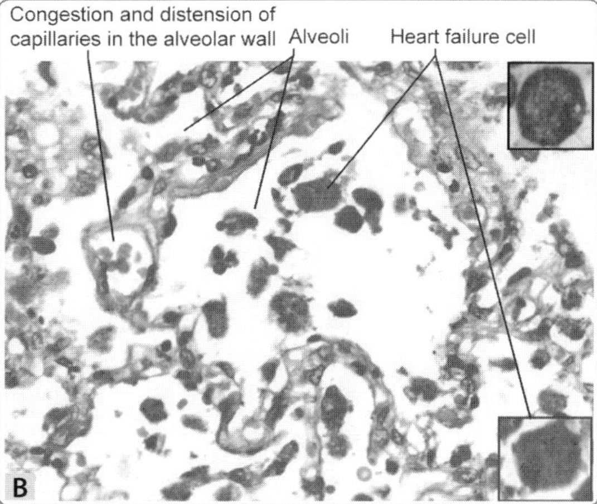

Figs 7.1A and B: Chronic venous congestion lung (A. diagrammatic and B. H and E) with thickened alveolar walls and hemosiderin laden macrophages (heart failure cells) in the alveolar lumen Inset of B, lower right-hemosiderin laden macrophage and upper left-Perl's stain imparting blue-black color to hemosiderin in the cytoplasm

(For color version, see Plate 3)

Microscopy (Fig. 7.1)

- **Distension** and **congestion of capillaries** in the alveolar septa of lung.
- **Thickened alveolar septa** due to increase in the fibrous connective tissue → responsible for the firm consistency of the lung.
- **Heart failure cells** are seen in the alveoli.

Chronic Passive Congestion of Liver

Q. Write short note on causes, gross and microscopic features of chronic venous congestion of liver/ CVC liver/nutmeg liver.

Causes

- **Right-sided heart failure** is the most common cause.
- **Rare:** Constrictive pericarditis, tricuspid stenosis and obstruction of inferior vena cava and hepatic vein.
- **Mechanism:** Dilatation of central veins → transmission of increased venous pressure to the sinusoids → dilatation of sinusoids → ischemic necrosis of hepatocytes in the centrilobular region.

Morphology

Gross

- **Liver increases in size** and weight and the **capsule appears tense.**
- **Cut section** shows **alternate** (combination of) **dark and light areas** (Fig. 7.2) and resembles cross-section of a nutmeg (**nutmeg liver**).
  - **Congested centrilobular regions** (with hemorrhage and necrosis) appear **dark red-brown.** Congestion is most prominent around terminal hepatic venule (central veins) within hepatic lobules.
  - **Periportal** (better oxygenated) **region** of the lobules appear **pale** and may show fatty change.

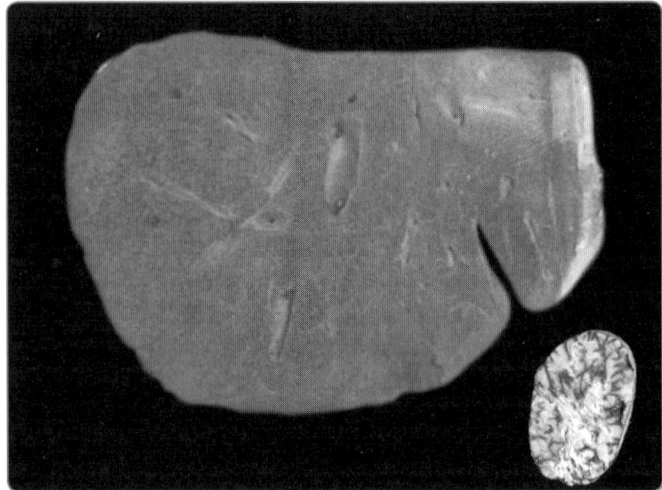

Fig. 7.2: Gross appearance of chronic venous congestion of liver, which shows alternate dark and light area and resembles the cut surface of a nutmeg (inset)

(For color version, see Plate 3)

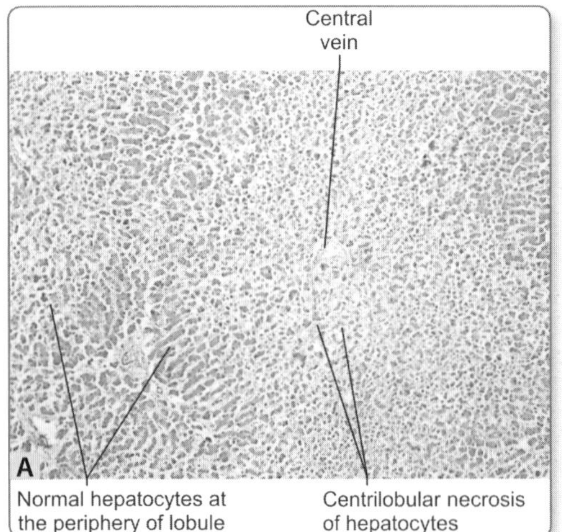

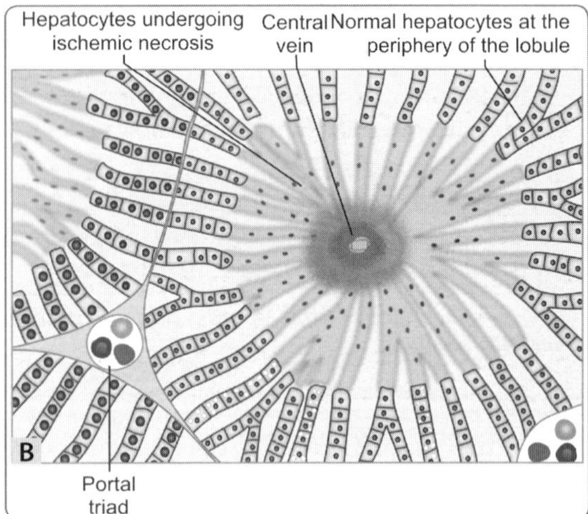

Figs 7.3A and B: Chronic venous congestion liver shows centrilobular necrosis with degenerating hepatocytes surrounded by apparently normal hepatic parenchyma in the periportal region. A. Photomicrograph; B. Diagrammatic

(For color version, see Plate 4)

Q. Causes and pathology of nutmeg liver

Microscopy (Fig. 7.3)

- **Centrilobular region:**
  - **Congestion and hemorrhage** in the central veins (terminal hepatic venule) and adjacent sinusoids.
  - The **severe central hypoxia may produce centrilobular hepatocyte necrosis.**
  - **Thickening of central veins and fibrosis** in prolonged venous congestion.
  - **Cardiac sclerosis/ cardiac cirrhosis** may occur with sustained chronic venous congestion (e.g. due to constrictive pericarditis or tricuspid stenosis).
- **Periportal region:** It shows **fatty change** in hepatocytes.

Congestive Splenomegaly (CVC Spleen)

Q. Write short note on CVC spleen/Gamna-Gandy bodies.

Congestion and enlargement of spleen is called as congestive splenomegaly.

Causes

- Chronic obstruction to the outflow of venous blood from spleen leads to higher pressure in the splenic vein.
  - **Intrahepatic obstruction to blood flow**: **Cirrhosis of the liver** is the main cause (e.g. alcoholic cirrhosis, pigment cirrhosis).
  - **Extrahepatic disorders**:
    - **Systemic or central venous congestion:** for example, tricuspid or pulmonic valvular disease, chronic cor pulmonale, right heart failure or following left-sided heart failure. Splenomegaly is only moderate and rarely exceeds 500 g in weight.
    - **Obstruction of the extrahepatic portal vein or splenic vein:** Due to spontaneous portal vein thrombosis, which is usually caused by intrahepatic obstructive disease, or inflammation of the portal vein (pylephlebitis). Thrombosis of the splenic vein can also develop by infiltrating tumors arising in neighboring viscera, such as carcinomas of the stomach or pancreas.

Morphology

Gross

- Spleen is **enlarged, firm and tense.** In long-standing chronic splenic congestion, spleen is markedly enlargement (1000–5000 g). **Capsule is thickened.**
- Cut section oozes dark blood.
- May show **Gamna-Gandy bodies,** which consist of **iron-containing, fibrotic, and calcified foci of old hemorrhage.**
- Enlarged spleen **may show excessive functional activity** termed as **hypersplenism** → leads to hematologic abnormalities (e.g. thrombocytopenia pancytopenia).

Microscopy

- **Red pulp**
  - **Dilatation and congestion** in the early stages.
  - Hemorrhage and fibrosis in later stages.
  - **Capillarization of sinusoids** may occur, in which sinusoids get converted into capillaries.
- **Thickened fibrous capsule and trabeculae.**
- **Slowing of blood flow** from the cords to the sinusoids → prolongs the exposure of the blood cells to macrophages in the spleen → leads to **excessive destruction of blood cells (hypersplenism).**

EDEMA

Q. Define edema.

Definition: An abnormal accumulation of fluid in the interstitial space within tissues is called edema.

Special forms of edema are listed in Table 7.1

Table 7.1: Special forms of edema

Terminology	Body cavity involved
Hydrothorax	Pleural cavity
Hydropericardium	Pericardial cavity
Hydroperitoneum (ascites)	Peritoneal cavity

Types of Edema Fluid

The edema fluid may be either transudate or exudate. The differences between transudate and exudate are presented in Table 3.3.

Q. Tabulate the differences between transudate and exudate.

1. **Transudate:** It is protein-poor fluid caused by increased hydrostatic pressure or reduced plasma protein.
   - **Causes:** Transudate is observed in heart failure, renal failure, hepatic failure, and certain forms of malnutrition.
2. **Exudate:** It is **protein-rich fluid** produced due to increased vascular permeability and is seen in **inflammation**.

Pathophysiologic Categories of Edema (Table 7.2)

Q. Define different pathophysiological categories of edema.

Edema may be localized or generalized in distribution.

Table 7.2: Pathophysiologic categories of edema

Mechanism	Causes
Increased hydrostatic pressure	Impaired venous return • Generalized – Congestive heart failure – Constrictive pericarditis • Regional – Ascites in cirrhosis – Obstruction (e.g. thrombosis) or compression of veins (e.g. external mass) – Arteriolar dilation: Heat
Decreased plasma osmotic pressure (Hypoproteinemia)	Nephrotic syndrome Ascites in cirrhosis of liver Malnutrition Protein-losing gastroenteropathy
Lymphatic obstruction	Inflammatory Neoplastic Postirradiation Postsurgical
Inflammation	Acute and chronic inflammation
Sodium retention	Excessive salt intake with renal insufficiency Increased tubular reabsorption of sodium: for example, increased renin-angiotensin-aldosterone secretion

Local/Localized Edema

Q. Pathogenesis of edema.

Q. Write short note on different types of edema.

- It is **limited to an organ or part** (for example, arm, leg, epiglottis, larynx).
  - **Obstruction of vein or lymphatic**: for example, edema of limb (usually the leg) develops due to venous or lymphatic obstruction caused by **thrombophlebitis, chronic lymphangitis, resection of regional lymph nodes, filariasis,** etc.
  - **Inflammation:** It is the **most common cause** of local edema.
  - **Immune reaction**: for example, urticaria (hives), or edema of the epiglottis or larynx (angioneurotic edema).

Generalized Edema

- It is **systemic** in distribution and affects visceral organs and the skin of the trunk and lower extremities.
  - **Causes**: Disorder of fluid and electrolyte metabolism.
    - **Heart failure**
    - **Nephrotic syndrome** (renal diseases with massive loss of serum proteins into the urine)
    - **Cirrhosis of the liver.**

Mechanism/Pathogenesis of Edema (Fig. 7.4)

- The movement of water and salts between the intravascular and interstitial spaces is controlled mainly by two opposite effect of **Starling forces.**
- The force that drives the fluid out of circulation is **vascular hydrostatic pressure** and the force which drives the fluid into circulation is **plasma colloid osmotic pressure**.

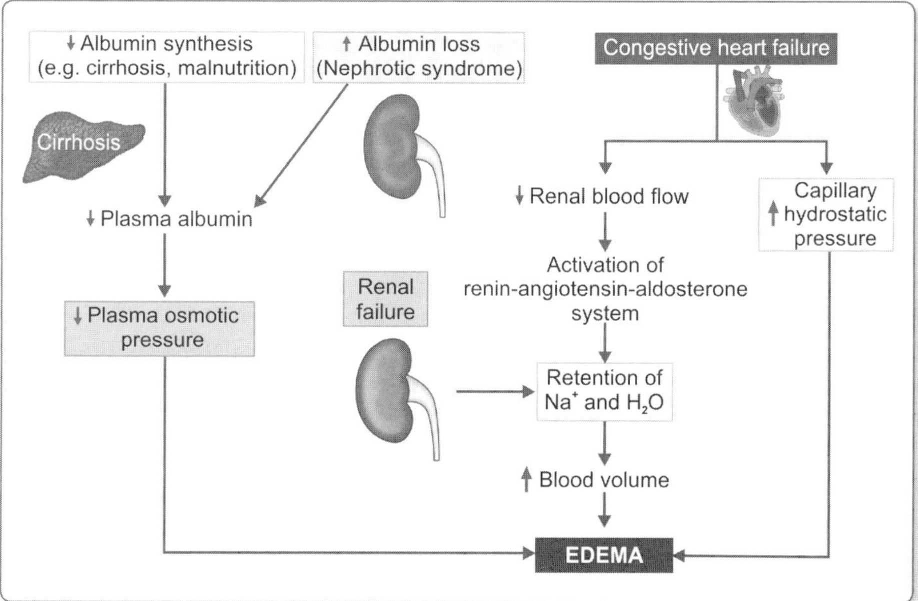

Fig. 7.4: Pathogenesis of systemic edema from congestive heart failure, renal failure, or reduced plasma osmotic pressure

Normal Fluid Balance

- Normally the fluid flows out from the arteriolar end of the microcirculation into the interstitium.
- This is balanced by flowing in of the fluid at the venular end.
- A small amount of fluid, which may be left in the interstitium, is drained by the lymphatic vessels, and it reaches the bloodstream via the thoracic duct.

Mechanism of Edema

- Any mechanism, which interferes with the normal fluid balance, may produce edema.
- **Increased capillary hydrostatic pressure or decreased colloid osmotic pressure** produces increased interstitial fluid.
- If the movement of fluid into tissues (or body cavities) exceeds lymphatic drainage, the fluid accumulates in the interstitial tissue.
- These mechanisms may operate singly or in combinations.

Increased Hydrostatic Pressure

Hydrostatic pressure at the capillary end of microcirculation drives the fluid out of the capillary into the interstitial tissue space. Any conditions, which increase the hydrostatic pressure, can produce edema. The increased hydrostatic pressure **may be regional or generalized**.

- **Local increase in hydrostatic pressure:** It can be due to **local impairment in venous return**. Examples,
  - **Deep venous thrombosis** in a lower extremity may produce localized edema in the affected leg.
  - **Postural edema** may be seen in the feet and ankle of individuals who stand in erect position for long duration.
- **Generalized increase in hydrostatic pressure**: It produces generalized edema. Most common cause is **congestive heart failure (CHF)**.
  - Congestive heart failure may be failure of the left ventricle, right ventricle or both.
  - **Right-sided heart failure** results in pooling of blood on the venous side of the circulation → increases the hydrostatic pressure in the venous circulation → increases movement of fluid into the interstitial tissue spaces → shows characteristic **peripheral pitting edema**.
  - **Left-sided heart failure** results in increased hydrostatic pressure in the pulmonary circulation → produces **pulmonary edema**.

Decreased Plasma Osmotic Pressure

Q. Write short note on pathogenesis of renal edema

Plasma osmotic pressure normally tends to draw the fluid into the vessels. The **plasma osmotic pressure is dependent on plasma proteins, mainly on albumin** (major plasma protein). Decreased plasma osmotic pressure may be due to:

- **Reduced albumin synthesis:** Occurs in **severe liver diseases** (e.g. cirrhosis) or **protein malnutrition** (due to decreased intake of proteins).
- **Loss of albumin**: May occur in the **urine or stool. Nephrotic syndrome** is an important cause of loss of albumin in urine. **Malabsorption and protein losing enteropathy** are characterized by loss of protein in the stool.

Consequences of decreased plasma osmotic pressure

- **Decreased plasma osmotic pressure** → **increased movement of fluid** from circulation **into the interstitial tissue spaces** → **reduced intravascular volume** → **decreased renal perfusion** → activates **increased** production of **renin, angiotensin, and aldosterone** → results in **salt and water retention**.
- These mechanisms cannot correct the reduced plasma volume because the persistence of primary defect of decreased serum protein.

Sodium and Water Retention

Increased **retention of sodium salt is invariably associated with retention of water**. Sodium and water retention may be a primary cause of edema.

- **Mechanism**
  - **Increased hydrostatic pressure** due to increased plasma volume
  - **Decreased plasma colloid osmotic pressure** due to dilution effect on albumin.
- **Causes**: May be primary or secondary
  - **Primary:** It is associated with disorders of kidney such as renal failure, glomerulonephritis.
  - **Secondary:** It develops in disorders that decrease renal perfusion, most important cause being congestive heart failure.

Q. Mention the mechanism of cardiac edema.

- **Mechanism of edema in congestive heart failure**
  - **Decreased cardiac output** → causes **decreased flow of blood to the kidney** → **activates the renin-angiotensin system** → **retention of sodium and water**.
  - Other adaptations also occur, which includes increased vascular tone and elevated levels of antidiuretic hormone (ADH).
- **Water retention by ADH mechanism**
  - ADH is released from the posterior pituitary, when there is reduced plasma volume or increased plasma osmolarity.
  - Primary retention of water can occur due to the increased release of ADH.
  - **Increased secretion of ADH** is seen in association with **lung cancer** and **pituitary disorders**.
  - This can lead to hyponatremia and cerebral edema.

Lymphatic Obstruction

Lymphatic obstruction causes impaired drainage of lymph and produces localized edema, called as **lymphedema**.

Causes of lymphatic obstruction:

- **Chronic inflammation of lymphatics** associated with fibrosis: for example, lymphedema occurring at scrotal and vulvar region due to **lymphogranuloma venereum**
- **Invasive malignant tumors**: for example, **lymphedema of breast** due to blockage of subcutaneous lymphatics **by malignant cells** gives rise to **orange skin (peau d' orange) appearance** to the involved region of skin in the breast
- **Pressure over lymphatic drainage** from outside: for example, tumors obstructing thoracic ducts
- **Damage by surgery/radiation**: Patients with breast cancer may develop severe edema of the upper arm as a complication of **surgical removal and/or irradiation of the breast** and **associated axillary lymph nodes**.

- **Parasitic infestations**: In **filariasis** (caused by *Wuchereria bancrofti)*, the parasite may cause extensive obstruction of lymphatics and lymph node fibrosis. If the block is in the inguinal region, it can produce edema of the external genitalia and lower limbs (upper arm if axillary region is involved) which may be massive and resemble the leg of an elephant and is known as **elephantiasis.**
- **Hereditary disorder**: **Milroy's disease** is a hereditary disorder characterized by abnormal development of lymphatics. The edema may be seen in one or both lower limbs.

Through lymph, proteins in the interstitial space are returned to the circulation. So, **edema fluid** produced due to lymphatic obstruction has a **high protein** concentration. The increased protein content may **stimulate fibrosis** in the dermis of the skin and is responsible for the induration found in lymphedema.

Morphology

Edema can be **easily detected on gross examination**. It may involve any organ or tissue, but is **most common in subcutaneous tissues, the lungs,** and the **brain**. Microscopically, edema appears as a clear space, which separates the extracellular matrix.

Generalized Edema

It is seen mainly in the subcutaneous tissues.

- **Subcutaneous edema:** It may be diffuse or more easily noticed in regions with high hydrostatic pressures. In most cases, the distribution of **edema is dependent on gravity** and is termed **dependent edema**. Thus, it is prominent in the legs when standing, and in the sacrum when recumbent. **If pressure is applied** by a finger over substantially edematous subcutaneous tissue, it **displaces the interstitial fluid and leaves a depression.** This sign is called as **pitting edema.**
- **Edema of renal origin**: It can **affect all parts of the body**. Initially, it is observed **in tissues with loose connective tissue matrix**, such as the **eyelids and scrotal region**. Edema in the eyelids is called **periorbital edema** and is a characteristic of severe renal disease.

Pulmonary Edema

- **Gross:** The **weight of lungs is increased** 2 to 3 times of normal weight. **Cut section** shows frothy, **blood-tinged fluid** (due to mixture of air, edema, and extravasated red cells) **oozing from the lung**.
- **Microscopy:** The edema fluid is seen in the alveolar septa around capillaries and reduces the diffusion of oxygen. Edema fluid present in the alveolar spaces favors bacterial infection.

Cerebral Edema

It may be **localized or generalized**. In generalized edema, the brain is grossly swollen with **distended gyri and narrowed sulci**. The ventricular cavities are compressed and the brain expands, it may herniate.

THROMBOSIS

Q. Define thrombus/thrombosis.

Definition: Thrombosis is defined as the **process of formation of a solid mass** in the **circulating blood from the constituents of flowing blood**.

The **solid mass formed** is called as **thrombus** and it consists of an aggregate of coagulated blood containing platelets, fibrin, and entrapped cellular elements of blood.

Etiology

Q. Describe the etiopathogenesis of thrombus.

Q. What is Virchow's triad?

Three primary abnormalities can lead to formation of a thrombus and constitute Virchow's triad (Figs 7.5A to C). These include:

1. **Injury to endothelium** (changes in the vessel wall)
2. **Stasis or turbulent blood flow** (changes in the blood flow)
3. **Hypercoagulability of the blood** (changes in the blood itself).

Injury to Endothelium (Changes in the Vessel Wall)

Endothelial injury may be either physical damage or endothelial dysfunction (or activation).

Physical Endothelial Injury

It is important for formation of thrombus in the **heart or the arterial circulation**. The endothelial cell injury **promotes adhesion of platelets at the site of injury**.

Causes:

- **Heart:**
  - Chambers of heart: for example, endocardial injury due to myocardial infarction with damage to the adjacent endocardium, catheter trauma.
    - **Valves:** Small thrombi on the valves are called as vegetations.
      - ◊ **Infective endocarditis:** Thrombi on valves (e.g. mitral, aortic valve) damaged by a bloodborne bacteria or fungi
      - ◊ **Damaged valves:** for example, due to rheumatic heart disease, congenital heart disease.
- **Arteries:** for example, ulcerated **atherosclerotic plaques**, traumatic or inflammatory vascular injury **(vasculitis)**.

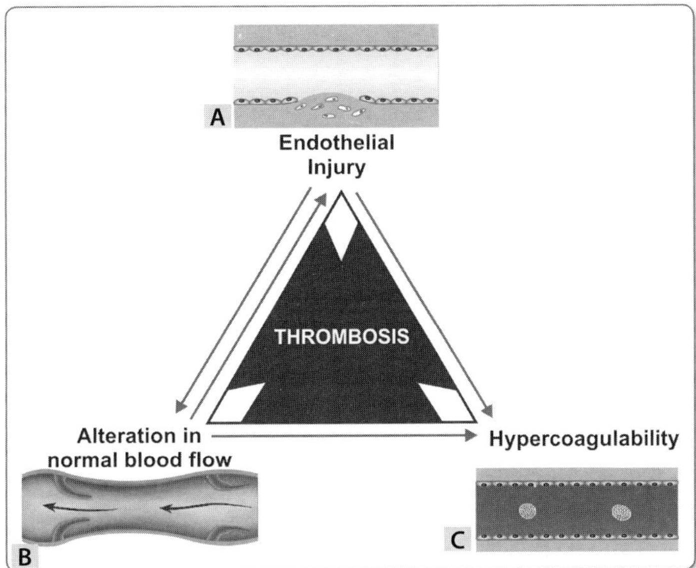

Figs 7.5A to C: Virchow's triad in thrombosis. A) Endothelial injury is the most important factor, B) Alteration in blood flow (stasis or turbulence) and C) Hypercoagulability

- **Capillaries:** Causes include **acute inflammatory lesions**, vasculitis and disseminated intravascular coagulation **(DIC)**.

Endothelial Dysfunction

Definition: Endothelial dysfunction is defined as an **altered state, which induces an endothelial surface that is thrombogenic or abnormally adhesive to inflammatory cells**. Thus, thrombus can develop without any denudation or physical disruption of endothelium.

Causes: Hypertension, turbulent blood flow, toxins (e.g. bacterial endotoxins, toxins from cigarette smoke), radiation injury, metabolic abnormalities (e.g. homocystinemia or hypercholesterolemia).

Alterations in Normal Blood Flow

Normal blood flow is **laminar**, in which **platelets** (and other blood cellular elements) **flow centrally**, separated from endothelium by a slower moving layer of plasma.

Causes

- **Turbulence** (disturbed movement of blood): It can produce thrombus in the arteries and heart.
- **Stasis**: It is a **major cause for venous thrombosis**.
- **Clinical disorder associated with turbulence and stasis**:
  - **Heart**
    - **Acute myocardial infarction**
    - **Arrhythmias/atrial fibrillation:** for example, **rheumatic mitral stenosis** in conjugation with disordered atrial rhythm (atrial fibrillation), it predisposes to mural thrombi in atria.
    - **Dilated cardiomyopathy**
  - **Arteries**
    - **Ulceration of atherosclerotic plaques**
    - **Aneurysms:** They cause local stasis.
  - **Veins:** Thrombi develop in the saphenous veins with varicosities or in deep veins.
- **Other causes**
  - **Hyperviscosity,** e.g. with **polycythemia vera**
  - **RBC disorders,** e.g. **sickle cell anemia** can cause vascular occlusions and stasis.

Hypercoagulability

Definition: Hypercoagulability state (also known as thrombophilia) is defined as a **systemic disorder associated with increased tendency to develop thromboembolism.**

Causes: It is a less frequent cause of thrombosis. Causes can be divided into primary (genetic) and secondary (acquired) disorders (Table 7.3).

Secondary/acquired disorders (Table 7.3): The pathogenesis of acquired thrombophilia is usually multifactorial.

Terminology

- **Mural thrombus:** It is **attached to the wall** and projects into the lumen, **without complete occlusion of the lumen**. It occurs in heart chambers or in the aortic lumen.
- **Occlusive thrombus**: It **occludes the lumen of the blood vessel** and prevents the flow of blood. It usually occurs in veins or smaller or medium sized arteries.
- **Vegetation**: It is a **thrombus on heart valve** and appears as polypoid mass projecting into the lumen (e.g. infective endocarditis).

Table 7.3: Major causes of hypercoagulable state

A. Primary (genetic)
Deficiency of antithrombotic (anticoagulant) factors 1. Antithrombin III deficiency 2. Protein C deficiency 3. Protein S deficiency 4. Methylene tetrahydrofolate reductase (MTHFR) gene mutation
Increased prothrombotic factors 1. Activated protein C (APC) resistance (factor V mutation/ factor Va/ factor V Leiden) 2. Excessive levels of prothrombin (prothrombin G20210A mutation) 3. High levels of factors VII, XI, IX, VIII; von Willebrand factor; fibrinogen 4. Homocystinuria
B. Secondary (acquired)
1. Antiphospholipid antibody syndrome
2. Venous stasis - Prolonged immobilization - Congestive cardiac failure - Prolonged bed rest
3. Increased platelet activation - Hematological disorders: Myeloproliferative neoplasms (polycythemia vera, essential thrombocythemia, myelofibrosis), paroxysmal nocturnal hemoglobinuria - Cancer - Nephrotic syndrome - Atrial fibrillation - Myocardial infarction - Heparin-associated thrombocytopenia - Thrombotic thrombocytopenic purpura (TTP)
4. Increased hepatic synthesis of coagulation factors and reduced anticoagulant synthesis - Oral contraceptive pill - Hyperestrogenic states (pregnancy and postpartum)
5. Release of procoagulant substances: Disseminated cancers
6. Tissue injury: Surgery, fracture, extensive burns
7. Reduced endothelial PGI_2: Old age

Types of Thrombi

Thrombi may be **arterial or venous type**. Differences between arterial and venous thrombus are shown in Table 7.4.

Morphology of Thrombi

- **Layers in thrombus:**
  - **First** layer of the thrombus on the endothelium/endocardium is a **platelet layer**.
  - **On top of the platelet layer, fibrin** is precipitated to **form upstanding laminae** which anastomose to form an intricate structure which **resembles coral** (coralline thrombus). In **between the upstanding laminae** and anastomosing fibrin meshwork, the **red blood cells get trapped. Retraction of fibrin produces a ribbed appearance** on the surface of thrombus.

Q. Write briefly on lines of Zahn.

- **Lines of Zahn**: Both gross and microscopy of thrombus show **alternating light** (pale or white) area of platelets held together by fibrin, **and dark retracted area** of fibrin meshwork with trapped RBCs. These alternating laminations of light and dark are known as **lines of Zahn (Fig. 7.6)**.

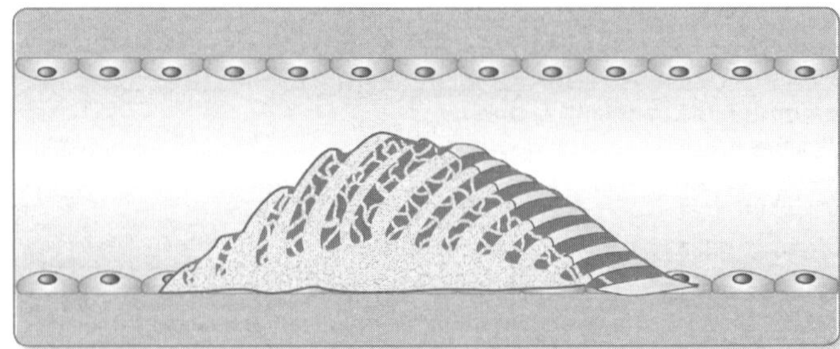

Fig. 7.6: Diagrammatic appearance of thrombus showing alternating dark and light areas (lines of Zahn)

Site and Types

Thrombi can develop anywhere in the cardiovascular system.

- **Heart:**
  - **Cardiac thrombi:** Usually develops at sites of turbulence or endocardial injury.
  - **Valves:** Thrombi on heart valves are called **vegetations**. They are more common on **mitral or aortic valves**.
- **Blood vessels:**
  - **Arteries:** Arterial thrombi tend to be **white**.
    - Aorta or larger arteries usually develop mural thrombi.
    - Thrombi developing in the medium or smaller arteries are frequently **occlusive**. They develop (in decreasing order of frequency) in the coronary, cerebral and femoral arteries.
  - **Veins:**
    - **Venous thrombi (phlebothrombi)** are usually **occlusive**, and form a long cast of the lumen. They occur usually at sites of stasis, and contain more trapped RBCs (and relatively few platelets). They are therefore known as **red,** or **stasis thrombi.**
- **Upper layer:** It is **poor in cells and is yellow-white**. It is firm representing coagulated plasma without red blood cells. It is called **chicken fat** because of its color and consistency.

Fate of the Thrombus (Fig. 7.7)

Q. Write short note on fate of a thrombus.

- **Dissolution/lysis:** of thrombi without any consequences.
  - **Recent thrombi may totally disappear** due to activation of fibrinolysis.
  - **Old thrombi** are **more resistant to lysis**.
- **Propagation of thrombi**: It is the **process in which thrombi grow and increase in size**. The thrombus which was initially **mural, may become occlusive** thrombus. The propagating portion of a thrombus is poorly attached to the wall and therefore **prone to fragmentation and embolization**.
  - **Arterial thrombi grow retrograde** from the point of attachment
  - **Venous thrombi extend in the direction of blood flow.**
- **Embolization:** Thrombi may get detached from its site of origin and form emboli. These emboli can travel to other sites through the circulation and lodge in a blood vessel away from the site of thrombus formation. The **consequences depend on the site of lodgment**. Large venous thrombi may get detached and travel to the pulmonary circulation to the lungs as pulmonary emboli.

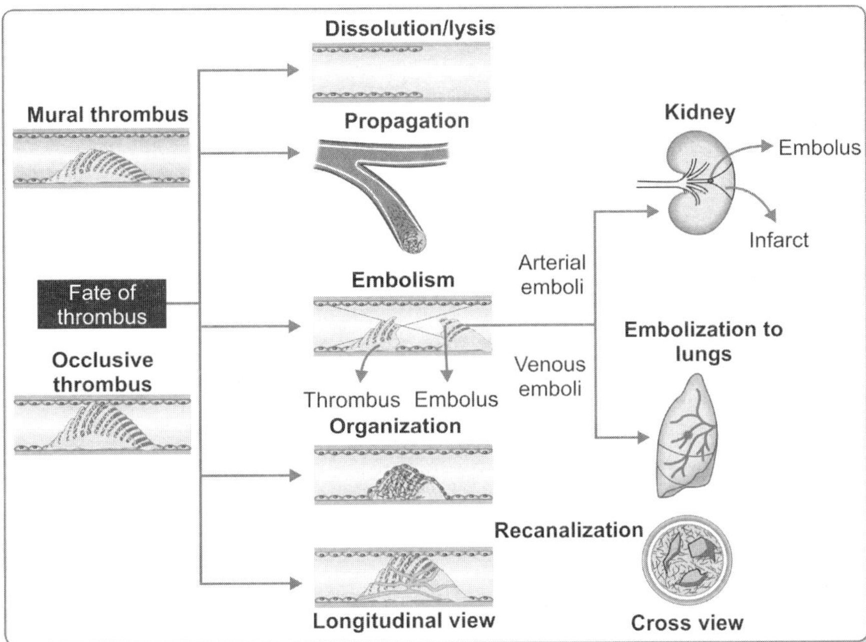

Fig. 7.7: Fate of thrombus

- **Organization:** If thrombi are not dissolved (either spontaneously or by therapy), these older thrombi become organized **by the ingrowth of endothelial cells, smooth muscle cells, and fibroblasts**. Small, organized thrombi may be incorporated into the vessel wall.
- **Canalization/recanalization**: New lumen/channels lined by endothelial cells may form in an organized thrombus. These capillary channels may form thoroughfare channels and can restablish the continuity of the original lumen.

Consequences of Thrombi

It depends on the site of the thrombosis.

- **Obstruction of involved vessel:** Thrombi can cause obstruction of involved arteries and veins.
  - **Arterial thrombi:** They may cause **infarctions** in the region supplied by the involved vessel. Occlusion at a certain locations (e.g. a coronary artery) can be life threatening.
  - **Venous thrombi:** Small venous thrombi may cause no symptoms. Larger thrombi can cause **congestion and edema in region distal to obstruction** by thrombus. Forced dorsiflexion of the foot produces tenderness in the calf associated with DVT and is known as **Homan sign**.
- **Embolization:** Arterial, cardiac and venous thrombi can undergo fragmentation and detach to form emboli. It is the major complication and these are called as thromboemboli. The consequences of embolism depends on: 1) site of lodgement of emboli, 2) tissue affected and 3) source of thromboemboli.
  - **Arterial and cardiac thromboemboli:** The commonest sites of lodgment of emboli are the brain, kidneys, and spleen because of their rich blood supply.
  - **Venous emboli:** They may lodge in the lungs causing various consequences of **pulmonary embolism.**

EMBOLISM

Q. Define embolus/embolism.

Definition: An embolus is a **detached intravascular** solid, liquid, or gaseous **mass** that is **transported in the blood to a site distant from its point of origin**. The process is called embolism.

Types of Emboli

Q. Mention different types of emboli.

Classification: Depending on

1. **Physical nature of the emboli:**
   - **Solid**: **Thromboemboli**, atheromatous material, **tumor emboli**, tissue fragments, bacterial clumps or parasites, foreign bodies.
   - **Liquid**: **Fat**, bone marrow and amniotic fluid.
   - **Gaseous**: **Air** or other gases.
2. **Whether infected or not**
   - **Bland**: Sterile.
   - **Septic**: Infected.
3. **Source (Fig. 7.8)**: The emboli may be **endogenous** (form within the body) or **exogenous** (introduced from outside).
   - **Cardiac emboli:** Usually, they arise from left side of the heart. For example, emboli from: 1) atrial appendage, 2) left ventricle in **myocardial infarction**, 3) vegetations on the valves in **infective endocarditis**.
   - **Vascular emboli**
     - **Arterial** emboli: for example, atheromatous plaque, aneurysms.
     - **Venous** emboli: for example, deep vein thrombus, tumor emboli.
     - **Lymphatic** emboli: for example, tumor emboli.

A. Write short note on paradoxical embolism.

4. **Flow of emboli:**
   - **Paradoxical emboli:** They are rare and the **emboli originate** in the **venous circulation** and **bypass the lungs** by traveling **through a right-to-left shunt** such as an atrial septal defect (incompletely closed/patent foramen ovale) or interventricular defect. Then, they **enter the left side of the heart** and **block the blood flow to the systemic arteries.**
   - **Retrograde emboli: Emboli**, which **travel against the flow of blood** are known as retrograde emboli. For example, **prostatic carcinoma metastasis to the spine**.

Pulmonary Embolism (PE)

Q. Write short note on pulmonary embolism.

Definition: It is defined as an **embolism in which emboli occlude pulmonary arterial tree.**

Site of Origin of Emboli (Fig. 7.8)

- **Deep leg veins**: DVTs are the source in more than 95% of cases of pulmonary emboli. Deep leg veins include **popliteal, femoral or iliac veins.**

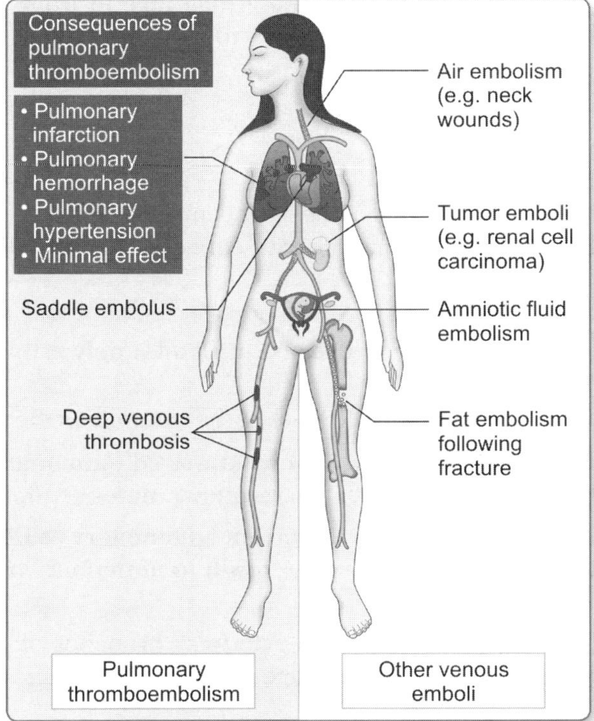

Fig. 7.8: Sources and effects of venous emboli

Risk of pulmonary embolism: Major risk factor is after surgery. The risk increases with advancing age, obesity, prolonged operative procedure, postoperative infection, cancer, and pre-existing venous disease.

Mechanism: DVTs undergo fragmentation → these thromboemboli are carried through progressively larger vascular channels → into the right side of the heart → right ventricle → they enter into the pulmonary arterial vasculature.

Fate of Pulmonary Embolism

Fate depends on the size of the embolus.

1. **Resolution or organization**: **Small** pulmonary **emboli** may travel into the smaller, branches of pulmonary arteries and may **resolve completely**. Most (60–80%) of them are clinically **silent**. With passage of time they become **organized** and are incorporated into the wall of pulmonary vessel.
2. **Massive pulmonary embolism**: When emboli **obstruct 60% or more of the pulmonary circulation**, it is known as massive pulmonary embolism.
   - **Saddle embolus:** It is a **large pulmonary embolus** which **lodges at the bifurcation of the main pulmonary artery**.
   - **Effects:**
     - **Acute right ventricular failure.**
     - **Shock.**

3. **Multiple recurrent pulmonary emboli**: These **may fuse to from** a **single large mass.** Usually, the patient who has had one PE is likely to have recurrent emboli.
4. **Paradoxical embolism**.

Consequences (Fig. 7.8)

1. **Pulmonary infarction**:
   - Most (about 75%) small pulmonary emboli do not produce infarcts. However, an embolus can **produce infarction in the patients with congestive heart failure or chronic lung disease**.
   - **Gross**:
     - **Type:** Usually **hemorrhagic type, because of blood supply to the infarcted (necrotic) area by the bronchial artery**.
     - **Shape: Pyramidal** in shape with the base of the pyramid on the pleural surface.
2. **Pulmonary hemorrhage: Obstruction of medium-sized pulmonary arteries** by emboli and subsequent rupture of these vessels can **result in pulmonary hemorrhage.**
3. **Pulmonary hypertension: Multiple recurrent pulmonary emboli → may cause mechanical blockage of the arterial bed → result in pulmonary hypertension → right ventricular failure**.
4. **Minimal effect:** Obstruction of **small end-arteriolar branches** of pulmonary artery by emboli usually **neither produces hemorrhage nor infarction**.

Systemic Thromboembolism

Definition: It is defined as an embolism in which **emboli occlude systemic arterial circulation**. Systemic arterial embolism **usually produces infarcts** in the region supplied by the involved vessel.

Sources of Systemic Emboli (Fig. 7.9)

Q. Write short note on thromboembolism

- **Heart**: Most common source of thromboemboli.
  - **Intracardiac mural thrombi**: Most common source. Examples
    - **Myocardial infarct of left ventricular wall**
    - In mitral stenosis, dilatation of left atrium and atrial fibrillation predisposes to thrombus and embolization.
  - **Valvular source**: Examples, **bacterial endocarditis** (valvular vegetation from aortic or mitral valves) or prosthetic valves
- **Blood vessels**: Thrombi on **ulcerated atherosclerotic plaques** or from aortic **aneurysms**
- **Unknown origin**.

Consequences

- The arterial emboli can travel to a wide variety of sites. This is in contrast to venous emboli, which lodge mainly in one vascular bed namely the lung.
- The arterial emboli tend to pass through the progressively narrow arterial lumen and lodge at points where the vessel lumen narrows abruptly (e.g. at bifurcations or in the area of an atherosclerotic plaque).

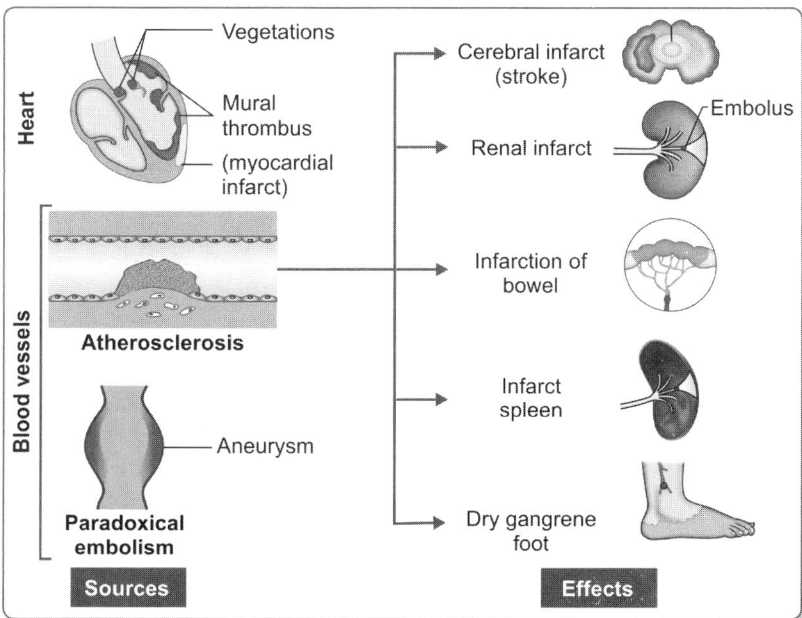

Fig. 7.9: Common sources and effects of systemic arterial emboli. It usually arises from the left side of the heart or from major arteries. Usual consequence is either infarction or gangrene at the site of lodgment

- **Fate of thromboembolus at the site of arrest:**
  - **Propagation and obstruction:** Thromboemboli may grow (propagate) locally at the site of arrest and produce severe obstruction leading to **infarction of the affected** tissues.
  - **Fragmentaion and lysis.**

Major Sites Affected by Arterial Thromboemboli (Fig. 7.9)

1. **Lower extremity** (75%): Embolism to an artery of the leg may produce **gangrene**.
2. **Brain**: Arterial emboli to the brain may produce **ischemic necrosis** in the brain (strokes).
3. **Intestine**: Emboli in the mesenteric vessels may produce **infarction of the bowel**.
4. **Kidney**: Renal artery embolism may cause small peripheral **infarcts** in the kidney.
5. **Blood vessels**: Emboli originating from bacterial vegetation may cause inflammation of arteries and produce **mycotic aneurysm**.
6. **Other sites**: Spleen and upper extremities are less commonly affected.

Fat and Marrow Embolism

Q. Write short note on fat embolism.

Fat and marrow embolus **consists of microscopic globules of fat with or without bone marrow** elements. Release of these elements into the circulation produces fat embolism.

Causes

- **Trauma to adipose tissue with fracture**: Severe trauma to adipose tissue, particularly accompanied by **fractures of bone** release fat globules or fatty marrow (with or without associated hematopoietic marrow cells) into ruptured blood vessels. Fat embolism occurs in about 90% of individuals with **severe skeletal injuries**, but less than 10% of them have clinical findings.

- **Soft tissue trauma and burns.**
- **During vigorous cardiopulmonary resuscitation.**

Manifestation

In **most of the cases,** it is **asymptomatic. Sometimes**, it may manifest as potentially **fatal fat embolism syndrome.**

Fat embolism syndrome: It is the term applied when the patients develops **symptoms due to severe fat embolism**. It develops in only minority of patients.

Pathogenesis

Fat embolism syndrome involves both mechanical obstruction and biochemical injury.

- **Mechanical obstruction**:
  - Trauma to adipose tissue associated with **fracture releases** emboli consisting of **fat globules and/fatty marrow**. These fat microemboli along with red cell and platelet aggregates may **enter the capillaries** which are ruptured at the site of the fracture.
  - The trauma may also cause hemorrhage into the marrow and into the subcutaneous fat. This increases interstitial pressure above capillary pressure, and fat globules are forced into the circulation.
  - The emboli travel through the circulation and can **occlude the pulmonary and cerebral microvasculature**.
- **Biochemical injury**:
  - The chemical composition of the fat present in the lung in fat embolism is different from that in adipose tissue. The mechanical obstruction alone cannot explain this difference. So, pathogenesis probably involves mechanical obstruction associated with biochemical injury.
  - **Biochemical injury is produced by free fatty acids** that are released from the fat globules. Free fatty acids **produce local toxic injury to endothelium**. They cause platelet activation and granulocyte recruitment along with release of injurious free radical, protease, and eicosanoid. These biochemical injury increases the severity of the vascular damage produced by mechanical obstruction.

Consequences of Fat Embolism

It depends on the size and quantity of fat globules and whether the emboli are arrested in the pulmonary or systemic circulation.

- **Sites of arrest of fat emboli:**
  - Emboli in the venous side lodge **in the lungs**.
  - **If emboli pass into systemic circulation**, they may be arrested in **brain, kidneys** and other organs.
- **Demonstration of fat embolism:** Fat is dissolved during routine tissue preparations by the solvents (xylene/xylol) used in paraffin embedding. The microscopic demonstration of fat microglobules requires frozen sections and special stains for fat (e.g. Sudan III and IV, Oil Red O and osmic acid).

Clinical Presentation

The most severe form of fat embolism syndrome may be fatal.

- **Time of development:** It develops **1 to 3 days after the traumatic injury**.

- **Respiratory symptoms:** These include sudden onset of **tachypnea, dyspnea and tachycardia** which may lead to **respiratory failure**.
- **Neurologic symptoms:** These include **irritability, restlessness,** delirium and coma.
- **Hematological findings:**
  - **Thrombocytopenia:** Rapid onset of thrombocytopenia produces **diffuse petechial rash** (found in 20–50% of cases) and may be a useful **diagnostic** feature.
  - **Anemia**: It is due to aggregation of red cells and/or due to hemolysis.
- **Chest radiography:** It shows diffuse opacity of the lungs → may progress to an **opacification of lungs** (whiteout)-characteristic of **acute respiratory distress syndrome**.

Air Embolism

Q. Write short note on air/gas embolism/Caissons disease/decompression sickness.

Air embolism occurs when **air is introduced into venous or arterial circulation**.

Causes

- **Trauma/injury:** Air may enter the venous circulation through **neck wounds and chest wall injury**.
- **Surgery/invasive procedures:** These include invasive surgical procedures such as **thoracocentesis**, punctures of the great veins during **obstetric or laparoscopic procedures**, into the **coronary artery during bypass surgery**, cerebral circulation by neurosurgery in the "sitting position", or hemodialysis.
- **Criminal abortion**.

Amount of air required: It is usually **more than 100 cc** to have a clinical effect of air embolism.

Decompression Sickness

It is a form of gas embolism and may be acute or chronic.

Acute Decompression Sickness

Cause: It develops when individuals **exposed to sudden decrease in atmospheric pressure**. Risk factors include:

- Individuals when exposed to high atmospheric pressure, such as **scuba and deep-sea divers and underwater construction workers** (e.g. tunnels, drilling platform construction), during rapid ascent to low pressure.
- Individuals in **unpressurized aircraft** during rapid ascent.
- **Sport diving**.

Mechanism

- When air is breathed at **high atmospheric pressure** (e.g. during a deep-sea dive), **large amounts of inert gas** such as nitrogen or helium are **dissolved in the blood, body fluids and tissues**.
- When the individual **ascends gradually**, the dissolved gas (particularly nitrogen) comes out from solution in the blood and tissues and exhaled. **It does not produce any injury**.
- However, **if ascent is too rapid, gas bubbles form in the blood circulation and within tissues** → **obstruct the flow of blood** → injure the cells.

Effects: The gas bubbles within small vessel obstruct the blood supply bends and chokes.

- **Musculoskeletal system**: Small vessel obstruction → reduced blood supply to skeletal muscles and supporting tissues in and about joints → produces muscular and joint pain → patient doubles up in pain. This painful condition is called the **bends**.
- **Respiratory system**: Obstruction of blood vessels of the lungs causes edema, hemorrhage, and focal atelectasis or emphysema. This may lead to a form of respiratory distress called the **chokes**.
- **Nervous system**: It may cause coma or even death.

Chronic Decompression Sickness

Caisson Disease

- A chronic form of decompression sickness is known as **Caisson disease** (named for the pressurized vessels/diving bells used in the bridge construction).
- Workers in these pressurized vessels may develop both acute and chronic forms of decompression sickness.
- Characteristic features: Avascular necrosis: Gas embolus in vessel produces obstruction to blood flow → causes multiple foci of **ischemic (avascular) necrosis of bone.** The more commonly involved bone includes the head of the femur, tibia, and humerus.

Amniotic Fluid Embolism

Q. Write short note on amniotic fluid embolism.

Amniotic fluid embolism **develops when amniotic fluid along with fetal cells and debris enter the maternal circulation**. The entry occurs through open (ruptured) uterine and cervical veins or a tear in the placental membranes (Fig. 7.10).

Time of occurrence: It is a rare maternal threatening complication, which occurs **at the end of labor and the immediate postpartum period**.

Consequences: From the venous circulation, amniotic fluid emboli enter the right-side of the heart and finally rest in pulmonary circulation. Amniotic fluid has a high thromboplastin activity and initiates a potentially **fatal disseminated intravascular coagulation (DIC).**

Morphology

- **Amniotic fluid contents within pulmonary vasculature**: Amniotic fluid emboli are composed of squamous cells shed from fetal skin, lanugo hair, fat from vernix caseosa, and mucin derived from the fetal respiratory or gastrointestinal tract.
- **Other findings**: These include marked pulmonary edema, **diffuse alveolar damage**, and features of DIC.

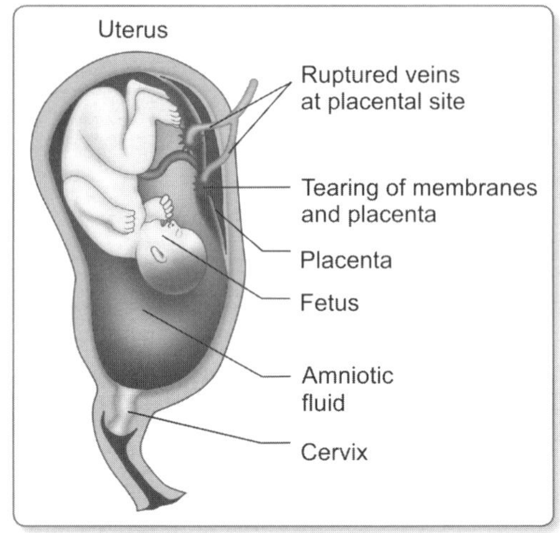

Fig. 7.10: Amniotic fluid embolism

Clinical Features

- **Abrupt onset**: It develops during immediate postpartum period, and is characterized by sudden onset of severe dyspnea, cyanosis, and neurologic impairment ranging from headache to seizures. Patient develops shock, coma and death.

- **Bleeding:** If the patient survives the initial acute crisis, patient develops bleeding due to disseminated intravascular coagulation (DIC).
- **Acute respiratory distress syndrome.**

INFARCTION

Q. Define Infarct/infarction.

Definition: An infarct is a **localized area of ischemic necrosis** caused by occlusion of either the arterial blood supply or the venous drainage. The **process** of producing infarct is known as **infarction**.

Mostly infarct is coagulative type of necrosis due to sudden occlusion of arterial blood supply. If the patient survives, the infarct heals with a scar.

Common and important infarcts are shown in Table 7.4.

Table 7.4: Common and important infarcts

Organ/tissue affected	Infarction
Heart	Myocardial infarction
Brain	Cerebral infarction
Lung	Pulmonary infarction
Bowel /intestine	Intestinal infarct
Extremities	Gangrene

Causes of Infraction

Q. What are the causes/etiology and effects of infarct.

- **Arterial causes:** most important
  - **Occlusions of lumen:** It is the most common cause and may be due 1) **thrombus** or 2) **embolus (Fig. 7.9).**
  - **Causes in the wall:** for example, local vasospasm, **hemorrhage into an atheromatous plaque** or thromboangiitis obliterans
  - **External compression of vessel:** Tumor.
- **Venous causes**
  - **Occlusions of lumen** may be due 1) thrombus or 2) embolus
  - **Extrinsic vessel compression:** tumor, torsion of a vessel (e.g. in testicular torsion or bowel volvulus), **strangulated hernia.**

Factors that Determine the Outcome of an Infarct

Q. Mention the factors that influence the development of an infarct.

The outcome of vascular occlusion may range from no or minimal effect to the death of a tissue or individual. The **major factors** that determine the outcome of infarct are:

1. **Nature of the vascular supply:**
   - **Dual/parallel blood supply:** Organs or tissues with double or parallel blood supply are **less likely to develop infarction**, e.g. lung, liver, hand and forearm.
   - **End-arterial blood supply:** Kidney and spleen has blood supply, which are end-arteries with little or no collaterals. Obstruction of vessels in these organs usually causes tissue death and **infarction.**

2. **Rate of occlusion: Slow occlusion** is **less likely to produce infarction than rapid occlusion**. This is because it provides time to develop alternate perfusion pathways.
3. **Vulnerability of tissue to hypoxia:**
   - **Neurons are highly sensitive to hypoxia**. They undergo necrosis even if the blood supply is occluded for 3 to 4 minutes.
   - In heart, myocardial cells are also quite sensitive to hypoxia, but less sensitive than neurons. Myocardial cells die after only 20 to 30 minutes of ischemia.
4. **Oxygen content of blood:** In a normal individual, partial obstruction of a small vessel may not produce any effect, but in a patient with anemia or cyanosis same may produce infarction.

Classification (Table 7.5)

Table 7.5: Classification of infarct

According to color	Presence or absence of infection	According to the age of infarct
• White/pale (anemic) • Red (hemorrhagic)	• Septic, when it is infected • Bland, when it is free of infection	• Recent or fresh • Old or healed

White/Pale Infarcts

They occur

1. With **arterial occlusions**
2. In **solid organs**
3. With **end-arterial circulation without a dual blood supply** (e.g. heart, spleen, and kidney)
4. **Tissue with increased density** which prevents the diffusion of RBCs from adjoining capillary beds into the necrotic area.

Red/Hemorrhagic Infarcts

They occur

1. With **venous occlusions**, e.g. ovary.
2. In **loose textured tissues**, e.g. lung: They allow red cells to diffuse through and collect in the necrotic zone.
3. In **tissues with dual blood supply**, e.g. lung and small intestine: It allows blood flow from an unobstructed parallel blood supply into a necrotic zone.
4. In **tissues previously congested** due to decreased venous drainage.
5. When **blood flow is re-established to a site of previous arterial occlusion** and necrosis, e.g. following coronary angioplasty of an obstructed coronary artery.

Q. Write short note on morphology of infarct.

Morphology

White/pale Infarcts

Organs involved includes **heart, kidneys, spleen,** and dry gangrene of the extremities.

Morphology

White/pale Infarcts

Organs involved includes **heart, kidneys, spleen,** and dry gangrene of the extremities.

Gross:

- Usually **wedge-shaped (Fig. 7.11).**
- **Occluded blood vessel** is seen **at the apex** and the **periphery/ surface** of the organ **forms the wide base.**
- **Acute infarcts** are **poorly defined** and **slightly hemorrhagic.**
- After 1 to 2 days, the infarct becomes soft, sharply demarcated, and light yellow in color.
- **Margins of infarct appear well defined** because of narrow rim of congestion caused by inflammation.
- **As time passes,** infarcts progressively become **paler** and more **sharply defined.**

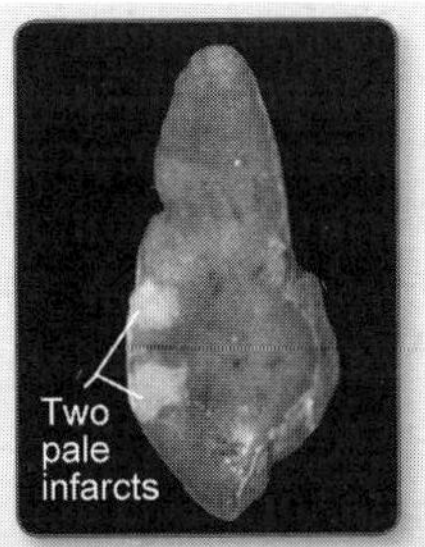

Fig. 7.11: Infarct spleen showing two wedge shaped pale/white infarct

Red/Hemorrhagic Infarcts

- Organs with a double blood supply: for example, **lung, liver**
- Organs with extensive collateral circulation: for example, **small intestine and brain**
- Reperfusion of infarcted area: for example, red infarct may occur in heart when the infarcted area is reperfused

Gross: Appear as **sharply circumscribed** area of necrosis, **firm** in consistency and **dark red to purple** in color.

Microscopy of Infarct

- **Both pale and red infarct** characteristically shows **ischemic coagulative necrosis.**
- Microscopic changes of **frank necrosis** appear after about **4 to 12 hours.**
- **Acute inflammation cells** infiltrate the necrotic area from the viable margins all-round the infarcts within a few hours. It becomes **prominent within 1 to 2 days.**
- Followed by a **reparative process,** which begins **at the preserved margins.** The **necrotic cells** in infarcts and extravasated red cells are **phagocytosed by macrophages.**
- In tissues composed of stable or labile cells, **parenchymal regeneration** can occur at the periphery where stromal architecture is preserved.
- **Granulation tissue** may **replace the infarcted area** which **matures to** form **scar tissue.**
- If the infarct is large (e.g. in heart or kidney), the necrotic center may persist for months.

Septic infarctions: They may occur in two situations:

- **Infection**: Infarct may get infected when it is **seeded by pyogenic bacteria**, e.g. infection of pulmonary infarct.
- **Septic emboli**: They contain organisms and can produce septic infarct, e.g. vegetations of bacterial endocarditis may cause septic infarct of spleen.

The organisms present in a **septic infarct** convert infarct into a frank **abscess.**

SHOCK

Q. Define shock.

Introduction: Shock is the most common, important, and very serious medical condition. It is the final common pathway for several clinical events, which are capable of causing death. These events include severe hemorrhage, extensive trauma or burns, large myocardial infarction, massive pulmonary embolism, and severe microbial sepsis.

Definition: Shock is a **pathological process** that results from inadequate tissue perfusion, **leading to cellular dysfunction and organ failure**.

Characteristic features: Extreme and widespread failure of the circulatory system (either due to decreased cardiac output or reduced effective circulating blood volume) → **systemic hypotension** (either due to reduced cardiac output or to reduced effective circulating blood volume) → **life-threatening inadequate/impaired tissue perfusion (hypoperfusion)** → tissue hypoxia a → **reversible** cellular injury → **irreversible tissue injury and organ failure** → **death**.

Classification

Q. Classify shock.

Q. List the main types of shock with suitable examples.

According to etiology (cause) shock can be classified into three major general categories (Table 7.6).

Table 7.6: Major types of shock

Type of shock	Principal mechanisms	Clinical example
Hypovolemic shock		
Loss of blood/plasma/ fluid → decreased circulating blood volume → low cardiac output → hypotension, and shock	Loss of blood volume	Massive hemorrhage, trauma
	Loss of plasma volume	Massive burns
	Loss of fluid	Vomiting, diarrhea, severe gastroenteritis
Cardiogenic shock		
Direct myocardial damage or a mechanical abnormality of the heart → low cardiac output → reduced cardiac output and blood pressure	Myocardial damage	Myocardial infarction Myocarditis Ventricular rupture
	Mechanical	Valvular failure (stenosis or incompetence) Hypertrophic cardiomyopathy Ventricular septal defect
	Arrhythmic	Ventricular arrhythmias
Septic shock	Endothelial activation/injury; leukocyte-induced damage, activation of cytokines, and disseminated intravascular coagulation	Overwhelming microbial infections (bacterial, fungal, viral, rickettsial)
Others		
Neurogenic shock	Result of loss of vascular tone and peripheral pooling of blood	Anesthetic accident or a spinal cord injury
Anaphylactic shock	Acute widespread systemic vasodilation and increased vascular permeability results in tissue hypoperfusion and hypoxia	IgE–mediated hypersensitivity reaction

Etiology and Pathogenesis

Q. Describe the etiology and pathogenesis of shock.

Q. Write short note on hypovolemic shock.

Hypovolemic Shock

Hypovolemic shock results from low cardiac output due to:

- **Loss of blood:** for example, **massive hemorrhage**.

- **Loss of plasma:** for example, **severe burns**.
- **Loss of fluid: Vomiting, diarrhea, severe gastroenteritis**, e.g. cholera.

Inadequate blood or plasma volume and fluid loss → hypovolemia → low cardiac output → hypotension → inadequate perfusion of tissue.

Cardiogenic Shock

Q. Write short note on cardiogenic shock.

Cardiogenic shock results from low cardiac output due to:

- **Intrinsic myocardial damage:** for example, **massive myocardial infarction**, ventricular arrhythmias.
- **Obstruction to the outflow blood from ventricles:** for example, pulmonary embolism.

The various causes of cardiogenic shock produce → severe dysfunction of left ventricule → **decreases cardiac output** → decreased tissue perfusion of tissue. The left-sided heart failure also reduces the entry of blood from pulmonary vein into the left atrium. This leads to movement of fluid from pulmonary vasculature into the pulmonary interstitial space and into the alveoli resulting in **pulmonary edema**.

Septic Shock

Q. Describe the pathogenesis of septic (endotoxic) shock.

Definition: Septic shock is defined as **shock due to severe sepsis with hypotension**, which **cannot be corrected by infusing fluids**.

Septic shock results from vasodilation and peripheral pooling of blood and is associated with dysfunction of multiple organs distant from the site of infection.

Causative Organisms:

- Septic shock may be caused by **gram-positive** (most common) **or gram-negative bacteria, fungi**, and, very rarely, protozoa or *Rickettsiae*.
- The common gram-positive bacteria include ***Staphylococcus aureus,*** **enterococci,** ***Streptococcus pneumoniae,*** and gram-negative bacilli which are resistant to usual antibiotics.

Major Pathogenic Pathways in Septic Shock

- **Trigger**: Most of septic shocks are triggered by bacteria or fungi that normally do not produce systemic disease in immunocompetent hosts.
- **Hallmark** of septic shock: It is **tissue hypoperfusion** due to **decrease in peripheral vascular resistance** as a result of **systemic vasodilation** and **pooling of blood in the periphery**. Cardiac output may be normal or even increased in early stages.
- **Initiation of shock**: Diverse microorganisms can cause septic shock indicates that a variety of microbial constituents can trigger the process of shock.
- **Major factors** contributing to the pathogenesis of septic shock (Fig. 7.12) are: 1) inflammatory and counter-inflammatory responses, 2) endothelial cell activation and injury, 3) organ dysfunction 4) metabolic abnormalities and 5) immune suppression.

1. **Inflammatory and counter-inflammatory responses: Microbial components** can **activate innate immune responses.**

   Innate immunity: Several substances derived from microorganisms recognize and are activate cells (e.g. macrophages, neutrophils, dendritic cells, endothelial cells) and soluble components of the innate immune system (e.g. complement). Once activated, these cells and factors of innate immune system initiate a number of inflammatory responses to

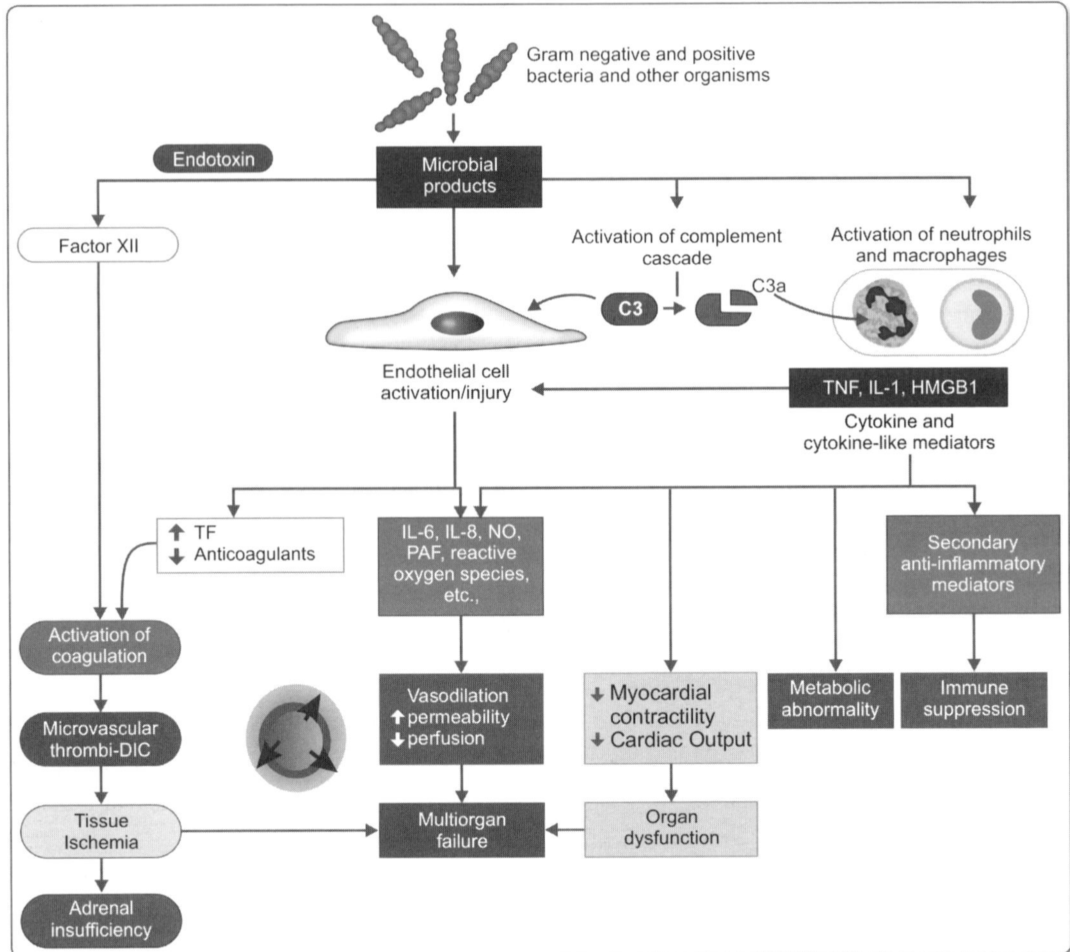

Fig. 7.12: Pathogenesis of septic shock. Microbial products initiate endothelial cell activation/injury activates endothelial cells, complement activation, activation of neutrophils and macrophages, factor XII. These initiating events lead to end-stage multiorgan failure.

Abbreviation: DIC—disseminated intravascular coagulation; HMGB1—high mobility group box 1 protein; NO—nitric oxide; PAF—platelet activating factor; TF—tissue factor.

produce septic shock and multiorgan dysfunction. Its activation leads to **production of proinflammatory mediators** which **produces endothelial cell activation/injury**.

- **Triggering of innate immune response**: **Leukocytes** (neutrophils and macrophages) and other cells of the innate immune system express pathogen receptors (e.g. toll-like receptor-TLR), which recognize a variety of microbe-derived substances containing pathogen-associated molecular patterns (PAMPs). Activation of these receptors **triggers innate immune response**.
- **Production of inflammatory mediators by** activated inflammatory cells:
  i. Proinflammatory cytokines: **TNF-α**, **IL-1**, IFN-γ, IL-12, and IL-18.
  ii. Cytokine-like mediators: for example, **high-mobility group box-1 protein (HMGB-1)**.
  iii. **Other mediators: Reactive oxygen species,** prostaglandins and platelet activating factor (**PAF**).

- **Effect of inflammatory mediators**: The inflammatory mediators induce endothelial cells (and other cell types) to upregulate adhesion molecule expression and further stimulate cytokine and chemokine production.

Activation of the complement cascade: Microbial components can also activate complement system and its components **have proinflammatory effect**: anaphylatoxins (C3a, C5a), chemotactic fragments (C5a), and opsonins (C3b). The hyperinflammatory state initiated by sepsis also activates counter-regulatory immunosuppressive mechanisms. This may involve both innate and adaptive immune cells. Thus, during the clinical course patients with septic shock may oscillate between hyperinflammatory and immunosuppressed states.

2. **Endothelial cell activation and injury:**

   Endothelial cell activation/injury is caused by either **microbial constituents or leukocyte-derived inflammatory mediators.**

   Sequelae of endothelial activation/injury

   a. **Activation of coagulation system and thrombosis**: Septic shock activates the coagulation system → forms **fibrin-rich thrombi in small vessels** → lead to the **hypoperfusion** of tissues throughout the body. It **produces dangerous complication DIC** in about 50% of septic patients.

      Factors activating coagulation system in sepsis:

      - **Increased production of tissue factor (TF) through endothelial injury** by pro-inflammatory cytokines (e.g. IL-6).
      - **Decreased production of anticoagulant factors**: These include tissue factor pathway inhibitor, antithrombin, thrombomodulin, and protein C and S.

   b. **Increased vascular permeability:** The proinflammatory state and endothelial cell activation associated with sepsis produces widespread vascular leakage and tissue edema. This decreases both delivery of nutrient and waste removal.

   c. **Vasodilation:** It is due to nitric oxide (NO) and vasoactive inflammatory mediators.

      - NO**:** It is produced due to increased expression of nitric oxide synthetase.
      - **Vasoactive inflammatory mediators:** These include C3a, C5a, and PAF.

The **systemic vasodilation and pooling of blood in the periphery** produces **hypotension** and **decreased perfusion of tissue (hypoperfusion).** This leads to **dysfunction of multiple organs**.

3. **Organ dysfunction**
   - **Decrease supply of oxygen and nutrients to the tissues**: Due to systemic hypotension, interstitial edema, and thrombi in the small vessels.
   - **Decreased contractibility of myocardium and cardiac output:** It is due to increased levels of cytokines and secondary mediators. This along with increased vascular permeability and endothelial injury can lead to the **adult respiratory distress syndrome**.
   - **Multiorgan failure:** It affects, particularly the **kidneys**, **liver**, **lungs**, and **heart**.

4. **Metabolic abnormalities:** These may be observed in patients with septic shock.
   - **Insulin resistance**: It is due to the action of proinflammatory cytokines.
   - **Hyperglycemia**: It is due to gluconeogenesis stimulated by cytokines such as TNF and **IL-1, stress-induced hormones** (such as glucagon, growth hormone, and glucocorticoids), and catecholamines. Hyperglycemia suppresses bactericidal activity of neutrophil.

- **Decreased glucocorticoid production:**
  - Initially, there is increased glucocorticoid production, and is later followed by decreased production due to adrenal insufficiency.
  - **Adrenal necrosis may also develop due to DIC (Waterhouse-Friderichsen syndrome).**
5. **Immune suppression:** It occurs in patients with septic shock. It is probably **due to**:
   - **Production of anti-inflammatory mediators** (e.g. soluble TNF receptor, IL-1 receptor antagonist, and IL-10).
   - **Widespread apoptosis of lymphocytes.**

Stages of Shock

Q. Describe 3 different stages of shock.

Shock is a progressive disorder, which if not treated, leads to death. It can be divided into three phases.

1. **Nonprogressive (compensated/reversible) phase**: During the initial phase, homeostatic compensatory mechanisms **redistribute the blood supply** in such a way that the effective **blood supply to the vital organs is maintained**. This is achieved by neurohumoral mechanisms, which try to maintain cardiac output and blood pressure.

   Compensatory changes: The neurohumoral mechanism produces the following compensatory changes:
   - **Widespread vasoconstriction** except vital organs. **Coronary and cerebral vessels** usually **maintain relatively normal blood flow, and oxygen delivery**. Cutaneous vasoconstriction → produces the coolness and pallor of the skin.
   - **Fluid conservation by kidney**.
   - **Tachycardia**.
2. **Progressive phase**
   - **If the underlying causes are not corrected**, shock **passes to the progressive phase**.
   - Characterized by **widespread tissue hypoperfusion** and **hypoxia** → intracellular aerobic respiration replaced by **anaerobic glycolysis** → **increased** production of **lactic acid** → metabolic **lactic acidosis** → **decreases** the tissue **pH** → dilatation of arterioles → peripheral **pooling of blood into the microcirculation** → **decreases** the **cardiac output** → produces **anoxic injury** to endothelial cell → favors development of **DIC** → widespread tissue hypoxia and **damage of vital organs**.
3. **Irreversible phase**:
   - **Without intervention, the shock eventually** enters an **irreversible stage**.
   - At this phase, **cellular and tissue injury is so severe** that even if the hemodynamic defects are corrected, **survival is not possible**.
   - Widespread cell injury results in leakage of lysosomal enzymes, which aggravate the shock state.
   - **Myocardial contractile function worsens** partly due to nitric oxide synthesis.
   - If ischemic intestine allows microbes from the intestinal flora to enter into the circulation it. This may lead to **superimposed bacteremic shock.**
   - The patient develops **acute tubular necrosis** and results in death.

Q. Describe the morphological changes in various organs in shock.

Q. Mention renal changes in shock.

Q. Write short note on lung changes in shock/diffuse alveolar damage.

Morphology (Table 7.8)

Changes in Cardiogenic or Hypovolemic Shock:

These are mainly due to hypoxic injury. Morphological changes are particularly evident in adrenals, kidneys, lungs, brain, heart, and gastrointestinal tract.

- **Adrenal**:
  - **Lipid depletion in cortical cell:** It is due to conversion of the relatively inactive vacuolated cells to metabolically active cells. The active cells utilize stored lipids for the synthesis of steroids.
  - **Focal hemorrhage:** It occurs in the inner cortex of adrenal in **severe** shock.
  - **Massive hemorrhagic necrosis** of the entire adrenal gland is found in the Waterhouse-Friderichsen **syndrome**, which is **associated with severe meningococcal septicemia**.
- **Kidney: Acute tubular necrosis** (acute renal failure) is a major complication of shock.
  - **Gross:** Kidney is **enlarged, swollen**, **congested**, and the **cortex may appear pale**. Cut section shows blood pooling in the outer region of the medulla.
  - **Microscopy:**
    - **Tubules:** Dilation of the proximal tubules and **focal necrosis of tubular epithelial cells**. Frequently, the tubular lumen may show **pigmented casts** formed due to leakage of hemoglobin or myoglobin.
    - **Interstitium**: It shows **edema** and **mononuclear cells** in the interstitium and within tubules.
- **Lungs**
  - Lungs are relatively resistant to hypoxic injury and are usually not affected in pure hypovolemic shock.
  - However, when shock is due to bacterial sepsis or trauma, it shows **diffuse alveolar damage** which can leads to acute respiratory distress syndrome (ARDS) also known as shock lung.
  - **Gross:** The lung is **firm and congested. Cut surface** shows **oozing out** of **frothy fluid.**
  - **Microscopy:**
    - **Edema:** It first develops around peribronchial **interstitial** connective tissue and later in the **alveoli**.
    - **Necrosis**: Endothelial and alveolar epithelial cells undergo necrosis and leads to formation of **intravascular microthrombi**.
    - **Hyaline membrane**: It is usually seen lining the alveolar surface. It may also line alveolar ducts and terminal bronchioles.
- **Heart**
  - **Gross:** It shows **petechial hemorrhages** in the epicardium and endocardium.
  - **Microscopy**: **Necrosis** of the myocardium is seen which may range from minute focus to large areas of necrosis. Prominent **contraction bands** are seen by light microscopy.
- **Liver**
  - **Gross:** Liver is enlarged. Cut section shows a **mottled** (blotched) appearance due to marked pooling of blood in the centrilobular region.
  - **Microscopy**: The centrilobular region of the liver shows **congestion and necrosis.**
- **Brain**: Encephalopathy (ischemic or septic) and cortical necrosis.
- **Gastrointestinal tract**: Shock produces **diffuse gastrointestinal hemorrhage. Erosions of the gastric mucosa** and superficial **ischemic necrosis** in the intestine lead to gastrointestinal bleeding.

Changes in Septic Shock

- Septic shock can lead to **DIC** which is characterized by **widespread** formation of fibrin-rich **microthrombi**, particularly in the brain, heart, lungs, kidney, adrenal glands, and gastrointestinal tract.
- The utilization of platelets and coagulation factors in DIC produces **bleeding manifestations**. It may show **petechial hemorrhages** on serosal surface and the skin.

Table 7.8: Summary of main morphological features of shock

Organ	Changes
Adrenal	Lipid depletion in the cortical cells
Kidney	Acute tubular necrosis
Lungs	Relatively resistant to hypoxic injury. However, in septic shock shows diffuse alveolar damage (shock lung) with hyaline membrane
Heart	Coagulative necrosis and contraction band necrosis
Liver	Congestion and necrosis of centrilobular region of the liver
Brain	Encephalopathy (ischemic or septic) and cortical necrosis
Gastrointestinal tract	Diffuse gastrointestinal hemorrhage. Erosions of the gastric mucosa and superficial ischemic necrosis in the intestine

Clinical Consequences

Q. Write short note on clinical consequences (end result) of shock

The clinical features of shock depend on the cause.

- **Hypovolemic and cardiogenic shock**: Usually, present with features of hypotension and hypoperfusion. The features include **altered sensorium, cyanosis, oliguria, weak rapid pulse, tachypnea**, and **cool, clammy extremities**.
- **Septic shock:** The **skin initially may be warm and flushed** because of peripheral vasodilation.

The initial underlying cause that precipitated the shock may be life threatening (e.g. myocardial infarct, severe hemorrhage, or sepsis). Later, the organ dysfunction involving **cardiac, cerebral, and pulmonary** function worsen the situation. The **electrolyte disturbances and metabolic acidosis** may further exacerbate the situation.

Patients who survive the initial complications may develop **renal insufficiency** characterized by a progressive decrease in urine output and severe fluid and electrolyte imbalances.

Prognosis

The prognosis depends on the cause and duration of shock.

- Patients with hypovolemic shock may survive with appropriate management.
- Septic shock, or cardiogenic shock associated with massive myocardial infarction, usually have high mortality rate.

Chapter 8

Nutritional Disorders

Chapter Outline

- Common vitamin deficiencies
- Fat-soluble vitamins
- Water-soluble vitamins-vitamin B complex

COMMON VITAMIN DEFICIENCIES

Vitamins are vital organic substances required in limited amounts with key roles in certain metabolic pathways.

Categories

Thirteen vitamins are necessary for health and are categorized as:

- **Fat soluble vitamins**: These include A, D, E, and K. Fat-soluble vitamins are stored in the body, but their absorption may be poor in fat malabsorption disorders or in disturbances of digestive functions.
- **Water-soluble vitamins:** All other vitamins (vitamins of the B complex group and vitamin C).

Sources

- Endogenous: Few vitamins can be synthesized endogenously. Examples include vitamin D from precursor steroids, vitamin K and biotin by the intestinal microflora, and niacin from tryptophan (essential amino acid).
- Exogenous: Dietary supply of all vitamins is essential for health.

Deficiency

A deficiency of vitamins may be:

- Primary: Deficient intake in the diet.
- Secondary: Due to disturbances in intestinal absorption, transport in the blood, tissue storage, or metabolic conversion.

FAT-SOLUBLE VITAMINS

Q. List vitamin A deficiency states

Q. Write short note on clinical features of vitamin A deficiency

Vitamin A (retinol)

Vitamin A (retinol) is part of the family of retinoids which is present in food and the body as esters combined with long chain fatty acids.

- **Vitamin A:** It is the name given to a group of related compounds and include:
  - **Retinol** (vitamin A alcohol): It is the chemical name given to vitamin A. It is the transport form and, as retinol ester, also the storage form.
  - **Retinal** (vitamin A aldehyde)
  - **Retinoic acid** (vitamin A acid)
- **Retinoids:** It is the generic term that encompasses vitamin A in its various forms and both natural and synthetic chemicals that are structurally related to vitamin A, but may not necessarily have vitamin A-like biologic activity.

Sources

- **Animal derived foods**: Pre-formed retinol is found only in foods of animal origin. The richest food source is liver, but it is also found in fish, milk, eggs, butter, and cheese.
- **Yellow and green leafy vegetables**: Vitamin A can also be derived from carotenoids (most important is β-carotene) which are provitamins that contribute approximately 30% of the vitamin A in human diets. Beta-carotene is the main carotenoid found in green vegetables, carrots, squash, spinach and other yellow and red fruits. They can be converted to active vitamin A in the body. Other carotenoids, lycopene and lutein, are of little quantitative importance.

Functions

Vitamin A has several metabolic roles. The main functions of vitamin A in human are as follows:

- **Maintenance of normal vision***:* It is one of the **major functions of vitamin A.** The visual process involves vitamin A-containing pigments. Retinaldehyde in its *cis* form is found in the opsin proteins in the rods **(rhodopsin) and cones (iodopsin) of the retina. Light causes retinaldehyde to change to its *trans* isomer, and this leads to changes in membrane potentials that are transmitted via neurons from the retina to the brain.**
  - Rhodopsin: *11-cis retinaldehyde* is part of the photoreceptor complex in rods of the retina. It is the most light-sensitive pigment and is important in reduced light.
  - Iodopsins: It is responsive to specific colors in bright light.
- **Regulation of cell growth and differentiation:** It is one of the major functions of vitamin A. Retinol and retinoic acid are involved in the **control of proliferation and differentiation of epithelial cells**. Vitamin A and retinoids play an important role in the orderly differentiation of mucus-secreting epithelium. In vitamin A deficiency, mucus-secreting cells are replaced by keratin-producing cells and this process is known as **squamous metaplasia.**
- **Regulation of lipid metabolism**: It is a key regulator of fatty acid metabolism, including fatty acid oxidation in fat tissue and muscle, adipogenesis, and lipoprotein metabolism. Retinyl phosphate is a cofactor in the synthesis of most glycoproteins containing mannose.
- **Host resistance to infections:**
  - Advantages of vitamin A supplementation

    - **Reduces morbidity and mortality in diarrhea: Can reduce morbidity and mortality from some forms of diarrhea. This may be due to the maintenance and restoration of the integrity of the epithelium of the gut.**
    - **Improves clinical outcome in preschool children with measles.**
  - **Immune function**: Vitamin A has ability to stimulate the immune system. Retinoids are needed for normal growth, fetal development, fertility, hematopoiesis and immune function.
  - **Antioxidant**: Retinoids, β-carotene, and some related carotenoids act as photoprotective and antioxidant agents.
- Signal for appropriate morphogenesis in the developing embryo.

Uses

- Skin disorders: Retinoids are used for the treatment of skin disorders (e.g. severe acne and certain forms of psoriasis)
- Treatment of acute promyelocytic leukemia and childhood neuroblastoma.

Deficiency

Causes: Due to general undernutrition or as a secondary deficiency as a consequence of malabsorption of fats.

- In children: The stores of vitamin A are depleted by infections, and vitamin A absorption is poor in newborn infants.
- In adults: Malabsorption syndromes, such as celiac disease, Crohn disease, and colitis, may cause vitamin A deficiency (in conjunction with deficiency of other fat-soluble vitamins). Bariatric surgery and, in elderly, continuous use of mineral oil as a laxative may produce vitamin A deficiency.

Pathologic Effects (Clinical Features) of Vitamin A Deficiency (Fig. 8.1)

- **Effects in the eye:**
  - **Night blindness**: Vitamin A is a component of rhodopsin and other visual pigments. Hence, one of the earliest manifestations of vitamin A deficiency is impaired vision, particularly impaired adaptation to the dark *(night blindness)*.
  - **Xerophthalmia:** Vitamin A is necessary for maintaining the differentiation of epithelial cells. Persistent deficiency produces **epithelial metaplasia** and **keratinization**. In the eyes it produces keratinization of the cornea—**xerophthalmia** (dry eye). Initially, there is dryness of the conjunctiva (xerosis conjunctivae) because of the replacement of the normal lacrimal and mucus-secreting epithelium by keratinized epithelium. Subsequently, there is a buildup of keratin debris in small opaque plaques gives rise to characteristic **Bitot spots** that progresses to erosion of corneal surface, softening and destruction of the cornea (**keratomalacia**), scarring and irreversible blindness.
- **Effects on other epithelia**: The epithelium lining the upper respiratory passage and urinary tract also undergoes **squamous metaplasia**.
  - Upper respiratory tract: Loss of the mucociliary epithelium of the airways predisposes to secondary pulmonary infections.
  - Urinary tract: Desquamation of keratin debris in the urinary tract predisposes to renal and urinary bladder stones.
  - Skin: Hyperplasia and *hyperkeratinization of the epidermis* with plugging of the ducts of the adnexal glands may cause follicular or papular dermatosis.

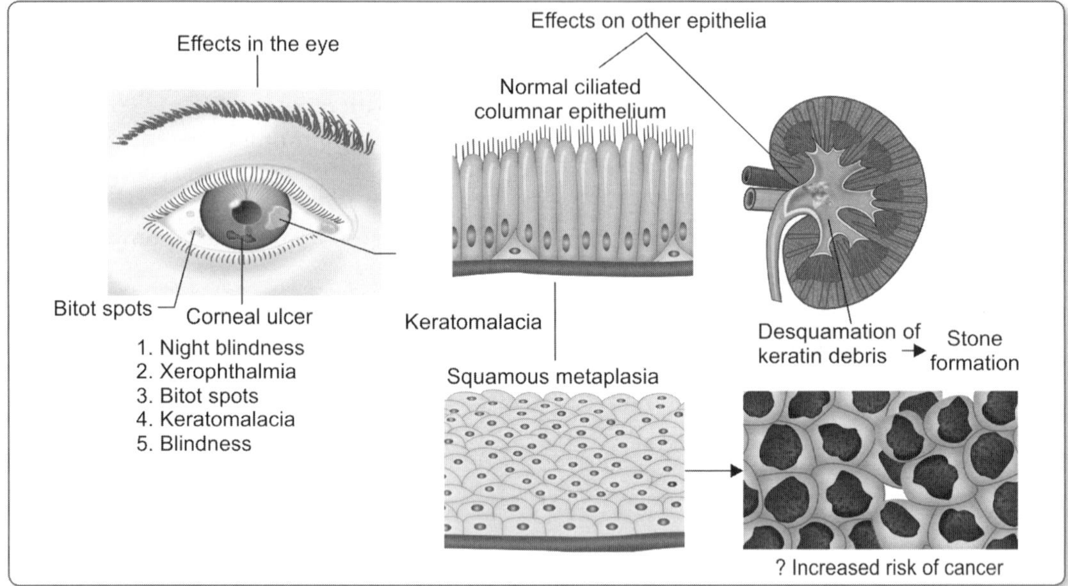

Fig. 8.1: Pathological effects of vitamin A deficiency

- **Immune deficiency**: It is responsible for higher mortality rates from common infections such as measles, pneumonia, and infectious diarrhea.
- Follicular hyperkeratosis.

Vitamin A Toxicity

- Both short- and long-term excesses of vitamin A may produce toxic effects.
- **Acute vitamin A toxicity**: It produces symptoms such as nausea, headache, dizziness, vomiting, skin desquamation, stupor, increased intracranial pressure and blurred vision. These symptoms may be confused with those of a brain tumor **(pseudotumor cerebri)**.
- **Chronic vitamin A toxicity**: It produces weight loss, anorexia, nausea, vomiting, and bone and joint pain. Retinoic acid stimulates osteoclast production and activity, leading to increased bone resorption and high risk of fractures. Repeated moderate or high doses of retinol can cause liver damage.
- **Retinol is teratogenic**: Synthetic retinoids should be avoided in pregnancy because of its teratogenic effects.

Vitamin D

Q. Write short note on vitamin D deficiency

Q. Write short note on rickets

Q, Write short note on osteomalacia

Q. Write short note on causes of vitamin D deficiency

- Vitamin D is a fat-soluble vitamin.
- It is required for the maintenance of adequate plasma levels of calcium and phosphorus to support metabolic functions, bone mineralization, and neuromuscular transmission.

Physiology

Vitamin D exists in 2 activated sterol forms.

1. Vitamin D3 (Cholecalciferol)
   - Produced in skin with direct sunlight, cod liver oil
   - Preferred form of supplementation
2. Vitamin D2 (Ergocalciferol)
   - Less effective as precursor to 1,25(OH)2-Vit D.

Sources

- **Endogenous synthesis:** About 80% of body's vitamin D is endogenously synthesized in the skin from a precursor, 7-dehydrocholesterol, by the action of solar or artificial UV light in the range of 290 to 315 nm (UVB radiation). This reaction synthesizes *cholecalciferol (vitamin D3).* However, dark skinned persons generally have a lower level of vitamin D production because of melanin pigmentation.
- **Exogenous source:** Dietary sources include deep-sea fish, fish-oils, plants, and grains, and their absorption depends on adequate intestinal fat absorption. In plants, vitamin D is present in a precursor form (ergosterol).

Metabolism of Vitamin D (Fig. 8.2)

- Main steps of vitamin D metabolism:
  - **Two sources of vitamin D**: (1) Photochemical synthesis of vitamin D from 7-dehydrocholesterol in the skin and (2) absorption of vitamin D from diet in the gut.
  - **Binding**: Vitamin D derived from both of the above mentioned sources bind to plasma α1-globulin *(D-binding protein or DBP)* and transported to the liver.
  - **Conversion**:
    - **In liver: Vitamin D (D_3) is converted into 25-hydroxycholecalciferol (25-OH-D) in the liver, by the action of 25-hydroxylases, including CYP27A1 and other CYPs.**
    - **In kidney: 25-OH-D is converted into** *1,25-dihydroxyvitamin D,* **[1α,25(OH)2D3] by the enzyme 1α-hydroxylase in the kidney.**

Functions

1,25-dihydroxyvitamin D mediates its biologic effects by binding to a member of the nuclear receptor superfamily, the vitamin D receptor (VDR). Vitamin D receptors for 1,25-dihydroxyvitamin D are present in most cells of the body.

1. **Regulation of plasma levels of calcium and phosphorus**: The main functions of 1,25-dihydroxyvitamin D on calcium and phosphorus homeostasis are:
   - **Stimulates intestinal absorption of calcium:** 1,25-dihydroxyvitamin D stimulates intestinal absorption of calcium in the duodenum through the interaction of 1,25-dihydroxyvitamin D with nuclear vitamin D receptor.
   - **Stimulates calcium reabsorption in the kidney:** 1,25-dihydroxyvitamin D increases calcium influx in distal tubules of the kidney.
   - **Interaction with PTH in the regulation of blood calcium**:
   - **Mineralization of bone**: Vitamin D plays a role in the mineralization of osteoid matrix and epiphyseal cartilage in both flat and long bones. Vitamin D stimulates osteoblasts to produce the calcium-binding protein osteocalcin, which is involved in the deposition of calcium during development of bone.

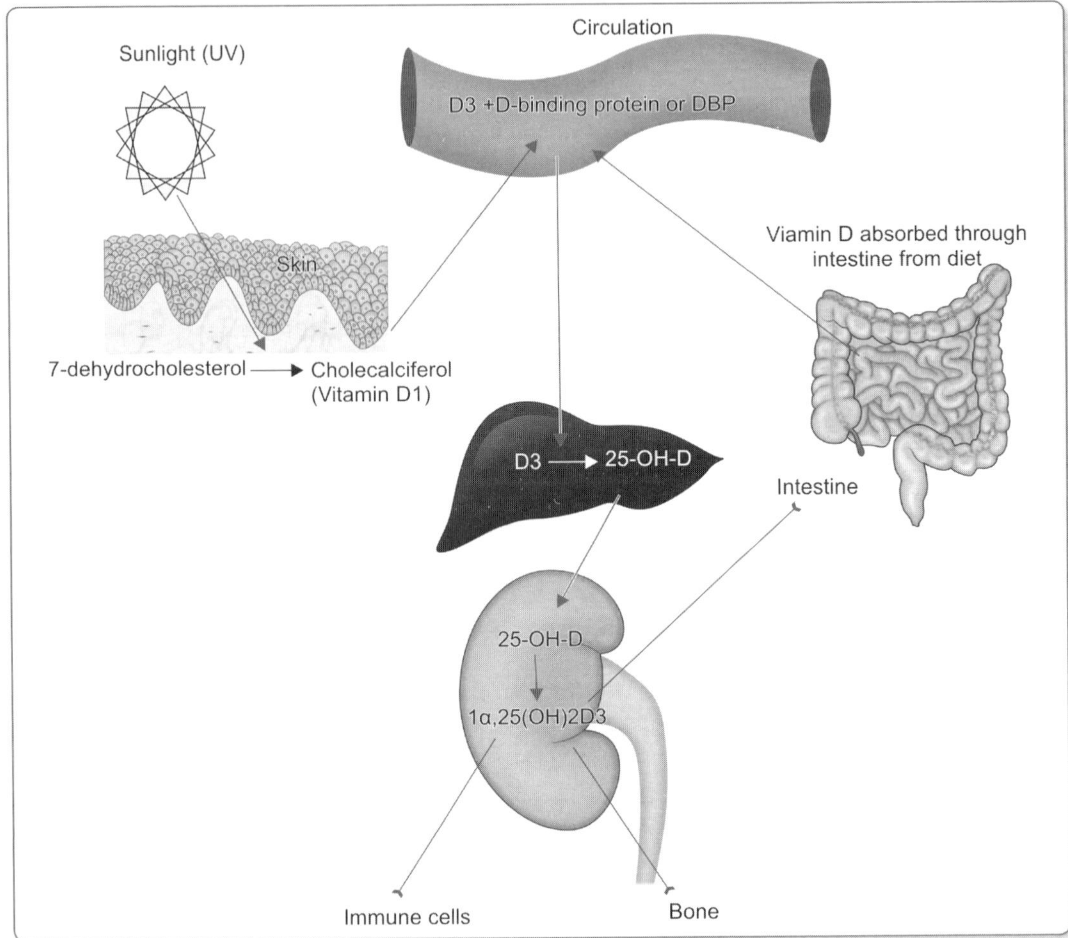

Fig. 8.2: Vitamin D synthesis and activation. Vitamin D is synthesized in the skin in response to ultraviolet radiation present in the sunlight and also is absorbed from the diet. It is then transported to the liver, where it undergoes 25-hydroxylation. 25(OH) D is the major circulating form of vitamin D. The final step in hormone activation, 1α-hydroxylation in the kidney

2. **Antiproliferative effects**: The VDR is expressed in the parathyroid gland, and $1,25(OH)_2D$ has an antiproliferative effect on parathyroid cells and it suppresses the transcription of the parathyroid hormone gene.
3. **Immunomodulatory:** Vitamin D is involved in the innate and adaptive immune system.

Deficiency

Causes

- Impaired cutaneous production due to limited exposure to sunlight
- Dietary absence: Diets deficient in calcium and vitamin D
- Malabsorption.

Milder forms of vitamin D deficiency is also called as **vitamin D insufficiency**, leads to an increased risk of bone loss and hip fractures in older adults.

Skeletal Effects of Vitamin D Deficiency

Rickets in Children (Fig. 8.3)

In children, before the closure of epiphyses, vitamin D deficiency causes retardation of growth associated with an expansion of the growth plate known as **rickets.** In the normal growth plate, there are three layers of chondrocytes namely (1) the reserve zone, (2) the proliferating zone, and (3) the hypertrophic zone. Rickets due to impaired vitamin D action is characterized by expansion of the hypertrophic chondrocyte layer. In vitamin D deficiency, the hypophosphatemia due to secondary hyperparathyroidism is responsible for the development of the rachitic growth plate.

Gross skeletal changes in rickets: It depends on the severity and duration of the vitamin D deficiency and also the stresses to which individual bones are subjected.

During the nonambulatory stage of infancy:

1. **Head:**
   - **Craniotabes:** The head and chest are subjected to the greatest stresses. The softened occipital bones become flattened, and the parietal bones buckle inward by pressure; with the release of the pressure, elastic recoil snaps the bones back into their original positions (craniotabes). The skull appears square and box-like. Delayed closure of anterior fontanelle.
   - **Frontal bossing:** Excess of osteoid produces **frontal bossing** and a **squared appearance to the head**.
2. **Chest**
   - **Rachitic rosary:** Overgrowth of cartilage or osteoid tissue at the costochondral junction causes deformation of the chest producing the **"rachitic rosary."**
   - **Pigeon breast/chest deformity:** The weakened metaphyseal areas of the ribs are subject to the pull of the respiratory muscles and thus bend inward. This creates anterior protrusion of the sternum producing **pigeon breast deformity** (pectus carinatum).
   - **Hrrison's sulcus/groove:** It is due to indrawing of ribs on inspiration.

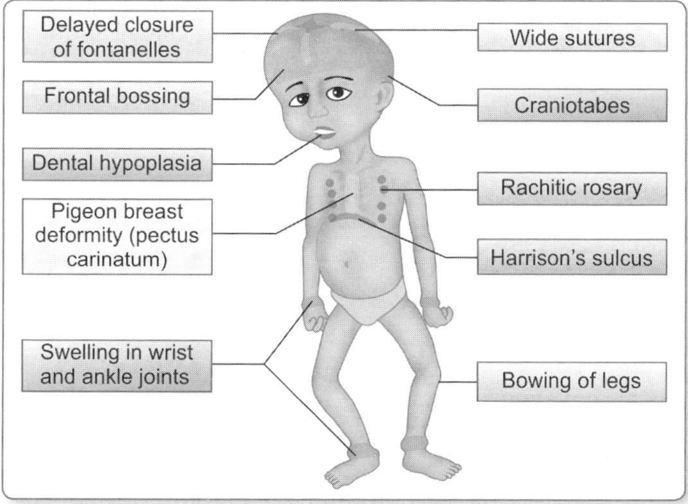

Fig. 8.3: Features of rickets

During the nonambulatory stage

- **Lumbar lordosis:** This occurs when an ambulating child develops rickets. It is characterized by deformities affecting the spine, pelvis, and tibia.
- **Bowing of the legs:** Due to affection of tibia.

Osteomalacia in Adults

Vitamin D deficiency in adults is accompanied by hypocalcemia and hypophosphatemia which result in impaired (hypo/under/inadequately) mineralization of bone matrix proteins, a condition known as osteomalacia. This hypomineralized bone matrix is biomechanically inferior (weak) to normal bone. This bone is prone to bowing of weight-bearing extremities and gross skeletal fractures or microfractures which are most likely to affect vertebral bodies and femoral necks.

Proximal Myopathy

It is observed in both in children and in adults with severe vitamin D deficiency. It is rapidly resolves by vitamin D treatment.

Hypocalcemic Tetany

Calcium is required for normal neural excitation and the relaxation of muscles. Hypocalcemic tetany is a convulsive state caused by an insufficient extracellular concentration of ionized calcium.

Non-skeletal Effects of Vitamin D

Vitamin D receptor is also present in various cells and tissues that are not involved in calcium and phosphorus homeostasis. Many cells such as macrophages, keratinocytes, and tissues such as breast, prostate, and colon can produce 1,25-dihydroxyvitamin D.

- Low levels of 1,25-dihydroxyvitamin D (<20 ng/mL) may increase in the incidence of cancers of colon, prostate, and breast cancers, but whether vitamin D supplement can reduce cancer risk has not known.

Vitamin D Toxicity

Prolonged exposure to normal sunlight does not produce an excess of vitamin D, but oral administration of mega doses of vitamin can lead to hypervitaminosis.

- In children: Hypervitaminosis D may cause metastatic calcifications of soft tissues (e.g. kidney).
- In adults: It can cause bone pain and hypercalcemia. Insufficiently large doses of vitamin D are a potent rodenticide.

Vitamin C (Ascorbic Acid)

Q. Write short note on clinical features of vitamin C deficiency

Q. Write short note on scurvy

It is a water-soluble vitamin.

Functions

- **Hydroxylation of procollagen**: It is necessary for the formation of collagen from procollagen. It is involved in the hydroxylation of proline and lysine in procollagen to hydroxyproline and hydroxylysine in mature collagen.
- **Antioxidant properties:** Ascorbic acid is the most active powerful reducing agent controlling the redox potential within cells. Vitamin C can scavenge free radicals directly and can act indirectly by regenerating the antioxidant form of vitamin E.

- It is involved in intracellular electron transfer.
- Promotion of nonheme iron absorption.

Sources

- Ascorbic acid is not synthesized endogenously in humans; therefore, we depend entirely on the diet for this vitamin.
- Vitamin C is present in milk and some animal products (liver, fish).
- Vitamin C is present in all fresh fruit and vegetables.
- Unfortunately, ascorbic acid is very easily destroyed by heat (e.g. cooking), increased pH, exposure to copper or alkalis and light.
- It is very easily soluble in water; hence traditional cooking methods reduce or eliminate it.

Deficiency

Causes

- Ascorbic acid is present in abundance in many foods. Hence, it is rare.
- Rarely, it may occur as a secondary deficiency, particularly among older persons who live alone, and chronic alcoholics.
- Occasionally, scurvy occurs in patients undergoing peritoneal dialysis and hemodialysis. It may develop in infants who are maintained on formulas of evaporated milk without supplementation of vitamin C.

Effects of deficiency (Fig. 8.4)

Scurvy: It is characterized by:

- **Bone disease**: More common in growing children. It is characterized by deranged formation of osteoid matrix.
- **Hemorrhages:** Marked tendency to bleed into the skin (petechiae, ecchymoses, perifollicular hemorrhages), bleeding into muscles, joints and underneath peritoneum.
- **Delayed wound healing**
- **Anemia**
- **Gums**: Inflamed and bleeding gums.

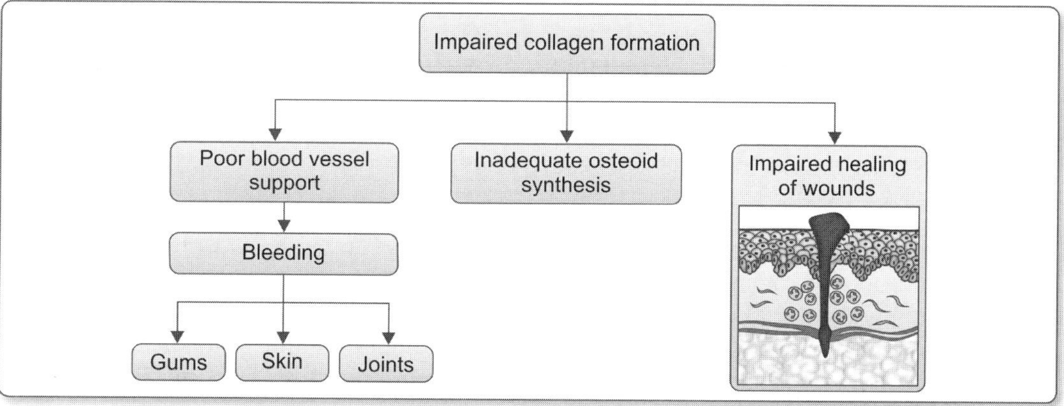

Fig. 8.4: Major consequences of vitamin C deficiency caused by impaired formation of collagen

Vitamin C Excess

- High/mega doses (1–2 g daily) vitamin C probably improves immune function (including prevention/resistance to the common cold). However, slight relief of cold is probably due to the mild antihistamine action of vitamin C.
- Vitamin C supplements may prevent atherosclerosis and cancer.

Vitamin E

Vitamin E is a collective name for 8 stereoisomers of tocopherols and tocotrienols. The most important dietary form is α-tocopherol.

Functions

- **Antioxidant:** It prevents oxidation of low-density lipoproteins (LDLs) and polyunsaturated fatty acids in cell membranes by free radicals. Other antioxidants (e.g. vitamin C, glutathione) and enzymes maintain vitamin E in a reduced state. Acts in conjunction with other antioxidants such as selenium.
- It helps maintain cell membrane structure.
- It affects DNA synthesis and cell signaling.
- Anti-inflammatory: Vitamin E also inhibits prostaglandin synthesis and the activities of protein kinase C and phospholipase A_2.
- Immune systems.

Sources

- Vitamin E is high in sunflower oil, safflower oil, and wheat germ oil; γ-tocotrienols are notably present in soybean and corn oils. Vitamin E is also present in meats, nuts, and cereal grains, and small amounts are present in fruits and vegetables.

Deficiency

- Dietary deficiency of vitamin E is very rare.
- Vitamin E deficiency is seen in only in premature infants and in severe and prolonged malabsorption diseases, such as celiac disease, or after small-intestinal resection.
- It can cause mild hemolytic anemias, ataxia and visual scotomas.

Vitamin K

Forms of vitamin K: There are two natural forms: vitamin K1 (phylloquinone) derived from vegetable (green leafy vegetables such as kale and spinach) and animal sources (liver), and vitamin K_2 (menaquinone) which is synthesized by bacterial flora in the colon and in hepatic tissue. Phylloquinone can be converted to menaquinone in some organs.

Functions

- **Coagulation**: Vitamin K is a co-factor for carboxylation of glutamic acid which is necessary for the production of carboxyglutamate (gla). Gla residues are found in four of the coagulation factor proteins (II, VII, IX and X). Thus it is involved in coagulation process.
- **Others:** Other important gla proteins include osteocalcin (in bone) and matrix gla protein (vascular smooth muscle) that are important in mineralization of bone. However, the importance of vitamin K for mineralization of bone and prevention of vascular calcification is unknown.

Deficiency

Causes

- In adults:
  - **Chronic small-intestinal disease**: e.g. celiac disease, Crohn's disease
  - **Obstruction of biliary tracts**: In obstructive jaundice, dietary vitamin K is not absorbed and it is necessary to administer the vitamin in parenteral form before surgery.
  - After small-bowel resection.
  - **Broad-spectrum antibiotics**: They can precipitate vitamin K deficiency by reducing gut bacteria, which synthesize menaquinones, and by inhibiting the metabolism of vitamin K.
  - **Warfarin and related anticoagulants**: Warfarin-type drugs prevent the conversion of vitamin K to its active hydroquinone form.
- **Deficiency in newborn**: It is because of (1) low fat stores, (2) low breast milk levels of vitamin K, (3) sterility of the infantile intestinal tract, (4) liver immaturity, and (5) poor placental transport.

Effects of Deficiency

- Vitamin K deficiency leads to **delayed coagulation and bleeding**. Hence, the symptoms of vitamin K deficiency are due to hemorrhage.
- **Newborn**: In breast-fed newborns it may cause **hemorrhagic disease of the newborn**. Intracranial, gastrointestinal and skin bleeding, can occur in vitamin K-deficient infants 1–7 days after birth. Thus, vitamin K (1 mg IM) is given routinely to newborn babies to prevent hemorrhagic disease.

WATER-SOLUBLE VITAMINS-VITAMIN B COMPLEX

Thiamine (Vitamin B_1)

- Thiamine was the first B complex vitamin identified and is referred to as vitamin B_1.

Functions

- Thiamine functions as a coenzyme in many α-ketoacid decarboxylation and transketolation reactions. Inadequate thiamin results in inadequate adenosine triphosphate synthesis and abnormal carbohydrate metabolism, respectively.
- May have an additional role in neuronal conduction.

Sources

- Yeast, organ meat, pork, legumes, beef, whole grains, and nuts.
- Milled rice and grains contain little or no thiamine. Thus, thiamine deficiency is more common in individuals who rely heavily on a rice-based diet.
- Tea, coffee (regular and decaffeinated), raw fish, and shellfish contain enzyme thiaminases, which can destroy thiamine. Thus, drinking large amounts of tea or coffee lower thiamine body stores.

Deficiency

Causes

- Most dietary deficiency of thiamine is due to **poor dietary intake**. Alcoholism, chronic renal dialysis and chronic illnesses such as cancer are common precipitant factors. High carbohydrate intake increases need for B1. Alcohol interferes with the absorption of thiamine and with the synthesis of thiamine pyrophosphate.

- Women with prolonged hyperemesis gravidarum. Maternal thiamine deficiency can lead to infantile beriberi in breast-fed children
- Anorexia
- Patients
  - with overall poor nutritional status on parenteral glucose
  - after bariatric bypass surgery
  - on chronic diuretic therapy due to increased urinary thiamine losses.

Effects of Deficiency

- **Mild deficiency**: Thiamine deficiency in its early stage is characterized by irritability, decrease in short-term memory, anorexia, fatigue, and headaches.
- **More severe deficiency-beriberi:** Prolonged thiamine deficiency causes beriberi. It is classically categorized as wet or dry or combination of two. It is the classic deficiency syndrome observed in individuals consuming polished rice diet. It shows combinations of peripheral neuropathy, cardiovascular dysfunction, and cerebral dysfunction.
  - Peripheral neuropathy: Complain of pain and paresthesia associated with diminished reflexes. The neuropathy affects the legs most markedly, and these patients have difficulty rising from a squatting position.
  - Cardiovascular dysfunction ("wet beriberi"): Congestive heart failure and low peripheral vascular resistance.
  - Cerebrovascular dysfunction:
    - **Wernicke's encephalopathy:** Acute appearance of nystagmus, ophthalmoplegia, ataxia and psychotic symptoms. The acute symptoms are reversible when treated with thiamine. However, if untreated, they may be followed by a prolonged and largely irreversible condition, called Korsakoff syndrome.
    - **Korsakoff syndrome:** Characterized clinically by hallucinations, disturbances of short-term memory, and confabulation. The syndrome is common in chronic alcoholics but may also be seen with thiamine deficiency resulting from gastric disorders, including carcinoma, chronic gastritis, or persistent vomiting.
- *Wet beriberi* presents primarily with cardiovascular symptoms.
- *Dry beriberi* presents with a symmetric peripheral neuropathy of the motor and sensory systems with diminished reflexes.

Riboflavin (Vitamin B_2)

- It is important for the metabolism of fat, carbohydrate, and protein. It also plays a role in drug and steroid metabolism, including detoxification reactions.
- Serves as a coenzyme for a diverse array of biochemical reactions and as an electron donor.
- The primary coenzymatic forms of riboflavin are flavin mononucleotide (FMN) and flavin adenine dinucleotide (FAD) and are known as *flavoenzymes* (e.g. succinic acid dehydrogenase, monoamine oxidase, glutathione reductase).

Sources

- Important dietary sources of riboflavin include milk, other dairy products and enriched breads and cereals.
- Other sources: Lean meat, fish, eggs, broccoli, and legumes.
- Riboflavin is extremely sensitive to light.

Deficiency

Causes: Almost always is due to dietary deficiency and is usually seen in conjunction with deficiencies of other B vitamins.

Effects of Deficiency

- Nonspecific and mainly manifests as **lesions of the mucocutaneous surfaces of the mouth and skin.** These include **hyperemia and edema of nasopharyngeal mucosa, cheilosis, angular stomatitis, glossitis and seborrheic dermatitis.** Other lesions include corneal vascularization, normochromic-normocytic anemia, and personality changes.

Niacin (Vitamin B_3)

- The term *niacin* refers to nicotinic acid and the corresponding amide, nicotinamide and their biologically active derivatives.
- Nicotinic acid and nicotinamide serve as precursors of two coenzymes, nicotinamide adenine dinucleotide (NAD) and NAD phosphate (NADP), which are important in numerous oxidation and reduction reactions.
- NAD and NADP are active in adenine diphosphate-ribose transfer reactions involved in DNA repair and calcium mobilization.

Sources

- Nicotinic acid and nicotinamide are absorbed from the stomach and small intestine. Sources of niacin include beans, milk, meat, and eggs. The essential amino acid tryptophan is a precursor of niacin.

Deficiency

Pellagra

- Niacin deficiency causes **pellagra.** It is found mostly in populations in which corn is the major source of energy in parts of China, Africa, and India.
- Early symptoms: Loss of appetite, generalized weakness and irritability, abdominal pain, and vomiting.
- Early signs: Bright red glossitis, stomatitis, vaginitis, esophagitis, vertigo, and burning dysesthesias
- Advanced stages: Characteristic skin rash develops that is pigmented and scaling that develops in in skin areas exposed to sunlight. This rash is known as *Casal's necklace* because it forms a ring around the neck.
- Four Ds: **D**iarrhea (in part due to proctitis and in part due to malabsorption), **d**epression, seizures, and **d**ementia (or associated symptoms of anxiety or insomnia) leading to **d**eath and **d**ermatitis, are part of the pellagra syndrome.

Pyridoxine (Vitamin B_6)

- *Vitamin B_6* refers to several derivatives of pyridine that include pyridoxine (PN), pyridoxal (PL), and pyridoxamine (PM), which are interconvertible in the body. The coenzymatic forms are pyridoxal-5-phosphate (PLP) and pyridoxamine-5-phosphate (PMP). 5'-Pyridoxal phosphate (PLP) is a cofactor for more than 100 enzymes involved in amino acid metabolism.
- Vitamin B_6 is also involved in synthesis of heme and many neurotransmitters and in the metabolism of glycogen, lipids, steroids, sphingoid bases, and several vitamins, including the synthesis of niacin from tryptophan.

Sources

- Plants contain vitamin B_6 in the form of pyridoxine.
- Animal tissues contain PLP and pyridoxamine phosphate.
- Rich food sources: Legumes, nuts, wheat bran, and meat.

Deficiency

- Deficiency usually seen in conjunction with other water-soluble vitamin deficiencies.
- Certain medications, such as isoniazid, cycloserine, penicillamine, l-dopa, ethanol, and theophylline can inhibit B_6 metabolism. Pyridoxine should be given concurrently with isoniazid to avoid neuropathy. Because vitamin B_6 interferes with the action of l-dopa, it should not be given with this drug.

Effects of Deficiency

- Stomatitis, angular cheilosis, glossitis, irritability, depression, and confusion occur in moderate to severe depletion
- Microcytic hypochromic anemia is due to diminished hemoglobin synthesis, since the first enzyme involved in heme biosynthesis. It may also produce normochromic-normocytic anemia.
- In infants: diarrhea, seizures/convulsions, and anemia.
- Severe vitamin B_6 deficiency: Peripheral neuropathy and abnormal electroencephalograms.

Vitamin B_{12}

A group of closely related cobalamine compounds.

Sources

- Microorganisms are the ultimate source of all naturally occurring vitamin B_{12}.
- Human beings are totally dependent on animal products in the diet for vitamin B_{12} requirement. Vitamin B_{12} is not present in food from vegetable sources. Therefore, strict vegetarians do not get an adequate quantity of vitamin B_{12}. A balanced diet (not rigid vegetarian!) contains significantly large amounts of vitamin B_{12} which accumulates in the body (liver) and is enough for several years. Due to this adequate storage, if there is any dietary deficiency or malabsorption of vitamin B_{12}, its clinical manifestations appear only after about 2 to 4 years. Vitamin B_{12} is a complex compound known as cobalamin.

Functions

Vitamin B_{12} is indirectly required for DNA synthesis in various metabolic steps and its deficiency impairs DNA synthesis. The two active coenzyme forms are deoxyadenosylcobalamin and methylcobalamin.

- Methylcobalamin is the main form of vitamin B_{12} in plasma, and is an essential coenzyme for conversion of homocysteine to methionine and formation of tetrahydrofolate (THF) from methyl THF.
- Vitamin B_{12} is also required for conversion of methylmalonyl CoA to succinyl malonyl CoA.

Deficiency

Causes (refer Table 12.5)

- Dietary inadequacy is a rare cause of deficiency except in strict vegetarians.
- Mostly due to loss of intestinal absorption. These include pernicious anemia, pancreatic insufficiency, atrophic gastritis, small bowel bacterial overgrowth, or ileal disease.

Effects of Deficiency

- Hematological changes: Megaloblastic anemia (refer chapter 12) and megaloblastic changes in other epithelia.
- Neurologic complications: Demyelination of peripheral nerves, posterior and lateral columns of spinal cord, and nerves within the brain. Altered mentation, depression, and psychoses occur.

Folic Acid

- Folates are a group of related pterin compounds. The fully oxidized form is called folic acid, which is not found in nature but is the pharmacologic form of the vitamin.

Source

- Entirely dependent on dietary sources. Green vegetables, yeast, legumes, fruits and animal proteins are the richest sources and most normal diets contain sufficient amounts of folic acid.
- The folic acid in these foods is largely in the form of polyglutamates. Polyglutamates are sensitive to heat (thermolabile); boiling, steaming or frying and cooking destroys most of the folic acid.

Functions

- All folate functions relate to its ability to transfer one-carbon groups.
- The active form of folic acid is tetrahydrofolate [THF] which is the biologic "middleman" involved in metabolic processes which synthesize DNA.

Deficiency

Causes (refer Table 12.5)

Effects of Deficiency

Megaloblastic anemia (refer chapter 12), diarrhea.

Vitamins and their principal clinical manifestations are summarized in Table 8.1.

Table 8.1: Vitamins and their principal clinical manifestations

Vitamin	Clinical finding
Thiamine	**Beriberi** (dry or wet): neuropathy, muscle weakness and wasting, cardiomegaly, edema, ophthalmoplegia, confabulation
Riboflavin	Magenta tongue (glossitis), angular stomatitis, seborrhea, cheilosis, and seborrheic dermatitis
Niacin	**Pellagra**: Pigmented rash of sun-exposed areas, bright red tongue, diarrhea, apathy, memory loss, disorientation
Vitamin B_6	Seborrhea, glossitis, convulsions, neuropathy, depression, confusion, anemia
Folate	Megaloblastic anemia, atrophic glossitis
Vitamin B_{12}	Megaloblastic anemia, loss of vibratory and position sense, abnormal gait, dementia
Vitamin C	Scurvy: Petechiae, ecchymosis, inflamed and bleeding gums, joint effusion, poor wound healing, fatigue
Vitamin A	Xerophthalmia, night blindness, Bitot's spots, follicular hyperkeratosis, immune dysfunction
Vitamin D	Rickets in children: Skeletal deformation, rachitic rosary, bowed legs Osteomalacia in adults
Vitamin E	Peripheral neuropathy, spinocerebellar ataxia, skeletal muscle atrophy, retinopathy
Vitamin K	Elevated prothrombin time, bleeding

Chapter 9

Hypertension

Chapter Outline

- Hypertension

HYPERTENSION

WHO definition of hypertension: Hypertension is defined as **systolic** pressure **above 160 mm Hg and/or diastolic** pressure **above 90.**

Causes of Hypertension (Table 9.1)

- **Primary/essential/idiopathic** hypertension: It constitutes about 95% of cases.
- **Secondary** hypertension: It forms about 5% of cases and there is an identifiable cause.

Table 9.1: Major causes of hypertension (systolic and diastolic)

Primary/Essential Hypertension (~ 95% of cases)
Secondary Hypertension
Renal • Acute glomerulonephritis • Chronic renal disease • Polycystic kidney disease • Renal artery stenosis (renovascular hypertension) • Renin producing tumors • Obstructive uropathy
Endocrine • Adrenal disorders: Cushing's syndrome, primary aldosteronism • Pheochromocytoma • Others: Hypothyroidism (myxedema), hyperthyroidism (thyrotoxicosis), hypercalcemia, acromegaly
Cardiovascular • Coarctation of aorta • Polyarteritis nodosa • Increased cardiac output • Increased intravascular volume
Neurologic • Psychogenic • Increased intracranial pressure • Sleep apnea
Pre-eclampsia/eclampsia
Medications • High-dose estrogens, adrenal steroids, decongestants, nonsteroidal anti-inflammatory agents

The prevalence and vulnerability to complications of hypertension increase with age.

Regulation of Normal Blood Pressure

Normal blood pressure is essential for survival; it causes damage when it increases continuously above the normal range.

Factors Determining Blood Pressure

- The major factors include age, sex, body mass index and diet, particularly sodium intake, exertion, emotional state and others.
- Blood pressure depends on two hemodynamic variables namely **cardiac output** and **peripheral vascular resistance**. These two, in turn, are influenced by many genetic, environmental and demographic factors.
  - **Cardiac output**: It depends on blood volume, which in turn is influenced by the sodium homeostasis.
  - **Peripheral vascular resistance**: It is determined by functional and anatomic changes in small arteries and arterioles. It is affected by neural and hormonal factors.

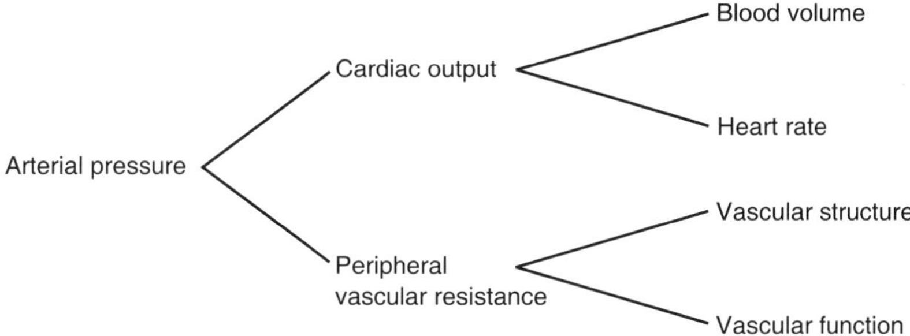

Role of Kidney

The kidneys **play an important role in the regulation of blood pressure**.

- **Renin-angiotensin system:** Kidney influences both peripheral vascular resistance and sodium homeostasis (thereby blood volume) through the renin-angiotensin system.
  - **Renin:** Whenever there is a fall in blood pressure, renin is secreted by the juxtaglomerular cells of the kidney and released into the blood circulation. It **cleaves plasma angiotensinogen to angiotensin I**, which is then converted **to angiotensin II** by angiotensin converting enzyme.
  - **Angiotensin II**: It raises blood pressure by **increasing both peripheral resistance** (direct action on vascular smooth muscle cells and causes vasoconstriction) **and blood volume** (by stimulating secretion of aldosterone by the adrenal zona glomerulosa, and increased reabsorption of sodium in distal tubules).
- **Antihypertensive substances**: The kidney also produces substances which causes vasodilatation and have antihypertensive effect. These include prostaglandins and nitric oxide (NO). They counterbalance the vasoconstriction produced by angiotensin II.
- **Sodium homeostasis and blood volume**:
  - **When blood volume is reduced,** the glomerular filtration rate falls → leads to increased reabsorption of sodium by proximal tubules of kidney → thereby conserves sodium and expands blood volume.
  - **When blood volume increased**, natriuretic factors (natriuretic peptides) are secreted by atrial and ventricular myocardium. They inhibit sodium reabsorption in distal tubules and cause excretion of sodium and diuresis. Natriuretic peptides also cause vasodilation and may be considered as endogenous inhibitors of the renin-angiotensin system.

Pathogenesis of Hypertension

Q. Write short note on pathogenesis of hypertension.

Mechanisms of Essential Hypertension

Essential hypertension is a **complex** and **multifactorial disorder**. Specific trigger is not known. Probable factors that play a significant role includes:

1. **Decreased renal sodium excretion***:* It is probably the **key feature**. Decreased excretion of sodium by kidney → leads to an **increase in fluid volume, cardiac output, and peripheral vasoconstriction** → raises the blood pressure.
2. **Raised vascular resistance:** Factors that produce vasoconstriction or stimuli that cause structural changes in the vessel wall → result in an increase in peripheral vascular resistance → cause primary hypertension.
3. **Genetic factors**: They play an important role in the development of hypertension. The genetic defects may be in the enzymes involved in aldosterone metabolism, sodium reabsorption and smooth muscle cell growth.
4. **Environmental factors:** These include stress, obesity, smoking, lack of physical activity and heavy intake of sodium salt.

Consequences of Hypertension

- **Risk factor**: Hypertension is one of the major modifiable risk factors for **atherosclerosis**.
- **Lesions/diseases produced:** Cardiac hypertrophy, congestive heart failure (hypertensive heart disease) and ischemic heart disease (IHD), multi-infarct dementia, aortic dissection, stroke, subarachnoid hemorrhage, hypertensive encephalopathy, retinal ischemia/infarction and renal failure.
- **Accelerated or malignant hypertension:** It is characterized by **rapid rise in blood pressure** (i.e. systolic pressure over 200 mm Hg, diastolic pressure over 120 mm Hg) → **renal failure, and retinal hemorrhages** and exudates, **with or without papilledema**.
  - It may develop in normotensive individuals but more common in patients with pre-existing benign hypertension (essential or secondary).
  - It develops in ~5% of hypertensive persons. If not treated, death occurs within a year or two.

Effects in Various Organs

Q. Write short note on vascular pathology in hypertension.

Vascular Pathology

Large and Medium Vessel Disease: Atheroscleosis

- Hypertension is one of the **major modifiable risk factors** for **atherogenesis.**
- **Causes degenerative changes in the walls** of large and medium arteries.
- Predisposes to: (1) **Aortic dissection** and (2) **Cerebrovascular hemorrhage**.

Small Vessel Diseases

Two forms can occur in hypertension: (1) Hyaline arteriolosclerosis, and (2) hyperplastic arteriolosclerosis.

1. ***Hyaline arteriolosclerosis:*** It is seen in the arterioles in patients with benign hypertension.
   - **Microscopy:** It shows **thickening of the wall due to homogeneous, pink hyaline material** and **narrowing of the lumen** (Fig. 9.1A).

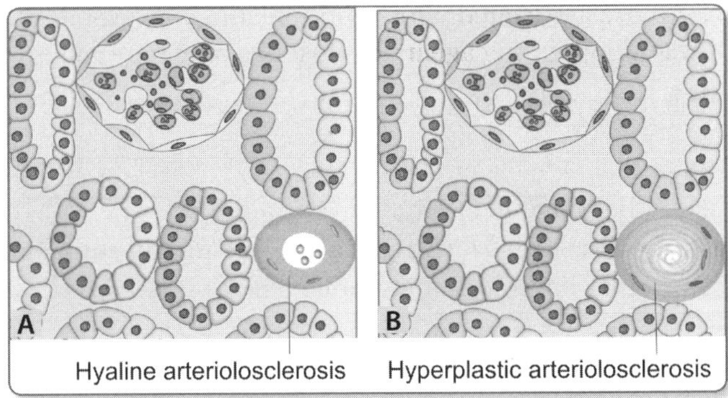

Figs 9.1A and B: Vascular changes (in renal blood vessels) in hypertension. A. Hyaline arteriolosclerosis in benign hypertension: The arteriolar wall is thickened, hyalinized, and the lumen is narrowed; B. Hyperplastic arteriolosclerosis in malignant hypertension: Shows onion-skinning with obliteration of arteriolar lumen

- **Consequence:** The arteriolar narrowing → impaired blood supply to kidney → produces **ischemia and glomerular scarring**. The kidney changes in benign hypertension are called **benign nephrosclerosis.**

2. ***Hyperplastic arteriolosclerosis:*** It occurs in **severe (malignant) hypertension**.
    - **Microscopy:** The blood vessels show "**onion-skin,**" **concentric, laminated thickening of the arteriolar walls** and narrowing of the arteriolar lumen (Fig. 9.1B). It may also show **fibrinoid deposits and necrosis** of vessel wall **(necrotizing arteriolitis)**, particularly in the kidney.

Hypertensive Heart Disease

- Systemic hypertension can increase the demands on the heart and cause pressure overload and left ventricular hypertrophy. It is termed as hypertensive heart disease (HHD).

Systemic (left-sided) hypertensive heart disease

- Hypertrophy of the heart develops as an adaptive response to the pressure overload produced by chronic hypertension. However, compensatory hypertrophy can ultimately lead to myocardial dysfunction, cardiac dilation, congestive heart failure (CHF).
- Pathologic criteria for the diagnosis of HHD
    - Left ventricular hypertrophy
    - Clinical history or pathologic evidence of hypertension in other organs (e.g. kidney).

Morphology of heart

- Hypertension produces left ventricular pressure overload hypertrophy. The left ventricular wall is thickened and may exceed 2.0 cm.
- Microscopically, there is increase in the size of myocardial fibers and their nuclei.

Nephrosclerosis

- ***Nephrosclerosis*** **is the term used for the renal pathology associated with sclerosis of renal arterioles and small Arteries. It is strongly associated with hypertension and can be divided into benign and malignant nephrosclerosis.**

Benign Nephrosclerosis

- **Definition:** Benign nephrosclerosis is defined as the **renal pathology associated with sclerosis of renal arterioles and small arteries**.

- Benign nephrosclerosis is associated with hypertension. However, it may also be observed in diabetes mellitus and increasing age in the absence of hypertension.

Morphology of Kidney

- Gross
  - Involvement: Bilateral.
  - **Size:** Kidneys are either **normal or smaller** (atrophic).
  - **Outer surface**: It shows a **fine, even granularity** resembling grain leather.
- **Microscopy** (refer vascular pathology mentioned above).

Malignant Hypertension and Accelerated Nephrosclerosis

- **Definition:** Malignant nephrosclerosis is defined as **renal disease associated with the malignant or accelerated phase of hypertension.**
- Malignant or accelerated phase of hypertension is relatively uncommon. It is often superimposed on preexisting **essential benign hypertension, secondary forms of hypertension,** or an underlying chronic renal disease, particularly glomerulonephritis or reflux nephropathy.

Morphology

- **Gross**
  - Size of the kidney depends on the duration and severity of the hypertension.
  - **Flea-bitten kidney:** It is characterized by the presence of **small, pinpoint petechial hemorrhages on the cortical surface** due to **rupture of arterioles or glomerular capillaries.**
- **Microscopy**
  - Histological changes of blood vessels → narrowing of vascular lumens → ischemic atrophy.
  - **Fibrinoid necrosis of arterioles:** It is characterized by **eosinophilic granular change in the wall of the blood vessel.**
  - **Onion-skinning** (hyperplastic arteriolitis): It is seen in **the interlobular arteries and arterioles.** It is characterized by **intimal thickening due to concentric proliferation of smooth muscle cells + fine concentric layering of collagen, proteoglycans and plasma proteins.**

Hypertensive Cerebrovascular Disease

The most important effects of hypertension on the brain are

- Lacunar infarcts
- Slit hemorrhages
- Hypertensive encephalopathy
- Massive hypertensive intracerebral hemorrhage.

Chapter 10

Diabetes Mellitus

Chapter Outline

- Diabetes mellitus
- Type 1 diabetes (T1D)
- Type 2 diabetes (T2D)
- Pathogenesis of the complications of diabetes

DIABETES MELLITUS

Diabetes mellitus is a **group of metabolic disorders having features of hyperglycemia.**

The prevalence of diabetes is increasing sharply in the developing countries because of more sedentary lifestyles. India and China have the largest prevalence of diabetics.

Diagnosis (Table 10.1)

Table 10.1: Levels of blood glucose in normal, pre-diabetes and diabetes

	Euglycemic	Pre-diabetes	Diabetes
Fasting glucose level	Less than **100** mg/dL	Greater than **100** mg/dL but less than **126** mg/dL	Greater than **126** mg/dL on more than one occasion
OGTT	Less than **140** mg/dL	Greater than **140** mg/dL but less than **200** mg/dL	Greater than **200** mg/dL

Normally the **blood glucose levels** are maintained in a very narrow range of **70 to 120 mg/dL.**

A. **Euglycemic:** Individuals are considered to be euglycemic, when
   1. **Fasting glucose** level is **less than 100 mg/dL**, or
   2. Glucose level **less than 140 mg/dL** following an **OGTT**.

B. **Pre-diabetes:** It is defined as condition in which there is **impaired glucose tolerance**, but elevated **blood sugar does not reach the criterion accepted for an outright diagnosis of diabetes.** The criteria for diagnosis are:
   - **Fasting glucose** level is **greater than 100 mg/dL but less than 126 mg/dL.**
   - **GTT** values **greater than 140 mg/dL but less than 200 mg/dL.**

   Risks in pre-diabetes: (1) **Progression to frank diabetes** over time and (2) **cardiovascular disease.**

C. **Diabetes:** Any **one of three criteria** can be used for the **diagnosis of diabetes:**
   1. A **random glucose** level **greater than 200 mg/dL, with classical signs and symptoms.**
   2. A **fasting** glucose level **greater than 126 mg/dL on more than one occasion.**
   3. **An abnormal oral glucose tolerance test** (OGTT), in which the **glucose level is greater than 200 mg/dL, 2 hours after a standard carbohydrate load.**

Classification

Q. Classify diabetes mellitus.

Diabetes is classified according to etiopathogenesis into different groups (Table 10.2) but **majority of cases fall into one of two** broad classes namely: **type 1 and type 2.**

Table 10.2: Classification of diabetes mellitus

1. **Type 1 diabetes:** Immune-mediated or idiopathic
2. **Type 2 diabetes**
3. **Genetic defects of β-cell function:** Maturity-onset diabetes of the young (MODY), neonatal diabetes
4. **Genetic defects in insulin action**
5. **Exocrine pancreatic defects:** Chronic pancreatitis, hemochromatosis
6. **Endocrinopathies:** Acromegaly, Cushing syndrome, hyperthyroidism, pheochromocytoma
7. **Infections:** Cytomegalovirus, coxsackie B virus
8. **Drugs:** Glucocorticoids, thyroid hormone
9. **Genetic syndromes associated with diabetes:** Down syndrome, Klinefelter syndrome, Turner syndrome
10. **Gestational diabetes mellitus**

TYPE 1 DIABETES (T1D)

- Accounts for ~ **5–10%** of all cases.
- **Age:** Most common in **childhood (younger than 20 years** of age). Since, it can develop at any age, the term "juvenile diabetes" should be avoided.

Cause

- **Autoimmune disease** characterized by:
  - **Pancreatic β-cell destruction**
  - **Absolute deficiency of insulin.**
- **Idiopathic:** It is a rare form in which there is no evidence for autoimmunity.

Pathogenesis of Type 1 Diabetes Mellitus (Fig. 10.1)

Q. Write short note on pathogenesis of type 1 diabetes mellitus.

Involves interplay of both genetic susceptibility and environmental factors.

- **Genetic susceptibility:**
  - Incidence of type 1 diabetes is greater in twins of affected individuals than in the general population, and greater in monozygotic than in dizygotic twins.
- **Environmental factors:**
  - **Viral infections:** They **may trigger islet cell destruction** and associations have been found between type 1 diabetes and infection with ***mumps, rubella, coxsackie B, or cytomegalovirus.*** **Three different mechanisms** explain the role of viruses in the induction of autoimmunity.

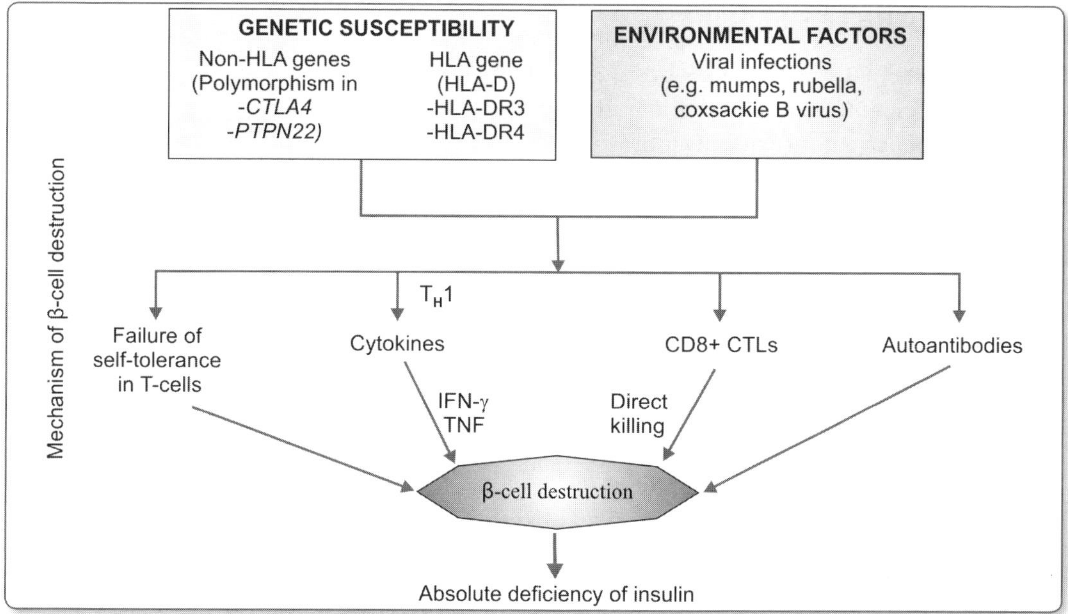

Fig. 10.1: Pathogenesis of type 1 diabetes mellitus

1. **Release of hidden or sequestered antigens**: Viral infections cause islet injury and inflammation, thereby release the sequestered β-cell antigens and **activates autoreactive T cells.**
2. **Molecular mimicry**: **Viruses** can **produce proteins that mimic** β-**cell antigens**. The **immune response** produced against the viral protein may **cross-reacts with the self-tissue** (β-**cell antigens**).
3. **Sharing of antigen epitopes:** First viral infections by a **predisposing virus**, during early in life might persist in the β-cells. Subsequent **re-infection** with a related virus known as **precipitating virus**, that shares antigenic epitopes may leads to an immune response against the β-cells.

Mechanisms of β-Cell Destruction

The autoimmune damage starts many years before the disease becomes clinically evident. **Hyperglycemia and ketosis occur after more than 90% of the** β **cells have been destroyed**. Various mechanisms include:

1. **Failure of self-tolerance in T-cells**: It is the **basic abnormality** in type 1 diabetes.
2. **Through cytokines**: T_H1 cells may destroy β cells by secreting cytokines, including **IFN**-γ and **TNF**.
3. **Directly by cytotoxic T cells**: The CD8+ CTLs may directly kill β cells.
4. **Autoantibodies against** β **cell antigens** (e.g. islet antigens β cell enzymes): They are found in 70–80% of patients with type 1 diabetes, and in asymptomatic family members. It is not known whether autoantibodies cause injury or are result of islet injury.

TYPE 2 DIABETES (T2D)

Q. Write short note on pathogenesis of type 2 diabetes mellitus.

- Accounts for ~ **90–95% of diabetic patients**.
- **Majority** of patients are **overweight**.
- Though known as "adult-onset," it is now found in children and adolescents also.

Pathogenesis of Type 2 Diabetes Mellitus (Fig. 10.2)

Type 2 diabetes is a **multifactorial disease**.

- **Environmental factors** play a role and includes:
  - **Sedentary lifestyle**
  - **Dietary habits and associated obesity**.
- **Genetic factors**:
  - Type 2 diabetes has a **concordance rate of 35% to 60% in monozygotic twins compared with 17% to 30% in dizygotic twins**.
  - **Lifetime risk** for type 2 diabetes in an offspring is more than double **if both parents are affected**.
  - **Diabetogenic genes** have been found.
  - There is **no evidence of an autoimmune basis**.

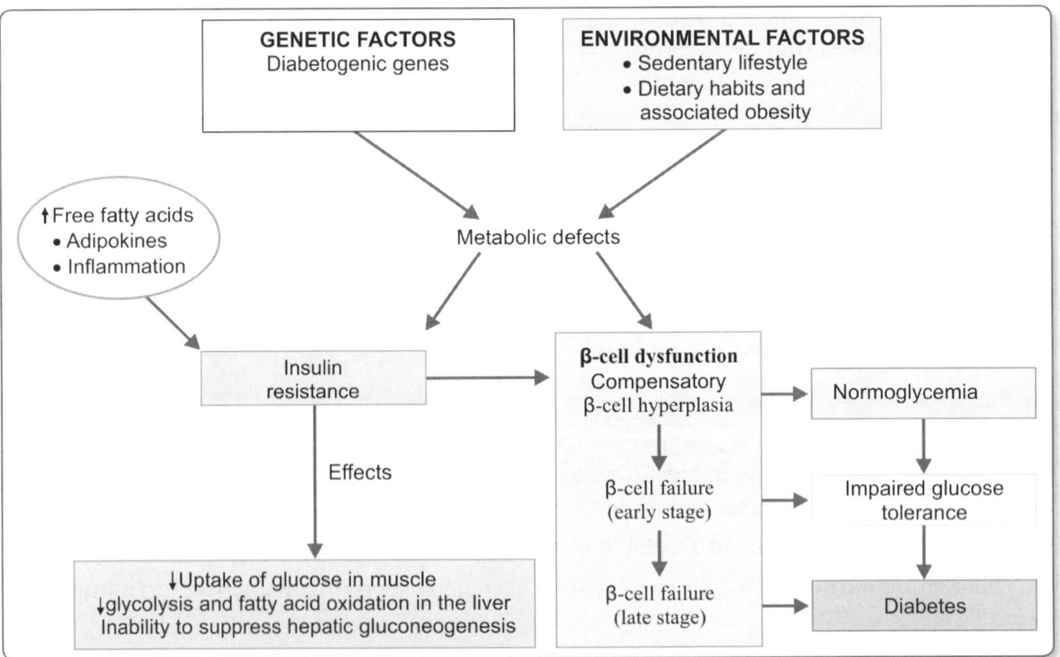

Fig. 10.2: Pathogenesis of type 2 diabetes. Insulin resistance associated with obesity is induced by free fatty acids, adipokines, and chronic inflammation in adipose tissue. Insulin resistance causes β cells of pancreas to undergo compensatory hyperplasia and the resulting hypersecretion of insulin maintains normoglycemia. However, at some point, β-cell compensation is followed by β-cell failure, and diabetes develops

Metabolic Defects in Type 2 Diabetes

Two important metabolic defects are:

Insulin Resistance

Definition: Insulin resistance is **the decrease/failure of target (peripheral) tissues to insulin action. Main factors** in the development of insulin resistance is **obesity**.

a. **Obesity and insulin resistance**: Obesity is associated with type 2 diabetes and the **visceral obesity is found in more than 80% of patients**.
   - **Distribution of body fat:** It has an effect on insulin sensitivity. **Central obesity** (abdominal fat) is **more associated with insulin resistance than are peripheral** (gluteal/ subcutaneous) fat depots.

b. **Consequences of insulin resistance:**
   i. **Decreased uptake of glucose in muscle**.
   ii. **Reduced glycolysis** and **fatty acid oxidation** in the liver.
   iii. **Inability to suppress hepatic gluconeogenesis**.

β-Cell Dysfunction

In type 2 diabetes, β-cell dysfunction manifests as **inadequate insulin secretion by the pancreatic β cells (relative insulin deficiency)** in association with insulin resistance and hyperglycemia. β-cell dysfunction is multifactorial in origin.

a. **Obesity and β-cell dysfunction:**
   - **Compensatory β-cell hyperplasia: Pancreatic β cells initially respond** to long-term demands of peripheral insulin resistance **by undergoing compensatory hyperplasia leading to increased insulin secretion (hypersecretion)**.
   - **β-cell failure (early stage):** However, at some point, β cells exhaust their capacity to adapt. β-cell compensation **cannot maintain normal blood sugar level**. This stage, the patient develop impaired glucose tolerance.
   - **β-cell failure (late stage):** The early stage of β-cell failure is followed by decreased insulin secretion, hyperglycemia and frank diabetes develops.
   - **Direct toxicity by amyloid deposits**: In long-standing type 2 diabetes, amyloid deposits in islets is seen in more than 90% of cases. The islet **amyloid protein may be directly cytotoxic to islets** causing β-cell dysfunction. This may be similar to amyloid plaques involved in the pathogenesis of Alzheimer disease.

PATHOGENESIS OF THE COMPLICATIONS OF DIABETES

Q. Write short note on pathogenesis of complications in diabetes mellitus.

Pathogenesis is multifactorial and includes:

- Hyperglycemia (glucotoxicity) is the main mediator
- Insulin resistance (described already)
- Obesity (described already).

Hyperglycemia

- **Control of blood sugar level** (glycemic control) **can reduce the long-term complications** of diabetes.
- **Glycemic control is assessed by** estimation of **glycosylated hemoglobins (HbA1C)**. HbA1C is formed by addition of glucose to hemoglobin in red cells. HbA1C should be maintained

below 7% in diabetic patients and its **measurement is helpful in knowing the glycemic control over the lifespan of a red cell** (120 days).

Organ Damage by Hyperglycemia

- The chronic hyperglycemia and the metabolic disorders cause secondary **damage in multiple organ** systems.
- Common organs damaged are **kidneys** (end-stage renal disease), **eyes** (adult-onset blindness), **nerves,** and **blood vessels (**gangrene of lower extremity).

Effects Hyperglycemia

Harmful effects of persistent hyperglycemia on peripheral tissues can be brought out by **three distinct metabolic pathways.**

Formation of Advanced Glycation End Products (AGEs) (Fig. 10.3)

In diabetics, glucose binds to proteins nonenzymatically and **is termed nonenzymatic glycosylation**.

- **Initial products:** The initial products of nonenzymatic glycosylation are chemically known as Schiff bases **are labile and can dissociate rapidly.**
- **Later products:** The initial labile products form → **stable advanced glycation end products** (AGEs). **The rate of AGE formation is markedly increased in the presence of hyperglycemia**.
- **Effects of AGEs:** It may be brought out by binding of AGEs to its specific receptor (RAGE-receptor for AGE) or by its direct action.
  - Releases pro-inflammatory cytokines and **growth factors** from intimal macrophages
  - Production of reactive oxygen species in endothelial cells
  - **Increases** procoagulant activity on endothelial cells and macrophages
  - **Increases** proliferation of vascular smooth muscle cells and synthesis of extracellular matrix

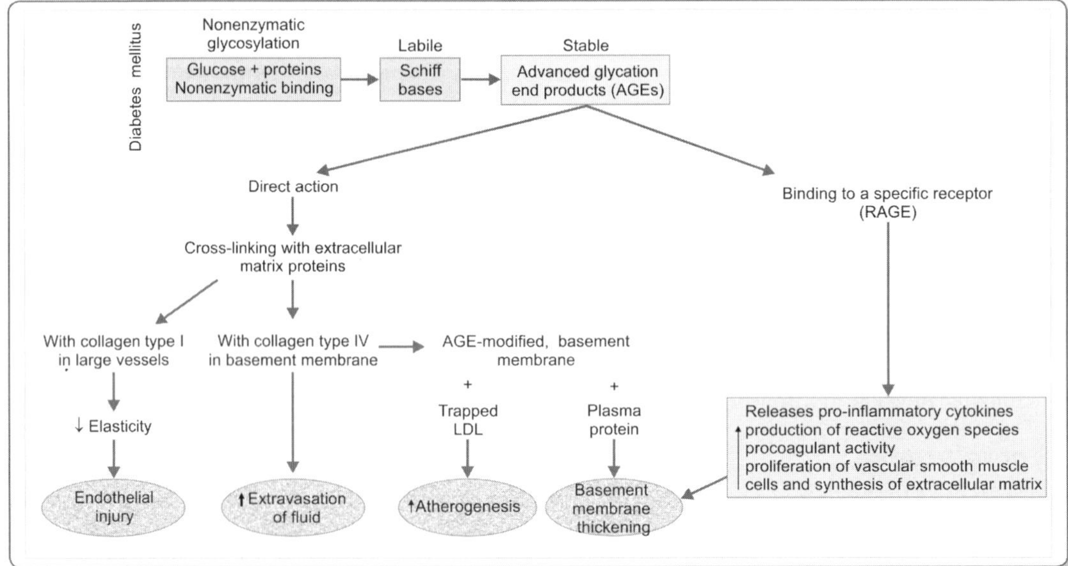

Fig. 10.3: Pathogenetic mechanism of injury advanced glycation end products (AGEs) in diabetes mellitus
RAGE=Receptor for AGE: LDL-Low density lipoproteins

- Resist proteolytic digestion → results in decreased removal and increased deposition of protein → **trapping of proteins in the glycosylated collagen of the basement membrane thickening**.
- **Trapping of LDL in the intima → accelerating atherogenesis.**

Activation of Protein Kinase C (PKC)

In patients with hyperglycemia, **intracellular hyperglycemia stimulates synthesis of diacyl glycerol (DAG) from glycolytic intermediates.** DAG **activates intracellular protein kinase C.**

Consequences of PKC activation: It produces:

- **Proangiogenic molecules** such as **vascular endothelial growth factor (VEGF)** → causes **neovascularization** characteristic of **diabetic retinopathy**.
- **Profibrogenic factors** (e.g. **TGF-β**) → results in **increased production of extracellular matrix and basement membrane material**.
- Plasminogen activator inhibitor (PAI-1) → **reduces fibrinolysis** and **favors vascular occlusion** (by forming atherosclerotic plaques or thrombus).

Disturbances in Polyol Pathways

- **Some tissues** (e.g. nerves, lenses, kidneys, blood vessels) **do not require insulin for glucose transport.**
- **Persistent hyperglycemia increases** the **intracellular glucose in these tissues → excess intracellular glucose is metabolized by the enzyme aldose reductase → to sorbitol (polyol)** → to fructose.
- This **reaction uses NADPH** (the reduced form of nicotinamide dinucleotide phosphate) as a cofactor.
- NADPH is also necessary for the regeneration of reduced glutathione (GSH). GSH protects against injury by free radicals.
- Reduced NADPH → decrease in GSH → increases cells **susceptibility to oxidative stress.**

Morphology

Pancreas

Lesions of pancreas are **not diagnostic** and are more common with type 1 than with type 2 diabetes. The morphological changes include:

- **Reduced number and size of islets:** It is seen in type 1 diabetes which is mild in type 2 diabetes.
- **Infiltration of islets (insulitis):** Mainly by T lymphocytes predominantly in type 1 diabetes.
- **Amyloid deposition within islets:** It is observed in and around capillaries and between cells in type 2 diabetes. In advanced stages, the islets may be virtually obliterated and may show fibrosis.
- **Increase in the number and size of islets.**

Blood Vessels

- **Hyaline arteriolosclerosis:** It can be found in hypertension, elderly nondiabetics without hypertension and more severe degree in diabetics also.
- In diabetics, it is **related to the duration of diabetes and the level of blood pressure.**
- It is characterized by **amorphous, hyaline thickening of the wall of the arterioles**, which may **narrow the lumen** of the vessel (refer Fig. 9.1A).
- **Diabetic microangiopathy:** It is characterized by **diffuse thickening of basement membranes,** which is **mostly seen in the capillaries of the skin, skeletal muscle, retina, renal glomeruli, and renal medulla.**
- Though **capillaries show basement membrane thickening, they are leakier to plasma proteins than normal.**
- The microangiopathy results in diabetic nephropathy, retinopathy, and some forms of neuropathy.

Diabetic Nephropathy—Renal Changes in Diabetes

Q. Write short note on renal changes in diabetes mellitus (diabetic nephropathy).

Diabetic nephropathy is the term used for **collective lesions that often occur together in the diabetic kidney**. Diabetic nephropathy can develop in both insulin-dependent type 1 diabetes and type 2 diabetes.

- The **kidneys** are **main targets** of diabetes.
- **Renal failure** is second only to myocardial infarction as a **cause of death** in diabetes.

Q. Write short note on KW lesion.

Renal lesions in diabetes can involve any component. Four lesions are encountered namely:

1. **Glomerular lesions**
2. **Renal vascular lesions (mainly arteriolosclerosis)**
3. **Pyelonephritis (including necrotizing papillitis)**
4. **Tubular lesions.**

1. Glomerular Lesions (Figs 10.4 and 10.5)

They are most **important and common renal lesions.** These include: (a) Thickening of capillary basement membrane (GBM), (b) diffuse mesangial sclerosis and (c) nodular glomerulosclerosis (Kimmelstiel-Wilson nodules).

a. **Diffuse** widespread **thickening glomerular capillary basement membrane.**
b. **Diffuse mesangial sclerosis**: It is characterized by **diffuse increase in PAS-positive mesangial matrix and mesangial cells.**
c. **Nodular glomerulosclerosis**: It is also called as **intercapillary glomerulosclerosis or Kimmelstiel-Wilson disease** and **are pathognomonic.**
    i. Glomerular lesion consists of **ovoid or spherical**, often laminated, **nodules of mesangial matrix** seen within the mesangial core and **situated in the periphery of the glomerulus.** These nodules can be surrounded by peripheral capillary loops with patent or dilated lumen. The nodules are **PAS-positive.** As the disease advances, the individual nodules increase in size → compress the surrounding capillaries.
d. **Insudative lesions**:
    i. **Fibrin caps**: These are **prominent subendothelial** accumulations of **hyaline material** in/along capillary loops.
    ii. **Capsular drops**: They consists of **round nodules adherent to Bowman's capsules** and are **seen between Bowman's capsule and the parietal epithelium.**

2. Renal Vascular Lesions

a. **Hyaline arteriosclerosis** (hyalinosis): It involves **both the afferent and the efferent arteriole** at the hilum of glomeruli. **Arteriolosclerosis efferent arteriole is rare in nondiabetics.**
b. **Renal atherosclerosis**: It involves arteries and arterioles and are similar to those found in other parts of the body.

Glomerular and arteriolar lesions together produce **renal ischemia** → leads to atrophy of tubules, interstitial fibrosis, and contraction of kidney.

3. Pyelonephritis

It is a tubulointerstitial inflammation of the kidneys.

a. Both the **acute and chronic pyelonephritis** occurs in nondiabetics as well as in diabetics. It is **more common** and tends to **more severe** in diabetics than in the general population.
b. **Necrotizing papillitis** (or papillary necrosis): It is one **special pattern of acute pyelonephritis** and is much more frequent in diabetics compared to nondiabetics. **Hyaline arteriolosclerosis** narrows blood vessels → **reduces the blood supply** to the renal medulla → ischemia → causes **necrosis of the tips of papillae** (papillary necrosis).

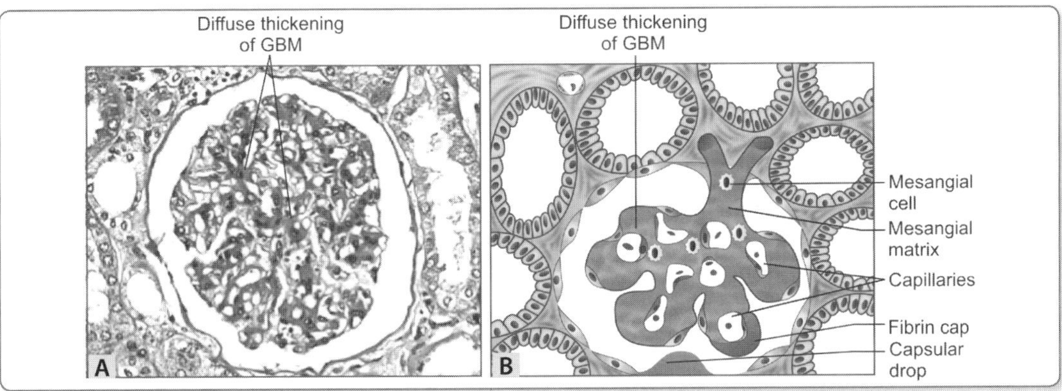

Figs 10.4A and B: Diabetic nephropathy (A. H and E stain and B. diagrammatic), glomeruli with diffuse widespread thickening glomerular capillary basement membrane and insudative lesions (fibrin cap and capsular drop)

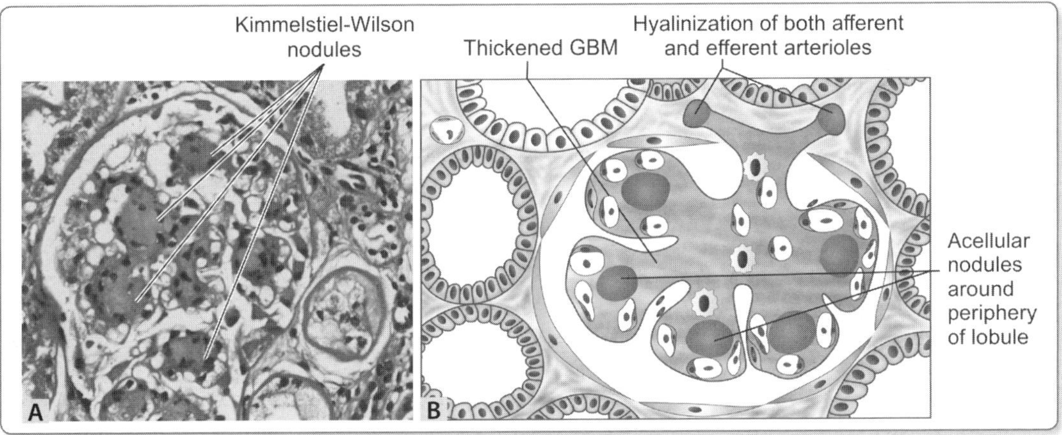

Figs 10.5A and B: Diabetic nephropathy (A. H and E stain and B. diagrammatic), nodular glomerulosclerosis shows oval nodules of mesangial matrix at the periphery of glomerulus

4. Tubular Lesions

The basement membrane of the tubules show thickening. In patients with high blood sugar level, the **epithelial cells of the proximal convoluted tubules show extensive deposits of vacuoles of glycogen**. These are known as **Armanni-Ebstein lesions**.

Electron Microscopy (Fig. 10.6)

- **Thickening of the lamina densa** of the glomerular basement membrane.
- **Increase in the mesangial matrix**, particularly in nodular lesions.
- **Insudative lesions** appear as electron-dense masses.

Immunofluorescence Microscopy

It reveals IgG, albumin, fibrinogen, and other **plasma** proteins in the GBM.

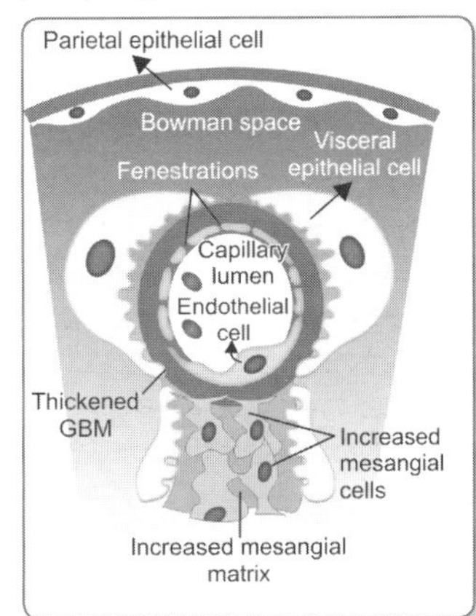

Fig. 10.6: Diagrammatic electron microscopic appearance of diabetic glomerulosclerosis showing thickened glomerular basement membrane, increased mesangial cells and mesangial matrix

Clinical Features of Diabetes (Fig. 10.7)

Type 1 Diabetes Mellitus

- **Age:** Type 1 diabetes can occur at any age.
- **Classical triad of diabetes**: It consists of **polyuria, polydipsia, polyphagia**, and **in severe cases ketoacidosis**, are due to metabolic derangements.
- **Insulin requirement:** In the **initial 1 or 2 years**, the exogenous insulin required may be **minimal** because of endogenous insulin secretion → **later**, its requirement suddenly **increases**.

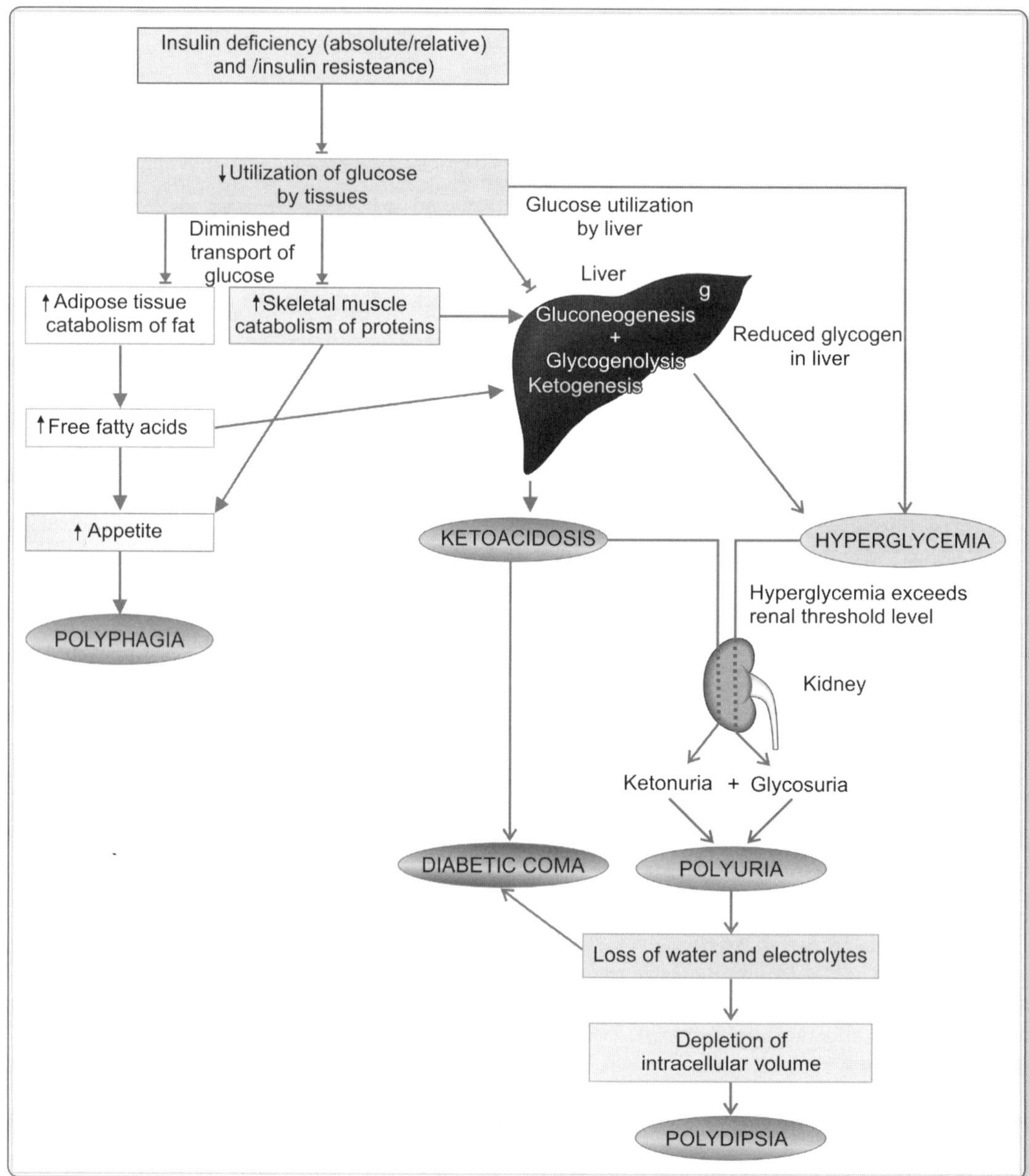

Fig. 10.7: Sequence of metabolic derangements underlying the symptoms and signs of uncontrolled hyperglycemia in diabetes mellitus

Consequences of Insulin Deficiency

Insulin is an anabolic hormone and its deficiency → results in a catabolic state, which affects glucose metabolism, fat and protein metabolism.

1. **Carbohydrate metabolism:**
   - **Diminished transport of glucose** into **muscle cells** and **adipose tissue**.
   - **Reduction of stored glycogen in liver and muscle** due to **glycogenolysis** → this **further aggravates the hyperglycemia**.
   - When **hyperglycemia exceeds the renal threshold** level → develops **glycosuria** → leads to osmotic diuresis → **increased quantity of urine known as polyuria,** with **loss of water and electrolytes**.
   - Water loss through urine + hyperosmolarity (due to hyperglycemia) → causes **depletion of intracellular water** → **stimulates** the osmoreceptors of the **thirst centers** of the brain → results in increased thirst known as **polydipsia**.
2. **Protein and fat metabolism:**
   - Insulin deficiency → causes **catabolism of proteins and fats** → produces a **negative energy balance** → leads to **increased appetite (polyphagia)**.
   - In spite of increased appetite, catabolic effects insulin results in paradoxical **loss of weight and muscle weakness**.
3. **Diabetic ketoacidosis:**
   - Serious complication of diabetes
   - More **common and marked in type 1 diabetes,** but may also occur in type 2 diabetes.
   - **Mechanism:**

   i. **Diuresis and dehydration: Marked insulin deficiency** + associated **epinephrine** release → stimulates the **secretion of glucagon** → leads to **decreased peripheral utilization of glucose** + **increased gluconeogenesis** → causes **severe hyperglycemia** (the blood glucose levels of 500 to 700 mg/dL) → osmotic **diuresis and dehydration** (characteristic features of ketoacidosis).

   ii. **Activation of the ketogenic machinery:**

      a. Insulin deficiency → **stimulates lipoprotein lipase** → which **breaks down fat stores** → **increases the free fatty acids levels.**

      b. **Free fatty acids** are **esterified to fatty acyl coenzyme A in the liver**.

      c. In the mitochondria of liver cells, **fatty acyl coenzyme A molecules are oxidized** to **ketone bodies (acetoacetic acid and β-hydroxybutyric acid).**

      d. When the **rate of production of ketone bodies exceeds the rate of utilization** by peripheral tissues, it results in **ketonemia** and **ketonuria**.

      e. If the excretion of ketone bodies in the urine is compromised by dehydration, it results in **systemic metabolic ketoacidosis**.

Type 2 Diabetes Mellitus

- **Age:** Usually occurs in older **above the age of 40 years** and frequently in **obese individuals.** Due to increase in obesity and sedentary lifestyle, it is now detected also in children and adolescents.
- **Presentation**: **Polyuria, polydipsia, unexplained weakness or weight loss. Ketoacidosis is infrequent** and presentation is usually mild.
- In **asymptomatic individuals**, the **diagnosis is made after routine blood or urine testing.**

Differences between type 1 and type 2 diabetes mellitus are listed in Table 10.3.

Q. List the differences between type 1 and type 2 diabetes mellitus.

Table 10.3: Differences between type 1 and type 2 diabetes mellitus

	Type 1 diabetes mellitus	Type 2 diabetes mellitus
Clinical		
Age of onset	Childhood and adolescence	Adult, also seen in childhood and adolescence
Weight	Normal or present with weight loss	Majority are obese
Insulin levels	Progressive decrease	Increased (early); normal or moderate decrease (late)
Circulating islet autoantibodies	Detected (anti-insulin, anti-GAD, anti-ICA512)	Not found
Diabetic ketoacidosis	Develops in absence of insulin therapy	Nonketotic hyperosmolar coma
Genetics		
HLA (human leukocyte antigen) association	Major linkage to MHC (major histocompatibility complex) class I and II genes HLA-DR3 and/-HLA-DR4	No HLA association
Non-HLA genes	Polymorphisms in *CTLA4* and *PTPN22*	Diabetogenic and obesity-related genes
Etiopathogenesis		
Mode of development	Autoimmune	Multifactorial
Mechanism	Breakdown in self-tolerance to islet auto-antigens	Insulin resistance in peripheral tissues, β-cell dysfunction
Morphology		
Insulitis (inflammation of islets)	Inflammatory infiltrate of T cells and macrophages in islets	No insulitis; amyloid deposition in islets
β -cell depletion	Moderate to severe	Mild

Complications (Fig. 10.8)

Q. Write short note on complications of type 1 diabetes mellitus.

- Complications are similar in both type 1 and type 2 diabetes.
- **Long-term complications of diabetes** usually develop about 15 to 20 years after the onset of hyperglycemia. They are responsible for the majority of the morbidity and mortality.

Diabetic Macrovascular Disease

The lesions of large- and medium-sized muscular arteries are the **most common causes of mortality** in long-standing diabetes. These include:

- **Atherosclerosis:** Diabetes is one of the major modifiable risk factor for atherosclerosis and other cardiovascular morbidities. The **atherosclerosis is more severe and occurs at earlier age**.
- **Myocardial infarction:** It is due to atherosclerosis of the coronary arteries and is the **most common cause of death in diabetics.** Diabetics have greater risk of coronary artery disease and cardiovascular complications than nondiabetics.
- **Gangrene of the lower extremities**: It results from advanced vascular disease and is more common in diabetics.
- **Renal vascular insufficiency**.
- **Cerebrovascular accidents** (stroke).

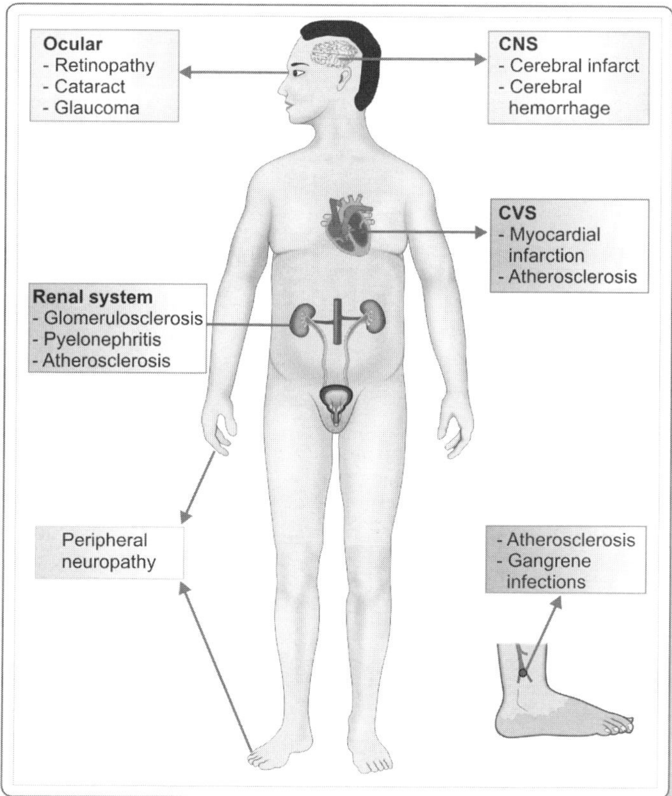

Fig. 10.8: Complications of diabetes

Microvascular Disease (Microangiopathy)

It involves small vessels and is characterized by capillary dysfunction in target organs and is mainly observed in kidneys (nephropathy), retina (diabetic retinopathy) and peripheral nerves (neuropathy).

- **Diabetic nephropathy:** About **30% to 40% of all diabetics** develop nephropathy (discussed above) and is **leading cause of end-stage renal disease**.
- **Diabetic retinopathy:** It develops in **~60% to 80% of diabetics, about 15 to 20 years after diagnosis**. The basic lesion of retinopathy is **neovascularization caused by hypoxia-induced overexpression of VEGF in the retina**. Diabetics have **increased risk for glaucoma** and **cataract formation**.
- **Diabetic neuropathy:** It may involve the **central and peripheral nervous systems**.

Diabetic Dyslipidemia

It is a condition in which there are **increased blood levels of triglycerides and LDL and decreased levels of the high-density lipoprotein** (protective).

Increased Susceptibility to Infections

Infections of the skin, tuberculosis, pneumonia, and pyelonephritis are common in diabetes.

Chapter 11

Neoplasia

Chapter Outline

- Classification
- Nomenclature of neoplasms
- Characteristics of benign and malignant neoplasms
- Carcinoma in situ
- Metastasis
- Precancerous conditions/lesions
- Molecular basis of cancer
- Steps in normal cell proliferation
- Hallmarks of cancer
- Etiology of cancer (carcinogenic agents)
- Laboratory diagnosis of cancer
- Clinical aspects of neoplasia
- Paraneoplastic syndromes
- Prognosis
- Common specific epithelial tumors
- Mesenchymal tumors

INTRODUCTION

Q. Define neoplasia.

Neoplasia literally means new growth, and a new growth formed is known as a neoplasm (Greek, *neo* = new + *plasma* = thing formed). The term tumor was originally used for the swelling caused by inflammation, but it is now used synonymously with neoplasm. Oncology (Greek *oncos* = tumor) is the study of tumors or neoplasms.

Willis Definition: "A neoplasm is an **abnormal mass of tissue**, the **growth of which exceeds and is uncoordinated with that of the normal tissues** and **persists in the same excessive manner after cessation of the stimuli which evoked the change."**

Salient General Features of Neoplasia

- **Origin:** Neoplasms arise **from cells** that normally maintain a **proliferative capacity**.
- **Genetic disorder:** Cancer is due to **permanent genetic changes** in the cell known as **mutations**. These mutations may occur in genes which regulate cell growth, apoptosis, or DNA repair.
- **Heritable:** The genetic alterations are passed down to the daughter tumor cells.
- **Monoclonal:** All the neoplastic cells within an individual **tumor originate from a single cell/or clone of cells that has undergone genetic change**. Thus, tumors are said to be monoclonal.

- **Carcinogenic stimulus:** The stimulus responsible for the uncontrolled cell proliferation **may not be identified or is not known**.
- **Autonomy:** In neoplasia, there is the **excessive** and **unregulated proliferation** of cells that do not obey the normal regulatory control. The cell proliferation is **independent of physiologic growth stimuli**. But tumors are dependent on the host for their nutrition and blood supply.
- **Irreversible:** Neoplasm is irreversible and **persist even after the inciting stimulus is withdrawn or gone**.
- **Differentiation**: It refers to the **extent to which the tumor cells resemble the cell of origin**. A tumor may show varying degrees of differentiation ranging from relatively mature structures that mimic normal tissues (well-differentiated) to cells so primitive that the cell of origin cannot be identified (poorly differentiated).

CLASSIFICATION

Q. Discuss the nomenclature and classification of tumors.

Tumors are classified as **benign and malignant, depending on** the **biological behavior** of a tumor.

1. **Benign tumors:** They have a relatively innocent microscopic and gross characteristic.
    - **Remain localized without invasion or metastasis.**
    - **Well differentiated**: Their cells **closely resemble their tissue of origin**.
    - **Prognosis:** It is **very good**, can be cured by surgical removal in most of the patients and the patient generally survives.
2. **Malignant tumors**: **Cancer is the general term** used for malignant tumors. The term cancer is derived from the Latin word for *crab*, because similar to a crab, malignant tumors adhere to any part that they seize on, in an obstinate manner.
    - **Invasion**: Malignant tumors invade **or infiltrate into the adjacent tissues or structures.**
    - **Metastasis:** Cancers **spread to distant sites** (metastasize), where the malignant cells reside, grow and again invade.
        - **Exception**: **Basal cell carcinoma** of the skin, which is histologically malignant (i.e. it invades aggressively), but **rarely metastasize** to distant sites. **Glioma** - Malignant tumor of CNS
    - **Prognosis:** Most malignant tumors cause death.

Microscopic Components of Neoplasms

Tumors (both benign and malignant) consist of two basic components:

1. **Parenchyma:** It is made up of neoplastic cells. The **nomenclature and biologic behavior of tumors** are **based primarily** on the **parenchymal component** of tumor.
2. **Stroma:** It is the **supporting, non-neoplastic tissue** derived **from the host**.
    - **Components: Connective tissue, blood vessels, and inflammatory cells** (e.g. macrophages and lymphocytes).
    - **Tumor consistency depends on amount of stroma**:
        - **Soft and fleshy:** These tumors have **scanty stroma**.
        - **Desmoplasia** (Fig. 11.1): **Parenchymal tumor cells may stimulate the formation of an abundant collagenous stroma** → referred to as desmoplasia. For example, some carcinoma in female breast have **stony hard consistency** (or **scirrhous**).

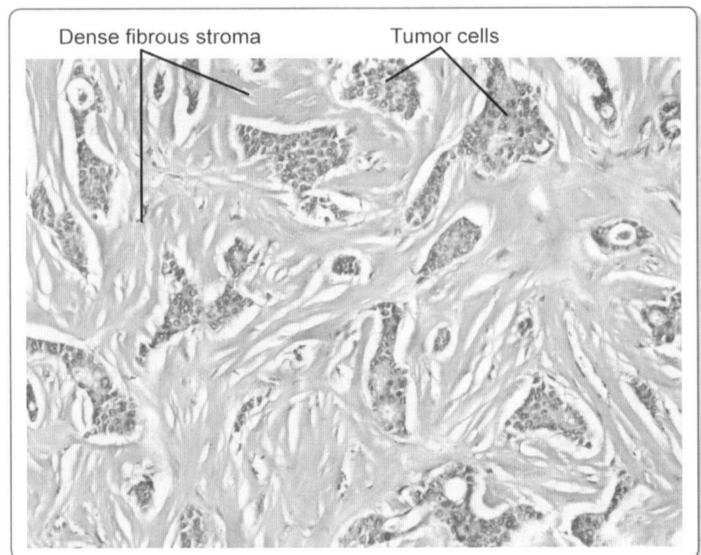

Fig. 11.1: Carcinoma of breast with abundant stroma separating malignant cells

(For color version, see Plate 4)

Table 11.1: Nomenclature of few benign and malignant mesenchymal tumors

Cell of origin	Benign	Malignant
Fibrous tissue	Fibroma	Fibrosarcoma
Fat cell	Lipoma	Liposarcoma
Blood vessel	Hemangioma	Angiosarcoma
Cartilage	Chondroma	Chondrosarcoma
Bone	Osteoma	Osteogenic sarcoma
Smooth muscle	Leiomyoma	Leiomyosarcoma
Skeletal muscle	Rhabdomyoma	Rhabdomyosarcoma

NOMENCLATURE OF NEOPLASMS

Benign Tumors

A tumor is said to be benign when its gross and microscopic appearances are innocent, remain localized, will not spread to other sites, and can be surgically removed locallly, the patient usually survives. They are generally **named by attaching the suffix "oma" to the cell of origin.**

1. Mesenchymal Tumors

They usually follow the above nomenclature (Table 11.1).

2. Epithelial Tumors (Fig. 11.2)

Their nomenclature is **not uniform but more complex**. They are classified in different ways:

a. Cells of origin
b. Microscopic pattern

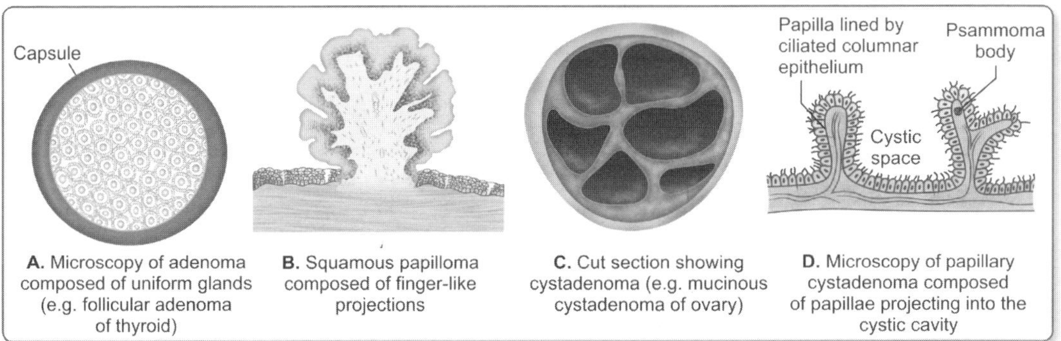

A. Microscopy of adenoma composed of uniform glands (e.g. follicular adenoma of thyroid)

B. Squamous papilloma composed of finger-like projections

C. Cut section showing cystadenoma (e.g. mucinous cystadenoma of ovary)

D. Microscopy of papillary cystadenoma composed of papillae projecting into the cystic cavity

Figs 11.2A to D: Morphological (gross/microscopic) appearance of some benign epithelial tumors

c. **Macroscopic architecture.**

- **Adenoma:** It is a **benign epithelial tumor arising from glandular epithelium**, although they **may or may not form glandular structures**.

  Example: Follicular adenoma of thyroid: It usually shows microscopically numerous tightly packed small glands (Fig. 11.2A).

- **Papilloma:** It is a **benign epithelial neoplasm** that produces microscopically or macroscopically **visible finger-like, exophytic or warty projections** from epithelial surfaces. Example: squamous papilloma (Fig. 11.2B).

- **Cystadenoma:** It is a tumor forming large cystic masses. Example: Serous cystadenoma of ovary (Fig. 11.2C).

- **Papillary cystadenoma**: It is a tumor which consists of papillary structures that project into cystic spaces. Example: Papillary serous cystadenoma of ovary (Fig. 11.2D).

A. Sessile polyp

B. Pedunculated polyp

Fig. 11.3: Gross types of polyps. A. Sessile polyp without a stalk and B. Pedunculated poly with stalk

Polyp (Fig. 11.3): It is a neoplasm that grossly produces **visible projection above a mucosal surface and projects into the lumen**. It may be either **benign or malignant**. It may have a stalk (**pedunculated** polyp) or may be without a stalk (**sessile** polyp). Example: Polyp of stomach or intestine.

Malignant Tumors

Malignant tumors can invade the adjacent structures and spread to distant sites (metastasize) and can cause death. They are termed as carcinoma or sarcoma depending on the parenchymal cell of origin.

1. Sarcomas

They are **malignant tumors arising in mesenchymal tissue**. These tumors have little connective tissue stroma and are fleshy (Greek *sar* = **fleshy**). Examples: Fibrosarcoma, liposarcoma, osteosarcoma. Malignant tumors arising from blood-forming cells are called *leukemias* (literally, white blood) or *lymphomas* (tumors of lymphocytes or their precursors).

2. Carcinomas

They are **malignant neoplasms arising from epithelial cell**, which may be derived from any of the three germ layers (Table 11.2).

Table 11.2: Nomenclature of carcinomas

Germ layer	Tissue/cell	Malignant tumor
Ectoderm	Epidermis	Squamous cell **carcinoma**
Mesoderm	Renal tubules	Adeno**carcinoma**
Endoderm	Lining of the gastrointestinal tract	Adeno**carcinoma**

Table 11.3: List of malignant tumors with suffix "oma"

Inappropriate terminology for malignant tumor	Site
Hepatoma	Liver
Melanoma	Skin
Seminoma/dysgerminoma	Testis/ovary
Lymphoma	Lymph nodes and extranodal lymphoid tissue

- **Undifferentiated malignant tumor**: It is a malignant tumor composed of undifferentiated cells, where the cell of origin cannot be made out on light microscopic examination.
- **Inappropriate terminology for malignant tumor** (Table 11.3): In certain malignant tumors, the terms suffix "oma" is inappropriately used and sounds like a benign tumor.

Mixed Tumors (refer Fig. 15.1)

They are **derived from a single germ layer** but show **divergent differentiation** along two lineages. Example: **Mixed tumor of salivary gland** (pleomorphic adenoma) is derived from a single clone (either myoepithelial or ductal reserve cell) and giving rise to two components, namely epithelial and myoepithelial cells (refer Chapter 15).

Teratomas

Q. Write short note on teratoma.

They are special types of mixed tumors **derived from totipotent germ cells** (normally present in **ovary, testis** and sometimes abnormally present in sequestered embryonic rest in midline). These cells have the capacity to **differentiate into any of the cell types** found in the adult body. Thus, teratoma contains recognizable **mature or immature cells** or tissues representative of more than one germ cell layer and sometimes all three. These cells or tissues are arranged in a helter-skelter fashion. The **tissues derivative from various germ cell layers** may include:

1. **Ectoderm** (e.g. skin, neural tissue, glia)
2. **Mesoderm** (e.g. smooth muscle, cartilage, bone, fat)
3. **Endoderm** (e.g. respiratory tract epithelium, gut, thyroid).

Hamartomas

- It is a **disorganized mass of benign-appearing cells**, **indigenous to the** particular **site**.
  Example: Pulmonary chondroid hamartoma consists of islands of disorganized, but histologically normal cartilage, bronchi, and vessels.

Choristoma

- It is an **ectopic island of normal tissue—heterotopic rest** (normal tissue in an abnormal site) and is a **congenital** anomaly.

Example: Presence of small nodular mass of normally organized pancreatic tissue in the submucosa of the stomach, duodenum, or small intestine.

Nomenclature of the more common forms of neoplasia is listed in Table 11.4.

CHARACTERISTICS OF BENIGN AND MALIGNANT NEOPLASMS

Q. Describe the characteristics of malignant tumors.

It is **very important to differentiate** benign from malignant tumors mainly because of the different prognostic outcome. In general, benign and malignant tumors can be distinguished on the basis of four fundamental features, namely: (1) differentiation and anaplasia, (2) rate of growth, (3) local invasion, and (4) metastasis.

Differentiation and Anaplasia

Differentiation

Defined as the **extent to which neoplastic parenchymal cells resemble** the corresponding **normal parenchymal cells.** This includes both morphological and functional differentiation. Differentiation **determines the grade of the tumor**.

Benign Tumors

- **Well differentiated:** The neoplastic cell **closely resembles the normal cell of origin**. It may be not possible to recognize it as a tumor by microscopic examination of individual cells (e.g. lipoma). Only the growth of these cells into discrete lobules discloses the neoplastic nature of the lesion (Fig. 11.4).
- **Mitoses:** They are **rare** and of normal configuration.

Malignant Neoplasms

Q. Write short note on histological features of malignant cell.

- Show a **wide range of differentiation** of parenchymal cells.
- Varies from **well differentiated to completely undifferentiated**.
- Cancers are usually graded either as well, moderately or poorly differentiated or numerically, often by strict criteria, as grade 1, grade 2 or grade 3.
- **Well-differentiated** tumors.
  - Well-differentiated adenocarcinomas of colon may form normal-appearing glands (Fig. 11.5).
  - Squamous cell carcinomas may show cells which appear similar to normal squamous epithelial cells (refer Figs 11.31A and B).
- **Poorly differentiated tumors**: They consist of cells that have little resemblance to the cell of origin.
- **Moderately differentiated:** These tumors show differentiation in between the well and poorly differentiated tumors.

Anaplasia

- Anaplasia **literally means "to form backward/backward formation"**, i.e. **reversal of differentiation of cell to a more primitive level**.
- Malignant neoplasms composed of undifferentiated cells are called as anaplastic tumors.

Table 11.4: Nomenclature of common tumors

Tissue of origin	Benign	Malignant
COMPOSED OF SINGLE PARENCHYMAL CELL TYPE		
Tumors of Mesenchymal Origin		
Connective tissue and derivatives	Fibroma	Fibrosarcoma
	Lipoma	Liposarcoma
	Chondroma	Chondrosarcoma
	Osteoma	Osteogenic sarcoma
Endothelial tissues		
Blood vessels	Hemangioma	Angiosarcoma
Peripheral nerve		
Nerve sheath	Neurofibroma, neurilemmoma	Malignant peripheral nerve sheath tumor
Blood Cells and Lymphoid Cells		
Hematopoietic cells		Leukemia
Lymphoid tissue		Lymphoma
Muscle		
• Smooth	Leiomyoma	Leiomyosarcoma
• Striated	Rhabdomyoma	Rhabdomyosarcoma
Tumors of Epithelial Origin		
Stratified squamous	Squamous cell papilloma	Squamous cell carcinoma
Basal cells of skin or adnexa		Basal cell carcinoma
Epithelial lining of glands or ducts or organs	Adenoma	Adenocarcinoma
	Papilloma	Papillary carcinoma
	Cystadenoma	Cystadenocarcinoma
	Papillary cystadenoma	Papillary cystadenocarcinoma
Transitional epithelium	Transitional-cell papilloma	Transitional-cell carcinoma
Tumors of melanocyte	Nevus	Malignant melanoma
MORE THAN ONE NEOPLASTIC CELL TYPE—MIXED TUMORS, DERIVED FROM ONE GERM CELL LAYER		
Salivary glands	Pleomorphic adenoma (mixed tumor) of salivary origin	Malignant mixed tumor of salivary gland origin
MORE THAN ONE NEOPLASTIC CELL TYPE DERIVED FROM MORE THAN ONE GERM CELL LAYER		
Totipotential cells in gonads or in embryonic rests	Mature teratoma, dermoid cyst	Immature teratoma

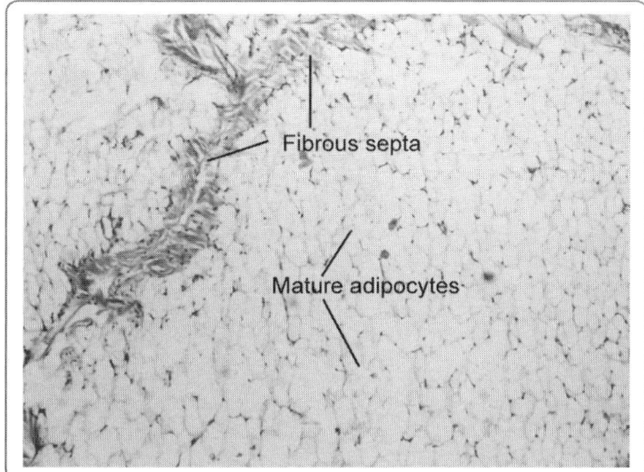

Fig. 11.4: Lipoma is a benign, well-differentiated tumor composed of lobules of fat cells that are identical in appearance to normal fat cells

(For color version, see Plate 5)

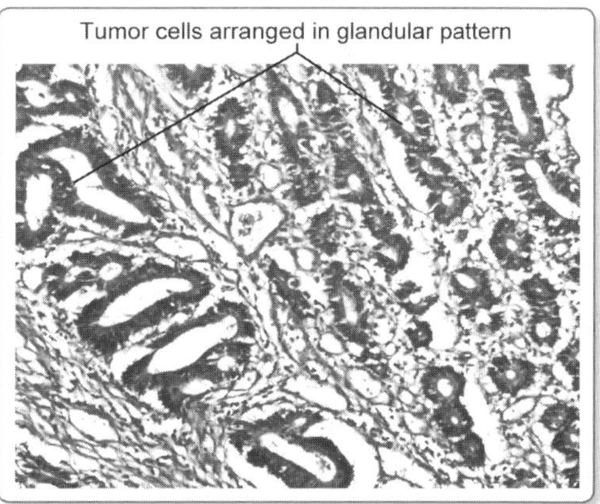

Fig. 11.5: Well-differentiated adenocarcinoma of the colon. It shows cancerous glands that are irregular in shape and size invading the muscular layer of the colon

(For color version, see Plate 5)

- **Lack of differentiation** (both structural and functional) **is called as anaplasia** and is **characteristic of malignancy**.
- The degree of anaplasia in a cancer cell correlates with the aggressiveness of the tumor.
- Thus, more anaplastic the tumor it becomes more aggressive.

Microscopic Features of Anaplasia (Figs 11.6A and B):

Q. Write short note on anaplasia.

- ***Pleomorphism:*** It is defined as **variation in the size and shape of cells and cell nuclei**. It is a feature of malignancy. Thus, cells within the same malignant tumor range from large cells (many times larger than the neighbor cells), to extremely small (primitive appearing) cells.

Q. Write short note on morphology of malignant cells.

- ***Abnormal nuclear morphology***:
  - **Extremely hyperchromatic nuclei** of tumor cells are **due to abundant chromatin** and **increased amount of DNA per cell** compared to that of a normal cell. Microscopically these **nuclei stain darkly (hyperchromatic nuclei)**.
  - **Nuclear shape and size is variable** and may be irregular. **Chromatin is coarsely clumped** and distributed along the nuclear membrane. **Large prominent nucleoli** are usually seen.
  - **Mitoses:** Presence of mitotic figures **indicates the higher proliferative activity** of the parenchymal cells
    - **Number of mitotic figures:** Compared to benign and few well-differentiated malignant tumors, undifferentiated tumors usually show **abundant (many) mitotic figures.**
    - **Atypical mitotic figures:** Normal mitosis produces bipolar spindles, and one cell divides into two. When the mitotic spindles are more than two, it is called as atypical. Presence of atypical bizarre mitotic figures is **important morphologic features of malignancy.**
- **Nuclear cytoplasmic (N : C) ratio**: In a normal cell N : C ratio is 1 : 4 or 1 : 6. In a malignant cell, the nuclei are enlarged, become disproportionately large for the cell, and the nuclear-to-cytoplasm ratio may be **increased** and may reach even up to 1 : 1.

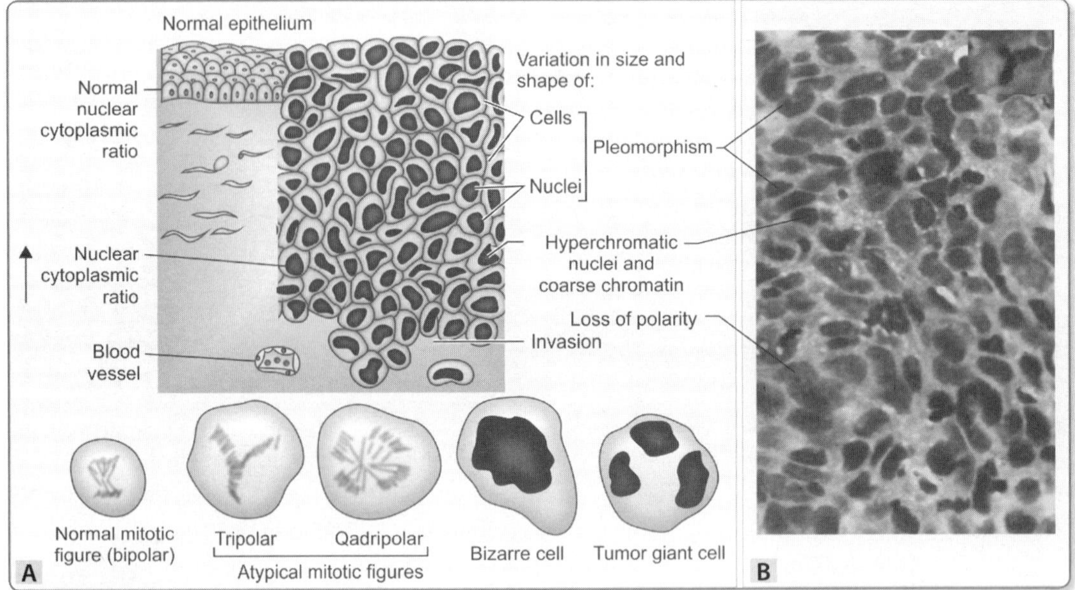

Figs 11.6A and B: Microscopic features of anaplasia. A. Diagrammatic, B. Photomicrograph showing nuclear and cytoplasmic pleomorphism, hyperchromatic nuclei, high nuclear cytoplasmic ratio and loss of polarity. Inset of B shows tripolar mitotic figure

- **Loss of polarity: Orientation of cells to one another** is known as polarity. The anaplastic cells lose the normal polarity → markedly disturbed orientation (architecture) of tumor cells.
- **Bizarre cells, including tumor giant cells**: Some tumors may show **bizarre cells with a single large polymorphic nucleus** and others having **two or more large, hyperchromatic nuclei** (Fig. 11.8).

Functional Changes

Well-differentiated tumors usually retain the functional characteristics. Function may be in the form of secretion and vary depending on the tumor type.

1. **Secretion of normal substances:**
   - **Hormones:** Benign tumors and **well-differentiated carcinomas of endocrine glands frequently secrete the hormones** characteristic of their cell of origin (e.g. steroid hormones from an adrenocortical adenoma).
   - **Normal product**: Example: **Well-differentiated squamous cell carcinomas** produce keratin → form characteristic **epithelial pearls**.
2. **Ectopic hormones**: Tumors may produce **substances** which are **not indigenous to the tissue of origin.** Example: Bronchogenic carcinomas may produce ACTH, parathyroid-like hormone, etc.

Rates of Growth

Factors Determining the Rate of Growth

1. **Degree of differentiation**
   - **Benign tumors** are well differentiated and **usually grow slowly.**
   - **Most malignant tumors grow more rapidly.**

2. **Dependency:** Growth also depends on:
   - **Hormonal stimulation**, e.g. uterine leiomyomas may suddenly grow during pregnancy and may undergo atrophy after menopause.
   - **Adequacy of blood supply.**

Local Invasion

Benign Tumors

1. **Localized:** Most benign tumors **grow as expansile masses** that remain localized to their site of origin.
   a. **No infiltration** into adjacent tissue or capsule (if present).
   b. **No metastasis.**
2. **Capsule** (Fig. 11.7): It is a rim of compressed connective tissue derived mainly from the extracellular matrix of the surrounding normal tissue.
   a. **Capsule → makes tumor palpable and movable mass** → can be surgically enucleated.
   b. **Benign tumors without capsule (unencapsulated)**. Examples: Hemangiomas, uterine leiomyoma.

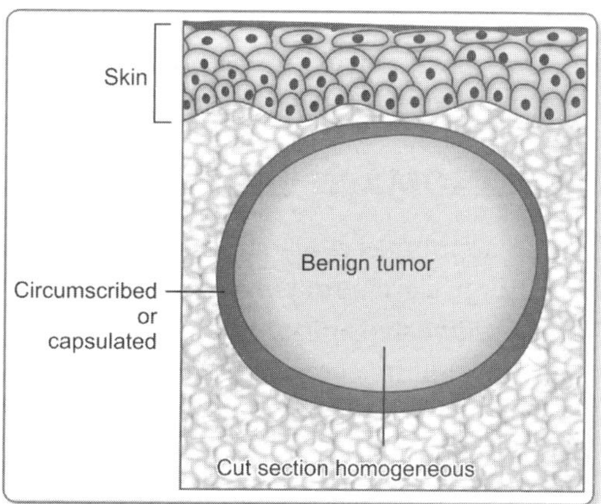

Fig. 11.7: Diagrammatic representation of a capsule in a benign tumor

Malignant Tumors

1. **Lack of capsule**: Malignant tumors are poorly demarcated from the surrounding normal tissue and lack true capsule.
2. **Invasion** (Figs 11.8 and 11.9)**: Two most reliable features** that differentiate malignant from benign tumors are **local invasion and metastases.**

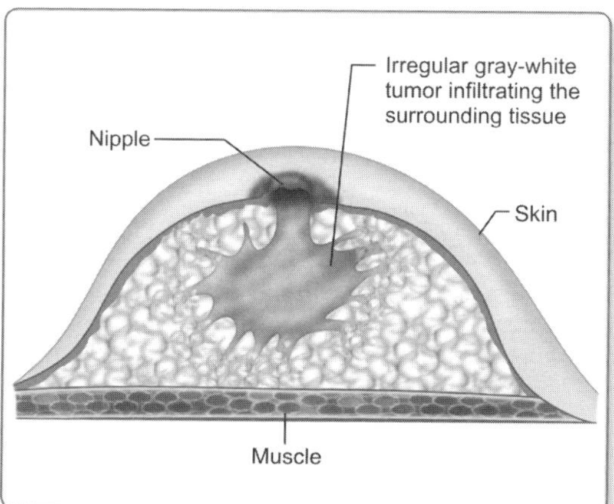

Fig. 11.8: Diagrammatic representation of cut section of an invasive ductal carcinoma of the breast

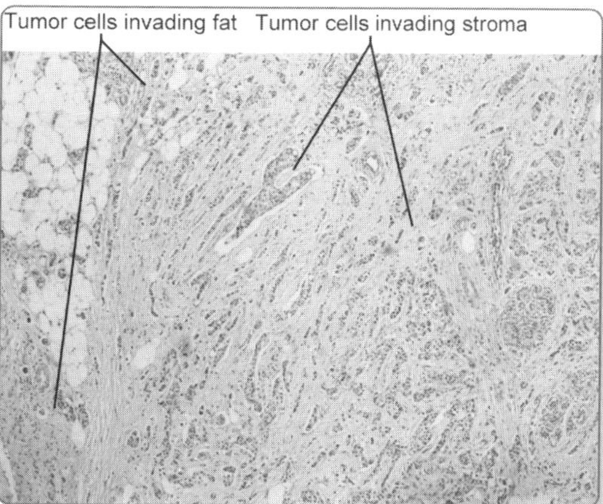

Fig. 11.9: Microscopic appearance of breast carcinoma showing invasion of breast stroma and fat by nests and cords of tumor cells

Local invasion:

a. **Invasion of adjacent tissue/organ:** The cancers may invade and destroy the adjacent tissues/ organ **progressive infiltration, invasion, and destruction of the surrounding tissue.**
b. **Tissues that resists invasion:** They include mature cartilage (e.g. epiphysis), elastic tissue of arteries.
c. **Invasion of blood vessels and lymphatics**
d. **Perineural invasion:** For example, cancer of prostate and pancreas, adenoid cystic carcinoma of salivary glands.

CARCINOMA IN SITU

Some carcinomas evolve from a **preinvasive stage** called as carcinoma in situ.

Definition: Carcinoma *in situ* is defined as:

1. A **preinvasive epithelial neoplasm.**
2. Shows **all the cytological features of malignancy.**
3. **Involves the entire thickness of the epithelium.**
4. Remains **confined within the epithelial basement membrane.**

The tumor cells cannot reach the potential routes of metastasis, such as blood vessels and lymphatics until the basement membrane has been breached or invaded.

Dysplasia

Q. Write short note on dysplasia.

The **cells that show cytological features of malignancy** and the term dysplasia is used for these changes (Fig. 11.10). It literally means disordered growth. The changes of dysplasia include:

1. **Cellular pleomorphism.**
2. **Large hyperchromatic nuclei.**
3. **High nuclear-to-cytoplasmic ratio.**
4. **Loss of polarity (architectural orientation).**

- **Classification of dysplasia: (1) mild, (2) moderate,** and **(3) severe** depending on the thickness of epithelium involved by the dysplastic cells.

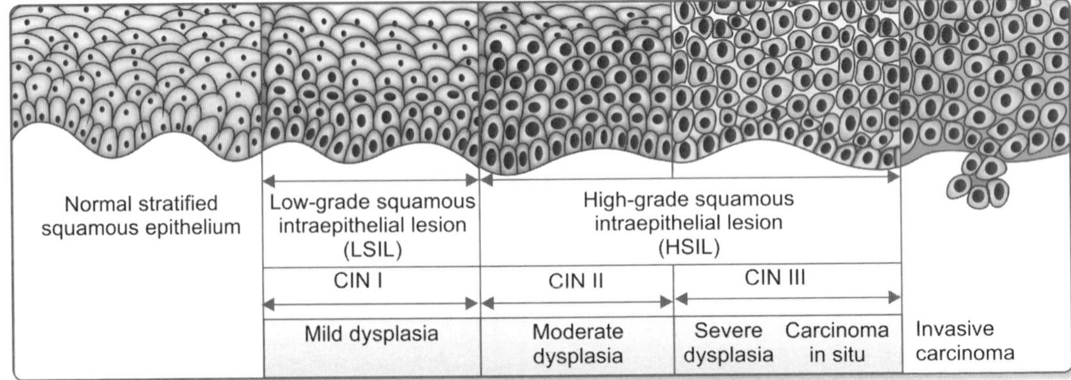

Fig. 11.10: Spectrum of dysplasia (e.g. cervix). CIN=cervical intraepithelial neoplasia

- **Fate:**
  - **Mild to moderate dysplastic changes**, which do not involve the entire thickness of epithelium **may be reversible**, if the cause is removed. Thus, **dysplasia need not progress to cancer**.
  - **Once the tumor cells breach the basement membrane,** the **tumor is said to be invasive** and carcinoma *in situ* may take years to become invasive. Most *in situ* tumor, with time penetrate the basement membrane and invade the subepithelial stroma.
- **Sites: Uterine cervix**, **skin**, and breast.
- **Asymptomatic:** In this stage, tumors are usually asymptomatic.

METASTASIS

Q. Define metastasis.

Definition: Metastases are tumor deposits that are physically discontinuous with the primary tumor and located in a distant tissue. This **process is known as metastasis** and the resulting **secondary deposits are called metastases.**

Significance

Q. Mode of spread of malignant tumors /Discuss the different modes of metastasis with examples.

1. Metastases clearly **identify a tumor as malignant** because benign neoplasms never metastasize. **Exceptions** include two malignant tumors, which are locally invasive, but rarely metastasize.
   - **Gliomas** (malignant neoplasms of the glial cells) in the central nervous system.
   - Basal cell carcinomas of the skin.
2. Metastases **strongly reduce the possibility of cure of cancer.**
3. Metastatic spread is the most **common cause of cancer death.**

Factors favoring metastasis*:* (1) poorly differentiated tumor, (2) more rapidly growing tumor, and (3) large primary tumor.

Morphological Appearance

- Microscopically, **metastases resemble the primary tumor**. But occasionally, they may be so anaplastic that their cell of origin cannot be made out.
- **Unknown primary: Sometimes metastases may appear without any clinically detectable primary tumor**.

Pathways of Spread

Invasiveness of cancers allows them to penetrate blood vessels, lymphatics, and body cavities. It provides an opportunity for spread/dissemination of cancers through the following pathways:

1. Lymphatic Spread

Q. Write short note on lymphatic spread of malignant tumors.

- **Most common pathway** of spread for carcinomas.
- **Regional node involvement**: Once the tumor cells gain access into the lymphatic vessels, they are carried to the regional draining lymph nodes.
- **Pattern of lymph node involvement follows the natural routes of lymphatic drainage**.
- **Sentinel lymph node** biopsy is done to know the presence or absence of metastatic lesions.

- **Skip metastasis**: When **local lymph nodes are bypassed** and **lymphatic metastases develop in lymph nodes distant from the site of the primary tumor**; these are called "skip metastasis". Example: **Abdominal cancers** may be **first detected by an enlarged supraclavicular node**.
- **Microscopic pattern of deposits:**
  - Initially, **tumor cells** are deposited in the **marginal sinus and later extend throughout the node**.
  - **Micrometastases consist of single tumor cells or very small clusters.**
- **Significance of lymph node metastases: Prognostic value**, e.g. in breast cancer, involvement of axillary lymph nodes is very important for assessing prognosis and for type of therapy.

2. *Hematogenous Spread*

Q. Write short note on hematogenous spread of malignant tumors.

Hematogenous spread is usual for sarcomas but is also found in carcinomas. Blood borne metastasis usually occurs in **osteosarcoma, choriocarcinoma** and **renal cell carcinoma.**

- **Vessels invaded:** Cancer cells easily invade **capillaries and venules**, but thick-walled arterioles and arteries are relatively resistant.
- **Tumors with affinity for venous invasion**
  - **Renal cell carcinoma:** It can invade the renal vein and grow in a snakelike fashion up the inferior vena cava, sometimes reaching the right side of the heart.
  - **Hepatocellular carcinoma:** It may invade branches of portal and hepatic vein and grow within the main venous channels.
- **Pattern of involvement**: With venous invasion, the pattern of metastases follow the venous flow.
- **Target organ for metastasis**:
  - **Liver and lungs:** They are the **most frequently involved** organs, because **all portal area drains to the liver**. Tumors which penetrate systemic veins, eventually drain into the vena cava. Since **all caval blood flows to the lungs**, it is the other common site for secondaries by hematogenous spread.
  - **Bone metastasis:** Cancer metastasizing to bone-prostate, lung, breast, liver, intestine, kidney and thyroid.
    - **Vertebral column is the common site and spread through the paravertebral plexus. Example: Carcinomas of the thyroid and prostate.**
  - **Other common sites: Brain** most common primary is lung cancer, kidney and adrenals.
  - **Organs relatively resistant**: For example, skeletal muscle and spleen.

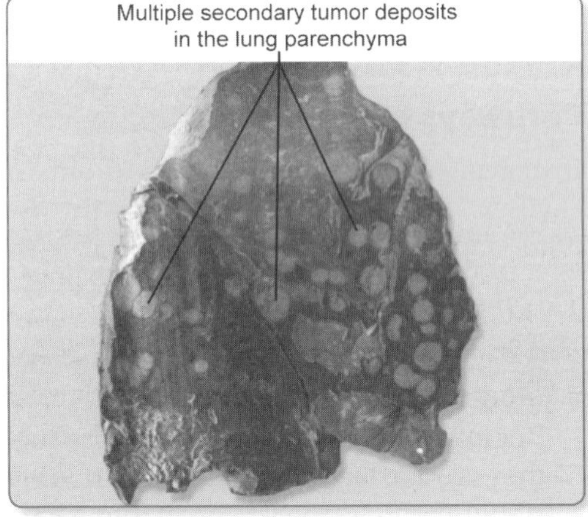

Fig. 11.11: Lung with multiple metastatic cancer

Morphology

- **Gross appearance** (Fig. 11.11): Appear as multiple round nodules of varying sizes found throughout the organ.
- **Microscopy:** The metastatic deposits generally resemble the structure of primary tumor.

3. Seeding of Body Cavities and Surfaces

1) **Transcelomic spread:**
   a. **Malignant tumor arising in organs adjacent to body cavities** (e.g. ovaries, gastrointestinal tract, and lung), **may seed body cavities.** The malignant cells may exfoliate or shed from the organ surfaces into the body cavities and cytological examination of this fluid may show malignant cells.
   b. Such body cavities include peritoneal (most common), pleural cavities (common), pericardial (occasionally), joint space, and subarachnoid space.
      i. **Peritoneal cavity:** Example: (1) **Ovarian tumors,** such as primary carcinomas of surface epithelial origin and (2) **Malignant GI tract tumors** may spread to involve peritoneal cavity → ascites.
      ii. **Pleural cavity**: Peripherally situated **lung tumors** → pleural effusions.
      iii. **Cerebrospinal fluid: Glioblastoma** commonly spread through CSF in the subarachnoid space to the spinal cord.
2) **Spread along the epithelial lined spaces**: It is not common. Examples:
   - Carcinoma endometrium may spread to ovary (or vice versa) through fallopian tube.
   - Carcinoma of kidney may spread to lower urinary tract via ureters.

4. Direct Transplantation

- Tumor cells may be directly transplanted (e.g. by surgical instruments like scalpel, needles, sutures) or implantation by direct contact (e.g. transfer of cancer of lower lip to the corresponding opposite site in the upper lip).
- Even though this method is theoretically possible, they are **rare**.

Differences between benign and malignant tumors are summarized in Table 11.5.

PRECANCEROUS CONDITIONS/LESIONS

Q. Write short note on precancerous lesions/premalignant neoplasms.

Precancerous conditions are **non-neoplastic disorders** in which there is a **well-defined association with an increased risk of cancer**. However, in majority of these lesions no malignant neoplasm develops except that they have an increased risk. Examples:

1. **Chronic atrophic gastritis** of pernicious anemia.
2. **Solar keratosis of the skin.**
3. **Chronic ulcerative colitis. It results from the accumulation of complementary mutations in a stepwise fashion over time.**
4. **Leukoplakia** (erythroplakia) of the oral cavity, vulva, and penis.
5. Barrett esophagus.
6. Squamous metaplasia and dysplasia of bronchial mucosa observed in chronic smokers.
7. Endometrial hyperplasia and dysplasia in women with unopposed estrogen stimulation.
8. Precancerous benign tumors: Few forms of benign tumors may transform into malignant. Example: Villous adenoma of the colon, as it increases in size, becomes malignant.
9. Benign develops occasionally into malignant: Most benign tumors do not become malignant. However, occasionally it may arise from benign tumors. Examples:
   - Leiomyosarcoma beginning in a leiomyoma.
   - Carcinoma developing in long-standing pleomorphic adenomas.
   - Malignant peripheral nerve sheath tumor in patients with neurofibromatosis.

Q. Discuss the differences between benign and malignant tumors.

Table 11.5: Differences between benign and malignant tumors

Characteristics	Benign	Malignant
A. MICROSCOPIC FEATURES		
1. Differentiation/anaplasia	Well differentiated	Well to poorly differentiated Anaplasia is characteristic
2. Pleomorphism	Usually not seen	Commonly present
3. Nuclear morphology	Usually normal	Usually hyperchromatic, irregular outline, and pleomorphic
4. Nucleoli	Usually absent	Usual and prominent
5. Mitotic activity	Rare and if present they are normal bipolar	High and may be abnormal or atypical (tripolar, quadripolar, multipolar)
6. Tumor giant cells	Not seen	May be seen and show nuclear atypia
7. Nuclear: cytoplasmic (N:C) ratio	Normal (1:4 to 1:6)	Increased (may be as much as 1:1)
8. Polarity	Maintained	Usually lost
9. Chromosomal abnormality	Not found	Usually seen
B. GROSS FEATURES		
1. Border/capsule	Mostly circumscribed or encapsulated	Usually poorly defined
2. Areas of necrosis and hemorrhage	Rare	Common, often found microscopically
C. CLINICAL FEATURES		
1. Rate of growth	Usually slow	Relatively rapid
2. Local invasion	Usually well-demarcated without invasion/infiltration of the surrounding normal tissues	Locally invasive, infiltrate surrounding normal tissue
3. Metastasis	Absent	Frequent
4. Biological behavior/prognosis	Usually prognosis is good	Prognosis is poor; usually death due to local invasion or metastatic complications

10. Congenital abnormalities may predispose to cancer. Example: The undescended testis is more prone to neoplasms than the normally located testis.

MOLECULAR BASIS OF CANCER

Fundamental Principles

1. **Cancer is a genetic disease** and arises through a series of somatic alterations in DNA that result in uncontrolled proliferation.
2. **Nonlethal genetic damage** (mostly in DNA) **known as mutations is essential for carcinogenesis**, because lethal damage cause death of cells. Mutation may be:
   - **Inherited** in the germ line and occurs in certain families.
   - **Acquired** by the action of environmental agents (e.g. chemicals, viruses or radiation) and result in sporadic cancers.
3. **Tumors are monoclonal,** i.e. they originate from a clonal proliferation of a **single type of progenitor cell that has undergone genetic damage**.

4. **Carcinogenesis is a multistep process.**
5. **Four classes of normal regulatory genes** are the **main targets of genetic damage**.
   - **Growth-promoting proto-oncogenes: Mutation of** normal cellular genes known as **proto-oncogenes** produces genes that leads to tumor formation and are known as **oncogenes**. They behave as **dominant genes**.
   - **Growth-inhibiting tumor suppressor genes:** They normally **prevent uncontrolled growth**.
     - Usually, **both normal alleles** of the **tumor suppressor genes must be damaged/ mutated** before transformation of cell can occur.
     - Two groups of tumor suppressor genes are: **(1) governors and (2) guardians**.
       - **Governor gene** mutations → **remove the brake for cellular proliferation** → neoplasia, e.g. *RB* gene.
       - **Guardian genes** sense the genomic damage and **prevents proliferation of cells with genetic damage** or if damage is too severe to be repaired → induces apoptosis e.g. p53.
   - **Genes involved in DNA repair:** Normally, they **repair nonlethal damage in other genes**, including proto-oncogenes, tumor suppressor genes, and genes that regulate apoptosis.
     - Mutations of DNA repair genes do not directly transform cells.
     - **Disability** in the DNA-repair genes **can predispose** cells to widespread mutations in the genome → **neoplastic transformation**.
   - **Genes that regulate programmed cell death** (apoptosis): They can behave as **proto-oncogenes** (loss of one copy is enough) or **tumor suppressor genes** (loss of both copies required).

STEPS IN NORMAL CELL PROLIFERATION

Normal cell follows a controlled proliferation. The different sequential steps (Fig 11.12) are:

1. **Growth factors binding** to its **specific cell surface receptor**.
2. **Transient and limited activation** of the **growth factor receptor** → activates signal-transuding proteins on the inner aspect of the cell membrane. Following this signaling, the receptor reverts to its resting state.
3. **Intracellular signal transduction:** Most of the signal-transducing proteins are located on the inner aspect of the plasma membrane. They **receive external signals** and get activated (by binding of growth factor to its growth factor receptors) and **transmit the growth signal across the cytoplasm → to the nucleus of the cell**. The most important signal-transducing protein belongs to **RAS family and ABL**.
4. **Transcription:** Activation of nuclear regulatory factors → initiates DNA transcription.
5. **Cell cycle:** Entry and progression of the cell into the cell cycle → resulting in cell division.

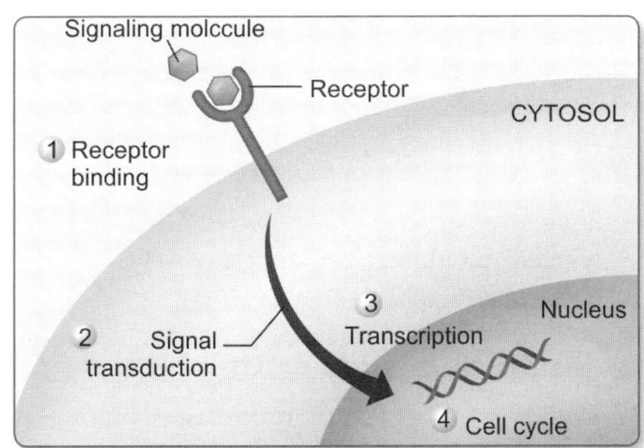

Fig 11.12: Steps in cell proliferation

HALLMARKS OF CANCER

Normal cell may undergo malignant transformation by corrupting any one of the normal steps involved in cell proliferation. **All cancers show eight fundamental changes in cell physiology. These are considered the hallmarks of cancer** and includes:

1. Self-sufficiency in growth signals.
2. Insensitivity to growth-inhibitory signals.
3. Altered cellular metabolism.
4. Evasion of cell death/apoptosis.
5. Limitless replicative potential.
6. Development of sustained angiogenesis.
7. Ability to invade and metastasize.
8. Ability to evade the host immune response.

1. Self-sufficiency in Growth Signals: Oncogenes

Q. Write short note on oncogene.

Proto-oncogenes are **normal cellular genes**, which encode a number of nuclear proteins that **regulate normal cell proliferation, differentiation, and survival**.

Oncogenes and Oncoproteins: Genes that promote autonomous cell growth in cancer cells are called **oncogenes** and are **altered/mutated versions of proto-oncogenes**.

- **Oncogenes** have the ability to **promote cell growth in the absence** of normal growth-promoting/**mitogenic signals**.
- **Products** of oncogenes → are called **oncoproteins**, which resemble the normal products of proto-oncogenes.
- **Oncoprotein production** is **not under normal regulatory control** → cells proliferate without the usual requirement for external signals and are freed from checkpoints → **growth becomes autonomous**.

Classification of oncogenes: Oncogenes can be classified according to the function of gene product (oncoprotein).

- Growth factors (e.g. *SIS* coding for platelet-derived growth factor)
- Growth factors receptors (e.g. *ERBB* coding for epidermal growth factor receptor)
- Signal transduction proteins (e.g. *RAS* and GTP)
- Nuclear-regulatory proteins (e.g. *MYC*)
- Cell cycle regulators (e.g. cyclins).

2. Insensitivity to Growth-Inhibitory Signals (Tumor Suppressor Genes)

Normally, the **products of tumor suppressor genes have a negative regulatory control of cell growth.** So, a second mechanism of **carcinogenesis results from** failure of growth inhibition, due to **deficiency of normal tumor suppressor genes** and **their products**.

General Characteristic Features of Tumor Suppressor Genes

Q. Define cancer suppressor genes.

1. **Apply brakes to cell proliferation**: Oncoproteins stimulate cell proliferation; whereas the products of tumor suppressor genes apply brakes and prevent uncontrolled cell proliferation. Two important tumor suppressor genes are ***RB*** and ***TP53*** gene.
2. **Mutations of tumor suppressor genes may be hereditary and spontaneous**.

Retinoblastoma Gene (RB gene)

***RB (RB1)* gene** was the **first discovered tumor suppressor gene**, which is present **on chromosome locus 13q14. Inactivation of *RB* gene was found in retinoblastoma**, which is a rare malignant childhood tumor derived from the retina. Retinoblastoma may occur either as a hereditary or sporadic form.

- **Method of inactivation of *RB* gene and associated tumors**:
  1. **Mutations/loss of *RB* gene:** It may be:
     - **Germline mutation,** e.g. in **retinoblastomas** and **osteosarcomas**.
     - **Acquired mutation,** e.g. in **glioblastomas, small-cell carcinomas of lung,** breast cancers, and bladder carcinomas.
  2. **Blocking of *RB* function:** It may occur even without *RB* mutation. Example: E7 protein of Human Papilloma Virus (HPV) bind to the hypophosphorylated *RB* → prevents binding of *RB* protein with E2F transcription factors → free E2F causes progression of cell cycle → cervical carcinomas.

TP53 Gene

TP53 is a **tumor suppressor gene located on small arm of chromosome 17(17p13).** Its protein product p53 is present in almost all normal tissues. ***TP53*** is one **of the most commonly mutated gene in cancer**.

Functions of p53

- **Guardian of the genome:** It functions as **critical gatekeeper genes**. It plays **main role in maintaining the integrity of the genome** and thus known as **guardian of the genome** or **"molecular policeman."**
- **Normal role of p53**: When there is **DNA damage, telomere shortening or other stresses** (e.g. hypoxia) → **activates p53** → **increases p53 levels** → leads to **arrest of cell cycle at G_1** phase. p53 also **induces DNA repair gene**. Cell cycle arrest gives time for the cells to repair DNA damage. During this time the damaged **DNA may be either repaired or damage may persist.**
- **Prevention of neoplastic transformation**: p53 prevents neoplastic transformation of cell by three interconnected mechanisms:
  1. Activation of **temporary cell cycle arrest** (quiescence)
  2. Activation of **permanent cell cycle arrest** (senescence)
  3. Triggering **programmed death of cells with damaged DNA (apoptosis).**

Method of inactivation of *p53* gene and associated tumors: **Most cancers have defect in p53 gene.**

1. **Mutations or deletion of *TP53* gene:** It allows cells with damaged DNA to progress through the cell cycle → neoplastic transformation.
2. **Blocking of p53 function:** Similar to *RB*, function of the p53 may be blocked even without mutation in *p53*. Example: Similar to *RB*, some DNA tumor viral products like HPV E6, promote p53 degradation.

3. Growth-Promoting Metabolic Alterations: The Warburg Effect

Cancer cells show a distinctive form of cellular metabolic alteration (even in the presence of adequate oxygen) characterized by high levels of glucose uptake and increased conversion of glucose to lactose (fermentation) via the glycolytic pathway. This is known as the Warburg effect or aerobic glycolysis. Warburg effect provides rapidly dividing tumor cells with metabolic intermediates that are needed for the synthesis of cellular components. This helps in promotion of tumor growth.

4. Evasion of Apoptosis

Apoptosis is a programmed cell death and **is one of the normal protective mechanism by which a cell with DNA damage (mutation) undergo cell death.** Mutations in the genes that regulate apoptosis may result in accumulation of neoplastic cells.

Methods of Evasion of Apoptosis and Associated Tumors

Tumor cells may escape or undergo reduced apoptosis. **Reduced apoptosis** may be **due to activation of either antiapoptotic proteins or reduced proapoptotic activity**.

1. **Activation of antiapoptotic Bcl-2**: Example, **follicular lymphomas** (about 85%) show a characteristic chromosomal translocation, t(14;18), causing **overexpression** of the **antiapoptotic Bcl-2 protein**. Neoplastic B lymphocytes are **protected from undergoing apoptosis** and survive for long periods.
2. **Reduced levels of proapoptotic BAX**: The p53 induces apoptosis of cells that are unable to repair DNA damage partly by transcriptional activation of **proapoptotic** BAX. **Mutation of p53 leads to reduced levels of BAX** resulting in decreased apoptosis.

5. Limitless Replicative Potential: Telomerase

All malignant tumors contain cells that are immortal and have limitless replicative potential.

- **Cancer Stem Cells**: A least few cells in all cancers have stem cell–like properties and are called as cancer stem cells. They may be formed either through transformation of a normal stem cell or through acquired genetic lesions that produces a stem-like state on a more mature cell.
- **Reactivation of telomerase**:
  - Most **normal cells** have a capacity to undergo **cell division for about 60 to 70 times.**
  - **Telomere is the special structure** present **at the ends of chromosomes. During each cell division**, a small section of the **telomere** is not duplicated resulting in **progressively shortening**, which is responsible for the limited replicative property of a cell. During the course of repeated cell cycles, there is progressive shortening of telomeres, which is prevented by an enzyme called telomerase.
  - **Telomere maintenance is seen in many types of cancers.** Cancer cells acquire lesions that inactivate senescence signals and reactivate telomerase, which act together to convey limitless replicative potential.

6. Development of Sustained Angiogenesis

- **Vascularization of tumor**: Solid tumors cannot grow without vascularization and is achieved mainly by **neoangiogenesis (common)** in which new vessels sprout from existing capillaries. **Angiogenesis is controlled by a balance between angiogenic promoters and inhibitors** that are produced by tumor and stromal cells. **In tumors this balance is tilted in favor of promoters.**
- **Effects of neovascularization**:
  - **Supplies nutrients and oxygen.**
  - **Secretion of growth factors** by newly formed endothelial cells, which stimulate the growth of adjacent tumor cells.
  - **Favor metastasis.**

7. Invasion–Metastatic Cascade (Molecular Events in Invasion and Metastasis)

Q. Discuss the mechanism of invasion and metastasis.

Invasion and metastasis are characteristic of malignant tumors.

Definition: Invasion-metastatic cascade constitutes the **entire sequence of events from** the beginning of **invasion** to the development of **metastasis**.

Phases

Invasion-metastatic cascade is a **complex multistep process**. It can be divided into two main phases namely: (A) **invasion of the extracellular matrix (ECM)** and (B) **metastasis (vascular dissemination and homing of tumor cells)**.

A. Invasion of Extracellular Matrix (Fig. 11.13)

Tumor cells must interact with ECM (includes basement membrane and interstitial tissue) at several steps in the invasion-metastaic cascade. Invasion of the ECM is an active process and consists of 4 steps:

i. **Loosening of tumor cells: Normal cells** are **attached to each other by** an adhesion molecules namely **E-cadherins.**
   - **Reduced/loss of E-cadherin function**: It is observed in most epithelial cancer (e.g. adenocarcinomas of the colon and breast) → **loosening of tumor cells.** The separated cells get **detached from the primary cancer**.

ii. **Local degradation/proteolysis of basement membrane and interstitial connective tissue:** Extracellular matrix is of two types namely: (1) basement membrane and (2) interstitial connective tissue.
   - **Secretion of degrading enzymes**: Malignant **tumor cells** and **stromal cells** (e.g. fibroblasts and inflammatory cells) **in the cancers secrete**/induce **many proteolytic enzymes** that **degrade ECM**. These enzymes includes: **Matrix metalloproteinases (MMPs), cathepsin, and urokinase plasminogen activator (u-PA)**.
   - **Local degradation of basement membrane and interstitial connective tissue:** This is achieved by proteolytic enzymes.

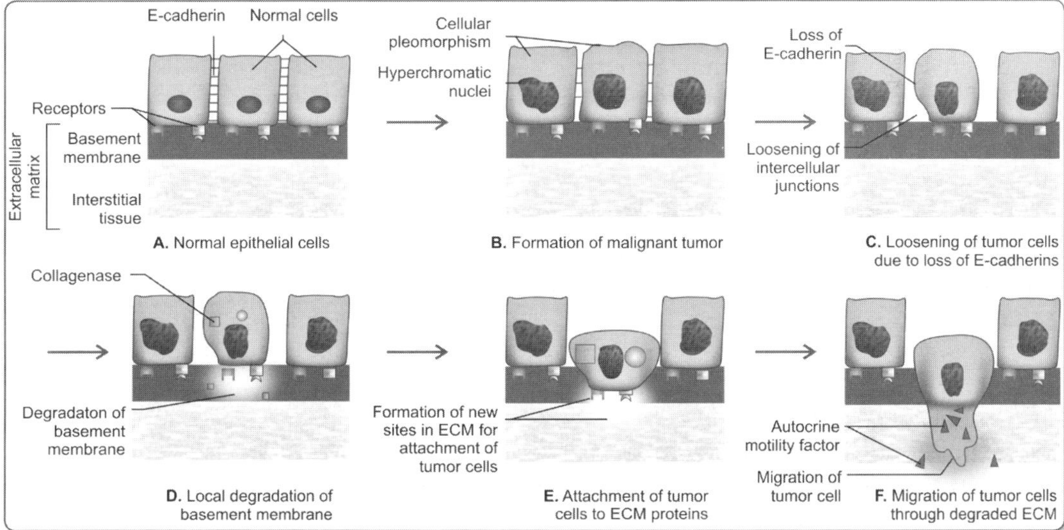

Fig. 11.13: Various steps in the invasion of extracellular matrix in invasion–metastasis cascades. (A) Normal cells. (B to F) Tumor cells loosen and detach from each other because of reduced adhesiveness. The tumor cells bind components of the extracellular matrix and secrete proteolytic enzymes that degrade the extracellular matrix. With binding to proteolytically generated new binding sites in the ECM, tumor cell migration follows. The tumor cells reach the nearby vessels to start the next phase, namely metastasis

iii. **Changes in attachment/adhesion of tumor cells to ECM proteins:** Normal epithelial cells have receptors (e.g. integrin) for basement membrane components (e.g. laminin and collagen) and are located at their basal surface.
   - **Generation of new sites**: Local degradation of basement membrane generates **new and strange sites** in the basement membrane.
   - **Adhesion of tumor cells to ECM**: The receptors on tumor cells attach to the new sites in the basement membrane.
   - **Stimulation of tumor cell migration**: It follows attachment/adhesion of tumor cells to ECM proteins.

iv. **Locomotion/migration of tumor cells through degraded ECM**: It is a multistep process.
   - **Locomotion/migration** drives the tumor cells **forward through the degraded basement membranes** and zones of proteolysis in the **interstitial connective tissue matrix**.
   - **Locomotion involves many receptors and signaling proteins**. The locomotion is potentiated by tumor cell-derived cytokines, such as **autocrine motility factors** (AMF) and other molecules.
   - **Migration through interstitial tissue**: The tumor cells invade and traverse through the surrounding interstitial connective tissue and ultimately **reach nearby blood and lymphatic vessels.** Cells gain access to the circulation by penetrating the basement membrane of vessels.

B. Metastasis (Vascular Dissemination and Homing of Tumor Cells)

Following the invasion of surrounding interstitial tissue, malignant cells may spread to distant sites by metastasis. Metastasis is **multistep process** by which tumor produces a secondary growth at a distant site or location. It has several steps (Fig. 11.14**).**

i. **Penetration of vascular or lymphatic channels (intravasation into the lumen of vessels)**: Malignant cells penetrate the basement membrane of blood vessels or lymphatic channels.

ii. **Invasion of the circulation and formation of tumor emboli**: **Tumor cells** that have entered the circulation **may be either destroyed** by host immune cells **or survives**. Survived tumor cells may aggregate to **form tumor emboli**.

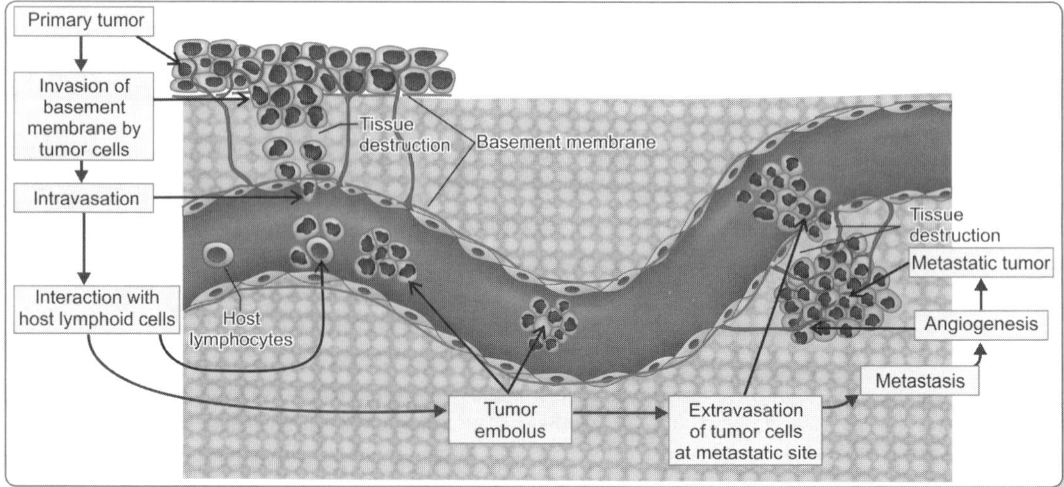

Fig. 11.14: Various steps involved in vascular dissemination and homing of tumor cells during the metastatic cascade

iii. **Transit through the circulation.**
iv. **Arrest within circulating blood or lymph**: It occurs at distant location away from primary tumor. At the site of arrest tumor cells adhere to endothelial cells.
v. **Exit from the circulation into a new tissue site**: Occurs through the basement membrane of lymphatics or blood vessel. The site at which circulating tumor cells leave the vessel or lymphatics must repeat the same events involved in invasion but in a reverse order.
vi. **Formation of micrometastases:** Tumor cells lodge at a distant new site to form micrometastases. Examples for favored sites of metastasis:
    - Prostatic carcinoma to the bone.
    - Bronchogenic carcinomas to the adrenals and to the brain.
    - Neuroblastomas to the liver and bones.
vii. **Angiogenesis.**
viii. **Local growth of micrometastases into macroscopic tumor**.

8. Evasion of Immune Surveillance (Host Defense)

- Immune system can identify the tumor cells as non-self and destroy those cells.
- Antitumor activity is mainly mediated by cell-mediated mechanisms.
- Different classes of tumor antigens include products of mutated proto-oncogenes, tumor suppressor genes, overexpressed or aberrantly expressed proteins, tumor antigens produced by oncogenic viruses, etc.
- Immunosuppressed patients have an increased risk for development of cancer, especially those produced by oncogenic DNA viruses.
- In immunocompetent patients, tumors may avoid the immune system by several mechanisms.

Genomic Instability as Enabler of Malignancy

The third class of genes in which mutations contribute to the pathogenesis of cancer are DNA repair genes. **DNA repair genes protect the integrity of the genome**.

Individuals with **inherited defects in DNA repair genes** are at **increased risk** of developing **cancer**. DNA-repair genes are not oncogenic by themselves, but their defect allows mutations in other genes to progress during cell proliferation. Usually, **genomic instability** develops **when both copies of the DNA repair genes are lost**. Different types of DNA repair genes defects and associated conditions are shown in Figure 11.15

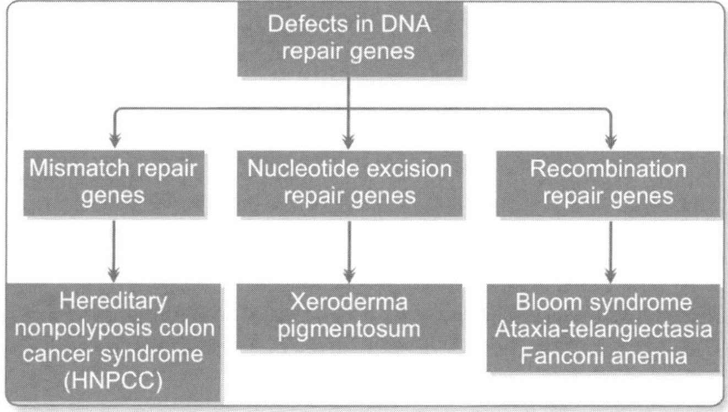

Fig. 11.15: Different types of DNA repair genes defects and associated conditions

ETIOLOGY OF CANCER (CARCINOGENIC AGENTS)

Q. Classify carcinogens /enumerate the types of carcinogens.

Definition: A **carcinogen** is an **agent known or suspected to cause tumors** and such agents are said to be **carcinogenic** (cancer causing). **Carcinogenic agents** (Fig. 11.16): (1) chemicals, (2) microbial agents, and (3) radiation.

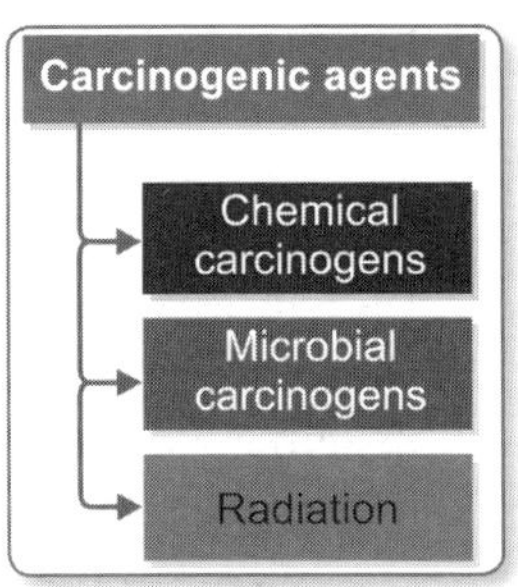

Fig. 11.16: Major types of carcinogenic agents

Chemical Carcinogenesis

Q. List major chemical carcinogens and describe in detail chemical carcinogenesis.

Sir Percival Pott (London surgeon) **first related scrotum skin cancer in chimney sweeps to a specific chronic chemical exposure to soot**. Based on this, a rule was made that chimney sweep members must bathe daily and this public health measure controlled scrotal skin cancer. Japanese investigators (Yamagiva and Ichikawa) experimentally produced skin cancers in rabbits by using coal tar. Subsequently, hundreds of chemical carcinogens were discovered.

Classification of Chemical Carcinogens

Chemical carcinogens may be classified into two categories: Direct acting and indirect acting. Major chemical carcinogens are listed in Table 11.6.

Table 11.6: Major chemical carcinogens

A. DIRECT-ACTING CARCINOGENS
1. ***Alkylating Agents***
– β-propiolactone – Anticancer drugs (cyclophosphamide, chlorambucil, nitrosoureas, etc.) – Dimethyl sulfate – Diepoxybutane
2. ***Acylating Agents***
– 1-Acetyl-imidazole – Dimethyl carbamyl chloride
B. INDIRECT-ACTING CARCINOGENS (PROCARCINOGENS)
1. ***Polycyclic and Heterocyclic Aromatic Hydrocarbons***
– Benz[*a*]anthracene – Benzo[*a*]pyrene – Dibenz[*a,h*]anthracene – 7,12-Dimethylbenz[*a*]anthracene – 3-Methylcholanthrene
2. ***Aromatic Amines, Amides, and Azo Dyes***
– 2-Naphthylamine (β-naphthylamine) – Benzidine – 2-Acetylaminofluorene – Dimethylaminoazobenzene (butter yellow)
C. NATURAL PLANT AND MICROBIAL PRODUCTS
– Aflatoxin B_1 – Griseofulvin – Betel nuts
D. OTHERS
– Nitrosamine and amides – Vinyl chloride – Metals : Nickel, chromium – Insecticides, fungicides – Asbestos.

A. Direct-acting Agents

Direct-acting chemical agents **do not require metabolic conversion** to become carcinogenic, but most of them are **weak carcinogens**. Some of the drugs (e.g. alkylating agents) used to cure, control, or delay recurrence of some cancer (e.g. leukemia, lymphoma), may produce a second form of cancer (e.g. acute myeloid leukemia) later.

- **Alkylating agents**:
  - **Source: Many cancer chemotherapeutic drugs** (e.g. cyclophosphamide, cisplatin, busulfan) are alkylating agents.
  - **Mechanism of action:** Alkylating agents **contain electron-deficient atoms** that **react with electron-rich atoms in DNA**. These drugs not only destroy cancer cells by damaging DNA, but also injure normal cells.
  - **Cancers produced**: Solid and hematological malignancies.

B. Indirect-acting Agents (Procarcinogens)

Q. Write short note on polycyclic hydrocarbons.

These chemicals **require metabolic activation** for conversion **to an active ultimate carcinogen**.

1. **Polycyclic aromatic hydrocarbons:** They are the **most potent** and extensively studied indirect-acting chemical carcinogens. Examples: benzo(a)pyrene, 3-methylcholanthrene, and dibenzanthracene.
   - **Source:**
     - Originally derived from coal tar, and fossil fuels.
     - **Cigarette smoke: Polycyclic aromatic hydrocarbons** are formed during high-temperature combustion of tobacco in cigarette smoking → responsible for lung cancer in cigarette smokers.
     - **Animal fats:** It may produce it during the process of broiling meats.
     - **Smoked food:** Examples, smoked meats and fish.
   - **Mechanism of action**:
     - **Polycyclic hydrocarbons** are metabolized by cytochrome P450-dependent mixed function oxidases to electrophilic (have electron-deficient atoms) epoxides.
     - Epoxides react with proteins and nucleic acids (DNA, RNA). Example: Polyvinyl chloride (used in plastic industry) is metabolized to an epoxide → causes hepatic angiosarcomas.
   - **Cancers produced**: The specific type of cancer produced depends on the route of administration. Examples: Cancers in the **skin**, **soft tissues**, **lung and breast**.
2. **Aromatic amines and azo dyes**: They are indirect-acting carcinogens.
   - **Source:**
     - In the past, the aromatic amines (β-naphthylamine) and azo dyes were used in the aniline dye and rubber industries.
     - Azo dyes were used for coloring food (e.g. butter and margarine, which give yellow color, scarlet red for coloring cherries).
   - **Mechanism of action**:
     - They are not carcinogenic at the point of application.
     - Both aromatic amines and azo dyes are mainly metabolized in the liver.
     - The aromatic amines are converted to active carcinogenic in the liver. However, can be detoxified immediately by conjugation with glucuronic acid in the liver.
     - The conjugated metabolite is excreted in the urine and deconjugated in the urinary tract by the enzyme glucuronidase. The urothelium is thus exposed to the active carcinogen (reactive hydroxylamine) which may cause bladder cancer.
   - **Cancers produced**: **Bladder cancer** (β-naphthylamine and benzidine) and **liver tumors** (azo dyes).

C. **Natural microbial product**

- **Aflatoxin B_1**
  - **Source:** Aflatoxin B_1 is a natural product of ***Aspergillus flavus***, a mold which grows on **improperly stored grains and peanuts**.
  - **Mechanism of action:** Metabolized to an **epoxide** and bind to DNA and also produces **mutations of *p53* gene**.
  - **Cancers produced :** Powerful liver carcinogen → **hepatocellular carcinoma**.

D. **Others**

- **Nitrosamines**: They are potent carcinogens.
  - **Source: Before the advent of refrigerator**, nitrites were added as **a preservative for meats and other foods.**
  - **Mechanism of action: Nitrites react with amines and amides** in the diet and are metabolized by commensal bacteria within the gut and converted to **carcinogenic nitrosamines**.
  - **Cancers produced**: Mainly **gastrointestinal neoplasms**.
- **Metals**: Compounds like arsenic, nickel, lead, cadmium, cobalt, chromium and beryllium can produce cancer. Most metal-induced cancers occur due to occupational exposure.
- **Asbestos**: Inhalation of asbestos fibers → results in asbestosis, pleural plaques, **mesothelioma** and **carcinoma of the lung**. Mesothelioma may involve pleura as well as peritoneum.

Mechanism of Action of Chemical Carcinogens

Molecular targets of chemical carcinogens: Most chemical carcinogens are mutagenic. A **mutagen** is an agent, which can **permanently alter the genetic constitution** of a cell.

- All direct and ultimate carcinogens (of indirect carcinogens) **contain highly reactive electrophilic groups → form adducts with DNA, RNA and proteins**.
- **Genes affected**: Any gene may be affected but commonly involved are proto-**oncogenes** (RAS) **and tumor suppressor genes** (p53).

Multistep Hypothesis (Fig. 11.17)

Chemical carcinogenesis is a **multistep** process. Once the tumor process is started, it does not require the continued presence of the carcinogen.

Four steps involved in chemical carcinogenesis are:

1. **Initiation**: It is the **first important step** that develops from **exposure of cells** to a sufficient dose of a **carcinogenic agent** (initiator).
   - **Reaction with DNA**: All initiators are highly reactive electrophiles (electron-deficient atoms) and can react with nucleophilic (electron-rich) sites in the cell. Sites of reaction of initiation are DNA, RNA, and proteins.
   - **Effect of initiation**: Initiators **produce nonlethal permanent (irreversible) alterations or damage to DNA (mutations)** in a cell. If damage is lethal or severe it causes cell death.
2. **Promotion**

Q. Promoters in carcinogenesis.

Q. Differences between initiators and promoters.

   - **Promoters**: They are **noncarcinogenic** agents and **cannot directly damage DNA** (mutation).
   - **Cell proliferation:** Promoters stimulate the initiated (with permanent DNA damage-mutated) **cells to enter into the cell cycle** → cell proliferation. Unlike initiators, the **cellular changes produces by promoters are reversible**.
   - **Produce changes only on initiated cell: Tumors develop only if the promoter is applied after the initiator** and not the reverse way.
   - **Examples of promoters includes**: phorbol esters, hormones, phenols, and drugs.
3. **Progression: Continuous proliferation** of initiated cells → **leads to secondary genetic abnormalities** → tumor growth becomes independent of the initiator or the promoter (i.e. autonomous). **Many accumulated mutations finally immortalize the cells.**

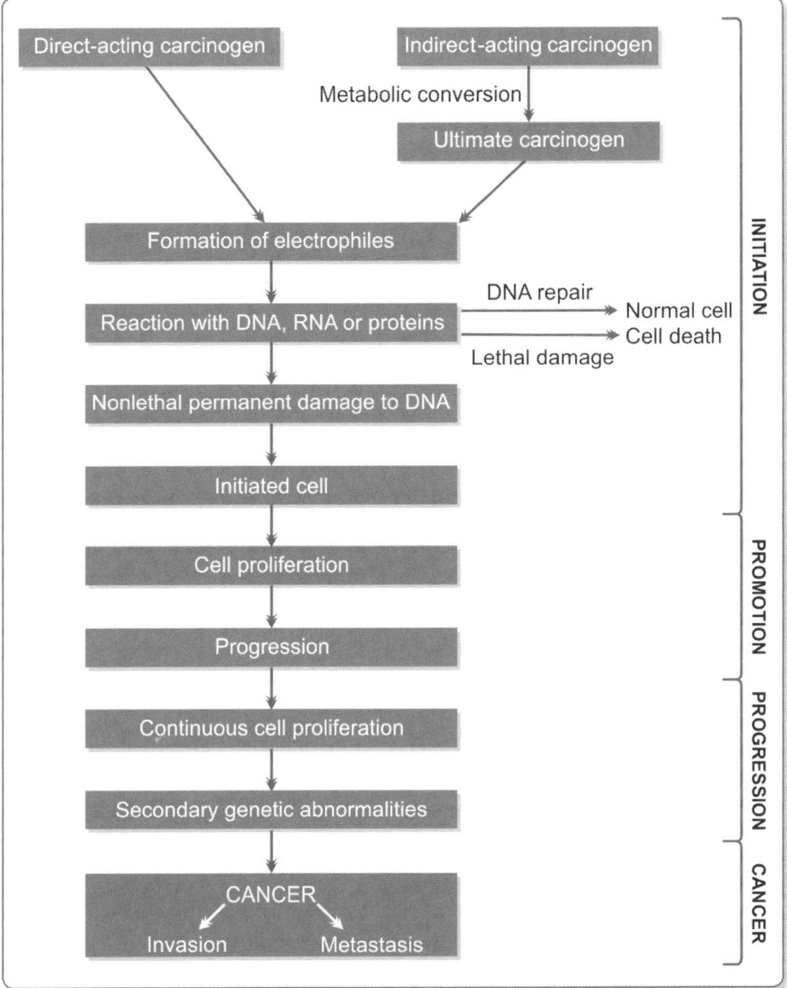

Fig. 11.17: Multistep theory of chemical carcinogenesis

4. **Cancer**: Final result of the different steps is the development of neoplasm → invasion → metastases.

Examples: The morphologic sequence of hyperplasia, dysplasia, and carcinoma in situ found in epithelium (e.g. skin, cervix, and colon) indicate multistep carcinogenesis.

Microbial Carcinogenesis

Viruses that cause tumors are called as oncogenic viruses. Many viruses have been proved to be oncogenic in animals, but only a few have been associated with human cancer.

Q. Classify/List oncogenic viruses.

Classification (Fig. 11.18): They are mainly classified depending on the genetic material into: (1) oncogenic **RNA viruses** and (2) oncogenic **DNA viruses**.

Oncogenic RNA Viruses

Human T-cell leukemia virus type 1: It is a retrovirus.

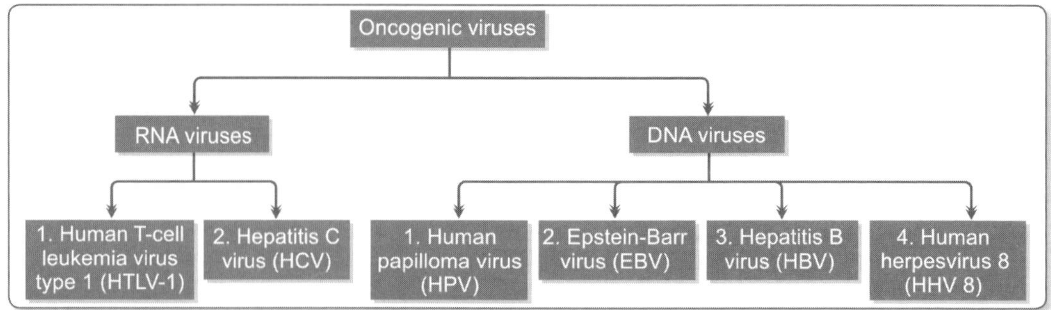

Fig. 11.18: Classification and types of oncogenic viruses

- **Major target** for neoplastic transformation: **CD4+ T lymphocytes.**
- **Tumor caused**: Adult **T-cell leukemia/lymphoma**—develops after a long latent period (20 to 50 years).
- **Mode of infection**: (1) sexual intercourse, (2) blood products, and (3) breast feeding.

Oncogenic DNA Viruses

Five DNA viruses can cause cancer. HCV is not a DNA virus and found to be associated with cancer.

1. Human Papilloma Virus (HPV)

Q. Write short note on oncogenesis by human papilloma virus.

- **Cell infected**: Human papilloma viruses (HPV) infects **only the immature squamous cells** but **its replication occurs in the maturing, nonproliferating squamous cells.** Thus, their full productive life cycle occurs only in squamous cells. The physical state of the virus differs in different lesions.
- **Types of HPV and associated lesions (Table 11.11):** More than 70 genetically different types of HPV have been identified. They are divided into **low-risk and high-risk HPVs.**

Mode of Action (Fig. 11.19)

Episomal form: In **benign lesions** such as benign warts, condylomata and most **precancerous lesions**; the HPV genome is present as nonintegrated, free (episomal) viral DNA.

Integration: In **cancers**, the HPV genome is integrated into the host genome and is essential for malignant transformation. **Integration results in overexpression of the two viral genes *E6* and *E7*.** Proteins products of E6 and E7 (oncoproteins) are important for the oncogenic effects of HPV.

- **Actions of E7 protein:**
  - **Inactivation of tumor suppressor *RB* gene**: **E7 protein binds** to the hypophosphorylated (active) form of ***RB* protein → releases its inhibitory effect on cell cycle progression** (Fig. 11.29).
  - **Inactivation of inhibitors of cell cycle:** For example, inactivation of CDKIs **(CDKN1A/ p21** and CDNK1B/p27) → **activates cell cycle**.
  - **Activation of cyclins (activators of cell cycle)**: These include cyclins E and A → facilitates G_2/M transition → **activation of cell cycle.**
- **Actions of E6 protein**: The E6 protein complements the effects E7.
  - **Inactivation of tumor suppressor *p53* gene**: E6 binds and degrades p53 → degrades BAX (a proapoptotic factor) → **prevents apoptosis.**

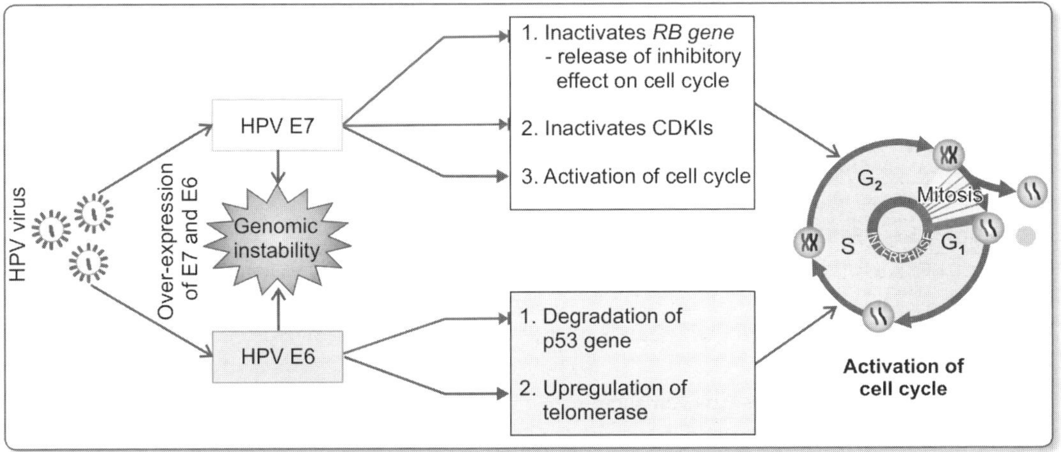

Fig. 11.19: Mode of action of HPV proteins E6 and E7 on the cell cycle

- **Activation of telomerase**: E6 up-regulates telomerase → prevents replicative senescence and **cell proliferation** continues.

- **Combined action of E6 and E7**: They induce centrosome duplication and **genomic instability**.

2. Epstein-Barr Virus (EBV)

EBV is a human **herpesvirus, which infects B lymphocytes**. Patients may manifest as a short-lived **infectious mononucleosis** or develop few human cancers. The **list of cancers** produced includes:

i. **African form of Burkitt lymphoma.**
ii. **B-cell lymphomas** in immunosuppressed (e.g. HIV infection or immunosuppressive therapy after organ transplantation).
iii. A subset of **Hodgkin lymphoma.**
iv. **Nasopharyngeal carcinoma (T cell tumor).**
v. **Some gastric carcinomas.**
vi. **Rare forms of T cell lymphomas and natural killer (NK) cell lymphomas.**
vii. Very rarely sarcomas.

3. Hepatitis B and C Viruses

HBV is a DNA virus whereas **HCV is RNA virus**. There is a strong association between chronic infection with HBV and HCV (chronic hepatitis and cirrhosis) with primary **hepatocellular carcinoma**.

4. Human Herpesvirus 8 (HHV 8)

It is a DNA virus, which **infects the spindle cells of Kaposi sarcoma** and is also **lymphocytes**.

Neoplasm produced:

- **Kaposi sarcoma:** It is a **vascular neoplasm**, which is the **most common neoplasm, associated with AIDS**. HHV 8 has also been found in Kaposi sarcoma from HIV-negative patients.
- **B-cell lymphoid malignancies**: Two uncommon lymphoid malignancies, namely, **primary effusion lymphoma** and **multicentric Castleman disease** are associated with HHV 8.

Various viruses implicated in human tumors are listed in Table 11.7.

Table 11.7: Various viruses implicated in human tumors and associated lesions

Type of virus	Lesions
ONCOGENIC RNA VIRUSES	
• Human T-cell Lymphotropic virus type-1	Adult T-cell leukemia/lymphoma
ONCOGENIC DNA VIRUSES	
1. Human Papilloma Virus	
A. Low-oncogenic risk HPV -benign lesions of squamous epithelium	
◆ HPV types 1, 2, 4, and 7	Benign squamous papilloma (wart)
◆ HPV-6 and HPV-11	Condylomata acuminata (genital warts) of the vulva, penis, and perianal region
	Laryngeal papillomas
B. High-oncogenic risk HPV- malignant tumors	
◆ HPV types 16 and 18	Squamous cell carcinoma of the cervix and anogenital region
	Oropharyngeal cancers (tonsil)
2. Epstein-Barr Virus	Burkitt lymphoma (requires cofactor-malaria)
	Nasopharyngeal cancer
3. Hepatitis B and C Viruses	Hepatocellular carcinoma
4. Human Herpes Virus-8	Kaposi's sarcoma
	Pleural effusion lymphoma, multicentric Castleman disease
5. Merkel Cell Polyoma Virus	Merkel cell carcinoma

Bacteria

Helicobacter pylori

Diseases caused by *H. pylori* are: (1) **peptic ulcers**, **(2) gastric adenocarcinomas, and (3) gastric lymphomas.**

Gastric lymphoma: *H. pylori* produces lymphoma of **B-cell origin** and are called as lymphomas of mucosa-associated lymphoid tissue, or **MALTomas**.

Radiation Carcinogenesis

Radiation is a **well-known carcinogen**.

Latency: **Extremely long latent period** is common and **it has a cumulative effect**. Radiation has also **additive or synergistic effects with other** potential **carcinogenic agents**.

Types of radiation: They are divided into two types, namely: (1) ultraviolet (UV) rays of sunlight, and (2) ionizing electromagnetic and particulate radiation.

Ultraviolet Rays

They are derived from the sunlight.

Tumors caused: **Skin cancer** namely: (1) **squamous cell carcinoma**, (2) **basal cell carcinoma**, and (3) **malignant melanoma**. They are more common on parts of the body regularly exposed to sunlight, and ultraviolet light (UVL).

Risk Factors

The amount of damage incurred depends on:

- **Type of UV rays**
- **Intensity of exposure**

- **Protective mantle of melanin**
  - **Melanin** absorbs UV radiation and has a **protective effect.**
  - Skin cancers are more common in fair-skinned people and those living in geographic location receiving a greater amount of sunlight (e.g. Queensland, Australia, close to the equator).

Pathogenesis

- UV radiation leads to → **formation of pyrimidine dimers in DNA**, which is a type of DNA damage which is responsible for carcinogenicity.
- **DNA damage is repaired by the nucleotide excision repair pathway.**
- With **excessive sun exposure**, the DNA **damage exceeds the capacity of the nucleotide excision repair pathway** and **genomic injury becomes mutagenic and carcinogenic.**
- **Xeroderma pigmentosum**: It is a rare **hereditary autosomal recessive disorder** characterized by **congenital deficiency of nucleotide excision repair DNA.** These individuals **develop skin cancers** (basal cell carcinoma, squamous cell carcinoma, and melanoma) due to impairment in the excision of UV-damaged DNA.

Ionizing Radiation

Electromagnetic (X-rays, γ rays) and particulate (α particles, β particles, protons, neutrons) radiations are all carcinogenic.

Cancers Produced

- **Medical or occupational exposure**, e.g. **leukemia, and skin cancers**
- **Nuclear plant accidents:** Risk of **lung cancers.**
- **Atomic bomb explosion**: Survivors atomic bomb explosion (dropped on Hiroshima and Nagasaki) → increased incidence of **leukemias** → mainly acute and chronic myelogenous leukemia after about 7 years. Subsequently, increased mortality due to **solid tumors** (e.g. breast, colon, thyroid, and lung).
- **Therapeutic radiation**: (1) **papillary carcinoma of the thyroid** follows irradiation of head and neck and (2) **angiosarcoma of liver** due to radioactive thorium dioxide used to visualize the arterial tree.

Mechanism: Hydroxyl free radical injury to DNA.

Tissues which are relatively resistant to radiation-induced neoplasia: Skin, bone, and the gastrointestinal tract.

LABORATORY DIAGNOSIS OF CANCER

Q. Write short note on laboratory diagnosis of cancer.

Confirmation of lesion as neoplastic usually requires cytological and/or histopathological examination of the suspected organ or tissue. Different laboratory methods available for the diagnosis of malignant tumors are:

1. Morphological Methods

Histopathological Examination

Histopathological diagnosis is based on the microscopic features of neoplasm and by this method of examination, **accurate diagnosis can be made in majority of cases.**

- **Clinical data**: It should be provided for accurate pathologic diagnosis. Examples:
  - Radiation causes changes in the skin or mucosa mimic changes seen in cancer.
  - Sections taken from the site of a healing fracture can mimic an osteosarcoma.
- **Adequate and representative** area of the **specimen** should be sent.
- **Proper fixation.**

Frozen Section

In this method, **tissue is frozen** and **sections are cut by special instrument** called **freezing microtome or cryostat**. Its **uses are**:

- **Rapid diagnosis:** Frozen section is used for quick histologic diagnosis (within minutes) and useful for determining the nature of a tumor (benign or malignant) lesion, especially when the **patient is still on the operation table**.
- **Evaluation of the margins of an excised cancer** to know whether excision of the neoplasm is complete.
- **Demonstration of fat** mainly in non-neoplastic lesions.

Various Techniques for Tissue Sampling

- **Needle biopsy**: Using cutting needle, a core of tissue 1 to 2 mm wide and 2 cm long is obtained. Tissue obtained is small and interpretation may be difficult.
- **Endoscopy biopsy:** It is performed through endoscopy. Usually performed for lesions in gastrointestinal, respiratory, urinary and genital tracts.
- **Incision biopsy:** In this representative tissue sample is obtained by incising the lesions.
- **Excision biopsy**: In this entire abnormal lesion is surgically removed.

Cytological Examination

It is performed on many tissues and usually done for identifying neoplastic cells.

Methods of Obtaining Cells

a. Exfoliative cytology: It is the **study of spontaneously exfoliated (shed) cells** from the lining of an organ into a body cavity.

- ***Sources of exfoliated cells:***
  1. **Surface of mucosal or epithelial lining: Cells may be shed naturally or obtained by artificial exfoliation.**
     - Female genital tract:
       - Cervix—cells can be obtained by cervical scrape
       - Vagina
     - Respiratory tract: Sputum and brush cytology by bronchoscopy
     - GI tract: Brush cytology by endoscopy
     - Urinary tract: Voided urine.
  2. **Body fluids:** Usually **cells are shed naturally into body fluids.**
     - Effusions: Pleural, peritoneal, pericardial
     - Other fluids: Synovial fluid, CSF and semen.

b. Fine-needle aspiration cytology (FNAC): It involves **aspiration of cells and attendant fluid with a small-bore needle**. The smears are prepared and stained, followed by microscopic examination of cells. It is **widely used, simple and quick procedure**.

- **Usual sites:** It is most commonly used for the assessment of **readily palpable superficial lesions** in sites such as the breast, lymph nodes, salivary gland, and thyroid. Presently due to **imaging techniques** this method is also used to lesions in **deep-seated structures** (e.g. pelvic lymph, and lesions in retroperitoneum, liver and pancreas).
- **Advantages:**
  - **Less invasive** and more **rapidly performed**
  - **Prevents surgery** and its associated risks
  - Extremely **reliable and useful**.

Method of Examination of Cytological Smears

- **Liquid-based cytology (thin prep):** This is a special technique for preparation of samples that provides uniform monolayered dispersion of cells on smears.

Fixatives Used

- For **Pap smears equal parts of ether and 95% ethanol or 95% ethanol alone**
- **Coating fixative** as aerosol sprays or with dropper to the surface of a freshly prepared smears

Pap smears are fixed immediately in fixative when smear is still wet and dry smears are fixed after the smear is air dried.

Cytological Characteristics of Cancer Cells

Cancer cells have decreased cohesiveness and show cellular features of **anaplasia**. Cytologically, differentiation can be made between normal, dysplastic, carcinoma in situ and malignant cells.

Disadvantages of Cytological Examination

- **Diagnosis is based on the features of individual cells** or a clump of cells, without the supporting evidence of loss of orientation.
- The **invasion** which is diagnostic of malignant tumor under histology **cannot be assessed** by cytology.

Histochemistry and Cytochemistry

These are stains, which identify the chemical nature of cell contents or their products. H and E staining cannot demonstrate certain specific substances/constituents of cells. This requires some special stains.

Immunohistochemistry

It is an immunological method of identifying the antigenic component in the cell or one of its components by using specific antibodies. It is widely used in the diagnosis or management of malignant neoplasms.

Uses of Immunohistochemistry

i. **To categorize undifferentiated cancers***:* Many malignant tumors of diverse origin resemble each other and are difficult to distinguish on routine hematoxylin and eosin (H and E) sections.
ii. **To determine the origin of poorly differentiated metastatic tumors**: It may be determined by using tissue-specific or organ-specific antigens.
iii. **For prognosis or to select the mode of treatment.**

Electron Microscopy

It helps in the **diagnosis of poorly differentiated/undifferentiated cancers**, which cannot identify the origin by light microscopy. Example: carcinomas show desmosomes

Table 11.8: Common tumor markers

Tumor marker	Associated tumors
1. **Hormones**	
– Human chorionic gonadotropin (hCG)	Trophoblastic tumors, nonseminomatous tumors of testis
– Calcitonin	Medullary carcinoma of thyroid
– Catecholamine	Pheochromocytoma
– Ectopic hormones	Paraneoplastic syndromes
2. **Oncofetal Antigens**	
– α-Fetoprotein (AFP)	Cancer of liver, nonseminomatous germ cell tumors of testis
– Carcinoembryonic antigen (CEA)	Carcinomas of the colon, pancreas, lung, and stomach
3. **Mucins and Other Glycoproteins**	
– CA-125	Ovarian cancer
4. **Isoenzymes**	
– Prostatic acid phosphatase (PAP)	Prostate carcinoma
– Neuron-specific enolase (NSE)	Small-cell carcinoma of lung, neuroblastoma
5. **Specific Proteins**	
– Immunoglobulins	Multiple myeloma and other gammopathies
– Prostate-specific antigen (PSA)	Prostate carcinoma
6. **New Molecular Markers**	
– p53, APC, RAS mutants in stool and serum	Carcinoma colon
– p53 and RAS mutants in sputum and serum	Lung cancer

and specialized junctional complexes, structures which are not seen in sarcomas or lymphomas.

Flow Cytometry

It quantitatively measures various individual cell characteristics, such as membrane antigens and the DNA content of tumor cells. Flow cytometry is useful for identification and **classification of tumors of T and B lymphocytes** and mononuclear-phagocytic cells.

2. Tumor Markers

Q. Write short note on tumor markers with examples.

Tumor markers are **products of malignant tumors** that can be detected in the cells themselves or in blood and body fluids.

Usefulness

- **Detection of cancer,** e.g. **PSA** is the most common and useful tumor markers used to screen **prostatic adenocarcinoma.** High levels of PSA are found in the blood of prostatic carcinoma patients but it also may be elevated in benign prostatic hyperplasia.
- **Determine the effectiveness of therapy**
- **Detection of recurrence.**

Types of markers (Table 11.8): These may be tumor-associated hormones, oncofetal antigens, specific proteins, mucin and glycoproteins, enzymes, and molecular markers.

3. Molecular Diagnosis

Molecular diagnosis can be done by different techniques such as FISH technique and PCR (polymerase chain reaction) analysis.

a. **Diagnosis of cancer:**
   - **Monoclonal** (malignant) **vs polyclonal (benign)**: To differentiate benign (polyclonal) proliferations of T or B cells from malignant (monoclonal) proliferations.
   - **Chromosomal alterations**: Many **hematopoietic neoplasms** (leukemias and lymphomas) and few solid tumors (e.g. Ewing sarcoma) are characterized by particular translocations that can be detected by FISH technique or by PCR analysis.

b. **Prognosis of cancer**: Certain genetic alterations are of prognostic value. They can be detected by routine cytogenetics and also by FISH or PCR assays. Example of poor prognostic feature is amplification of the N-*MYC* gene and deletions of 1p in neuroblastoma, and amplification of *HER-2/Neu* in breast cancer.

c. **Detection of minimal residual disease***:* PCR can detect minimal residual disease or the onset of relapse in patients who are treated for leukemia or lymphoma. For example, detection of *BCR-ABL* transcripts in treated patients with CML.

d. **Detection of hereditary predisposition to cancer***:* Germ-line mutations in many tumor suppressor genes are associated with increased risk for specific cancers. This will help in prophylactic surgery, and counseling of relatives at risk. For example, *BRCA1*, *BRCA2*, and the *RET* proto-oncogene.

e. **For therapeutic decision:** It is useful in target therapy.

   Molecular profiles of tumors: Present methods like DNA microarray technology can measure the expression **single gene to all genes** in the genome instead of only one gene at a time.

CLINICAL ASPECTS OF NEOPLASIA

Q. Clinical features of malignant tumors.

Both benign and malignant tumors may produce clinical features by its various effects on host.

Local Effects

These are due to encroachment on adjacent structures.

- **Compression**: Example, adenoma in the ampulla of Vater causing obstruction of biliary tract.
- **Mechanical obstruction**: It may be caused by both benign and malignant tumors. Example, tumors may cause obstruction or intussusception in the GI tract.
- **Endocrine insufficiency**: It is caused by destruction of an endocrine gland either due to primary or metastatic cancer.
- **Ulceration, bleeding and secondary infections:** It may develop in benign or malignant tumors in the skin or mucosa of the GI tract. Example:
  - Melena (blood in the stool) in neoplasms of the gut
  - Hematuria in neoplasms of the urinary tract.
- **Rupture or infarction of tumor.**

Functional Effects

These include:

- **Hormonal effects**: It may be observed both in benign and malignant tumors of endocrine glands. Example: β-cell adenoma of the pancreas may produce insulin → to cause fatal hypoglycemia.
- **Paraneoplastic syndromes:** Nonendocrine tumors may secrete hormones or hormone-like substances and produce paraneoplastic syndromes (explained below).

- **Fever:** It is most commonly associated with Hodgkin disease, renal cell carcinoma, and osteogenic sarcoma. Fever may be due to release of pyrogens by tumor cells or IL-1 produced by inflammatory cells in the stroma of the tumor.

Cancer Cachexia (Wasting)

It is defined as **progressive weight loss accompanied by severe weakness, anorexia, and anemia developing in patients with cancer**.

- **Mechanism:** It is poorly understood and may be due to **TNF and other cytokines**, like IL-1, interferon-γ, and leukemia inhibitory factor. They may be produced by macrophages in the tumor or by the tumor cells themselves.

PARANEOPLASTIC SYNDROMES

Q. Write short note on paraneoplastic syndrome.

Malignant tumors invade local tissue, produce metastasis and can produce a variety of products that can stimulate hormonal, hematologic, dermatologic, and neurologic responses.

Definition: Paraneoplastic syndromes are **symptom complexes in cancer patients** which are **not directly related to mass effects or invasion or metastasis or by the secretion of hormones indigenous to the tissue of origin**.

Frequency: Though they occur in 10% to 15% of patients, it is important because:

1. **May be the first manifestation** of an occult neoplasm.
2. **May be mistaken for metastatic disease** leading to inappropriate treatment.
3. May present clinical problems which **may be fatal**.
4. Certain tumor products causing paraneoplastic syndromes may be **useful in monitoring recurrence** in patients who had surgical resections or are undergoing chemotherapy or radiation therapy.

Some paraneoplastic syndromes, their mechanisms and common cancers causing them are listed in Table 11.9.

PROGNOSIS

Q. Write short note on prognostic factors of malignant tumors.

The prognosis of malignant tumors vary and is determined partly by the characteristics of the tumor cells (e.g. growth rate, invasiveness), and partly by the effectiveness of therapy.

Prognostic Indices

Prognosis and the treatment of a malignant tumor depend on:

1. **Tumor type**: It is usually identified from the growth pattern of the tumor and its origin by only histopathological examination.
   - **Prognosis depends on the histological type** (e.g. squamous cell carcinoma, melanoma, adenocarcinoma, leiomyosarcoma).
   - Some tumors like lymphomas require further subclassification into Hodgkin and non-Hodgkin's lymphoma, each of which is then further subclassified by the cell type.
2. **Grading of malignant tumors**: It is done by histological examination and is mainly based on the **degree of differentiation** of the tumor cells.
   - In general, there is a **correlation between histologic grade and biologic behavior**.

Table 11.9: Paraneoplastic syndromes

Clinical syndromes	Cause/mechanism	Example of associated cancer
1. Endocrinopathies		
Cushing syndrome	ACTH or ACTH-like substance	Small-cell carcinoma of lung
Syndrome due to inappropriate antidiuretic hormone secretion (SIADH)	Antidiuretic hormone or atrial natriuretic hormones	Small-cell carcinoma of lung
Hypercalcemia	Parathyroid hormone-related protein (PTHRP), TGF-α, TNF, IL-1	Squamous cell carcinoma of lung
		Renal carcinoma
Carcinoid syndrome	Serotonin, bradykinin	Bronchial carcinoid
Hypoglycemia	Insulin or insulin-like substance	Fibrosarcoma
Polycythemia	Erythropoietin	Renal carcinoma, hepatocellular carcinoma
2. Neurologic (neuromyopathic) syndromes		
Myasthenia	Immunological	Bronchogenic carcinoma
3. Cutaneous syndromes		
Acanthosis nigricans	Immunological; secretion of epidermal growth factor	Carcinoma of stomach, lung and uterus
Dermatomyositis	Immunological	Bronchogenic, breast carcinoma
Exfoliative dermatitis	Immunological	Lymphoma
4. Changes in osseous, articular, and soft-tissue		
Hypertrophic osteoarthropathy and clubbing of the fingers	Not known	Bronchogenic carcinoma
5. Vascular and hematologic syndromes		
Venous thrombosis (Trousseau syndrome)	Tumor products like mucins which activate clotting	Pancreatic carcinoma
		Bronchogenic carcinoma
Disseminated intravascular coagulation	Procoagulant substance: cytoplasmic granules (e.g. acute promyelocytic leukemia cells), or mucus (adenocarcinomas)	Acute promyelocytic leukemia, prostatic adenocarcinomas
Nonbacterial thrombotic endocarditis	Hypercoagulability	Advanced mucus secreting adenocarcinomas
6. Renal syndromes		
Nephrotic syndrome	Tumor antigens, immune complexes	Various cancers
7. Amyloidosis		
Primary amyloidosis	Immunological (AL protein)	Multiple myeloma
Secondary amyloidosis	AA protein	Renal cell carcinoma and other solid tumors

Abbreviations: ACTH, adrenocorticotropic hormone; IL, interleukin; TGF, transforming growth factor; TNF, tumor necrosis factor

- Most grading systems classify tumors into three or four grades of increasing malignancy. Low-grade tumors are well differentiated; high-grade ones tend to be anaplastic.
  - **Shortcomings: (1) less correlation with behavior**: In general, in soft-tissue sarcomas, grading is of less clinical value than staging; **(2) subjective:** Grading is subjective and the degree of differentiation can vary in different areas of the same tumor.

3. **Staging of tumors:** It **refers to the extent of spread of a malignant tumor** and is independent of grading. The **mode of treatment is determined by the stage of a cancer** than by its grade.

Q. Write short note on staging of cancer

- **Criteria:** Staging requires **both histopathological examination** of the resected tumor and **clinical assessment** of the patient [including additional non-invasive techniques like computed tomography (CT), magnetic resonance imaging (MRI) and positron emission tomography (PET)].
- The **criteria used** for staging **vary with different organs**. Commonly the staging of cancers is based on:
  - **Size and extent of local growth of the primary tumor**: Example: in colorectal cancer, the tumor which has penetrated into the muscularis and serosa of the bowel is associated with a poorer prognosis than with a tumor restricted to superficial mucosa/submucosa.
  - **Extent of spread to regional lymph nodes**: Presence of lymph node metastases indicates poor prognosis than without lymph node involvement.
  - **Presence of or absence of blood-borne (distant) metastases**: The presence of blood-borne distant metastases is bad prognostic sign and is a contraindication to surgical intervention other than for palliative measures.

TNM Staging Systems

Q. Grading and staging of cancer.

It is the cancer staging system widely used and it varies for each specific form of cancer. Its general principles are:

- **T** refers to the **size of the primary tumor**.
  - It is suffixed by a number which indicates the size of the tumor or local anatomical extent. The number varies according to the organ involved by the tumor. With increasing size, the primary lesion is characterized as T1 to T4. T0 is used to denote an in situ lesion.
- **N** refers to **lymph node status**.
  - It is suffixed by a number to indicate the number of lymph regional nodes or groups of lymph nodes showing metastases.
  - N0 would mean no nodal involvement, whereas N1 to N3 would denote involvement of an increasing number and range of nodes.
- **M** refers to the presence and anatomical extent of **distant metastases**.
  - M0 signifies no distant metastases, whereas M1 indicates the presence of metastases.

COMMON SPECIFIC EPITHELIAL TUMORS

Squamous Papilloma

Squamous papillomas are benign neoplasms.

Sites: Larynx, vulva and skin.

1. **Laryngeal squamous papillomas**
   - Usually located on the true vocal cords
   - Gross: Soft, raspberry-like proliferations rarely more than 1 cm in diameter. They are usually single in adults but may be multiple in children (referred to as juvenile laryngeal papillomatosis)
   - Microscopy: Composed of multiple slender, finger-like projections supported by central fibrovascular cores and covered by an orderly stratified squamous epithelium.

2. **Vulvar squamous papillomas**
   - Located on vulvar surfaces and may be single or numerous (vulvar papillomatosis).
   - Microscopy: Exophytic lesions covered by nonkeratinized squamous epithelium (Figs 11.20 and 11.2B).

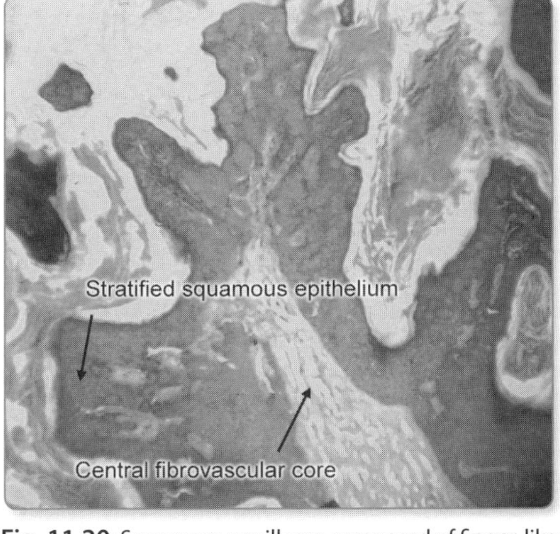

Fig. 11.20: Squamous papilloma composed of finger-like projections supported by central fibrovascular core and covered by an orderly stratified squamous epithelium.
(For color version, see Plate 6)

Adenoma

It is a **benign epithelial tumor arising from glandular epithelium**, although they **may or may not form glandular structures. Examples:**

- **Follicular adenoma of thyroid:** It usually shows microscopically numerous tightly packed small glands.
- **Adenomas of GIT:** Adenomas can be classified as **tubular**, **tubulovillous**, or **villous**.
  - **Tubular Adenomas (Adenomatous Polyps):** They constitute two thirds of the adenomas of large intestine.
    - **Gross:** Appear as small, smooth-surfaced, pedunculated polyps usually less than 2 cm in diameter (Figs 11.21A and B). Tubular adenoma over 2 cm has higher risk of invasive carcinoma.
    - **Microscopy:** Consists of closely packed small rounded or tubular glands (Fig.11.21C) embedded in a stroma (increase in the number of glands and cells per unit area compared to the normal mucosa). The cells lining the glands are crowded and contain enlarged hyperchromatic nuclei. May show variable degree of epithelial dysplasia.
  - **Villous Adenomas (Villous Papilloma)**
    - They constitute one tenth of colonic adenomas and are predominantly found in the rectosigmoid region.

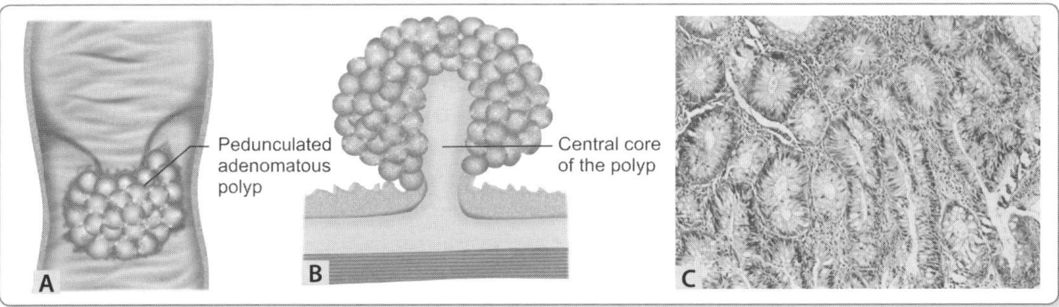

Figs 11.21A to C: Tubular adenoma (A and B diagrammatic). A. Shows a pedunculated tubular adenomatous polyp; B. Cut section of tubular adenoma shows a central core; C. Photomicrograph shows closely packed tubular glands with dysplasia of lining epithelium

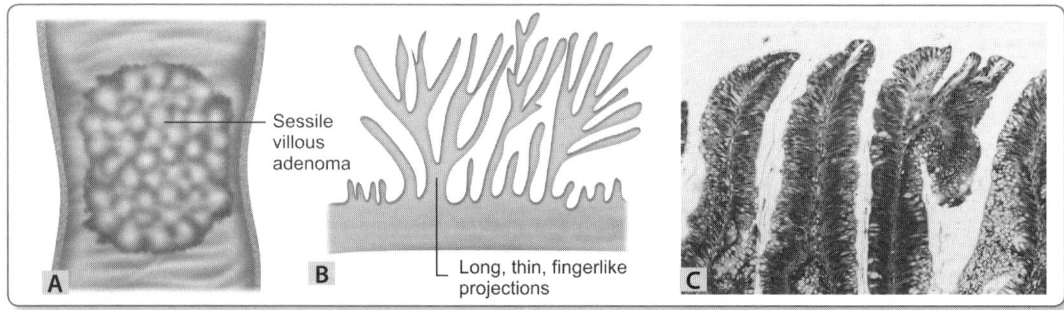

Figs 11.22 A to C: Villous adenoma (A and B diagrammatic) C. Thin, long, fingerlike projections covered by dysplastic epithelium

- **Gross:** Large, broad-based, sessile, elevated lesions with cauliflower-like surface (Figs 11.22A and B). Most are over 2 cm, but may be as large as 10 to 15 cm in diameter.
- **Microscopy:** Composed of thin, long, fingerlike projections (papillary, crown-like growth), which superficially resemble the villi of the small intestine (Fig. 11.22C). The lining epithelium shows dysplasia similar to tubular adenomas. However, villous adenomas (larger than 2 cm) likely contain foci of carcinoma more commonly than tubular adenomas.

- **Tubulovillous Adenomas**
  - **They show a mixture of both tubular and villous elements.** Polyps with more than 25% and less than 75% villous component are called as tubulovillous.

Squamous Cell Carcinoma

Q. Write short note on squamous cell carcinoma of skin.

- **Second most common tumor** arising **on sun-exposed sites**.
- **Sex:** More **common in men** than in women.
- **Clinical presentation:** Appear as sharply defined, red, scaling plaques.
- Sites: Skin, oral cavity, larynx, penis, cervix, esophagus, lung and sites wherever there is squamous epithelium.

Etiology and Pathogenesis

Risk Factors

- **Exposure to UV light:** It **may produce DNA damage** and is the **most important cause** of squamous cell carcinoma of skin. The risk is proportional to the degree of lifetime sun exposure.
- **Chronic immunosuppression:** It may be due to **chemotherapy or organ transplantation** and may contribute to carcinogenesis. The immunosuppression reduces host surveillance and increases the susceptibility of keratinocytes to infection and transformation by oncogenic viruses. These oncogenic viruses include human papilloma virus (HPV) subtypes 5 and 8. Apart from damaging DNA, sunlight can cause a defect in cutaneous immunity by reducing the immune surveillance function of epidermal Langerhans cells.
- **Other risk factors:**
  - **Industrial carcinogens**: **Tars and oils.**
  - **Chronic non-healing ulcers:** e.g. chronic osteomyelitis.
  - **Old burn scars (e.g. Marjolin's ulcers).**

- **Ingestion of arsenicals.**
- **Ionizing radiation.**
- Tobacco and betel nut chewing in the oral cavity.

Genetics of Squamous Cell Carcinoma

- **Mutations in tumor suppressor *p53* gene:**
  - **UV light** present in the sunlight damages DNA.
- **Mutations in DNA repair genes:**
  - **Xeroderma pigmentosum** is a disorder characterized by **inherited mutations in DNA repair genes,** and these **patients are susceptible to squamous cell carcinoma.**
- **Other genes**: Dysregulated RAS signaling may also be responsible.

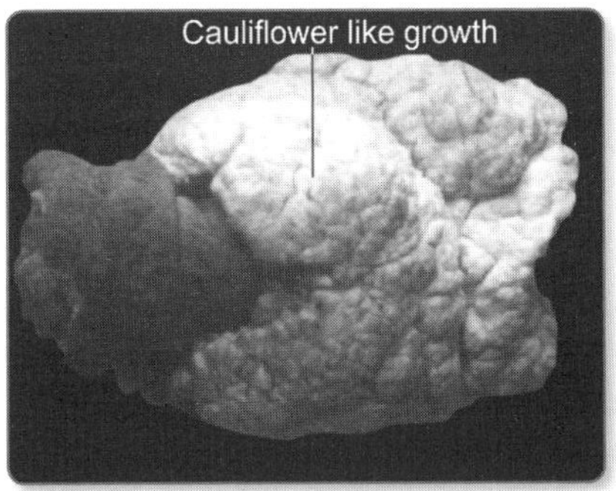

Fig. 11.23: Squamous cell carcinoma of penis with cauliflower-like appearance

Morphology

Squamous cell carcinoma in situ:

- Characterized by **cells with atypical** (enlarged and hyperchromatic) **nuclei involving all levels** of **epidermis.**
- **No invasion** through the basement membrane of the dermoepidermal junction.

Invasive squamous cell carcinoma:

Gross (Fig. 11.23)**:** Invasive lesions are more advanced lesions, which appear as **nodular growth and may ulcerate.** The ulcer is **surrounded by a wide, elevated, indurated border.**

Microscopy: Tumor consists of **irregular masses of epidermal cells** that **proliferate downward into the dermis.** They show variable degrees of differentiation, ranging from well to poorly differentiated.

- **Well differentiated squamous cell carcinoma** (Figs 11.24A and B): They are composed of **polygonal squamous tumor cells arranged in orderly lobules** and **produce large amounts of keratin.** Some of this keratin form **epithelial or squamous pearls** and are characteristically seen in well-differentiated tumors.
- **Moderately differentiated squamous cell carcinoma:** They consist of **anaplastic squamous cells, which show single-cell keratinization** (dyskeratosis). It may be associated with areas of geographic necrosis.
- **Poorly differentiated squamous cell carcinoma**: They consist of **highly anaplastic cells.** Poorly differentiated tumor **may require immunohistochemical stains for keratins to confirm the diagnosis.**

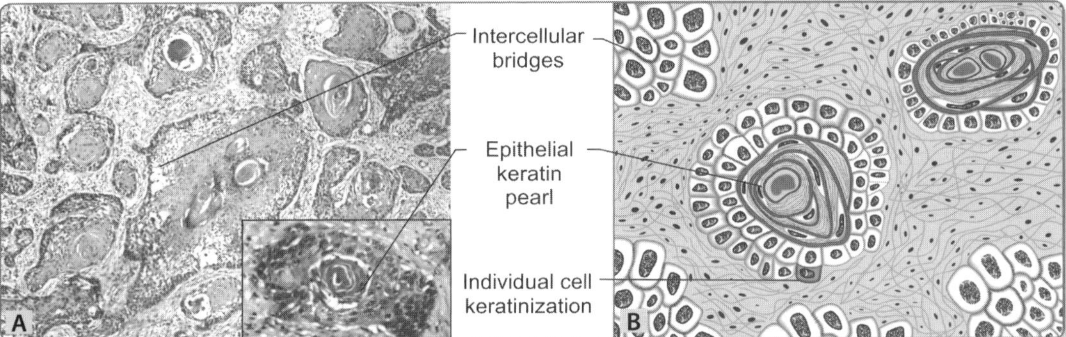

Figs 11.24A and B: A. Photomicrograph and B. Diagrammatic; Well-differentiated squamous cell carcinoma composed of polygonal squamous tumor cells arranged in orderly lobules and produce large amounts of keratin. Some of this keratin form epithelial or squamous pearls (inset of A)

(For color version, see Plate 6)

Basal Cell Carcinoma

Q. Write short note on basal cell carcinoma (rodent ulcer) of skin.

- Basal cell carcinoma is the most common, **slow-growing invasive cancer** that **rarely metastasizes.**
- **Sites:** Occur at **sun-exposed sites** and in fair skinned people. Usual site is **above a line drawn from angle of mouth to the pinna of the ear.**
- **Origin:** Basal cell carcinoma derives its name from the cytological similarity of the tumor cells to the normal basal cells of the epidermis. It is believed to be **primitive 'adnexal' carcinomas probably of indubitable hair follicle derivation.**

Etiology and Pathogenesis

- The incidence of basal cell carcinoma is also **more in patients with immunosuppression** and **inherited defects in DNA repair** such as **xeroderma pigmentosum.**

Genetics of Basal Cell Carcinoma

1. **Mutation in tumor suppressor gene:**
   - **Mutation in *PTCH*: *PTCH* acts as tumor suppressor gene.** Mutations of genes belonging to the *PTCH* signaling pathway are important for the development of both common **sporadic and inherited** form of basal cell carcinoma.
   - ***p53* mutations:** They occur in 40 to 60% of cases.
2. **Defect in DNA repair genes: Xeroderma pigmentosum** is a disorder of DNA repair, associated with increased incidence of basal cell carcinoma.

Clinical Presentation

- Appear as **pearly papules** often containing prominent, dilated subepidermal blood vessels.
- Some tumors may contain melanin and may resemble melanocytic nevi or melanomas.
- Advanced tumors **may ulcerate, and locally invade and erode the underlying bone or facial sinuses like a rodent** and are known as **rodent ulcers.**

Morphology

Gross

- **Appearance varies** and may be **nodular, ulcerative, superficial or erythematous.**
- **Nodulo-ulcerative** basal cell carcinoma is the **most common type** and present as a nodule that increases slowly in size and undergoes central ulceration. A **typical lesion** consists of a **slowly enlarging ulcer surrounded by a pearly, rolled border.** This represents the so-called rodent ulcer (**erodes the underlying structures similar to a rodent**).

Microscopy (Figs 11.25A and B)

- **Tumor cells:** They **resemble the normal basal cell layer** of the epidermis and referred to by some as basaloma (germinative) cells. The tumor cells are **deeply basophilic epithelial cells** and have a **large, oval, or elongated nucleus with narrow rim of cytoplasm.**
- **Arrangement:** Tumors cells are arranged in **nests** and are attached to the epidermis and protrude into the subjacent papillary dermis.
- **Peripheral palisading:** At the periphery of each nest, the **columnar cells are arranged radially with their long axes in parallel alignment** known as peripheral **palisading.**
- **Clefting artifact between tumor islands and adjacent stroma:** It may **sometimes help distinguish BCC from other adnexal neoplasms displaying basaloid cell proliferation.**
- **Two patterns of growth:**
  - **Multifocal growths:** These tumors originate from the epidermis and extend over several square centimeters or more of skin surface (multifocal superficial type).
  - **Nodular lesions:** These tumors grow deeply downward into the dermis as cords and islands of variably basophilic cells with hyperchromatic nuclei.

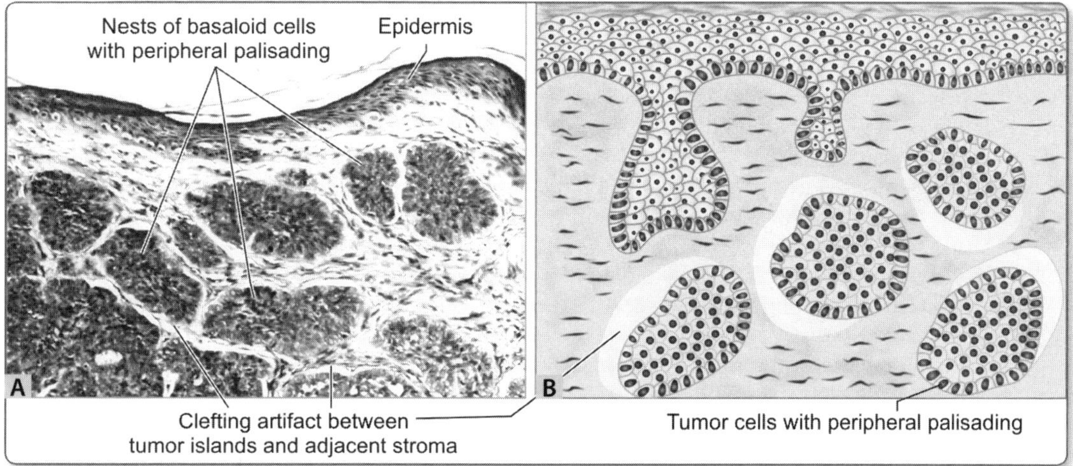

Figs 11.25A and B: Basal cell carcinoma. Composed of nests of uniformly atypical basaloid cells within the dermis, that are often separated from the adjacent stroma by thin clefts. A. Photomicrograph; B. Diagrammatic

(For color version, see Plate 6)

Melanoma

Q. Write short note on malignant melanoma.

Melanoma is a **relatively common** neoplasm.

- **Site:**
  - **Skin**: It is the most common site and may develop in the trunk, leg, face, sole, palm and nail beds.
  - **Other sites**: Oral and anogenital mucosal surfaces, esophagus, leptomeninges, eye, and the substantia nigra.
- **Cell of origin**: Melanocytes.

Etiology and Pathogenesis

Predisposing Factors

A. Sun Exposure

- **Melanomas most commonly develop on sun-exposed surfaces**, particularly the upper back in men and the back and legs in women.
- **Lightly pigmented individuals** are at **greater risk** than darkly pigmented individuals.

B. Inherited Genes

About 10 to 15% of melanomas are familial and the genetic abnormalities are:

1. **Mutations in tumor suppressor gene:**
   - **Mutations in *CDKN2A* gene:** It is observed in familial as well as in few sporadic melanomas.
   - **Mutations in *RB* gene**: These are common in both familial and sporadic melanomas.
   - **Silencing of *PTEN* gene.**
2. **Oncogene activation**: It may occur by **mutations in proteins involved in signal transduction.** Aberrant increases in RAS signaling may occur due to **mutations in** *RAS* or *BRAF*, which promote cell **growth and survival**.

Morphology (Figs 11.26A to C)

Q. Write short note on morphology of malignant melanoma.

Growth phases

1. **Radial growth phase:** During this phase, the **melanoma spread horizontally** within the **epidermis and superficial dermis.**
   - It represents the **initial stage** where the tumor cells **lack the capacity to metastasize.**
   - Tumors in radial growth phase **fall into different clinicopathologic classes.**
     a. **Lentigo maligna:** It usually **present as an indolent lesion** on the **face of older men.** The tumor may remain in the radial growth phase for **several decades.**
     b. **Superficial spreading:** It is the **most common type** of melanoma, and **usually** involves the **skin exposed to sun.**
     c. **Acral/mucosal lentiginous melanoma:** It is **not related to sun exposure** and usually seen in the **palm, sole or mucosa.**
2. **Vertical growth phase: After a variable and unpredictable period,** melanoma from the radial phase develops a **vertical growth phase.**
   - **Characteristics:** During this phase:
     - Tumor cells **invade downward** into the deeper dermis.
     - **Melanoma may appear as a nodule and develop clone of cells with metastatic potential.**
     - **Maturation is absent from the deep invasive portion** of melanoma.
     - **Risk of metastasis** correlates with the **depth of invasion,** which is the distance from the superficial epidermal granular cell layer to the deepest intradermal tumor cells. This measurement is known as the **Breslow thickness.**

Microscopy (Figs 11.27A and B)

1. **Tumor cells:** They have **similar appearance in both the radial and vertical phases** of growth.
   - **Size:** Tumor cells are usually **larger than normal melanocytes** or nevus cells found in melanocytic nevi.
   - **Nuclei:** They are **large with irregular contours, clumping of chromatin at the periphery** of the nuclear membrane, and **prominent red (eosinophilic) nucleoli. Mitotic figures** are often seen.
2. **Pattern of growth:** Tumor cells are arranged in **solid masses, sheets, islands,** etc. Tumor invades upper epidermis as well as deeper dermis.
3. **Melanin pigment:** It is **seen in melanoma.** The melanoma, **which does not show the pigment,** is known as **amelanotic melanoma.** Melanin is present **in the cytoplasm as uniform brown fine granules.**

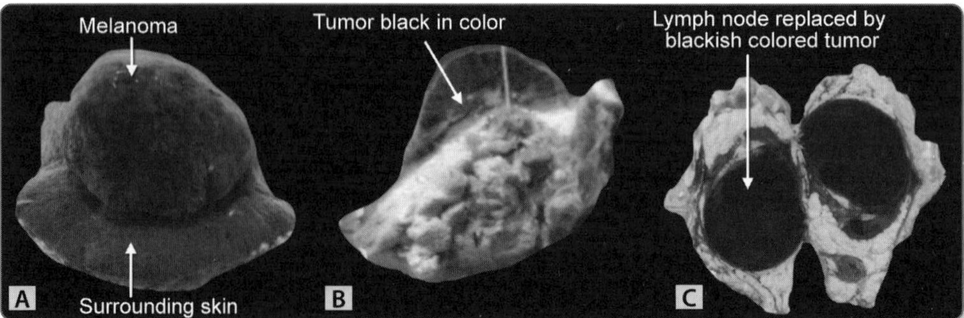

Figs 11.26A to C: Gross features of malignant melanoma. A. Nodular growth projecting from the skin; B. Cut section of the same shows blackish pigmentation in the tumor; C. Lymph node with extensive metastasis from malignant melanoma (black color)

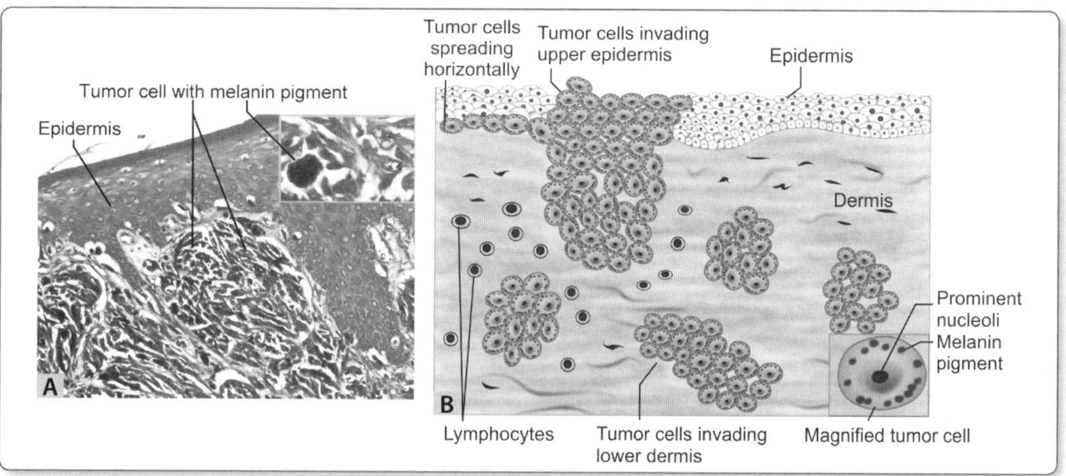

Figs 11.27A and B: A. Photomicrograph of malignant melanoma showing nests of tumor cells in the upper dermis containing melanin pigment. Inset shows tumor cell with melanin pigment; B. Diagrammatic microscopic appearance of malignant melanoma showing nests of tumor cells infiltrating epidermis (radial growth phase) and dermis (vertical growth phase)

Clinical Features

- Melanoma of the skin is **usually asymptomatic**, but may present with itching or pain at the site of lesion.
- **Changes in pigmented lesions**: These are the **most important clinical signs** of melanoma and include:
  - **Color:** Unlike benign nevi, **melanomas show variations in color**, ranging from shades of black, brown, red, dark blue, and gray.
  - **Size:** Majority are **larger than 10 mm** in diameter at the time of diagnosis. But, if a pigmented lesion is greater than 6 mm a diameter, any change in appearance, and new onset of itching or pain should raise the suspicion of malignancy.
  - **Shape:** The borders of melanomas are **irregular and often notched**, whereas they are smooth, round, and uniform in melanocytic nevi.

Adenocarcinoma

- Carcinoma arising from secretory/mucosal epithelial lining glands or ducts or organs is called adenocarcinoma.
- **Sites:** Stomach, colorectal region, gallbladder, pancreas, uterus, prostate and other glandular organs.
- Gross appearance varies with the site of adenocarcinoma.
  - The **tumor cells contain abundant mucin** which expand the cytoplasm and push the nucleus to the periphery creating **signet-ring cell** appearance.
  - If the signet-ring cells constitute **more than 50%** of the tumor, it is classified as **signet-ring cell carcinoma**.

Microscopy (Figs 11.28A and B and 11.5)

Adenocarcinoma may be **well differentiated, moderately or poorly differentiated**.

- Most of the tumors show **glands of variable size and configuration** separated by moderate amount of stroma. Mitotic figures are usually abundant.

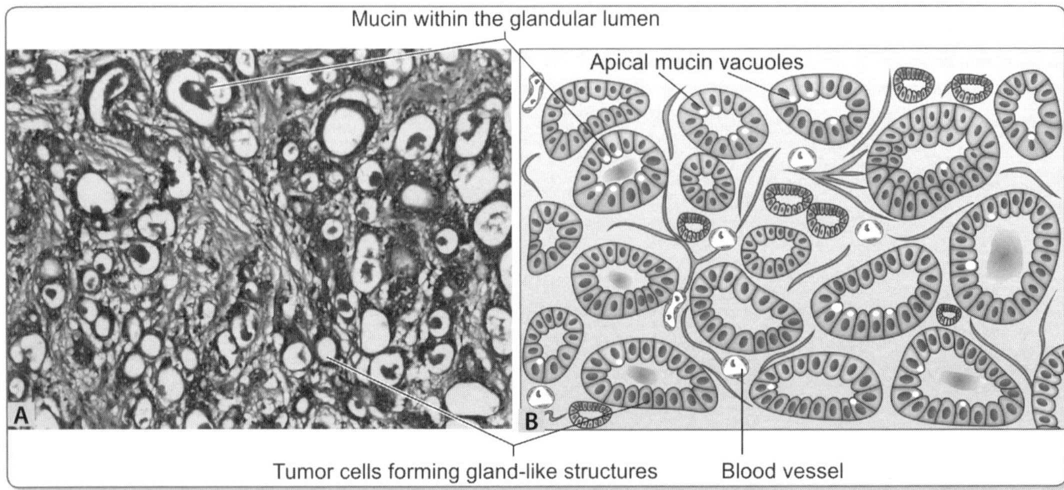

Figs 11.28 A and B: Microscopic appearance of adenocarcinoma carcinoma. A. Photomicrograph; B. Diagrammatic

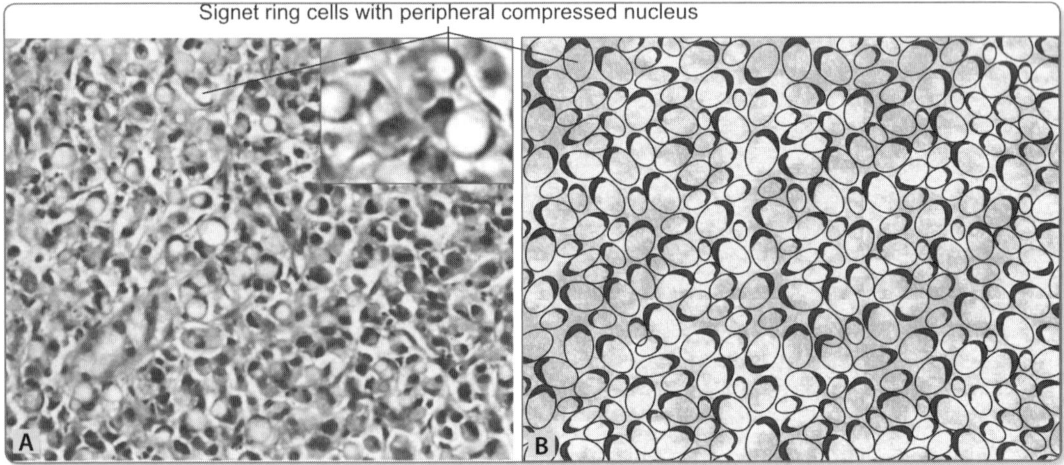

Figs 11.29 A and B: A. Microscopic appearance of signet ring carcinoma. Inset shows signet ring cells (upper right). B. Diagrammatic appearance of signet ring carcinoma

- Poorly differentiated carcinoma shows only few glands.
- **Mucinous adenocarcinomas:** They secrete abundant mucin and accumulate within the intestinal wall and are associated with poor prognosis.
- **Signet-ring carcinoma:** The **tumor cells contain abundant mucin** which expand the cytoplasm and push the nucleus to the periphery creating **signet-ring cell** (Figs 11.29A and B) appearance.

MESENCHYMAL TUMORS

Fibroma

A benign tumor arising in fibrous tissue is called a *fibroma*. True fibromas are uncommon in soft tissue. Combination of fibrous and other mesenchymal tissue is more often seen. These include neurofibroma, fibromyoma, dermatofibroma and fibrolipoma.

- **Oral cavity: Fibroma** is common in the oral mucosa. It is a reactive lesion rather than a neoplastic process. It is called as irritation fibroma (traumatic fibroma or focal fibrous hyperplasia).
  - **Gross:** It occurs as a submucosal nodular mass primarily on the buccal mucosa along the bite line or the gingiva.
  - **Microscopy:** It shows fibrous connective tissue stroma. It is thought to be a reactive proliferation caused by repetitive trauma.
- **Ovary**: Fibromas of ovary are relatively common benign tumors composed of fibroblasts. They constitute about 4% of all ovarian tumors.
  - **Gross:** They are predominantly unilateral in about 90% of cases. They are usually solid, spherical, encapsulated, gray-white tumors.
  - **Microscopy:** They consists well-differentiated fibroblasts and a scant interspersed collagenous stroma.
- **Dermis**: Benign fibrous histiocytoma (dermatofibroma) constitutes a heterogeneous family of benign dermal neoplasms of uncertain lineage. They are usually seen in adults and often on the legs of young and middle-aged women. They consist of mixture of both fibrous tissue and histiocytes.

Fibrosarcoma

Fibrosarcomas are very rare tumors because many of the tumors earlier diagnosed as fibrosarcomas presently belong to a group of tumors known as fibrous histiocytomas.

Fibrosarcoma is a slow growing malignant tumor arising from fibrous tissue. It is often found between 4th to 7th decades of life. Most commonly they occur in the lower extremity (thigh and around knee), upper extremity, trunk, head and neck, and retroperitoneum.

- **Gross:** They are circumscribed gray-white, firm and lobulated tumors. Cut section has a soft, fish flesh-like appearance. Areas of hemorrhage and necrosis are usually seen.
- **Microscopy:** The tumor consists of spindle-shaped fibroblasts arranged in intersecting fascicles (Fig 11.30). Well-differentiated fibrosarcomas show characteristic herring-bone pattern (herring = a type of sea-fish). Poorly-differentiated fibrosarcomas show pleomorphic fibroblasts with frequent mitotic figures.

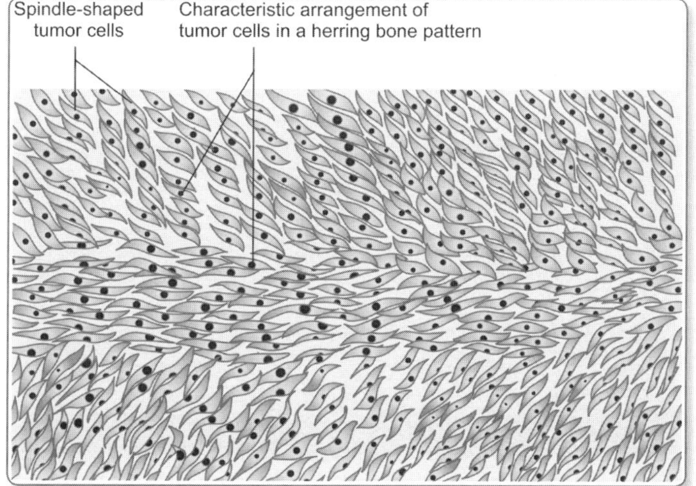

Fig 11.30: Fibrosarcoma composed of spindle-shaped fibroblasts arranged in intersecting fascicles (characteristic herring-bone pattern)

Tumors of Adipose Tissue

Lipoma

- Lipoma is the **commonest benign tumor of fat.**
- It is the **most common soft issue tumor of adulthood**.
- Occur most often during 4th to 5th (middle adulthood) decades of life.
- Lipomas are usually single, soft, mobile painless mass.
- Site: Usually arises in the subcutaneous tissues of the proximal extremities, neck, back, shoulder and trunk. Infrequently, lipomas are large and intramuscular.
- Gross (Fig 11.31): It is usually a well encapsulated (may be poorly circumscribed), small, round to oval mass. The cut surface is soft, yellow, greasy and often lobulated.
- Microscopy (Fig. 11.4): It shows lobules of mature adipocytes separated by delicate fibrous septa.
- A thin fibrous capsule is usually found surrounding the tumor.

Liposarcoma

- Liposarcoma is one of the most common soft tissue sarcomas of adulthood.
- Age: It occurs mainly during 5th to 6th decades of life.
- Sites: Deep soft tissues of the proximal extremities and in the retroperitoneum.

Gross:

- Liposarcomas appear as nodular masses of 5 cm or more in diameter. Tumors are usually appearing circumscribed but infiltrate into surrounding tissue. Cut section show gray-white to yellow color with myxoid and gelatinous appearance.

Microscopy

The cell required for the diagnosis of liposarcoma is lipoblast. These cells may be univacuolated or multivacuolated and uninucleated or multinucleated. Liposarcomas are histologically divided into four morphologic subtypes:

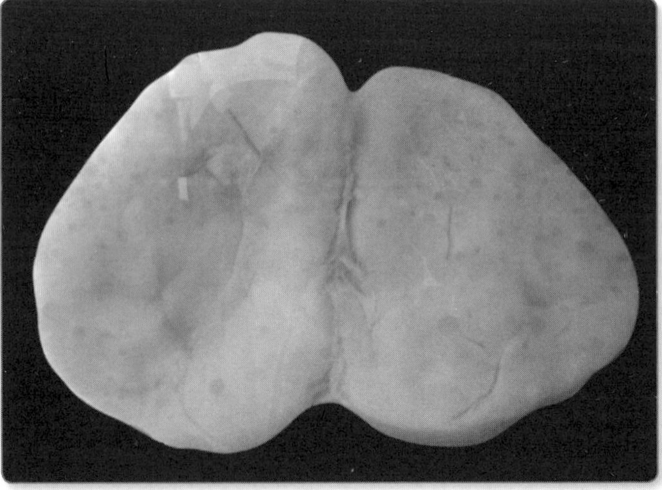

Fig. 11.31: Lipoma: well capsulated, lobulated and yellow benign tumor of fat

(For color version, see Plate 7)

1. Well-differentiated liposarcoma: Contains adipocytes with scattered atypical spindle cells and lipoblasts.
2. Myxoid liposarcoma: Most common histological subtype. Contains abundant basophilic extracellular matrix, arborizing capillaries (chicken-wire pattern) and primitive cells at various stages of adipocyte differentiation reminiscent of fetal fat.
3. Round cell liposarcoma: It consists of uniform, round to oval cells with central hyperchromatic nuclei. The cytoplasm shows multiple vacuoles.
4. Pleomorphic liposarcoma: It is highly undifferentiated/anaplastic liposarcoma and consists of sheets of anaplastic cells, bizarre nuclei and variable amounts of immature adipocytes (lipoblasts).

Behavior: All histological types of liposarcoma recur locally and often repeatedly unless adequately excised. Well-differentiated liposarcoma is relatively indolent; the myxoid/round cell liposarcoma is intermediate in its malignant behavior. The pleomorphic variant usually is aggressive and frequently metastasizes.

Chapter 12

Hematology

Chapter Outline

Disorders of Red Cells
- Anemia
- Iron deficiency anemia
- Megaloblastic anemia
- Pernicious anemia
- Aplastic anemia
- Hereditary defects in hemoglobin
- β-Thalassemia major
- Sickle cell anemia

Disorders of White Cells
- Normal differential leukocyte count (DLC)
- Quantitative disorders of leukocytes
- Acute leukemia
- Acute lymphoblastic leukemia/lymphoma
- Acute myelogenous leukemia
- Chronic myelogenous leukemia
- Chronic lymphocytic leukemia

Disorders of Hemostasis
- Normal hemostasis
- Classification of hemostatic disorders
- Immune thrombocytopenic purpura
- Coagulation disorders
- Hereditary coagulation disorders
- Hemophilia
- Acquired coagulation disorders

DISORDERS OF RED CELLS

ANEMIA

Definition

Q. Define anemia.

- **Decrease** below normal limit (below the reference level for the age and sex of the individual) of the **hemoglobin concentration (Hb)/RBC count/hematocrit (packed cell volume)**.
- **Reduction of the total circulating red cell mass** below normal limits.
- **Decrease in the oxygen-carrying capacity** of the blood, which leads to tissue hypoxia.

Anemia may be **absolute** (decreased RBC mass), or **relative** (associated with a higher plasma volume). Anemia is conventionally used for absolute anemia.

Classification of Anemia

Q. Classify anemia.

Q. Etiological classification of anemia.

1. **Morphological classification** (Table 12.1): it is based on:
   a. **Red cell size** (normocytic, microcytic, or macrocytic), and
   b. **Degree of hemoglobinization** (normochromic or hypochromic).
2. **Etiological classification:** The etiological classification of anemia is listed in Table 12.2.

Red Cell Indices

Q. Write short note on red cell indices.

Red cell indices are useful in morphological characterization and diagnosis of anemias. They are either directly measured or automatically calculated by specialized instruments. Red cell indices include:

1. **Mean Corpuscular Volume (MCV)**
   - MCV is indicative of average volume of the RBC and is expressed in femtoliters (fL).
   - It is used for classification and differential diagnosis of anemias.
   - **Normal range: 82–98 fL.**

$$\text{MCV} = \frac{\text{PCV} \times 1000}{\text{RBC count in millions}} = 0.45 \times 1000/5 = 90 \text{ fL}$$

2. **Mean Corpuscular Hemoglobin (MCH)**
   - MCH indicates the amount of Hb (weight) per RBC and is expressed as picograms (1 pg $= 10^{-12}$ g).
   - It is of limited value in differential diagnosis of anemias.

Table 12.1: Morphological classification of anemia

Type of anemia	Microcytic hypochromic	Normocytic normochromic	Macrocytic
Size of RBCs	Smaller than normal	Normal	Larger than normal
Central pallor in RBCs	More than 1/3	Normal	Normal
Mean corpuscular volume (MCV)	Reduced (<80 fL)	Normal (82–98 fL)	Increased (>100 fL)
Mean corpuscular hemoglobin concentration (MCHC)	Reduced (<30 g/dL)	Normal (31–36 g/dL)	Normal (31–36 g/dL)
Examples	Iron deficiency anemia, thalassemia	During blood loss, anemia of chronic diseases	Deficiency of vitamin B_{12} and folic acid
Morphology of RBC			

Table 12.2: Etiological classification of anemia

Impaired Red Cell Production
• **Disturbed proliferation and maturation of erythroblasts** – Defective DNA synthesis ◆ Megaloblastic anemias due to deficiency or impaired utilization of vitamin B_{12} and folic acid ◆ Anemia of renal failure due to deficiency of erythropoietin ◆ Anemia of chronic disease due to iron sequestration and relative erythropoietin deficiency ◆ Anemias of endocrine disorders – *Defective hemoglobin synthesis* ◆ Defective heme synthesis: Iron deficiency, sideroblastic anemia ◆ Defective globin synthesis: Thalassemias • **Marrow Replacement** – *Primary hematopoietic neoplasms*: Acute leukemia, myelodysplastic syndromes • **Marrow Infiltration (myelophthisic anemia)** – *Metastatic neoplasms* • **Disturbed Proliferation and Differentiation of Stem Cells** – Aplastic anemia, pure red cell aplasia
Increased Red Cell Destruction (Hemolytic Anemias)
• **Intrinsic (Intracorpuscular) abnormalities** – *Hereditary* ◆ Membrane abnormalities: Spherocytosis, elliptocytosis ◆ Enzyme deficiencies: Glucose-6-phosphate dehydrogenase, pyruvate kinase ◆ Disorders of hemoglobin synthesis ◊ Deficient globin synthesis: Thalassemia syndromes ◊ Structurally abnormal globin synthesis (hemoglobinopathies): Sickle cell anemia – *Acquired* ◆ Membrane defects: Paroxysmal nocturnal hemoglobinuria • **Extrinsic (Extracorpuscular) abnormalities** – *Antibody-mediated* ◆ Isohemagglutinins: Transfusion reactions, Rh disease of the newborn ◆ Autoantibodies: Idiopathic (primary), drug-associated, systemic lupus erythematosus – *Mechanical trauma to RBCs:* ◆ Microangiopathic hemolytic anemia: Disseminated intravascular coagulation – *Infections:* Malaria
Blood Loss
• **Acute: trauma** • **Chronic:** Lesions of gastrointestinal tract (e.g. carcinoma colon), gynecological disturbances

- **Normal range: 27–32 pg**

$$\text{MCH} = \text{Hb (in g/L)/RBC (in millions/}\mu\text{L)} = 15 \times 10/5 = 30 \text{ pg}$$

3. **Mean Corpuscular Hemoglobin Concentration (MCHC)**
   - MCHC denotes the average concentration of hemoglobin in the RBC taking volume into account. It is expressed as g/dL (earlier it was expressed as %).
   - It is a better indicator of hypochromasia than MCH.
   - **Normal range: 31–35 g/dL.**

$$\text{MCHC} = \text{Hb (in g/dL)/PCV} = 15/0.45 = 33 \text{ g/dL}$$

4. **Red Cell Distribution Width (RDW)**
   - RDW is a quantitative measure of anisocytosis.
   - **Normal RDW is 11.5% to 14.5%.**

- A normal RDW indicates that RBCs are relatively uniform in size. A raised RDW indicates that red cells are heterogeneous in size and/or shape. In early iron deficiency anemia, RDW increases along with low MCV while in thalassemia trait, RDW is normal with low MCV.

$$\text{RDW} = (\text{Standard deviation} \div \text{mean cell volume}) \times 100$$

IRON DEFICIENCY ANEMIA

Q. Discuss the etiopathogenesis of iron deficiency anemia.

Iron deficiency anemia (IDA) is the **most common nutritional disorder**.

Etiology (Table 12.3)

IDA is due to deficiency of iron causing **defective heme synthesis**.

Pathogenesis of Iron Deficiency Anemia

It is due to decreased synthesis of heme and can be divided into 3 stages.

- **Stage 1 (Iron depletion):** Iron adequate to maintain normal hemoglobin level and **only serum ferritin decreased.**
- **Stage 2 (Iron deficient erythropoiesis): Lowering of serum iron and transferrin saturation levels** without anemia (Hb, MCV and MCH within normal range). Bone marrow shows iron deficient erythropoiesis.
- **Stage 3 (Iron deficiency anemia):** Low serum iron, serum ferritin and transferrin saturation. Impaired hemoglobin production. Morphologically, **first reduction in the size (microcytic) and later increase in the central pallor (hypochromia) of RBCs.**

Laboratory Findings

Peripheral Blood

- **Hemoglobin and hematocrit (PCV): Decreased**

Table 12.3: Causes of iron deficiency anemia

- **Dietary deficiency/lack**
  - Milk-fed infants
  - Elderly with improper diet and poor dentition
  - Low socioeconomical sections
  - Vegetarians (contains poorly absorbable inorganic iron)
- **Impaired absorption**
  - Total/partial gastrectomy
  - Intestinal absorption is impaired in sprue, other causes of intestinal steatorrhea and chronic diarrhea
  - Specific items in the diet, like phytates of cereals, tannates, carbonates, oxalates, phosphates and drugs can impair iron absorption
- **Increased demand/requirement**
  - Growing infants, children and adolescents
  - Pregnancy and lactation
- **Chronic blood loss: Due to bleeding from the**
  - Gastrointestinal tract (e.g. peptic ulcers, gastric carcinoma, colonic carcinoma, hemorrhoids, hookworm infestation or nonsteroidal anti-inflammatory drugs)
  - Urinary tract (e.g. renal or bladder tumors)
  - Genital tract (e.g. menorrhagia, uterine cancer)
  - Respiratory tract (e.g. hemoptysis)

- **Red cell indices:**
  - **MCV:** <80 fL (normal 82–98 fL)
  - **MCH:** <25 pg (normal 27–32 pg)
  - **MCHC:** <27 g/dL(31–36 g/dL)
  - **RDW: Increased** and >15%. It is **earliest sign of iron deficiency** (normal 11.5–14.5%).

Q. Write short note on peripheral smear findings in iron deficiency anemia.

- **Peripheral smear (Figs 12.1 and 12.2):**
  - *RBCs:* **Microcytic** (small) and **hypochromic** (pale). Severe anemia shows ring/pessary cells. **Moderate anisocytosis** and **poikilocytosis** pencil/cigar-shaped cells.
  - *WBCs:* Normal; eosinophilia in hookworm infestation.
  - *Platelets:* Normal

- **Reticulocyte count:** Low for the degree of anemia.

Bone Marrow

- *Cellularity:* Moderately **hypercellular**.
- *M:E (Myeloid:Erythroid) ratio:* Varies from 2:1 to 1:2 (normal 2:1 to 4:1).
- *Erythropoiesis:* Hyperplasia and **micronormoblastic maturation.**
- *Myelopoiesis:* Normal.
- *Megakaryopoiesis:* Normal.
- ***Absence of bone marrow iron:*** "Gold standard" test, demonstrated by **negative Prussian blue reaction.**

Serum Iron Profile (Table 12.4)

Q. Hematological and biochemical investigations in iron deficiency anemia

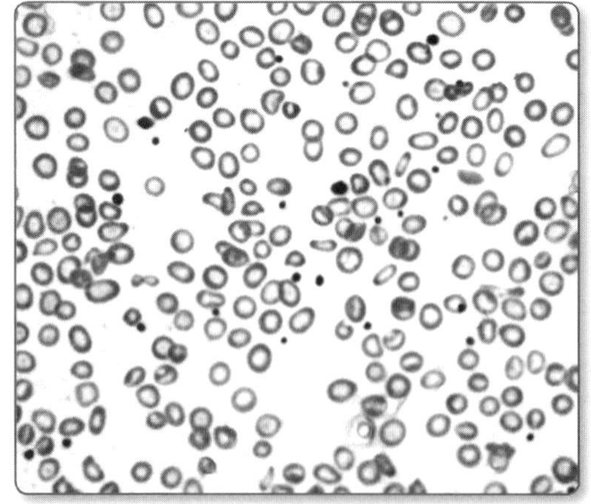

Fig. 12.1: Peripheral blood smear showing microcytic hypochromic red blood cells
(For color version, see Plate 7)

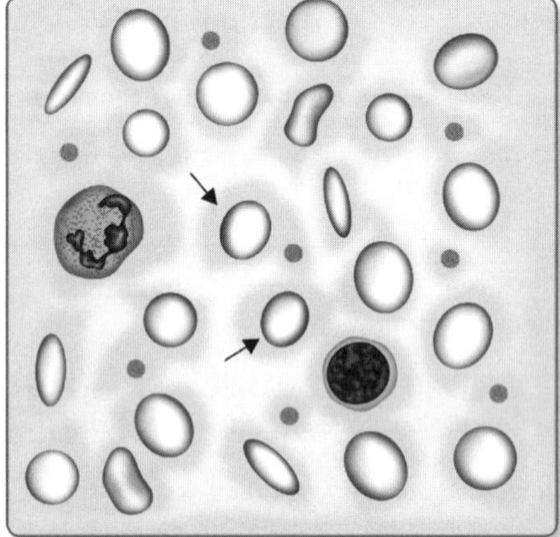

Fig. 12.2: Diagrammatic appearance of peripheral blood smear with microcytic hypochromic red blood cells (arrows)
(For color version, see Plate 7)

Table 12.4: Serum iron profile in IDA

	Normal range	Value in IDA	Observation
Serum ferritin	15–300 μg/L	<15 μg/L	↓
Serum iron	50–150 μg/dL	10–15 μg/dL	↓
Serum transferrin saturation	30–40%	<15%	↓
Total plasma iron-binding capacity (TIBC)	310–340 μg/dL	350–450 μg/dL	↑
Serum transferrin receptor (TFR)	0.57–2.8 μg/L	3.5–7.1 μg/L	↑
Red cell protoporphyrin	30–50 μg/dL	>200 μg/dL	↑

Reticulocyte Hemoglobin

It is **decreased** and is **an early feature of IDA**.

Clinical Features of IDA

Nonspecific and related to both severity and the cause of the anemia (e.g. gastrointestinal disease)

- **Onset:** Insidious.
- **Nonspecific symptoms: Fatigue, palpitations, breathlessness,** weakness and irritability.
- **Pharyngeal/esophageal webs** formed cause dysphagia.
- **Patterson-Kelly or Plummer-Vinson syndrome:**
  - Microcytic hypochromic anemia
  - Atrophic glossitis
  - Esophageal webs
- **Congestive heart failure in severe** anemia.
- **Central nervous system: Pica**-unusual craving for substances with no nutritional value like clay or chalk. **Craving for ice** (pagophagia) **specific to iron deficiency**. Pica may be the cause rather than effect of IDA.

Physical Findings

Diminished tissue enzymes cause characteristic epithelial changes of iron deficiency anemia.

- Angular stomatitis and glossitis
- Chronic atrophic gastritis
- Koilonychia (spoon nails)

Causes of Microcytic Hypochromic Anemia

Q. Enumerate the causes of microcytic hypochromic anemia.

- **Iron deficiency anemia**
- **Thalassemia major**
- **Anemia of chronic disorders**
- **Others:** Alcohol, lead poisoning and drugs
- Sideroblastic anemia (rare cause).

MEGALOBLASTIC ANEMIA

Q. Discuss the causes and pathogenesis of megaloblastic anemia.

Anemias characterized by **defective**/impaired **DNA synthesis** and **distinct megaloblasts in the bone marrow.** Megaloblastic anemias are common among anemias due to impaired red cell production.

Etiology of Megaloblastic Anemia (Table 12.5)

Table 12.5: Causes of megaloblastic anemia

Vitamin B_{12} Deficiency

• **Decreased intake:** Inadequate diet, "pure vegetarians" (vegans)
• **Impaired absorption**
  – Gastric: Deficiency of gastric acid or pepsin or intrinsic factor
    ◆ Pernicious anemia
    ◆ Post-gastrectomy
  – Intestinal
    ◆ Loss of absorptive surface
      ◊ Malabsorption syndromes
      ◊ Diffuse intestinal disease, e.g. lymphoma, systemic sclerosis
      ◊ Ileal resection, Crohn disease
    ◆ Bacterial or parasitic competition for vitamin B_{12}
      ◊ Bacterial overgrowth in blind loops and diverticula of bowel
      ◊ Fish tapeworm infestation
• **Increased demand:** Pregnancy, hyperthyroidism, disseminated cancer

Folic Acid Deficiency

• **Decreased intake:** Inadequate diet—alcoholism, malnutrition
• **Impaired absorption**
  – Malabsorption states: Nontropical and tropical sprue
  – Diffuse infiltrative diseases of the small intestine (e.g. lymphoma)
  – Drugs: Anticonvulsant phenytoin and oral contraceptives
• **Increased loss:** Hemodialysis
• **Increased demand:** Pregnancy, infancy, disseminated cancer, markedly increased hematopoiesis
• **Impaired utilization:** Folic acid antagonists, such as methotrexate

Pathogenesis of Megaloblastic Change

1. **Impaired DNA synthesis:** Megaloblastic anemia is commonly due to deficiency of **vitamin B_{12} (cyanocobalamin) or folic acid.** Both vitamins are coenzymes necessary for the synthesis of thymidine (one of the four bases found in DNA).
   a. **Delayed maturation of nucleus.** The **nuclear maturation lags behind the cytoplasmic maturation** and results in **abnormally large** nucleated **erythroid precursors** named as **megaloblasts.**
   b. Cytoplasm matures normally. RBCs are larger than normal → **macrocytes**.
   c. Affects all rapidly dividing cells of the body (including skin, GI tract, and bone marrow).
2. **Ineffective erythropoiesis:** Megaloblast precursors undergo intramedullary destruction.

Laboratory Findings of Megaloblastic Anemia

Q. Write short note on the laboratory findings in megaloblastic anemia.

Blood findings in vitamin B_{12} and/or folic acid deficiency are similar.

Peripheral Blood

Q. Peripheral smear and bone marrow findings in megaloblastic anemia

- **Hemoglobin and hematocrit (PCV): Reduced**
- **Red cell indices**
  - ↑ **MCV:** Above 100 fL (normal 82–98 fL)
  - ↑ **MCH** (normal 27–32 pg)
  - **Normal MCHC** (31–36 g/dL)

- **Peripheral smear (Figs 12.3 and 12.4): Pancytopenia** (decreased RBC, WBCs and platelets).
  - *RBCs:*
    - Macrocytic and oval (**egg-shaped macro-ovalocytes**)-**diagnostic**.
    - Most macrocytes **lack the central pallor** (Figs 12.3 and 12.4).
    - **Marked** variation in the size and shape of red cells **(anisopoikilocytosis**).
    - Evidence of dyserythropoiesis: Basophilic stippling, (precipitated ribosomal RNA). Cabot ring nuclear remnants and Howell Jolly bodies nuclear remnants.
  - *WBCs:*
    - **Decreased** WBC count (leukopenia).
    - **Hypersegmented neutrophils** (more than five nuclear lobes): First and specific morphological sign of megaloblastic anemia. These neutrophils are also larger than normal (**macropolys**).
  - *Platelets:* **Decreased**.

- **Reticulocyte count:** Normal or low.

Dimorphic Anemia

- **Combined vitamin B_{12}/folic acid and iron deficiency.**
- Peripheral smear shows two populations of RBCs namely: Macro-ovalocytes and microcytic hypochromic (Fig. 12.5).

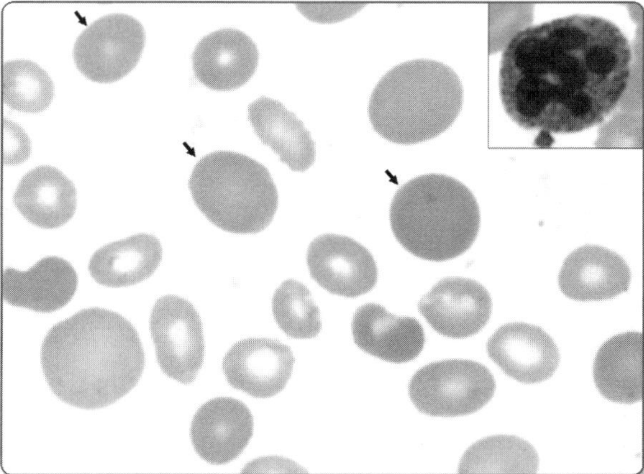

Fig. 12.3: Peripheral blood smear showing macro-ovalocytes (arrows) and hypersegmented neutrophil (inset)

(For color version, see Plate 7)

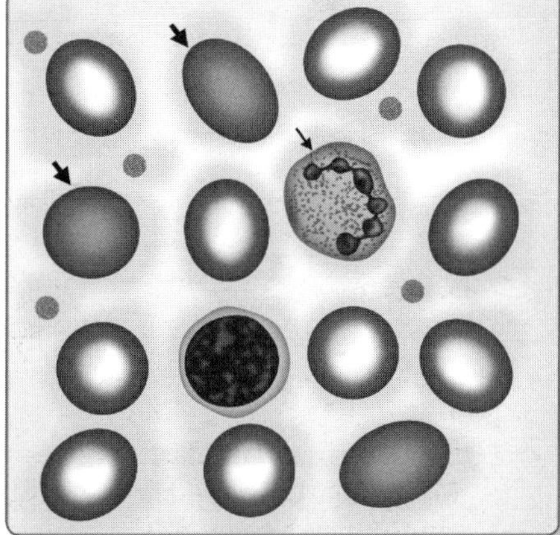

Fig. 12.4: Diagrammatic peripheral blood smear showing macro-ovalocytes (thick arrows) and hypersegmented neutrophil (thin arrow)

(For color version, see Plate 7)

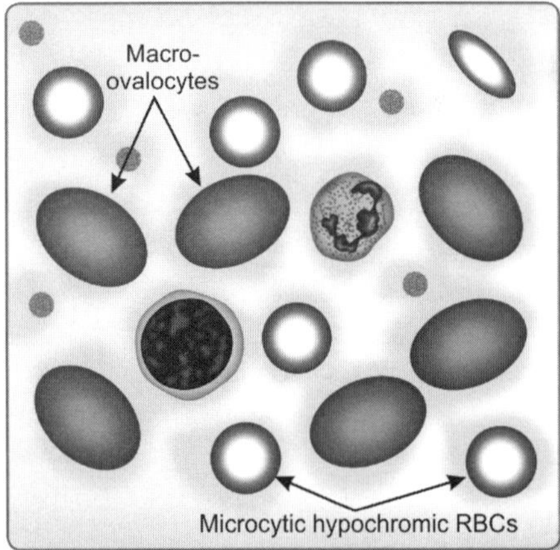

Fig. 12.5: Diagrammatic peripheral blood smear of dimorphic anemia showing macro-ovalocytes and microcytes

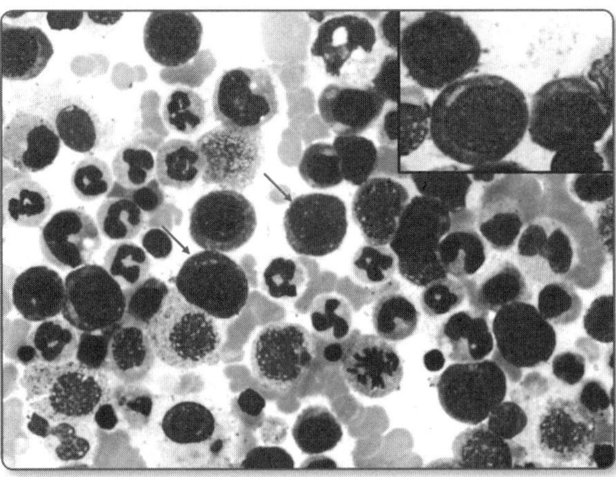

Fig. 12.6: Bone marrow aspirate showing megaloblastic precursors (arrows) in varying stages of maturation (inset shows early megaloblast)
(For color version, see Plate 8)

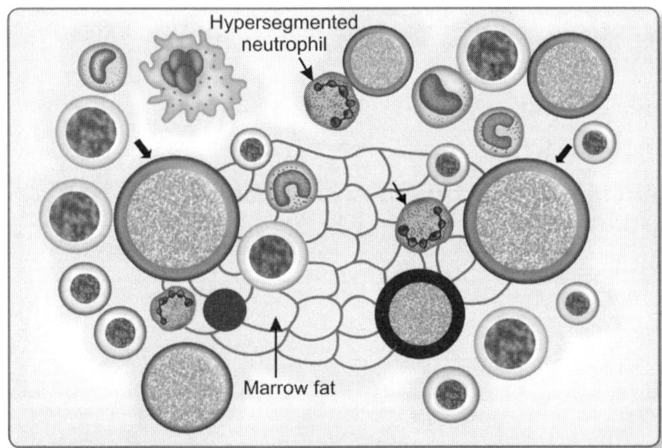

Fig. 12.7: Diagrammatic picture of bone marrow aspirate showing megaloblastic precursors (thick arrows) in varying stages of maturation
(For color version, see Plate 8)

Bone Marrow

- *Cellularity:* Moderately to **markedly hypercellular.**
- *M: E ratio:* Due to marked erythroid hyperplasia, M: E ratio is reversed ranging from 1:1 to 1:6 (normal 2:1 to 4:1).
- *Erythropoiesis:* **Megaloblastic type** (Figs 12.6 and 12.7)
  - **Megaloblasts: Large, abnormal counterparts of normal normoblasts.** Megaloblast shows **asynchrony of nuclear and cytoplasmic maturation.** The cytoplasm shows normal hemoglobinization.
  - **Ineffective erythropoiesis:** Developing megaloblasts die in marrow (intramedullary hemolysis).
- *Myelopoiesis:*
  - Myeloid cells adequate in number.
  - Granulocytic precursors display nuclear-cytoplasmic asynchrony in the form of **giant metamyelocytes and band forms.**
- *Megakaryopoiesis:* Normal or increased in number.
- *Bone marrow iron:* Moderately increased.

Biochemical Tests for Megaloblastic Anemia

Common for both vitamin B_{12} and folic acid deficiency

Deoxyuridine suppression test: It is a sensitive measure of deficiency of 5, 10-methylene THF, which occurs in both folic acid and vitamin B_{12} deficiency.

- ↑ Serum homocysteine
- ↑ Serum bilirubin: Mild increase causes mild jaundice
- ↑ Serum iron and ferritin
- ↑ Plasma lactate dehydrogenase (LDH)
- **Serum vitamin B_{12}/folate decreased.**

Diagnostic tests for vitamin B_{12} deficiency

- Serum vitamin B_{12} levels: Decreased
  - ↑ Serum methylmalonic acid
  - ↑ Urinary excretion of methylmalonic acid
- **Schilling test** for vitamin B_{12} absorption (Refer page).

Specific tests for folic acid deficiency

- **Serum folic acid levels:** Decreased
- **FIGLU in urine: Excessively excreted.**

PERNICIOUS ANEMIA

Q. Discuss the etiopathogenesis and morphology of pernicious anemia.

Pernicious anemia (PA) is an autoimmune disease due to **deficiency of intrinsic factor** causing **impaired absorption of vitamin B_{12}** and megaloblastic anemia.

Rare in India. A genetic predisposition is suspected.

Age: Older age—**fifth to eighth decades** of life

Sex: Females are more involved than males (F: M is 1.5: 1).

Etiopathogenesis

- An **autoimmune** disease due to destruction of gastric mucosa.
- Stomach shows **damage to parietal cells**, dense infiltration by lymphocytes and plasma cells → **chronic atrophic gastritis** → **failure of production of intrinsic factor**.
- **Presence of autoantibodies: Two major types** of autoantibodies—
  - **Anti-intrinsic factor (IF) antibody**
    - **Type I (blocking) antibody:** Blocks the binding of vitamin B_{12} to IF. Present in 50–75% of the cases.
    - **Type II (binding) antibody:** Attaches to the IF–vitamin B_{12} complex and prevent its binding to receptors in the ileum. Present in about 40% of patients.
  - **Parietal cell (Type III) antibody:** Neither specific for PA nor other autoimmune disorders. It is found in 90% of patients.

Morphology

Alimentary System

- **Atrophic glossitis:** Tongue shiny, glazed and beefy.

- **Stomach:**
  - **Diffuse chronic atrophic gastritis** and impaired secretion of hydrochloric acid, pepsin and intrinsic factor.
  - **Intestinal metaplasia.**

Central Nervous System

Found in 75% of cases.

- **Demyelination in the dorsal and lateral tracts:** Subacute combined degeneration
- Peripheral neuropathy.

Laboratory Findings (Fig. 12.8)

Q. Write short note on laboratory findings in pernicious anemia.

Blood, bone marrow and biochemical test findings are similar to those described earlier for megaloblastic anemias.

Specific Diagnostic Tests for Pernicious Anemia

- **Schilling test for vitamin B_{12} absorption: Abnormal**
  - Radioactive vitamin B_{12} is used to assess the status of intrinsic factor (IF) and vitamin B_{12}.

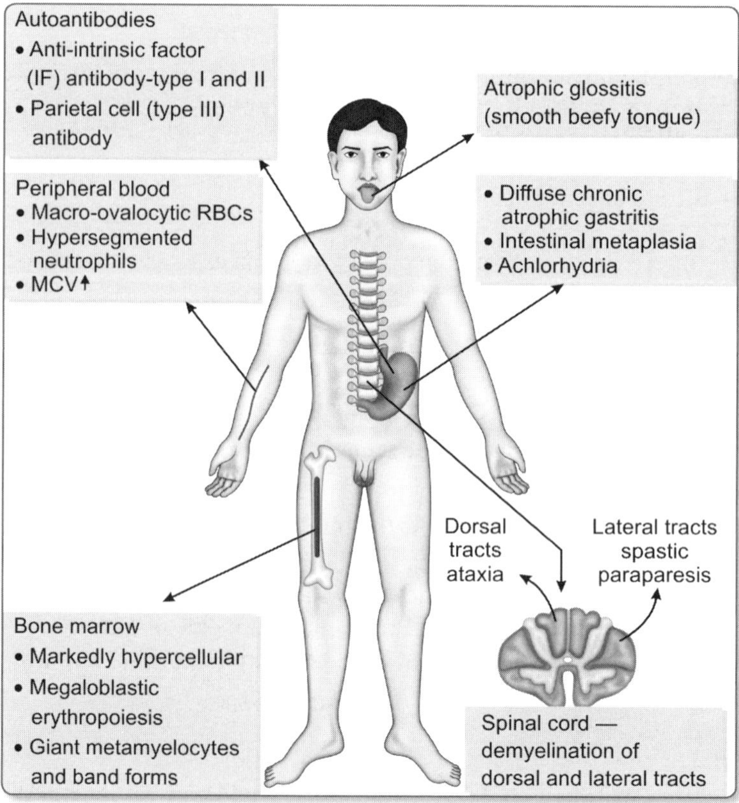

Fig. 12.8: Clinical features and laboratory findings in pernicious anemia

- Helps in distinguishing megaloblastic anemia due to IF deficiency (pernicious anemia) from other causes of vitamin B_{12} deficiency.
- **Serum antibodies to intrinsic factor** are highly specific for pernicious anemia.
- **Achlorhydria** with histamine/pentagastrin stimulation.
- Severe **deficiency of intrinsic factor**.

Clinical Features of Megaloblastic Anemia

Q. Mention the various clinical features of megaloblastic anemia.

The clinical features of vitamin B_{12} deficiency anemia and pernicious anemia are:
- **Onset: Insidious** and progresses slowly.
- **Classic triad of presentation:** Weakness, sore throat and paresthesias.
- **Tongue:** Painful red **"beefy"** tongue.
- **Neurological manifestations:**
  - **Bilateral peripheral neuropathy:** Glove and sock distribution of **numbness or paresthesia.**
  - **Demyelination of spinal cord: Subacute combined demyelination/degeneration of dorsal and lateral tracts—ataxia**, uncoordinated gait, impairment of vibration and position sense.
- **Atherosclerosis:** Serum homocysteine level is raised and is a **risk factor for atherosclerosis** and thrombosis.

APLASTIC ANEMIA

Q. Write short note on aplastic anemia.

Hematopoietic stem cell (HSC) disorder characterized by:
- **Pancytopenia** (anemia, neutropenia and thrombocytopenia).
- With **markedly hypocellular bone marrow** (less than 30% cellularity).

Etiology

The most common causes associated with aplastic anemia are shown in Table 12.6.

Table 12.6: Common causes of aplastic anemia

Acquired	
Idiopathic	
• Acquired defects in stem cell	
• Immune mediated	
Secondary	
Chemical agents	
• Cytotoxic drugs: Alkylating agents, antimetabolites	• Benzene
• Inorganic arsenicals	• Chloramphenicol
Idiosyncratic	
• Chloramphenicol	• Phenylbutazone
• Penicillamine	• Carbamazepine
• Gold salts	• Organic arsenicals
• Methylphenylethyl hydantoin	
Physical agents: Whole-body irradiation	
Viral infections: Hepatitis virus, Epstein-Barr virus, cytomegalovirus, herpes zoster (Varicella zoster), HIV	
Inherited: Fanconi anemia, telomerase defects	

Clinical Features

- Any age of both sexes
- Insidious
  - Progressive weakness, pallor and dyspnea due to anemia.
  - Frequent (mucocutaneous bacterial infections) or fatal infections due to neutropenia.
  - Bleeding manifestations in the form of petechiae, bruises and ecchymoses due to thrombocytopenia.

Laboratory Findings

Peripheral Blood

- ↓ **Hemoglobin**
- ↓ **PCV**
- ↓ **Reticulocyte count:** Markedly decreased.

- **Peripheral smear: Pancytopenia**, i.e. decreased red cells, neutrophils and platelets.
  - *RBCs:* Normocytic normochromic anemia
  - *WBCs:* Total leukocyte count decreased. **Neutrophils markedly diminished** and neutropenia is a reflection of the severity of aplasia. Initial stages, lymphocytes normal in number as the disease progresses their count decreases.
  - *Platelets:* Count is decreased.

Bone Marrow

- **Marrow aplasia**—best appreciated in a **bone marrow (trephine) biopsy**
  - *Cellularity:* Marked **hypocellularity.**
  - *Hematopoiesis:* **Paucity of all erythroid, myeloid and megakaryocytic precursors.**
  - *Other cells:* **Lymphocytes and plasma cells are prominent.**

No Splenomegaly

Diagnosis: Diagnosis is made with **peripheral blood** and **bone marrow biopsy findings.**

Prognosis: Unpredictable.

HEREDITARY DEFECTS IN HEMOGLOBIN

Classification

Q. Classify hereditary disorders of hemoglobin.

Hemoglobin defects may be quantitative (reduced production of normal hemoglobin) or qualitative (production of abnormal hemoglobin).

- ***Quantitative defect:*** Characterized by reduced of α-globin or β-globin chain (e.g. thalassemia). It leads to net reduction of hemoglobin.
- ***Qualitative defect:*** Characterized by production of abnormal hemoglobin (e.g. sickle cell anemia).

Thalassemia Syndrome

- These are group of inherited disorders due to **abnormality of globin production**.

- It is characterized by **decreased or absence of synthesis** of either **α or β-globin** chain of adult hemoglobin, HbA ($\alpha_2\beta_2$).

Classification

They are mainly classified as:
- **β-Thalassemia syndromes: Impaired synthesis of β-chains** of globin.
- **α-Thalassemia syndromes: Impaired synthesis of α-chains** of globin.
- **Miscellaneous thalassemia syndromes**.

β-Thalassemia

- **Autosomal recessive** hereditary disorder.
- **Diminished synthesis** of **β-globin chains** and normal synthesis of α-chains. It may be classified as β thalassemia major, intermedia and minor.
- β-globin chains are encoded by a single gene.
- The molecular errors over 200 genetic defects leading to β-thalassemia have been identified.
- Different types of **mutations in β-globin gene.**

β-THALASSEMIA MAJOR

Q. Write short note on β-thalassemia major.

- It is a **hereditary hemolytic anemia** due to **absence of synthesis of β-globin** chain of hemoglobin. The **synthesis of α-globin** chain **is not affected**.
- Homozygous form of β^0/β^0 or β^+/β^+ or double heterozygous β^0/β^+
- Most common in Mediterranean countries, parts of Africa and South East Asia.
- **Hemolytic anemia** is of **severe degree**.

Pathophysiology of β-thalassemia Major (Fig. 12.9)

Consequence of Defective or Absent β-chains

- **Severe hemolytic anemia** due to:
  1. **Absence of β-globin chain**.
  2. **Ineffective erythropoiesis: Unpaired and excess α-chains aggregate** into insoluble precipitates, which bind to and **damage the membrane of erythroid precursors**. These erythroid precursors fail to mature and **undergo apoptosis** in the marrow.
  3. **Extravascular hemolysis:** RBCs with α-chain inclusions are removed by macrophages of spleen (extravascular hemolysis).
- **Synthesis of fetal hemoglobin (HbF):** The Υ-globin chain synthesis continues even 6 months after birth and combines with α-globin leading to **increased levels of HbF** ($\alpha_2\Upsilon_2$). The level of HbF varies from 30% to 90%.

Consequences of Ineffective Erythropoiesis

- **Changes in bone marrow: Marked erythroid hyperplasia.**
- **Changes in bone:**
  - **Skull X-ray: Hair on end ("crew-cut") appearance**
  - **Typical facies: Thalassemic facies**—prominent forehead, cheekbones and upper jaw.
- **Extramedullary hematopoiesis:** in **liver and spleen** → consequent hepatosplenomegaly.
- **Cachexia:** Develops in untreated patients.

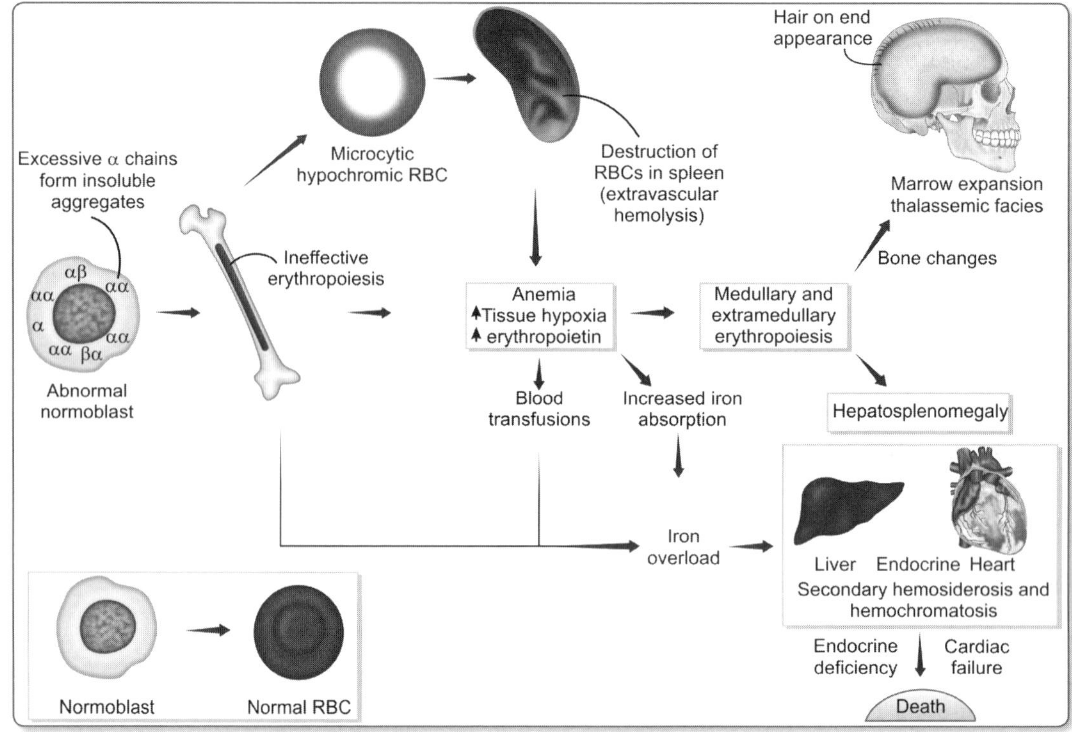

Fig. 12.9: Pathogenesis of β-thalassemia major and its consequence

Iron Overload and its Consequences

- **Causes of iron overload:**
  1. **Increased absorption of dietary iron** from duodenum
  2. **Hemolysis**
  3. **Repeated transfusions** (usual mode of treatment).
- **Consequences:** Iron overload produces **hemosiderosis** and **secondary hemochromatosis** and damages to parenchyma of organs (e.g. **heart**, **liver** and **pancreas).**

Clinical Features

- **Age:** Infants develop **moderate to severe anemia** 6–9 months after birth.
- **Growth and development:** Untreated/untransfused children **fail to thrive** and die within 4–5 years of age.
- **Bone changes:** Those who survive longer develop distortion of skull and facial bones. X-ray **skull** shows **hair on end appearance** (Fig. 12.11) and face shows a characteristic **thalassemic facies**.
- **Marked splenomegaly:** Up to 1500 grams due to hyperplasia and extramedullary hematopoiesis.
- **Extramedullary hemopoiesis: Liver and lymph nodes** may show **extramedullary hematopoiesis.**
- **Iron overload:** Multiple blood transfusions may lead to iron overload and result in **hemosiderosis and secondary hemochromatosis (**heart, liver and pancreas).

Laboratory Findings

Peripheral Blood

Q. Mention the laboratory findings in β-thalassemia major.

- **Hemoglobin** (ranges from 3 to 8 g/dL) **and hematocrit** (ranges from 8 to 23%)**: Markedly reduced.**
- **RBC count increased/normal (**in contrast to iron deficiency anemia).
- **Reticulocyte count increased** and in the range of 5 to 15%.
- **Red cell indices:**
  - **MCV decreased** and in the range of 45–70 fL (normal range 82–98 fL).
  - **MCHC decreased** and in the range of 22–30 g/dL (normal range 31–35 g/dL).
  - **MCH decreased** and in the range of 20–28 pg (normal range 27–32 pg).
  - **RDW-within normal limits** (in contrast to iron deficiency anemia where it is increased).

Q. Write short note on peripheral smear findings in β-thalassemia major.

- **Peripheral smear:**
  - *RBCs:*
    - **Microcytic hypochromic** anemia
    - Moderate to marked anisocytosis and poikilocytosis
    - Many **target cells** (Figs 12.10 and 12.11)
    - Basophilic stippling
    - **Nucleated red cell precursors** (normoblasts) in variable numbers (5–40%).
  - *WBCs:* Leukocytosis with mild left shift.
  - *Platelets:* Normal.

Bone Marrow

- *Cellularity:* **Markedly hypercellular**.
- *M: E ratio:* Reversed to 1:1 to 1:5 depending upon the degree of erythroid hyperplasia.
- *Erythropoiesis:* **Normoblastic with marked erythroid hyperplasia**.
- *Myelopoiesis:* Normal.
- *Megakaryopoiesis:* Normal.
- *Bone marrow iron:* **Markedly increased** due to increased dietary absorption and hemolysis.

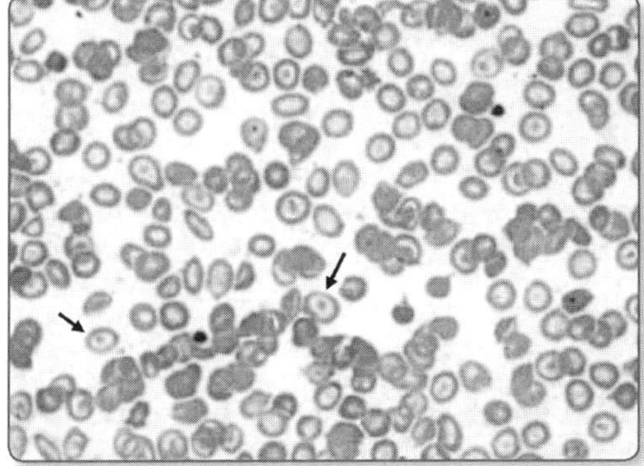

Fig. 12.10: Peripheral blood smear in β-thalassemia showing target cells (arrows)

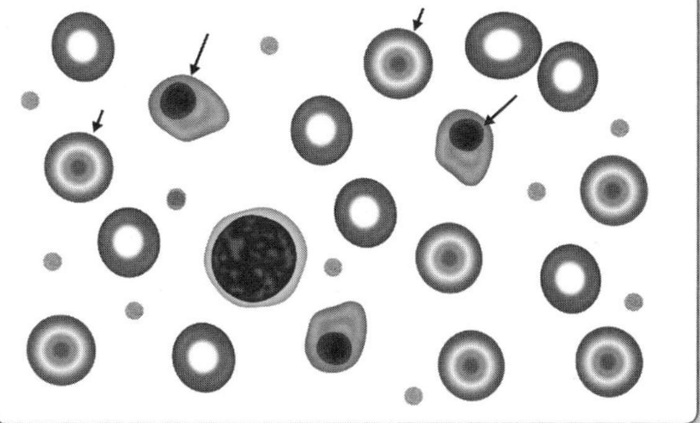

Fig. 12.11: Diagrammatic appearance of peripheral blood smear in β-thalassemia showing target cells (short arrows) and nucleated red cells (long arrows)

SICKLE CELL ANEMIA

Sickle cell anemia is a **hereditary disorder** of hemoglobin characterized by **production of defective hemoglobin** called **sickle hemoglobin (HbS).** On low oxygen tension or deoxygenation, HbS imparts **sickle shape to RBCs**. HbS is produced due to **qualitative defect** in hemoglobin production caused by **mutation in β-globin gene**.

Characteristic Features

- **Autosomal recessive disorder** manifests early in life.
- **Homozygous state** (SS) caused by a **mutation in the β-globin gene.**
- **HbS** constitutes **more than 70% of hemoglobin** in their RBCs with no HbA.

Etiopathogenesis

Q. Discuss the etiopathogenesis of sickle cell anemia.

- **Production of abnormal hemoglobin** called **sickle hemoglobin (HbS).**
- **Missense point mutation:** In HbS, there is **substitution of glutamic acid by valine in the 6th position the β-globin** chain of hemoglobin. It alters the solubility or stability of the hemoglobin and **produces hemolytic anemia**.
- HbS is responsible for the characteristics of the disease.

Molecular Basis of Sickling

- During **low O_2 tension or deoxygenation, HbS** molecules **undergo aggregation and polymerization.**
- If deoxygenation continues, the **aggregated HbS** molecules **form long needle-like fibers** (or pseudocrystalline structures known as **tactoids**) within RBCs.
- The **tactoids grow** in length beyond the diameter of RBCs and **distort RBC shape**.
- **RBC** become elongated and assumes a **shape** like **sickle** (or crescent moon or holly-leaf or boat) and **predisposes to stasis and vascular occlusion**.
- **When** the **oxygen tension returns** to normal, the **sickled red cell returns to normal shape**.
- **Recurrent sickling** causes red cell membrane damage and these RBCs become **irreversibly sickled cells (ISC)**.

Clinical Features

- Presence of **HbF in the first 6 months** of life has a **protective** role.
- **Symptoms appear after 6 months** of age as the HbF disappears.
- **Infants and children present with** acute problems like **severe infection**, **acute chest syndrome, splenic sequestration** and **stroke**.
- **Chronic hypoxia** in children is responsible for generalized **impairment of growth** and development. **Adults manifest with chronic organ damage**.

Chronic Hemolytic Anemia

- **Lifelong hemolysis** (mainly extravascular) and causes **chronic hemolytic anemia**, which is of **moderate degree**. This produces **raised unconjugated (indirect) bilirubin**, and predisposes to **pigment** bilirubin **gallstones** (cholelithiasis) and **cholecystitis**.

Crises

Four types of crises are encountered. These are:

1. **Sickling crisis (vaso-occlusive/pain/painful/infarctive crisis)**
   - Most common
   - **Blockage of microcirculation** by sickled red cells produces **hypoxic injury and infarction**.
   - **Bone:** Manifest as the **hand-foot syndrome, dactylitis** of the bones of the hands or feet or both.
   - **Lung: Acute chest syndrome (dangerous)**.
   - **Spleen: Acute abdominal pain** due to infarcts of abdominal viscera caused by occlusion of vessels. **Recurrent splenic infarction** results in **autosplenectomy.**
2. **Hemolytic crisis**
   - Rare type and presents with **marked increase in hemolysis**.
3. **Aplastic crisis**
   - Associated **with parvovirus B19**.
   - Reticulocytopenia.
4. **Sequestration crisis**
   - Usually occurs in **children.**
   - **Sudden trapping of blood** in spleen or liver causes rapid enlargement of the organ and **drop in hematocrit** leading to **hypovolemic shock**.

Increased Susceptibility to Infections

- Common infections are **pneumonia** due to ***Pneumococcus***, **meningitis** due to ***S. pneumoniae*** and **osteomyelitis** due to ***Salmonella***. Increased frequency of osteomyelitis is due to bone infarcts, which act as a nidus for infection.
- **Septicemia** and **meningitis** are the most common causes of death in children.

Chronic Organ Damage

Particularly seen in the spleen, bones, kidneys, heart, lungs, brain and skin.

- **Spleen**
  - Children after 6 months of life present with splenomegaly (up to 500 g).
  - After 5–6 years of age, the spleen gets fibrosed and **gradually reduces in the size** due to **multiple infarcts**.
  - Gradual **loss of splenic function** secondary to infarcts results in **autosplenectomy**.
- **Bone:** Osteomyelitis, particularly with *Salmonella typhimurium*.
- **Extremities: Skin ulcers** over the lower extremities.

Laboratory Findings in Sickle Cell Anemia

Peripheral Blood

Q. Laboratory findings in sickle cell anemia.

- **Hemoglobin: Decreased**.
- **Hematocrit (PCV): Decreased.**
- **ESR: Reduced**.
- **Reticulocyte count: Increased** and range from 3 to 10%.

- **Peripheral smear**
  - *RBCs:*
    - Normocytic normochromic to mildly hypochromic.
    - Moderate to severe degree of **anisopoikilocytosis**.
    - **Characteristic cell is** the **sickle cell**—appear as long, curved cells with pointed ends (Figs 12.12 and 12.13); may also show **target cells** (due to red cell dehydration) **and ovalocytes**.
    - **Polychromatophilia due to reticulocytosis**.
  - *WBCs:* Mildly increased with shift to left.
  - *Platelets:* Mildly increased.

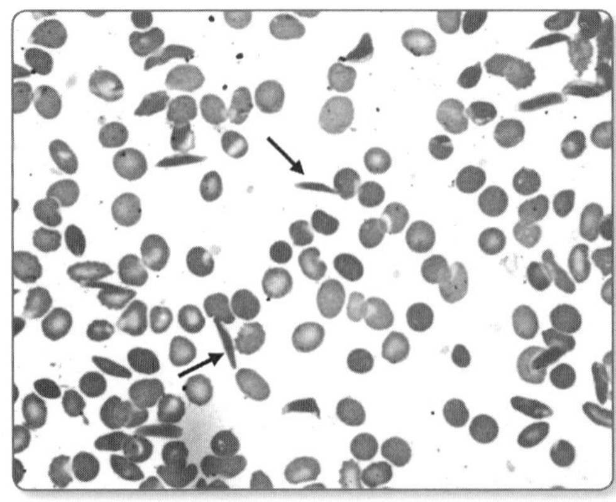

Fig. 12.12: Peripheral blood smear with sickle cells (arrows)

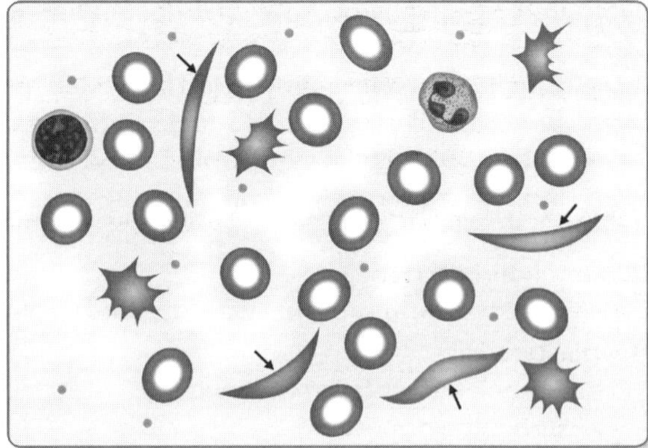

Fig. 12.13: Diagrammatic peripheral blood smear with sickle cells (arrows)

Bone Marrow

- *Cellularity:* **Hypercellular.**
- *Erythropoiesis:* **Compensatory normoblastic erythroid hyperplasia**, which expands the marrow and causes resorption of bone and secondary new bone formation.
- *Myelopoiesis:* Normal.
- *Megakaryopoiesis:* Normal.
- *Iron stores:* Usually increased.

Serum Findings

- **Serum bilirubin: Raised** and **predisposes to** pigment **gallstone**s.
- **Iron status: Raised** serum iron, serum ferritin and transferrin saturation.
- **Serum haptoglobin: Reduced.**
- **Urine Urobilinogen: Increased.**

Diagnostic/Confirmatory Tests

- **Sickling test:**
  - **Sickling** is **induced** by adding a **reducing** (oxygen-consuming) **agent** like 2% sodium metabisulfite or sodium dithionite to blood sample.
  - Red cells with HbS show **sickled** (Fig. 12.14) **and holly leaf** appearance.
  - It is **diagnostic** of sickle cell anemia.
- **Hemoglobin electrophoresis:** HbS is a slow moving compared to HbA and HbF.
- **Estimation of HbF:** In homozygous state constitutes about 10–30% of hemoglobin.
- **HPLC:** Useful for confirmation of diagnosis.
- **Prenatal diagnosis:** By analysis of fetal DNA obtained by amniocentesis or chorionic villous biopsy, to detect the point mutations.

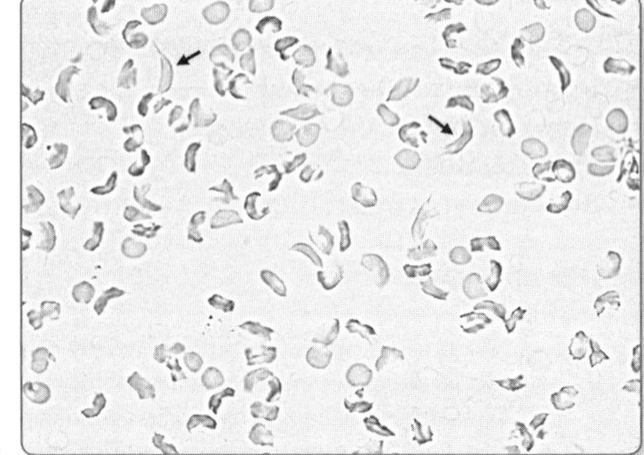

Fig. 12.14: Sickling test. Sickled red cells (arrows) induced by reducing agent (2% sodium metabisulfite)

DISORDERS OF WHITE CELLS

NORMAL DIFFERENTIAL LEUKOCYTE COUNT (DLC)

The normal range of DLC in an adult is presented in Table 12.7.

Table 12.7: Normal range of different leukocytes in an adult

Type of white blood cell	Normal range
Neutrophils	40–70% (2.0–7.0 × 10^9/L)
Lymphocytes	20–40% (1.0–3.0 × 10^9/L)
Monocytes	2–10% (0.2–1.0 × 10^9/L)
Eosinophils	1–6% (0.02–0.5 × 10^9/L)
Basophils	Less than 1% (0.02–0.1 × 10^9/L)

QUANTITATIVE DISORDERS OF LEUKOCYTES

Leukocytosis

Q. Define leukocytosis and list its causes.

An increase in the **total** number of **leukocytes** in the blood **more than 11,000/cu mm** (11 × 10^9/L).

Causes: Common causes of leukocytosis are shown in Table 12.8.

Table 12.8: Common causes of leukocytosis

• Infections – Bacterial – Viral infections (e.g. infectious mononucleosis)
• Leukemia – Acute – Chronic: Chronic lymphocytic leukemia and chronic myeloid leukemia
• Leukemoid reactions
• Physiological – Pregnancy – Exercise

Leukopenia

Total leukocyte count is less than 4,000/cu mm (4 × 10^9/L).
Causes: Common causes of leukopenia are shown in Table 12.9.

Table 12.9: Common causes of leukopenia

• Typhoid and paratyphoid
• Anemia – Aplastic anemia – Megaloblastic anemia
• Hypersplenism
• Drugs including cytotoxic drugs
• Radiation
• Rarely leukemia

Disorders of Neutrophils

Neutrophilia (Fig. 12.15)

Q. Define neutrophilia and mention its causes.

An absolute neutrophil count of more than 8,000/cu mm (8 × 10^9/L). Differential count shows more than 70% neutrophils and is usually accompanied by leukocytosis (15–30 × 10^9/L).

Causes of neutrophilia: Major causes of neutrophilia are shown in Table 12.10.

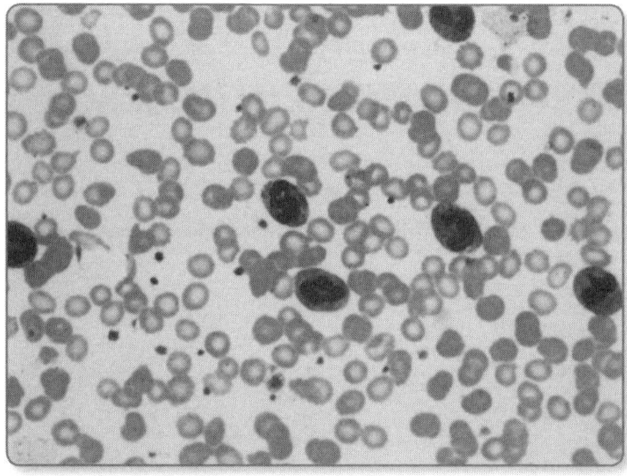

Fig. 12.15: Peripheral smear showing neutrophilia

Leukemoid Reaction

Benign leukocytic proliferation characterized by a **total leukocyte count of more than 25 × 10^9/L** with immature white cells (like band forms, metamyelocytes and myelocytes).

It is different from chronic myelocytic/myeloid leukemia (Table 12.11).

Neutropenia (Agranulocytosis)

Reduction in the absolute neutrophil count (total WBC × % segmented neutrophils and band forms) below 1.5 × 10^9/L (1,500/cu mm).

Etiology: The causes of neutropenia are presented in Table 12.12.

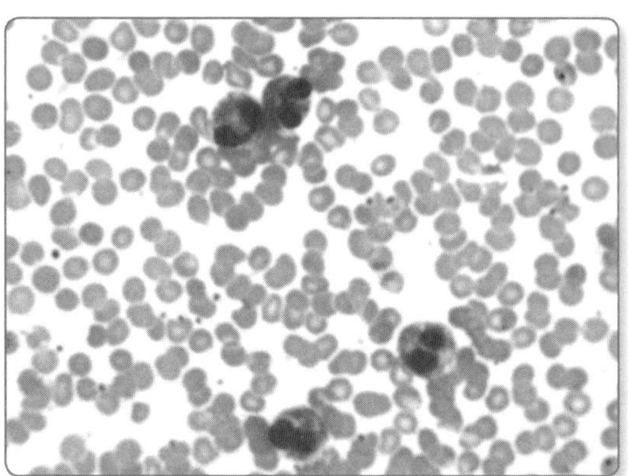

Fig. 12.16: Peripheral smear showing eosinophilia

Eosinophilia (Fig. 12.16)

Eosinophil count of more than 450/cu mm (0.45 × 10^9/L).

Causes of eosinophilia are presented in Table 12.13.

Table 12.10: Major causes of neutrophilia

• **Pathological:** – Acute bacterial and fungal infections: ◆ Localized: Pyogenic microorganisms causing infections, e.g. pneumonias, pyogenic meningitis, cellulitis, diphtheria, abscess, tonsillitis, etc. ◆ Generalized: Septicemia, acute rheumatic fever – Acute inflammatory processes: Inflammatory conditions (acute appendicitis), vasculitis – Tissue necrosis: Burns, myocardial infarction, gangrene, neoplasms (tumor necrosis) – Acute stress or hypoxic states: Following hemorrhage, hemolysis and surgery – Myeloproliferative neoplasms: Chronic myeloid leukemia, polycythemia vera – Metabolic: Uremia, acidosis, gout – Miscellaneous: Eclampsia, steroid therapy
• **Physiological:** – Exercise (shift from marginating pool to circulating pool), newborns, extremes of temperature, pain, emotional stress and during obstetric labor

Q. Tabulate the differences between leukemia and leukemoid reaction.

Table 12.11: Differences between leukemoid reaction and chronic myeloid leukemia

	Leukemoid reaction	Chronic myeloid leukemia
Clinical features	Features of causative disease	Splenomegaly, and bone pain are common
Peripheral blood findings		
WBC		
Total WBC count	Moderately increased, rarely exceeds $50 \times 10^9/L$	Markedly increased and usually 50 $\times 10^9/L$
Differential leukocyte count	Shift to the left with few immature forms. Toxic granulation seen	Shift to the left with numerous immature forms. Myelocyte and neutrophil peak
Eosinophilia and basophilia	Variable	Present
Leukocyte alkaline phosphatase (LAP)	Increased	Decreased
RBC		
Anemia	Usually minimal or absent	Severe and progressive
Platelets		
Number	Variable	Normal or increased
Extramedullary myeloid tumors	Absent	Present
Philadelphia chromosome	Absent	Present

Table 12.12: Causes of neutropenia

- **Inadequate production:**
  - ***Suppression of stem cells:*** In these disorders granulocytopenia represents a component of pancytopenia
    - Aplastic anemia
    - Marrow infiltration
    - Metastatic tumors
    - Granulomatous disorders
  - ***Suppression of committed granulocytic precursors***
    - Drugs and chemicals (e.g. sulfonamides, analgesics, arsenicals)
    - Ionizing radiation
  - ***Diseases associated with ineffective hematopoiesis***
    - Megaloblastic anemias: Vitamin B_{12} or folate deficiency
    - Myelodysplastic syndromes
  - ***Congenital:*** Kostmann syndrome (rare)
  - ***Severe infections***
    - Bacterial (e.g. typhoid, paratyphoid, septicemia)
    - Viral (e.g. influenza, infectious mononucleosis, hepatitis, measles)
    - Rickettsial (e.g. scrub typhus)
    - Protozoal (e.g. malaria, kala-azar)
- **Increased destruction of neutrophils:**
  - ***Immunologically mediated destruction***
    - Idiopathic
    - Secondary
      - ◊ Drugs
      - ◊ Autoimmune disorders, e.g. systemic lupus erythematosus
  - ***Splenic sequestration*** may be associated with pancytopenia
- **Shift from the circulating pool to marginating pool:**
  - Hemodialysis and cardiopulmonary bypass
- **Idiopathic: Mechanism not known**
  - Hodgkin and non-Hodgkin lymphoma
  - Chronic lymphocytic leukemia
  - Viral infections (HIV, hepatitis)
  - Cyclic neutropenia

Q. Define eosinophilia and list its causes.

Table 12.13: Causes of eosinophilia

• **Allergic/atopic conditions**	
– Asthma	– Urticaria
– Hay fever	– Drug reactions
– Allergic rhinitis	
• **Parasitic infestations (with tissue invasion)**	
– Roundworm infestation	– Hookworm infestation
– Filariasis	
• **Fungal infections** (e.g. coccidioidomycosis)	
• **Skin diseases**	
– Dermatitis (eczema)	– Pemphigus
– Scabies	– Dermatitis herpetiformis
• **Hematological diseases**	
– Chronic myeloid leukemia	– Polycythemia
– Hodgkin lymphoma	– Acute myelomonocytic leukemia
– Eosinophilic leukemia	
• **Miscellaneous**	
– Tropical eosinophilia	– Pulmonary eosinophilia
– Löeffler's syndrome	– Hypereosinophilic syndrome
– Eosinophilic granuloma	

Table 12.14: Causes of lymphocytosis

• **Acute infections**
– Viral infections: Infectious mononucleosis, mumps, measles, chickenpox, infectious hepatitis
– Toxoplasmosis
• **Chronic infections/inflammatory diseases**
– Tuberculosis
– Syphilis
– Brucellosis
– Inflammatory bowel disease: Crohn disease and ulcerative colitis
• **Hematologic malignancies**
– Acute lymphoblastic leukemia
– Chronic lymphocytic leukemia
– Non-Hodgkin lymphoma with spill over
– Adult T cell leukemia/lymphoma
– Hairy cell leukemia

Lymphocytosis

Lymphocyte (Fig. 12.17) count more than 4,000/cu mm (4×10^9/L) in adults and more than 8,000/cu mm (8×10^9/L) in child. Common causes of lymphocytosis are given in the Table 12.14

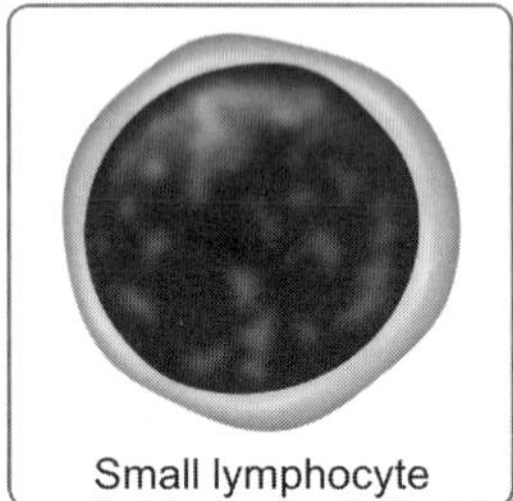

Small lymphocyte

Fig. 12.17: Diagrammatic appearance of lymphocyte

ACUTE LEUKEMIA

Definition

Q. Define and classify leukemia.

Acute leukemia is a malignant disease of the bone marrow stem cell and its characteristic features are:

- **Bone marrow: Diffuse replacement** with proliferating neoplastic blast cells that fail to mature. **Blast cells more than 20%** (WHO criteria) of the nucleated cells in the marrow.
- **Peripheral blood: Abnormal numbers and forms of immature white blood cells.**

Aleukemic/subleukemic leukemia is characterized by very few/no blasts in the peripheral blood.

Acute leukemia are mainly divided into two groups namely acute lymphoblastic leukemia (ALL) and acute myeloblastic leukemia (AML).

Etiology and Pathogenesis

Risk factors: Risk factors (Table 12.15) may cause mutations in the proto-oncogenes and tumor suppressor genes.

Table 12.15: Risk factors for acute leukemia

Environmental Factors
• **Ionizing radiation** • **Drugs:** – Alkylating agents—nitrogen mustard, chlorambucil, etc. – AML occurs in myeloma patients treated with melphalan – Leukemia follows chemotherapy of lung and ovarian cancer • **Chemicals:** Benzene (used in paint industry, plastic glues, etc.)
Genetic Disorders
Example: Down syndrome (ALL or AML), Fanconi anemia (AML), ataxia telangiectasia (ALL, NHL)
Acquired Disorders
• PNH and aplastic anemia may transform into acute leukemia • AML may develop de novo or secondary to myelodysplastic syndrome (MDS)

Classification

Q. Classify acute leukemia.

Traditional classification depending on microscopic appearance of the involved cell and the course of leukemias is presented in Table 12.16.

Table 12.16: Traditional classification of leukemia

• **Acute leukemia** – Acute myelogenous/myeloblastic/myelocytic/myeloid leukemia (AML) – Acute lymphoblastic/lymphocytic leukemia (ALL)
• **Chronic leukemia** – Chronic myeloid leukemia (CML) – Chronic lymphocytic leukemia (CLL)

FAB Classification of Acute Leukemias

- **First French, American and British (FAB)** classification (1976) was **based on the 1. morphological and 2. cytochemical characteristics of** blast cells.
- **Revised FAB classification** (Table 12.17): it includes
  1. **M:** Morphology and cytochemistry of blast cells
  2. **I:** Immunophenotyping
  3. **C:** Cytogenetics
  4. **M:** Molecular genetics.

Table 12.17: Revised French, American and British (FAB) classification of acute leukemias

Acute Lymphoid Leukemia	
L_1	Small homogenous cells with inconspicuous nucleoli
L_2	Large cells with variable size and 1–2 nucleoli
L_3	Large, homogeneous cells with finely stippled chromatin and prominent nucleoli. Cytoplasm is basophilic and vacuolated
Acute Myeloid Leukemia	
M_0	Minimally differentiated AML
M_1	AML without maturation
M_2	AML with maturation
M_3	Promyelocytic leukemia
M_4	Myelomonocytic leukemia
M_5	Monocytic leukemia
M_6	Erythroleukemia
M_7	Megakaryocytic leukemia

WHO Classification (2008) of Acute Leukemia (Table 12.18)

Table 12.18: WHO classification (2008) of acute lymphoblastic and myeloid leukemia

- **Acute Lymphoblastic Leukemia**
  - **Precursor**-B lymphoblastic leukemia/lymphoma
  - **Precursor** -T lymphoblastic leukemia/lymphoma

- **Acute Myeloid Leukemia (AML)**
  - AML with recurrent genetic abnormalities
    - AML with t(8;21)(q22;q22); *RUNX1-RUNX1T1*
    - AML with inv(16)(p13;1q22); *CBFB-MYH11*
    - APL with t(15;17)(q22;q12); *PML-RARA*
    - AML with t(9;11)(p22;q23); *MLLT3-MLL*
  - AML with MDS-related changes
  - Therapy-related myeloid neoplasms
  - AML not otherwise specified
    - AML minimally differentiated
    - AML without maturation
    - AML with maturation
    - Acute myelomonocytic leukemia
    - Acute monoblastic and monocytic leukemia
    - Acute erythroid leukemia
    - Acute megakaryoblastic leukemia
  - Myeloid sarcoma
  - Myeloid proliferation related to Down syndrome

Abbreviations: AML, Acute myeloid leukemia; APL, Acute promyelocytic leukemia; MDS, Myelodysplastic syndrome

Differences between Myeloblast and Lymphoblast (Table 12.19)

Q. List the differences between myeloblast and lymphoblast.

ACUTE LYMPHOBLASTIC LEUKEMIA/LYMPHOMA

- **Acute Lymphoblastic Leukemia/Lymphoma** (ALL) is a group of neoplasms consisting of **lymphoblasts.**

Table 12.19: Differences between myeloblast and lymphoblast based on morphology and cytochemistry

	Lymphoblast (Fig. 12.18)	**Myeloblast (Fig. 12.19)**
Size	2–3 times the size of lymphocyte	3–5 times the size of lymphocyte
Cytoplasmic characters		
Amount	Scanty (less cytoplasm than myeloblast)	Scanty to moderate (more cytoplasm than lymphoblast)
Color	Blue	Gray
Cytoplasmic granules	Agranular	May have cytoplasmic granules
Auer rod	Negative	Positive
Nuclear characters		
Nuclear chromatin	Uniform, coarse	Uniform, fine
Nucleoli	Inconspicuous or 1 to 2	3 to 5, prominent
N:C ratio	High	High
Accompanying cells	Lymphocytes	Promyelocytes, myelocytes, meta-myelocytes, band forms and neutrophils
Cytochemistry		
Myeloperoxidase	Negative	Positive
Sudan black	Negative	Positive
PAS	Block positivity	Negative
Nonspecific esterase	Negative	Positive in M4 and M5

- Lymphoblast is immature, precursor B (pre-B) or T (pre-T) lymphocyte.
- WHO classification (Table 12.18):
  - **Precursor B cells** ALL (about 85%) seen in **childhood** and present as **acute leukemias.**
  - **Precursor T cells** ALL (15%) present in adolescent males as **lymphomas**, often with involvement of mediastinum (thymus).

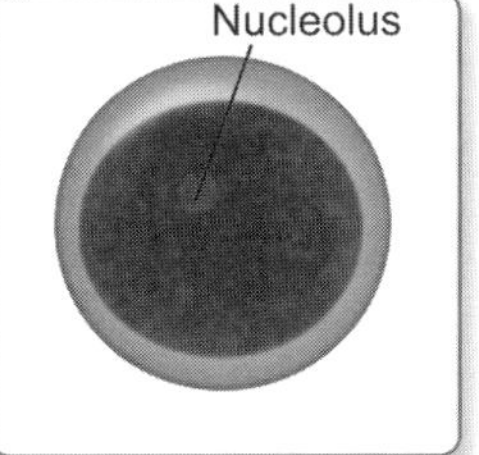

Fig. 12.18: Diagrammatic appearance of lymphoblast **(For color version, see Plate 8)**

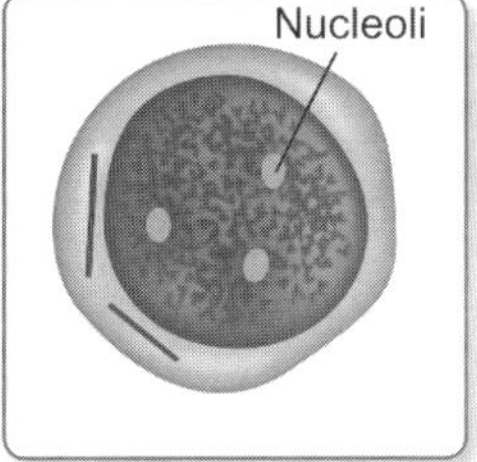

Fig. 12.19: Diagrammatic appearance of myeloblast **(For color version, see Plate 8)**

Molecular Pathogenesis

- Chromosomal abnormalities are found in about 90% of ALLs.
  - **Numerical abnormality:** Hyperploidy (>50 chromosomes) and hypoploidy.
  - **Structural abnormality:** Balanced chromosomal translocations (e.g. Philadelphia chromosome).

Classification of Acute Lymphoblastic Leukemia (Tables 12.17, 12.18)

Clinical Features

Age: Most common hematological malignancy of **children**. Most common between **1 and 5 years** of age and between **30 and 40 years.**

Sex: Slight male preponderance.

Onset: **Abrupt**.

Symptoms:

- **Bone marrow failure:**
  - Anemia: Causes **fatigue, weakness.**
  - Neutropenia: **Infections** by bacteria or opportunistic fungi. Develop sore throat and respiratory infections.
  - Thrombocytopenia: **Bleeding** into the skin and mucosa in the form of purpura or ecchymoses.
  - **Bone pain** and **sternal tenderness.**
- **Extramedullary infiltration:**
  - **Lymphadenopathy:** 75% of patients, usually involve **cervical lymph nodes.**
  - **Bone pain and tenderness.**
  - **Hepatosplenomegaly:** Splenomegaly is more common than hepatomegaly.
  - **Mediastinal thymic mass:** More common in T-ALL.
- **CNS involvement:** Spread into the meninges causes **leukemic meningitis** ALL (pre-B).
- **Testicular involvement** (ALL).

Laboratory Findings

Peripheral Blood

Q. Write short note on laboratory/peripheral smear findings in acute lymphoblastic leukemia.

- **Total WBC count: Markedly raised** ranging from 20×10^9/L to 200×10^9/L
- **Platelet count:** Reduced (thrombocytopenia).
- **Hemoglobin: Decreased** and may be as low as 3 g/dL.

- **Peripheral smear (Figs 12.20 and 12.21):**
  - *RBCs:* Normocytic normochromic anemia.
  - *WBCs:* Total count **markedly increased** and **20% or more lymphoblasts.**
    - **Morphology of lymphoblasts:**
      - ◊ **Larger than small lymphocyte**
      - ◊ **High N:C ratio**
      - ◊ **Nucleus with condensed chromatin and nucleoli are either absent or inconspicuous**
      - ◊ **Scant to moderate agranular basophilic cytoplasm.**
  - *Platelets:* Thrombocytopenia.

Cytochemistry of lymphoblasts

- PAS: Cytoplasmic aggregates of **PAS positive** (Figs 7.3 and 7.6) material **(block positivity).**
- Myeloperoxidase (MPO) negative.
- Sudan black B negative.

Q. Write short note on acute myeloid leukemia

Bone Marrow

- *Cellularity:* Markedly **hypercellular** due to proliferation of blasts.
- *Erythropoiesis and myelopoiesis:* Reduced.
- *Megakaryopoiesis:* Megakaryocytes gradually decrease.
- ***Blasts:* Constitute 20–100% of the marrow cells.**

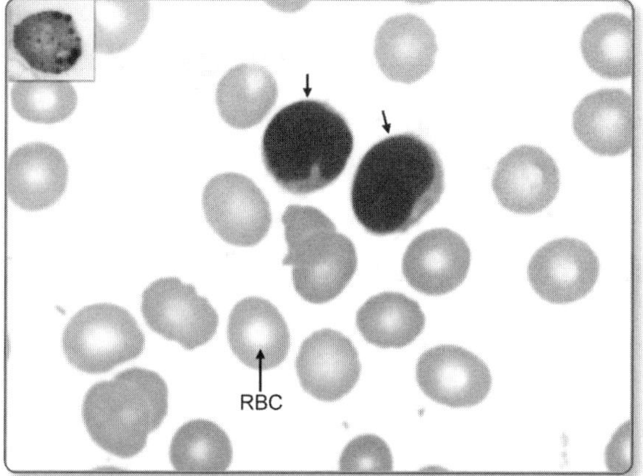

Fig. 12.20: Peripheral blood smears in acute lymphoblastic leukemia showing lymphoblasts (arrows). Inset shows lymphoblast with block positivity with PAS stain

(For color version, see Plate 9)

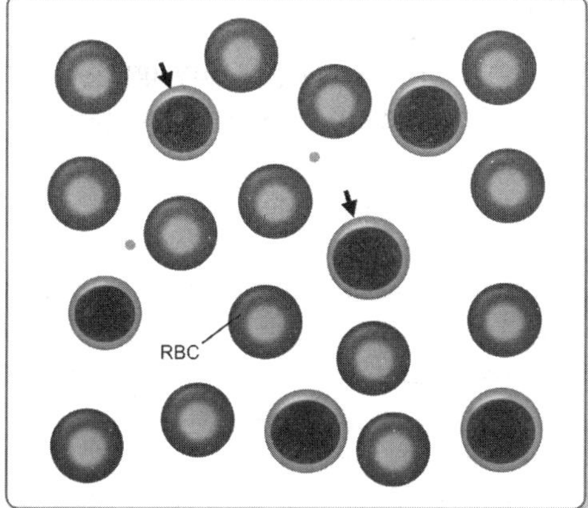

Fig. 12.21: Diagrammatic peripheral blood smear in acute lymphoblastic leukemia showing lymphoblasts (arrows)

(For color version, see Plate 9)

Immunophenotyping

Terminal-deoxynucleotidyl-transferase (TdT) + in pre-B and **pre-T** lymphoblasts.

- Immature B cells + positive for pan B cell marker CD19 and CD10 (CALLA—common ALL antigen).
- Precursor T ALL cells are positive for CD2, CD5 and CD8.

Biochemical Findings

- Serum uric acid: Raised due to destruction of leukemic cells during chemotherapy leading to hyperuricemia.
- LDH: Raised, because of increased turnover of leukemic cells.

CSF Examination

To know/rule out CNS involvement.

ACUTE MYELOGENOUS LEUKEMIA

Q. Write short note on classification of acute myeloid leukemia

Q. Write short note on acute myeloid leukemia

Definition: Neoplasm of hematopoietic progenitors characterized by proliferation resulting in **accumulation of immature myeloblasts in the marrow.**

Classification of acute myelogenous leukemia (AML): Refer Tables 12.17 and 12.18.

Molecular Pathogenesis

- Many recurrent genetic abnormalities can disrupt genes encoding transcription factors involved in normal myeloid differentiation.
- **Mutated tyrosine kinase activation** is a common.

Clinical Features

Age: AML may develop at **any age**, but is more **common in adults**.

Onset: Acute leukemias are **abrupt in onset**.

Symptoms: Related to depressed marrow function.

- ***Bone marrow failure*:**
  - Anemia: Fatigue and weakness.
  - Neutropenia: Life-threatening infections by bacteria or opportunistic fungi.
  - Thrombocytopenia: Bleeding, patient may also develop disseminated intravascular coagulation (DIC) in AML M3 and primary fibrinolysis.
  - Bone pain and tenderness.
- ***Extramedullary infiltration***
  - Gingival hypertrophy (M4 and M5) and infiltration of skin (leukemia cutis).
  - Hepatosplenomegaly: Usually more than in ALL.

Laboratory Findings

Peripheral Blood

Q. Write short note on laboratory/peripheral smear findings in AML.

- **Total WBC Count:** Markedly raised ranging from 20×10^9/L to 100×10^9/L.
- **Hemoglobin:** Decreased and ranges from 5 to 9 g/dL.

- **Peripheral smear (Figs 12.22 and 12.23):**
  - *RBCs:* Normocytic normochromic type of anemia.
  - *WBCs:* Total WBC **count markedly increased.**
    - Differential count: **More than 20% myeloid blasts.** May show more than one type of blast or blasts with hybrid features.
    - **Morphology of myeloblasts**
      - ◊ **3 to 5 times larger than the diameter of a small lymphocyte.**
      - ◊ **High N:C ratio.**
      - ◊ **Fine nuclear chromatin with 2-4 variably prominent nucleoli.**
      - ◊ **More cytoplasm than lymphoblasts—azurophilic, peroxidase-positive granules.**
      - ◊ **Presence of Auer rods is definitive evidence of myeloid differentiation.**
    - **Auer rods** are azurophilic needle-like peroxidase-positive structures in the cytosol of myeloblasts (M_2 and M_3 subtype).
  - *Platelets:* Moderate to severe thrombocytopenia and causes bleeding from skin and mucosa.

Cytochemistry of Myeloblasts

- **Stain positively** with **myeloperoxidase (MPO) and Sudan black B.**
- Monoblasts stain with nonspecific esterases.

Bone Marrow

- *Cellularity:* Markedly **hypercellular.**
- *Erythropoiesis:* **Markedly suppressed.**
- *Myelopoiesis:* Suppression of myeloid maturation and **myeloblasts constitute more than 20% of marrow cells.**
- *Megakaryopoiesis:* **Gradually decreased.**

Immunophenotyping

Diagnosis of AML is confirmed by using stains for myeloid specific antigens.

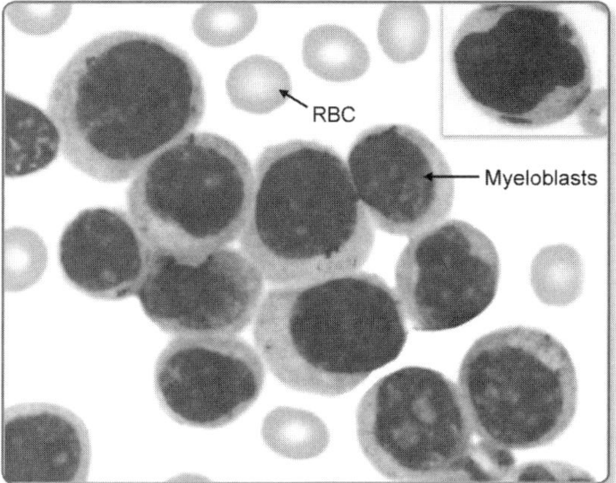

Fig. 12.22: Peripheral smear in AML with myeloblasts. Inset shows myeloblast with Auer rod

(For color version, see Plate 10)

Fig. 12.23: Diagrammatic peripheral blood smear in AML with myeloblasts. One myeloblast with two Auer rods (arrow)

(For color version, see Plate 10)

Cytogenetics

Very important in the WHO classification of AML (Table 12.18).

CHRONIC MYELOGENOUS LEUKEMIA

Definition

Chronic myelogenous leukemia (CML) is one of the myeloproliferative neoplasm (MPN) of **pluripotent hematopoietic stem cell** characterized by overproduction of cells of the myeloid series which results in marked splenomegaly and leukocytosis.

Distinguished from other myeloproliferative neoplasms by the presence of:

1. Chimeric fusion BCR-ABL gene.
2. Philadelphia (Ph) chromosome in more than 90% of cases.

Etiology and Pathogenesis

Q. Write short note on etiology of chronic myeloid leukemia

Risk factor: Exposure to ionizing radiation and benzene.

Molecular Pathogenesis

Philadelphia (Ph) Chromosome (Fig. 12.24)

Q. Write short note on Philadelphia chromosome and its clinical significance.

- Acquired chromosomal abnormality **in all proliferating hematopoietic stem cells** (erythroid, myeloid, monocytic and megakaryocytic precursors).
- **Balanced reciprocal translocation** between long arm of chromosome 9 and 22, i.e. **t (9; 22) (q 34; q 11.2).** It increases the length of chromosome 9 and shortening of 22. This **shortened chromosome 22** is known as Philadelphia chromosome (Fig. 12.24).

BCR-ABL Fusion Gene

- **ABL** proto-oncogene from chromosome 9 **joins** the **BCR** on chromosome 22.

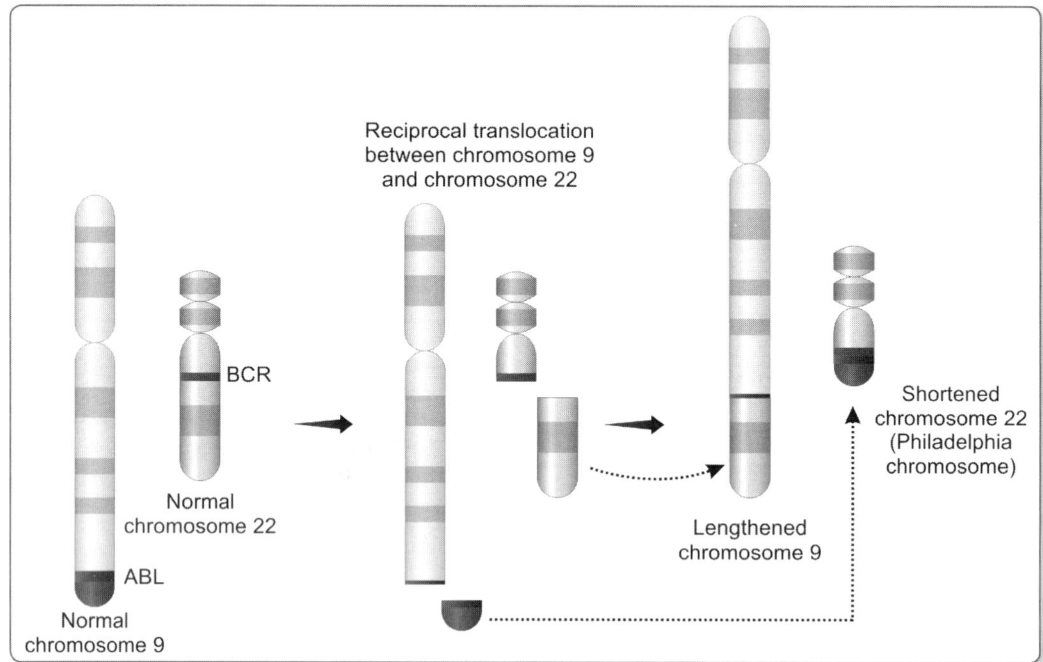

Fig. 12.24: Balanced reciprocal translocation between long arm of chromosome 9 and chromosome 22 resulting in shortened chromosome 22 known as Philadelphia chromosome

- It produces a new **chimeric (fusion) gene called BCR-ABL, thus converting ABL proto-oncogene into oncogene.** The product of the fusion gene plays a central role in the development of CML.
- The product of this oncogene, i.e. **oncoprotein** (e.g. **p210) causes cell division** and **inhibition of apoptosis.**

Clinical Features

Q. Write short note on clinical features of chronic myeloid leukemia

- *Age*: **Usually occurs between 40 to 60 years** of age.
- *Sex:* Males slightly more affected than females.
- ***Onset:* Insidious.**

Symptoms:

- **Nonspecific symptoms:** Fatigue, weakness, weight loss, anorexia.
- **Fullness of abdomen due to splenomegaly** (caused by leukemic infiltration and extra-medullary hematopoiesis). Splenomegaly is moderate to severe and is characteristic feature in majority (80–90%) of patients.
- **Hepatomegaly:** Mild or moderate seen in 60–70% of cases.

Natural History of Chronic Myeloid Leukemia

Three different phases: 1. chronic phase, 2. accelerated phase and 3. blastic phase.

Chronic/Stable/Indolent Phase (CP)

- **Most are diagnosed in this phase.**
- Lasts for 2 to 6 years.
- If not treated, progresses gradually to accelerated phase or abruptly to blastic phase.

Laboratory Findings

Peripheral blood

Q. Write short note on laboratory findings /peripheral smear in CML.

- **Hemoglobin:** Usually less than 11 g/dL.

- **Peripheral smear:**
  - *RBCs:* **Normocytic normochromic anemia**
  - *WBCs:*
    - **Marked leukocytosis** (12–600 × 10^9/L) total **leukocyte count** usually **exceeds 100 × 10^9/L (1,00,000/cu mm).**
    - **Shift to left (shift to immaturity)**—granulocytes at all stages of development (neutrophils, metamyelocytes, myelocytes, promyelocytes and an occasional myeloblasts).
    - **Predominant cells** are **neutrophils and myelocytes.**
    - **Blasts** are usually **less than 10%** of the circulating WBCs (Figs 12.25 and 12.26).
    - **Basophilia and eosinophilia.**
    - **Decreased NAP/LAP score:** NAP score in CML is decreased below 20 (normal score range is 40–100). Helpful in differentiating CML from leukemoid reaction.
  - *Platelets:* Platelets range from normal (150–450 × 10^9/L) to greater than 1000 × 10^9/L. Up to 50% have **thrombocytosis.**

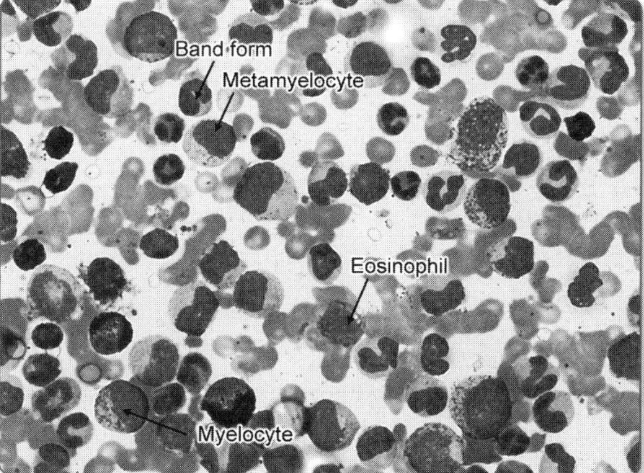

Fig. 12.25: Peripheral blood picture in chronic/stable phase of chronic myeloid leukemia

(For color version, see Plate 11)

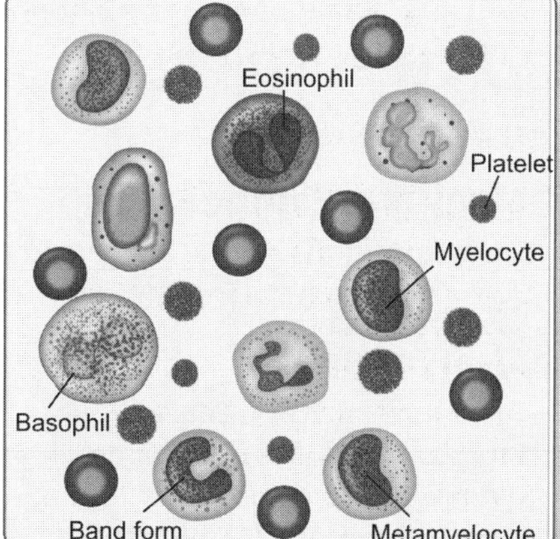

Fig. 12.26: Diagrammatic peripheral blood picture in chronic/stable phase of chronic myeloid leukemia

(For color version, see Plate 11)

Q. Write short note on bone marrow findings in chronic myeloid leukemia

Bone Marrow
- *Cellularity:* Markedly **hypercellular** due to **myeloid hyperplasia.**
- *M: E ratio:* Often exceeds **20:1**.
- *Erythropoiesis:* **Diminished erythropoiesis** as disease progresses.
- *Myelopoiesis:* **Marked hyperplasia. Blast** cells usually **less than 10%.** Basophils, eosinophils and their precursors are usually found.
- *Megakaryopoiesis:* Megakaryocytes are either normal or increased. **Dwarf megakaryocytes.**
- *Sea-blue histiocytes* **(Gaucher-like cells/pseudo Gaucher cells)** are seen.

Biochemical findings:
- Serum uric acid raised
- Serum LDH raised.

Philadelphia chromosome and ***BCR-ABL fusion gene: Demonstrated*** either by chromosomal analysis or **fluorescent in situ hybridization (FISH)** or PCR based tests.

Accelerated Phase (AP)
- **More aggressive** and lasts for few months.

Blast Phase/Crisis (BP)
- **Blood picture resembles acute leukemia** and has **poor prognosis.**

CHRONIC LYMPHOCYTIC LEUKEMIA

Definition

Q. Write short note on chronic lymphocytic leukemia.

Chronic lymphocytic leukemia (**CLL**)/small lymphocytic lymphoma (**SLL**) is a **tumor composed of monomorphic small B lymphocytes** in the peripheral blood, bone marrow and lymphoid organs (spleen and lymph nodes).
- Both CLL and SLL is a **single entity with different presentations**.
- **Small lymphocytic lymphoma** (SLL) is tissue equivalent of chronic lymphocytic leukemia (CLL).
- CLL/SLL tumor cells coexpress CD5 and CD23.

Etiology and Pathogenesis
- **Environmental factors:** Suggested but none proved.
- **Hereditary factors:** Families with higher risk of CLL or other lymphoid neoplasms.

Clinical Features
- ***Age:*** Between **50–60 years** of age.
- ***Sex:*** More in males than in females (2:1).
- ***Symptoms:***
  - **Asymptomatic** in about 25–30%
  - **Nonspecific symptoms: Fatigue,** loss of weight and anorexia
  - **Generalized lymphadenopathy**
  - **Immunological defects** either as i**mmune deficiency or autoimmunity.**

Laboratory Findings

Peripheral Blood
- **Hemoglobin: Decreased** and usually below 13 g/dL.
- **Total leukocyte count** is **increased (20–50 × 10⁹/L).**

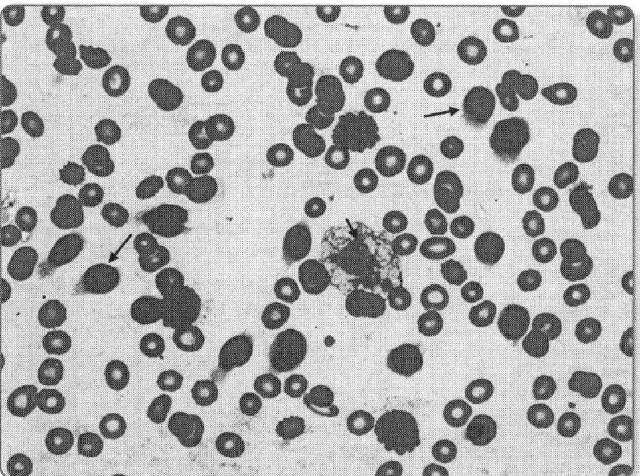

Fig. 12.27: Peripheral blood smears in chronic lymphocytic leukemia showing numerous small lymphocytes (long arrows) and few smudge cells (short arrow)

(For color version, see Plate 12)

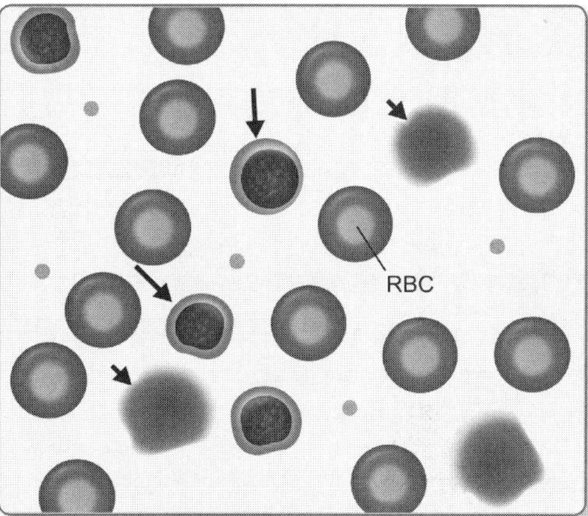

Fig. 12.28: Diagrammatic peripheral blood smears in chronic lymphocytic leukemia showing numerous small lymphocytes (long arrows) and few smudge cells (short arrows)

(For color version, see Plate 12)

- **Peripheral smear (Figs 12.27 and 12.28):**
  - *RBCs:* Normocytic normochromic anemia.
  - *WBCs:*
    - Differential leukocyte count shows **lymphocytosis** and constitutes **more than 50%** of the white cells.
    - **Lymphocytes mature type**—small with scant cytoplasm, **nuclei** round with clumped coarse chromatin **("soccer ball"/block-type chromatin).** Nucleoli absent.
    - **Smudge cells** or basket cells (fragile leukemic cells).
  - *Platelets:* Initially **normal** count and later may be decreased.

Bone Marrow

- *Cellularity:* **Hypercellular** marrow due to infiltration by mature lymphocytes.
- *Erythropoiesis:* Normal.
- *Myelopoiesis:* Normal.
- *Megakaryopoiesis:* Normal.
- *Lymphocytic infiltrate:* As the disease advances neoplastic lymphocytes replace the normal erythroid, myeloid and megakaryocytic series in the bone marrow resulting in anemia, neutropenia and thrombocytopenia.

Lymph Node

- Show loss of normal architecture
- Diffuse infiltration by monomorphic, small, round lymphocytes
- Lymphocytes have nuclei with coarse chromatin and scanty cytoplasm
- Small, nodular aggregates of medium to large-sized lymphocytes known as **proliferation centers or pseudo-follicles or growth centers** and when found are **pathognomonic for CLL/SLL.**

Course and prognosis: Median survival rate is 4 to 6 years. They may progress to B cell prolymphocytic transformation or into diffuse large B cell lymphoma (Richter syndrome).

DISORDERS OF HEMOSTASIS

NORMAL HEMOSTASIS

- Hemostasis is the **body's response to vascular damage/injury.**
- Includes several sequences of events at the site of vascular injury. They are as follows:

Primary Hemostatic Plug

Platelet adhere to subendothelial structures at the site of injury. The **platelets change their shape** and **release granule contents.** The released contents cause platelet **aggregation and form primary hemostatic plug.**

Secondary Hemostatic Plug

Exposure of tissue factor at the site of vascular injury **activates the extrinsic coagulation system. The fibrin formed develops into a secondary hemostatic plug.**

CLASSIFICATION OF HEMOSTATIC DISORDERS (TABLE 12.20)

Q. Classify bleeding disorders.

1. **Bleeding disorders (hemorrhagic disorders/hemorrhagic diathesis):** Bleeding disorders have an **abnormal tendency to bleed** (hemorrhage) due to failure of hemostasis.
2. **Thrombotic disorders:** They cause **thrombus formation.**

Bleeding Disorders Caused by Vessel Wall Abnormalities

Vascular purpura (nonthrombocytopenic purpura) is group of **disorders of blood vessels** that results in **bleeding.** They should be distinguished from bleeding disorders due to abnormalities of platelets.

Table 12.20: Classification of disorders of hemostasis

Classification
• **Bleeding disorders** – **Disorders of primary hemostasis** ◆ **Vessel wall abnormalities** ◊ Congenital, e.g. Ehlers-Danlos syndrome ◊ Acquired, e.g. Henoch-Schönlein purpura ◆ **Platelet abnormalities** ◊ Quantitative: Thrombocytopenia (e.g. ITP, drug-induced, congenital) ◊ Qualitative: Platelet function disorders - Inherited, e.g. Glanzmann thrombasthenia, Wiskott-Aldrich syndrome, Bernard Soulier syndrome - Acquired, e.g. Uremia, drugs – **Disorders of coagulation system (disorders of secondary hemostasis)** ◆ **Congenital:** Hemophilia A, B; von Willebrand disease; other coagulation factor deficiencies [XI, VII, II, V, X] ◆ **Acquired:** Vitamin K deficiency, liver disease, disseminated intravascular coagulation
• **Thrombotic disorders** – **Inherited** ◆ Deficiency of antithrombotic factors: Antithrombin III deficiency, protein C deficiency, protein S deficiency ◆ Increased prothrombotic factors: Activated protein C (APC) resistance (Factor V mutation/factor V Leiden) ◆ Prothrombin (G20210A mutation) – **Acquired:** Fibrinolytic system defects

Classification of bleeding disorders caused by vessel wall abnormalities are presented in Table 12.21.

Table 12.21: Classification of bleeding disorders caused by vessel wall abnormalities

• **Acquired disorders** – Due to decreased amount of connective tissue ◆ Senile purpura ◆ Scurvy ◆ Cushing syndrome and steroid therapy – Due to vasculitis ◆ Henoch-Schönlein purpura ◆ Infections ◆ Drug reactions – Associated with plasma cell neoplasms ◆ Amyloidosis – Miscellaneous ◆ Simple easy bruising
• **Congenital/inherited disorders** – Hereditary hemorrhagic telangiectasia – Ehlers-Danlos syndrome – Marfan syndrome

Bleeding Disorders Due to Abnormalities of Platelet

Classification of Platelet Disorders (Table 12.22)

Table 12.22: Classification of platelet disorders

Quantitative Platelet Disorders	
• **Thrombocytopenia** – Increased destruction – Sequestration • **Thrombocytosis**	 – Decreased production – Dilutional
Qualitative Platelet Disorders	
• **Hereditary** – Defective adhesion of platelets – Defective platelet aggregation • **Acquired**	 – Disorders of platelet secretion

Thrombocytopenia

- Decrease in the **platelet count below** the lower limit of **150,000/cu mm** (150×10^9/L).

Clinical Features of Thrombocytopenia

- Cutaneous bleeding appears as pinpoint hemorrhages (petechiae) and ecchymoses.
- Mucosal bleeding.
- Intracranial bleed (subarachnoid and intracerebral hemorrhage) rare but serious.

Severity of Bleeding

- **Post-traumatic** bleeding—when the platelet **count is 20,000 to 50,000/cu mm**.
- **Spontaneous** bleeding—when the platelet count falls **below 20,000/cu mm.**
- **Intracranial** bleeding—when platelet count is <**10,000/cu mm.**

Causes of Thrombocytopenia (Table 12.23)

Table 12.23: Causes of thrombocytopenia

• **Increased platelet destruction** – **Immune mediated** ◆ **Autoimmune** ◊ Primary: Immune thrombocytopenic purpura (acute and chronic) ◊ Secondary: Systemic lupus erythematosus, B cell lymphoid neoplasms ◆ **Alloimmune:** Post-transfusion or pregnancy ◆ **Drug-induced:** Quinidine, heparin, sulfa compounds ◆ **Infections:** HIV infection, infectious mononucleosis, cytomegalovirus – **Non-immune mediated** ◆ Disseminated intravascular coagulation ◆ Thrombotic thrombocytopenic purpura, hemolytic uremic syndrome ◆ Mechanical destruction: Prosthetic heart valves, malignant hypertension ◆ Microangiopathic hemolytic anemias
• **Decreased production of platelets** – **Generalized primary diseases of bone marrow:** Aplastic anemia (congenital and acquired) – **Bone marrow invasion/infiltration:** Leukemia, disseminated cancer – **Selective impairment of platelet production** ◆ Drug-induced: Alcohol, thiazides, cytotoxic drugs ◆ Infections: Measles, human immunodeficiency virus (HIV) – **Ineffective megakaryopoiesis** ◆ Megaloblastic anemia ◆ Myelodysplastic syndromes
• **Sequestration** – Hypersplenism
• **Dilutional**

IMMUNE THROMBOCYTOPENIC PURPURA

- Most common form of thrombocytopenia.
- **Due to increased destruction of platelets** by **immune mechanisms**—mainly **autoimmune** mechanism.

Types of Immune Thrombocytopenic Purpura (ITP)

Acute Immune Thrombocytopenic Purpura

Q. Write short note on immune thrombocytopenic purpura.

- **Self-limited** disease.
- **Children:** 2 to 4 years and seen equally in both sexes.
- Presents **1 to 3 weeks after viral** (measles, rubella, EBV) **infection.**
- Platelet destruction by **antiplatelet autoantibodies.**
- **Platelet count is decreased**, sometimes even below 10,000/cu mm (10×10^9/L).

Clinical Features

- **Sudden onset.**
- **Petechiae, gum bleeding, epistaxis** and mild fever.
- Usually **resolve** spontaneously **within 6 months.**
- **Excellent prognosis.**

Chronic Immune Thrombocytopenic Purpura

- Persistent **thrombocytopenia** for **more than 6 to 12 months.**
- Indolent, females are more affected than males (F:M = 3:1).
- **More common** and usually seen in **adults (20 to 40 years).**

Pathogenesis of ITP (Fig. 12.29)

- **Autoimmune disorder** characterized by formation of **antiplatelet antibodies**, directed against membrane glycoproteins (most often IIb-IIIa or Ib-IX of platelets).
- Antiplatelet antibodies in about 80% of patients and are of the **IgG type.**
- Antiplatelet antibodies act as opsonins and are recognized by IgG Fc receptors present on mononuclear phagocytes of RE system (mainly spleen) and are destroyed there resulting in thrombocytopenia.
- **Splenectomy causes marked improvement** in 75% to 80% of patients.

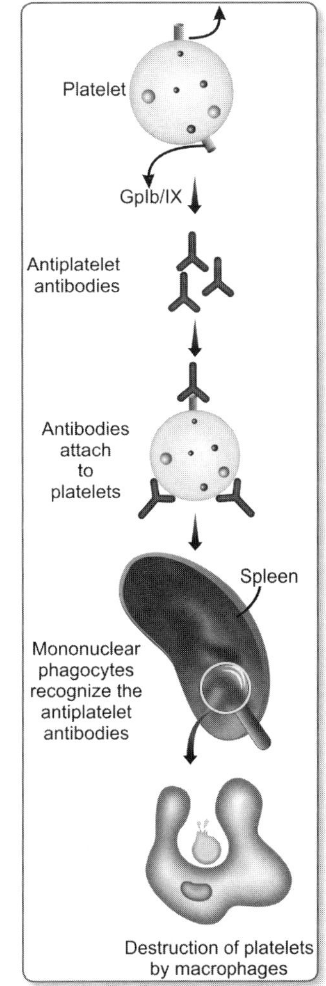

Fig. 12.29: Pathogenesis of idiopathic thrombocytopenic purpura

Clinical Features

- More common in **females** (F:M ratio is 3:1).
- Age between **20 and 40 years**.
- Clinical features are due to thrombocytopenia: **Skin bleeding, mucosal bleeding, menorrhagia** in females, etc.

Laboratory Findings

Peripheral Blood

Q. Write short note on laboratory findings in ITP.

- **Platelet count: Markedly reduced**—below 80,000/cu mm (80×10^9/L).
- **Hemoglobin:** Ranges from 7 to 12 g/dL.

- **Peripheral smear**
  - *Platelets:* **Markedly reduced** (thrombocytopenia) and **abnormally large sized platelets (mega-thrombocytes/giant platelets)**.
  - *RBCs:* **Chronic blood loss** (e.g. menorrhagia) due to ITP may **lead to microcytic hypochromic anemia.**
  - *WBCs:* Normal.

Bone Marrow

- *Cellularity:* **Hypercellular.**
- *Megakaryopoiesis:*
  - **Moderate increase in number** (Fig. 12.30) of both **immature and mature** forms of **megakaryocytes.**
  - **Immature megakaryocytes predominate-large nonlobulated single nuclei and basophilic cytoplasm.**

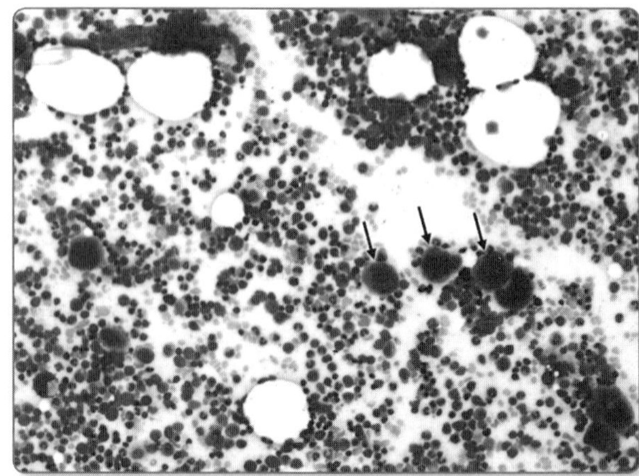

Fig. 12.30: Bone marrow in ITP showing moderate increase in number of megakaryocytes (arrows)

- *Erythropoiesis:*
  - **Prolonged bleeding** may cause anemia leading to **normoblastic erythroid hyperplasia**.
  - Constant bleeding leads to **iron deficiency** and **micronormoblastic erythroid hyperplasia.**
- **Myelopoiesis***:* Normal.
- **Storage iron***:* Severe and chronic bleeding causes iron deficiency with reduced iron stores.

- **Bleeding time (BT): Prolonged**, but PT and PTT are normal.
- **Tourniquet test: Positive.**
- **Clotting time (CT): Normal.**
- **Tests for platelet autoantibodies:** May be positive.
- **Spleen:** Normal size.

COAGULATION DISORDERS

Bleeding due to coagulation disorders must be distinguished from those due to platelet/ vascular disorders (Table 12.24).

Table 12.24: Distinguishing patterns of bleeding in platelet/vascular and coagulation disorders

Characteristics	Platelet/vascular disorders	Coagulation disorders
Onset	Spontaneous and develops immediately after trauma/surgery	Delayed bleeding after trauma/ surgery
Type of lesion	Petechiae, ecchymoses	Hematomas
Sites	Skin, mucous membrane	Deep tissues
• Mucous membrane	Common from nose, mouth, gastrointestinal and genitourinary tracts	Uncommon except from gastrointestinal or genitourinary tract
• Into the joint	Absent	Common in severe factor deficiencies
• Into the muscle	Following trauma	Spontaneous

Classification of Coagulation Disorders (Table 12.25)

Table 12.25: Classification of coagulation disorders

• **Hereditary coagulation disorders**	
– Hemophilia A	– Hemophilia B
– von Willebrand disease	– Others
• **Acquired (secondary) coagulation disorders**	
– Vitamin K deficiency	– Liver disease
– Others	

HEREDITARY COAGULATION DISORDERS

Usually, due to deficiency of single coagulation factor.

Factor VIII-vWF Complex

- **Factor VIII-vWF complex** has two components:
  - Plasma **factor VIII**
  - **von Willebrand factor.**
- **vWF protects factor VIII** and important for its stability. **Subendothelial vWF promotes platelet adhesion.**
- Whenever there is vascular endothelial injury, **plasma vWF** gets **adsorbed to exposed subendothelial matrix** and **augments adhesion of platelets.**

HEMOPHILIA

Q. Write short note on hemophilia

- Hemophilia **A and B** are **similar in both clinical and pathological features**, the **difference** being **in the deficient factor**.
- Both are **sex-linked recessive disorders** resulting in inherited deficiency of the clotting factor or synthesis of a defective clotting factor.
- **Males are affected** and **females are carriers**.

Hemophilia A (Factor VIII Deficiency)

- **Common hereditary X-linked recessive** disease.
- About 30% of hemophiliacs may be due to acquired mutations.
- **Reduced amount or** activity of **factor VIII** is associated with **life-threatening bleeding.**
- Bleeding is due to both inadequate coagulation and inappropriate clot removal (fibrinolysis).

Mode of Inheritance (Fig. 12.31)

- X-linked recessive disease. **Genes** for factor VIII are located **on the long arm of the X-chromosome**.
- Does not manifest when there is a normal copy of X-chromosome.
- **Males** with a defective/mutant factor VIII gene (hemophiliac gene) on their single X chromosome (X_H) **suffer** from hemophilia.
- **Heterozygous females are carriers** and do not express the full clinical disease because of the paired normal X-chromosome.
- However, females with two copies of the defective X_H chromosome may rarely suffer from hemophilia.

Clinical Features

Clinical severity **depends on the level of factor VIII activity with normal range expressed as percentage.** Severe cases have less than 1% residual factor VIII activity.

Common clinical presentations include:

- Frequent and spontaneous **hemorrhage into the joints**-hemarthrosis.
- Hemorrhage into **soft tissues.**
- **Prolonged bleeding** following trauma.

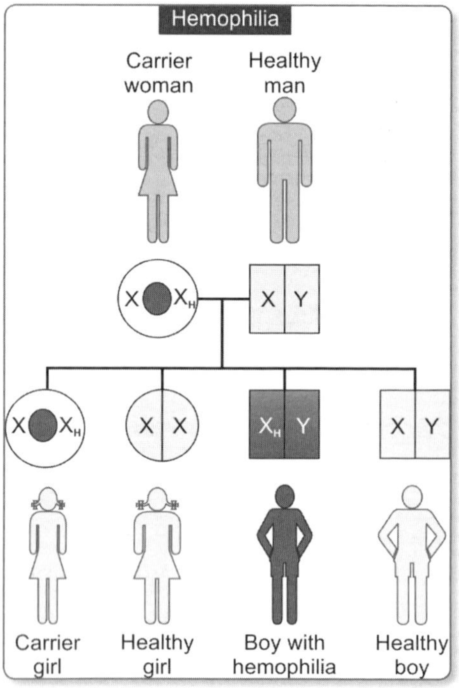

Fig. 12.31: Mode of inheritance in hemophilia

Laboratory Findings

- **Bleeding time: Normal**
- **Clotting time: Prolonged,** but is not a sensitive test
- **Platelet count: Normal**
- **Prothrombin time: Normal**
- **Activated partial thromboplastin time (APTT): Increased** (normal 30–40 seconds)
- **Factor VIII assay: Essential for the diagnosis** and to assess the levels and severity of disease.
- **Fibrinogen assay:** Normal
- **FDP:** Negative
- **Detection of carriers:** By DNA markers
  - To detect female carriers
  - Prenatal diagnosis of affected fetuses.

Complications

Due to Hemophilia

- **Deforming arthritis and contractures:** This is due to repeated bleeding into the joints. Organization and fibrosis of intramuscular hematomas → contractures of involved muscles.
- **Anemia:** Excessive, spontaneous or repeated bleeding leads to anemia.

Due to Therapy

- **Viral hepatitis: Hepatitis B, C and D** in patients who received multiple transfusions of FFP/ cryoprecipitate.
- **AIDS:** In individuals who received fresh frozen plasma (FFP) or cryoprecipitate, when screening tests for HIV were not available.
- **Factor VIII inhibitors:** Makes further management difficult.

Hemophilia B (Christmas Disease, Factor IX Deficiency)

- **Clinically indistinguishable from hemophilia A**
- **X-linked recessive** disorder
- **Variable clinical severity**

- Assay of factor IX should be done to diagnose Christmas disease (named after the first patient).

Laboratory Findings

Similar to hemophilia A.

- **Bleeding time:** Normal
- **Clotting time:** Prolonged
- **Platelet count:** Normal
- **Prothrombin time:** Normal
- **Activated partial thromboplastin time (APTT):** Increased (normal 30–40 seconds)
- **Factor IX assay:** Factor IX is decreased.

Von Willebrand Disease (vWD)

Q. Write short note on von Willebrand disease

- Most common **inherited** bleeding disorders.
- Most cases are **autosomal dominant disorders**.
- Variable clinical picture with more than 20 variants.

Categories

Grouped into two major categories:

- **Quantitative deficiency of vWF:** Decreased circulating vWF
  - Type 1- autosomal dominant, mild disorder and form about 75% of all cases.
  - Type 3-autosomal recessive, severe disorder and least common type.
- **Qualitative defects in vWF:**
  - Type 2-autosomal dominant, accounts for 25% with several subtypes.

Clinical Features

- Most cases are of **mild bleeding**
- Common symptoms
  - Spontaneous bleeding from mucous membranes (e.g. epistaxis)
  - Excessive bleeding from wounds or menorrhagia
- In severe cases, similar to hemophilia A.

Laboratory Findings

- **Platelet count:** Normal
- **Bleeding time:** Prolonged
- **Clotting time:** Prolonged
- **Tourniquet test (Hess test):** Positive due to defect in platelet adhesion
- **APTT:** Prolonged APTT
- **PT:** Normal
- **vWF assay:** Plasma level of active vWF is decreased
- **Platelet function test:** Defective ristocetin induced platelet aggregation test is diagnostic of vWF.

Laboratory tests in hereditary disorders are summarized in Table 12.26.

Table 12.26: Summary of laboratory tests in hereditary coagulation disorders

	Hemophilia A	Hemophilia B	von Willebrand disease
Bleeding time	N	N	Increased
APTT	Increased	Increased	Increased
Factor VIII	Decreased	N	Low or normal
Factor IX	N	Decreased	N
vWF	N	N	Decreased

Abbreviation: N, normal

ACQUIRED COAGULATION DISORDERS

Coagulation Factor Abnormalities

Usually characterized by multiple clotting abnormalities

- **Vitamin K deficiency:** In neonates, low levels of vitamin K levels may produce life-threatening hemorrhage during the first week of life known as ***hemorrhagic disease of the newborn.***
- **Liver disease:** Liver synthesizes all the clotting factors and severe liver disease is associated with a hemorrhagic diathesis.
- **Other causes:** Disseminated intravascular coagulation that involves deficiency of several coagulation factors.

Disseminated Intravascular Coagulation

Q. Write short note on DIC

Widespread disorder with **combination of thrombosis and hemorrhage.**

Etiology

Develops as a secondary complication of wide variety of disorders (Table 12.27).

Table 12.27: Major disorders associated with disseminated intravascular coagulation

• **Infections** – Gram-negative bacterial sepsis – Fungi, viruses, Rocky Mountain – spotted fever, malaria	– Meningococcemia and other bacteria
• **Obstetric complications** – Retained dead fetus – Abruptio placentae – Toxemia and pre-eclampsia	– Septic abortion – Amniotic fluid embolism
• **Neoplasms** – Carcinomas of pancreas, prostate, lung and stomach – Acute promyelocytic leukemia	
• **Massive tissue injury** – Traumatic – Fat embolism	– Burns – Surgery
• **Vascular disorders** – Aortic aneurysm, giant hemangioma	
• **Immunologic reactions** – Transfusion reactions	– Transplant rejection
• **Respiratory distress syndrome** – Miscellaneous ◆ Snakebite, liver disease, acute intravascular hemolysis, shock, heat stroke, hypersensitivity, vasculitis	

Clinical Features

- **Serious, often fatal**, clinical condition
- Signs and symptoms are related to:
  - **Hemorrhagic diathesis/bleeding:** Most common, manifest as ecchymoses, petechiae or bleeding from mucous membranes or at the sites of venipuncture.
  - **Microvascular thrombi:** Tissue hypoxia and infarction of the organ leading to multiorgan failure.

Laboratory Findings in DIC

Screening Assays

- **Coagulation abnormalities**
  - **APTT: Increased** as a result of consumption and inhibition of the function of clotting factors.
  - **Prothrombin time: Increased.**
  - **Thrombin time (TT): Increased** because of decreased fibrinogen.
  - **Fibrinogen:** Decreased.
- **Bleeding time: Increased** due to decreased platelet count.
- **Platelet count: Decreased** due to utilization of platelets in microthrombi.
- **Peripheral smear: Microangiopathic hemolytic anemia with schistocytes.**

Confirmatory Tests

- **Fibrinolysis abnormalitie**s
- **FDP** (fibrin degradation/split products): Secondary fibrinolysis results in **generation of FDPs**, which can be measured by latex agglutination
- **D-dimer test:** It is **specific for diagnosing DIC**.

Chapter 13

Lymph Nodes

Chapter Outline
- Lymphoid neoplasms
- Non-Hodgkin lymphoma
- Hodgkin lymphoma
- Metastatic carcinoma

LYMPHOID NEOPLASMS

Definition

- **Lymphomas** are malignant lymphoid neoplasms due to lymphoid tissue proliferations that arise as discrete tissue masses. Lymphomas are mainly subdivided into **Hodgkin lymphoma (HL)** and **non-Hodgkin lymphomas (NHLs)**.
- **Leukemias** are neoplasms that present with widespread involvement of the bone marrow and (usually, but not always) the peripheral blood.

Many "lymphoma" occasionally have leukemic presentations, and evolution to "leukemia" is not unusual during the progression of incurable "lymphomas." Conversely, few "leukemias" may sometimes arise as soft tissue masses without detectable bone marrow disease. Therefore, the terms leukemia and lymphoma reflect the usual tissue distribution of the disease at presentation.

Classification of Lymphoid Neoplasms (Table 13.1)

Table 13.1: WHO classification of the lymphoid neoplasms (2008)

• **Precursor Lymphoid Neoplasms** – B lymphoblastic leukemia/lymphoma – T lymphoblastic leukemia/lymphoma
• **Mature B Cell Neoplasms** – Chronic lymphocytic leukemia/small lymphocytic lymphoma – B cell prolymphocytic leukemia – Splenic B cell marginal zone lymphoma – Hairy cell leukemia – Lymphoplasmacytic lymphoma – Heavy chain disease

Contd...

Contd...

– Plasma cell neoplasm – Follicular lymphoma – Mantle cell lymphoma – Diffuse large B cell lymphoma – Burkitt lymphoma
• **Mature T and NK Cell Neoplasms** – T cell prolymphocytic leukemia – T cell large granular lymphocytic leukemia – Mycosis fungoides – Sézary syndrome – Peripheral T cell lymphoma, NOS – Angioimmunoblastic T cell lymphoma – Anaplastic large cell lymphoma – Adult T cell leukemia/lymphoma – Extranodal NK/T cell lymphoma, nasal type
• Hodgkin Lymphoma – **Classical Hodgkin lymphoma** ◆ Nodular sclerosis classical Hodgkin lymphoma ◆ Mixed cellularity classical Hodgkin lymphoma ◆ Lymphocyte-rich classical Hodgkin lymphoma ◆ Lymphocyte depleted classical Hodgkin lymphoma – Nodular lymphocyte predominance Hodgkin lymphoma

WHO classification of lymphoid neoplasms depends on clinicopathological and immunological profile (Table 13.2) and has clinical and therapeutic importance.

Table 13.2: Cell type and its antigens detected by monoclonal antibodies

Cell type	Antigen detected
T cell	CD1, CD3, CD4, CD5, CD8
B cell	CD10, CD19, CD20, CD21, CD23, CD79a
Monocyte or macrophage	CD11c, CD13, CD14, CD15, CD33, CD64
NK cell	CD16, CD56
Stem cell and progenitor cell	CD34
All leukocytes	CD45 (LCA)

Abbreviations: CD, cluster designation; NK, natural killer; LCA, leukocyte common antigen

NON-HODGKIN LYMPHOMA

Follicular Lymphoma (FL)

Q. Write short notes on follicular lymphoma.

Composed of follicle center (germinal center) **B cells** of lymphoid follicles (centrocytes and centroblasts).

Morphology

Gross

- Involves **lymph nodes**, spleen and bone marrow.
- **Architecture** of lymph node is **lost**; frequently infiltrate the perinodal tissue (Fig. 13.1).

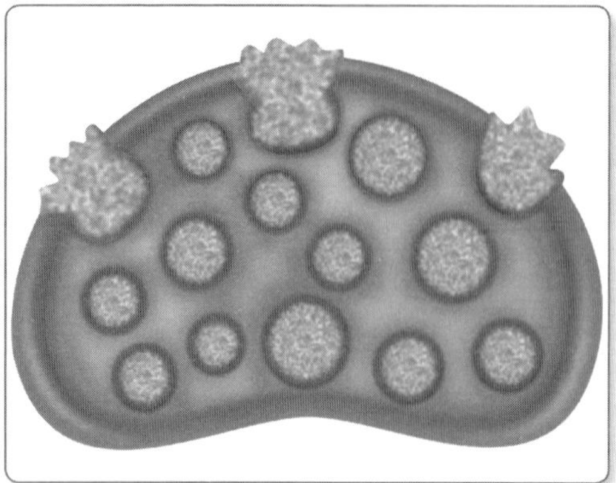

Fig. 13.1: Diagrammatic appearance of follicular lymphoma. Neoplastic follicles are seen in both the cortex and medulla and infiltration of the perinodal tissue

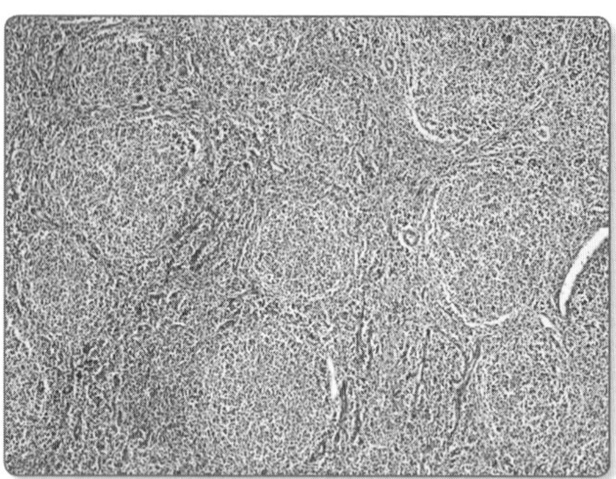

Fig. 13.2: Follicular lymphoma shows nodular aggregates of malignant lymphoid cells

Microscopy

- **Follicular** (nodular) growth pattern, **neoplastic follicles** are **poorly defined** (Fig. 13.2).
- **Two types of B cells.**
  - **Centrocytes** (small cleaved cells)
    - Cleaved nuclei
    - Inconspicuous nucleoli
  - **Centroblasts** (large non-cleaved cells)
    - Round or oval nuclei with open nuclear (vesicular) chromatin
    - Multiple (1 to 3) nucleoli
    - Usually 3 times the size of lymphocyte.

Immunophenotype: Expresses **CD19, CD20** (pan-B cell markers), **CD10** (CALLA), **surface immunoglobulin and BCL2 protein.**

Cytogenetics and molecular genetics: t (14; 18) (q32:q21), with IgH and BCL2 as partner genes and leads to constitutive **overexpression of BCL2** protein.

Clinical Features

- Peak in **sixth and seventh decades**.
- **Generalized lymphadenopathy**.

Diffuse Large B Cell Lymphoma (DLBCL)

Heterogeneous group of **aggressive**, neoplasm of large B cell with **diffuse** growth pattern. Constitutes about 20 to 30% of NHL and 60% to 70% of aggressive lymphoid neoplasms.

Microscopy

- **Loss of** lymph node **architecture** with **diffuse growth pattern.**
- **Neoplastic cells:**
  - **Large** round or oval cells, **4 to 5 times** of a **small lymphocyte.**
  - Moderate pale or basophilic cytoplasm.
  - **Nucleus** equals or larger than the **nucleus of a macrophage** with different appearances.

Immunophenotype

- Express pan-B cell markers such as **CD19, CD20, CD22 and CD79a**.
- Also express **germinal center markers** like CD10 and BCL6.
- **Negative for TdT.**

Cytogenetics and Molecular Profile

- **Translocation of BCL2 gene:** t (14; 18) translocation
- **Mutations of the BCL6 gene.**

Clinical Features

- More common between **65 and 70 years** of age.
- Slight **male** preponderance.
- Rapidly **enlarging** mass at a single or multiple **nodal or extranodal sites.**

Burkitt Lymphoma (BL)

Q. Write short notes on Burkitt lymphoma.

- **Highly aggressive B cell** neoplasm, often presents as **extranodal** lymphoma or as an acute leukemia.
- Composed of **medium-sized, monomorphic lymphoid cells** with basophilic **vacuolated cytoplasm.**

Clinical Variants

- **Endemic (African) Burkitt lymphoma (BL):**
  - Occurs in Africa, affects **children and adolescents.**
  - **Associated with Epstein-Barr virus infection and malaria**.
  - Usually involves the **jaw** and present as a mandibular mass.
- **Sporadic (nonendemic) BL:**
  - Occurs in **children or young adults.**
  - **Abdominal mass** and involves **ileocecum** and **peritoneum**.
- **Immunodeficiency-associated (HIV) BL:**
  - Involves lymph nodes and bone marrow.

Microscopy

- Burkitt lymphomas, irrespective of the categories, are **histologically similar**.
- Lymph node shows **loss of architecture**.
- Involved tissues show **diffuse** infiltrate of **monotonous medium-sized lymphoid cells** (Figs 13.3 and 13.4).
- **Appearance of neoplastic lymphoid cells:**
  - **Medium-sized cells**.
  - **Round or oval nuclei** having clumped **coarse chromatin** with **several (2 to 5) nucleoli.**
  - **Moderate** amount of deeply **basophilic cytoplasm, multiple, small**, **round lipoid** (clear) **vacuoles** which stain positive with oil red O.
  - **Numerous mitotic figures**.
- **Starry sky pattern:** Tumor cells undergo **apoptosis** and nuclear remnants of these apoptotic cells are phagocytosed and cleared by benign macrophages. These macrophages in the background of lymphoid cells creates **"starry sky"** appearance (Figs 13.3 and 13.4).

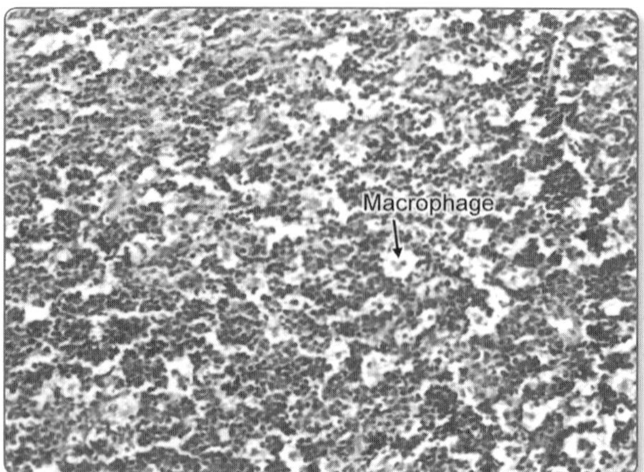

Fig. 13.3: Burkitt lymphoma composed of medium-sized lymphoid cells admixed with benign macrophages giving a "starry sky" appearance

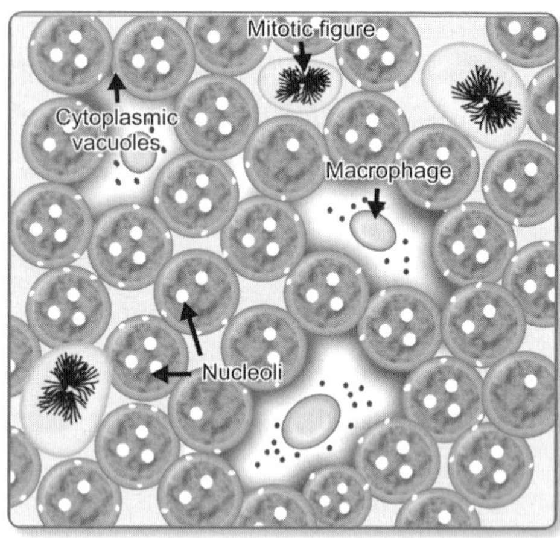

Fig. 13.4: Diagrammatic appearance of Burkitt lymphoma composed of medium-sized lymphoid cells admixed with benign macrophages giving a "starry sky" appearance

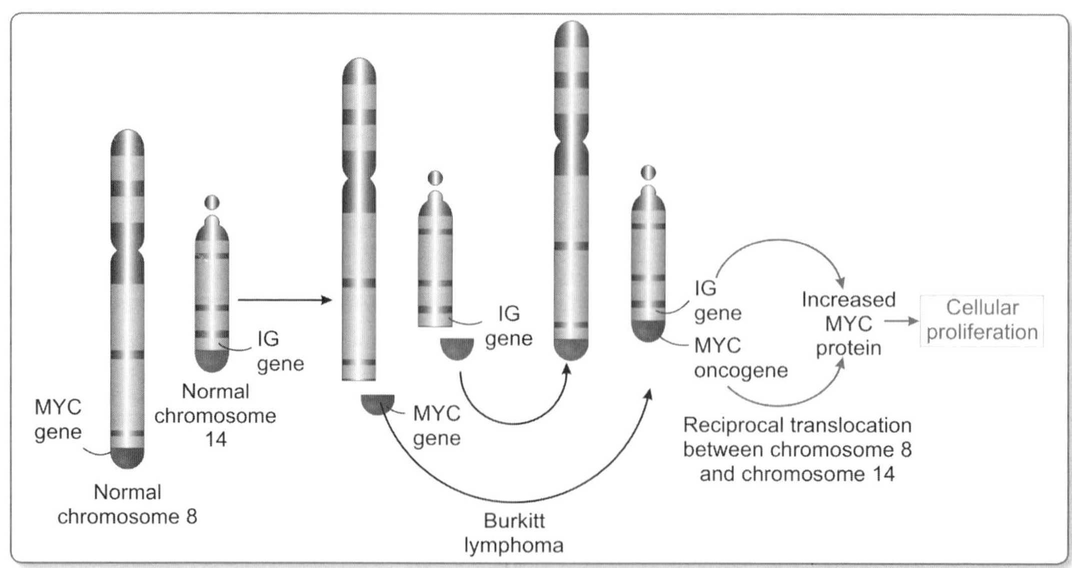

Fig. 13.5: Chromosomal translocation and activated MYC oncogene in Burkitt lymphoma

Immunophenotype

- Express surface **IgM, monotypic κ or λ light chain.**
- **Positive for common B cell antigens** (CD19, CD20, and CD22).
- **Positive for CD10 and BCL6.**
- BCL2 negative.

Cytogenetic and Molecular Genetic Features (Fig. 13.5)

Translocations of c-MYCgene

- MYC (c-MYC) is a **proto-oncogene**-on chromosome 8.
- **Most common translocation t (8:14) (q24; q32).**

- **Translocations of c-MYC gene,** converts proto-oncogene into **MYC** oncogene, which leads to **overexpression of MYC protein** (oncoprotein). This causes **uncontrolled cell proliferation** and stimulation of apoptosis.
- **Mutations inactivate p53.**
- **Poor prognostic factors:**
  - Involvement of blood, bone marrow and central nervous system.
  - Bulk of the disease-unresected tumor of more than 10 cm in diameter.
  - High serum LDH levels.
  - Presence of residual disease after excision.

Mature T Cell and NK Cell Neoplasms

Peripheral T Cell Lymphoma (PTCL), NOS

Mainly involves lymph node.

Microscopy

- **Lymph node** with **effacement of the normal architecture.**
- **Paracortical or diffuse infiltration** by neoplastic T cells.
- **Neoplastic T cells**
  - **Small, intermediate to large cells** with sparse or abundant; clear, eosinophilic or basophilic.
  - **Vesicular or hyperchromatic nuclei, prominent nucleoli.**

Immunophenotype

- Lack TdT (expressed by immature T cells).
- Express pan-T cell-CD2, C3, CD5 and either α β or γ δ T cell receptors (TCR).

Mycosis Fungoides

- **Cutaneous T cell lymphoma.**
- Lymphoid cells with **irregular nuclear outlines.**
- Limited to **skin.**

Age: Most are adults or elderly.

Microscopy

- **Epidermis (epidermotropism) and upper dermis** is infiltrated by neoplastic T cells.
- Groups of neoplastic cells in the epidermis—**Pautrier's microabscess.**
- Tumor cells have **convoluted (cerebriform) nuclear contours.**

Sézary Syndrome

Rare disease and is defined by the triad namely:

1. **Widespread exfoliative erythroderma**
2. **Generalized lymphadenopathy**
3. **Presence of characteristic Sézary cells** in the skin, lymph nodes and peripheral blood.

Prognosis: Aggressive disease and most die of opportunistic infections.

HODGKIN LYMPHOMA

Hodgkin Lymphoma(HL): Malignant lymphoid neoplasms with following characteristics:

- **Minority** (1–3%) **of specific neoplastic cells** (Hodgkin cells and **Reed-Sternberg cells**).

Table 13.3: WHO classification (2008) of Hodgkin lymphoma

• **Classical Hodgkin lymphoma (CHL)** – **Nodular sclerosis classical Hodgkin lymphoma (NSCHL)** – **Mixed cellularity classical Hodgkin lymphoma (MCCHL)** – **Lymphocyte-rich classical Hodgkin lymphoma (LRCHL)** – **Lymphocyte depleted classical Hodgkin lymphoma (LDCHL)**
• **Nodular lymphocyte predominant Hodgkin lymphoma (NLPHL)**

- **Majority background of** reactive **non-neoplastic cells.**
- Usually involves **lymph nodes.**
- Majority occurs in **young** adults.

Classification (Table 13.3)

Q. Classify Hodgkin lymphoma.

Hodgkin lymphoma (HL) is broadly divided into **two types**, which differ in clinical features, behavior, morphology and immunophenotype.

Cell of Origin and Immunophenotype

- **Classical Hodgkin lymphoma**
  - Cell of origin: **Germinal center or post-germinal center B cell**
  - Immunophenotype: **CD15** and **CD30 positive**
- **Nodular lymphocyte predominant Hodgkin lymphoma**
  - Cell of origin: **Germinal center B cell at the centroblastic stage** of differentiation.
  - Immunophenotype: **CD15** and **CD30 negative**.

Morphology of Neoplastic Cells

Q. Write short note on RS cell and its variants.

Reed-Sternberg (RS) Cells are neoplastic cells (Fig. 13.6) **pathognomonic** of Hodgkin lymphoma.

Appearance and description of diagnostic Reed-Sternberg cells and its variants are shown in Figure 13.7.

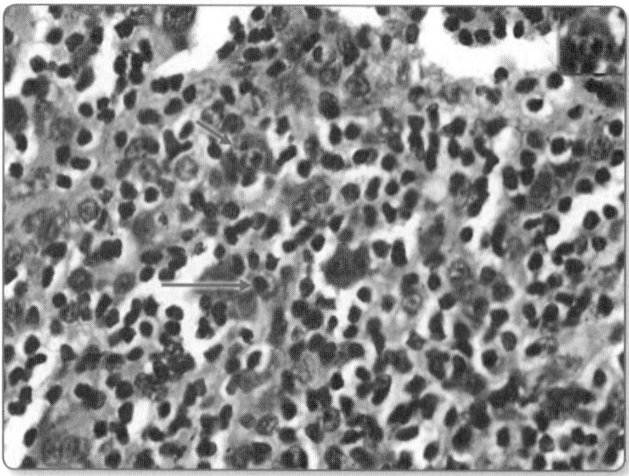

Fig. 13.6: Microscopic appearance of Hodgkin lymphoma showing RS cells (short arrow and inset) and Hodgkin cells (long arrow) within the background of mixed population of reactive cells

(For color version, see Plate 13)

DESCRIPTION	APPEARANCE
Large cells (20 to 60 μm in diameter) Abundant eosinophilic cytoplasm Nucleus: Typically two large nuclei -"mirror image" Prominent eosinophilic nucleolus surrounded by a halo	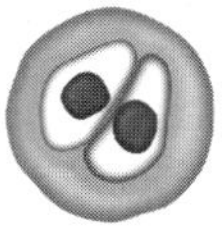 Classic RS cell
Single, large, round nucleus with a large eosinophilic inclusion-like nucleolus May be seen in any subtypes of CHL	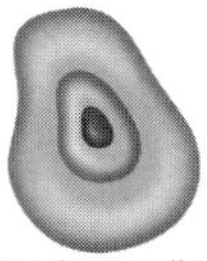 Mononuclear cell variant (Hodgkin cell)
Abundant, lightly acidophilic or water-clear cytoplasm Large folded or multilobed nucleus One or more prominent eosinophilic nucleoli Seen in nodular sclerosis of CHL	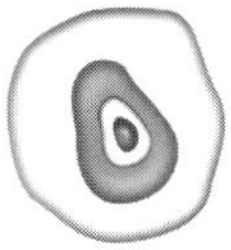 Lacunar cell variant
Dark eosinophilic cytoplasm with pyknotic nuclei Strongly indicate HL but not diagnostic	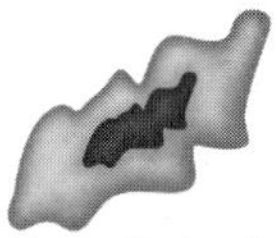 Mummified cell variant
Highly pleomorphic cells Large bizarre hyperchromatic nuclei Commonly found in lymphocyte-depleted CHL	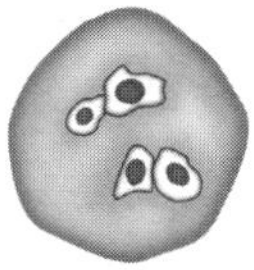 Anaplastic/pleomorphic variant
Abundant pale cytoplasm with popcorn nucleus Specific to the nodular lymphocyte predominance type of HL	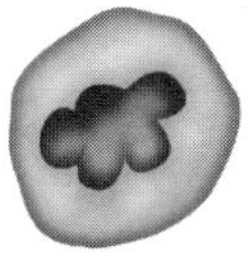 Lymphocyte predominant cell (LP cell)/popcorn cell

Fig. 13.7: Diagrammatic appearances and characteristic features of Reed-Sternberg cells and its variants

Various types of cells found in Hodgkin lymphoma are listed in Table 13.4.

Table 13.4: Types of cells found in Hodgkin lymphoma

Non-neoplastic cells	Neoplastic cells
• Reactive lymphocytes	• Reed-Sternberg cells (classical)
• Macrophages/histiocytes – **Granulocytes** – **Eosinophils** – **Neutrophils**	• Variants – **Mononuclear** – **Lacunar** – **Mummified** – **Anaplastic/pleomorphic** – **Lymphocyte predominant (LP) cell/popcorn**
• Plasma cells	

Classical Hodgkin Lymphoma

Classical Hodgkin lymphoma (CHL) account for **95%** of Hodgkin lymphomas and has 4 subtypes.

Nodular Sclerosis Classical Hodgkin Lymphoma (NSCHL)

Q. Write short note on nodular sclerosis HL.

Subtype of CHL characterized by **collagen bands** that surround **nodules** and have **lacunar cell variant of Reed-Sternberg cells.**

- Most common: **40% to 70%** of cases.
- Most between **20 and 30 years of age** with **equal** frequency in **males and females.**
- **Rarely associated with EBV.**
- Involves **mediastinal lymph nodes.**

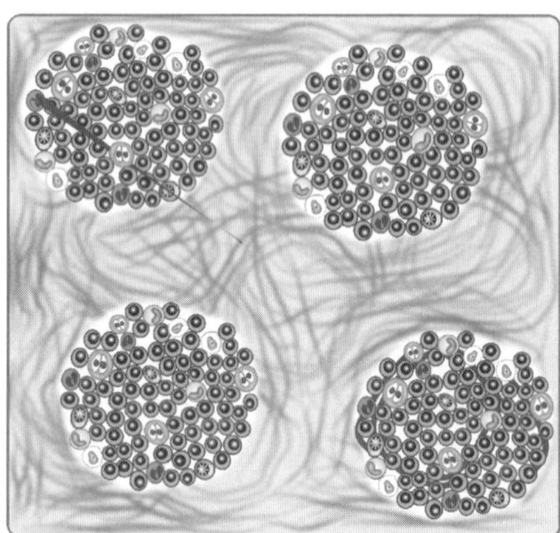

Fig. 13.8: Nodular sclerosis classical Hodgkin lymphoma with nodules separated by bands of collagen. Also seen are lacunar cells and RS cells in each nodule within the background of lymphocytes, eosinophils, plasma cells and macrophages

Microscopy of NSCHL (Fig. 13.8)

- **Loss of lymph node architecture.**
- **Sclerosis and nodules: Broad collagen** bands (sclerosis) divide the lymphoid tissue into **nodules of varying sizes and shapes.**
- **Presence of lacunar cell.**
- **Background: Small T lymphocytes, eosinophils, plasma cells, and macrophages.**

Immunophenotype

- RS cells are **CD15+ and CD30+; CD45- and T cell markers negative.**
- **EBV negative.**

Mixed Cellularity Classical Hodgkin Lymphoma (MCCHL)

Q. Write short note on Mixed cellularity HL.

- **Second common subtype:** 20% to 25% of cases
- **More common in males**
- **Strongly associated with EBV**
- **Older age**, with **systemic symptoms** (such as night sweats and weight loss) and **advanced tumor stage**
- Involves **peripheral lymph nodes.**

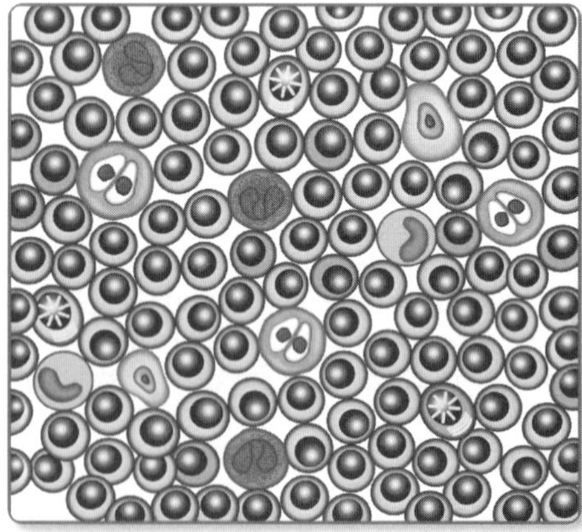

Fig. 13.9: Mixed cellularity classical Hodgkin lymphoma with classical RS cells, Hodgkin cells in the background of mixed cellular population consisting of lymphocytes, eosinophils, plasma cells and macrophages

Microscopy of MCCHL (Fig. 13.9)

- Lymph node architecture obliterated
- **Plenty of Reed-Sternberg cells** and Hodgkin cells
- **Back ground: Small lymphocytes, eosinophils (sometimes numerous), neutrophils, plasma cells and benign macrophages (histiocytes).**

Immunophenotype: RS cells are **CD15+, CD30+** and **EBV+** (about 70%).

Lymphocyte-rich Classical Hodgkin Lymphoma (LRCHL)

- Subtype of classical Hodgkin lymphoma with **scattered Hodgkin and RS cells**.
- **Uncommon**—about 5% of classical HL.
- More in **elderly** patients, associated with **EBV in 40%** of cases.
- Involves **peripheral lymph nodes**.

Microscopy of LRCHL (Fig. 13.10)

- **Growth patterns:** May show two patterns
  - **Nodular—**common
  - **Diffuse—**rare
- **Only few Reed-Sternberg cells and Hodgkin cells**
- **Background: Abundant reactive small lymphocytes.**

Immunophenotype: CD45–, CD20–, CD15+ and CD30+.

Lymphocyte-depleted Classical Hodgkin Lymphoma (LDCHL)

Subtype of classical Hodgkin lymphoma **rich in Hodgkin and RS cells** in a background depleted in non-neoplastic lymphocytes.

- **Rarest**—less than 5% of cases
- Predominantly in **older, HIV-positive patients**, often **EBV-associated** (over 90%)
- Predominantly **retroperitoneal lymph nodes, abdominal organs and bone marrow**.

Microscopy of LDCHL (Fig. 13.11)

- **Paucity of lymphocytes.**
- **Plenty of RS cells** or their **anaplastic/pleomorphic variants.**
- Histological types
  - **Reticular: Numerous Hodgkin and RS cells** with depletion of lymphocytes.
  - **Diffuse sclerosis/fibrosis:** Hypocellular infiltrate containing bizarre RS cells with fine fibrosis.

Immunophenotype: RS cells are **CD15+, CD30+; majority are EBV+.**

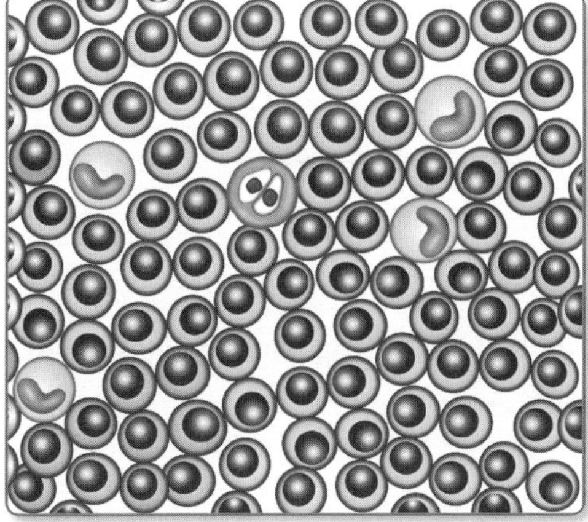

Fig. 13.10: Lymphocyte-rich classical Hodgkin lymphoma. One RS cell is seen in a background of many small lymphocytes and few histiocytes

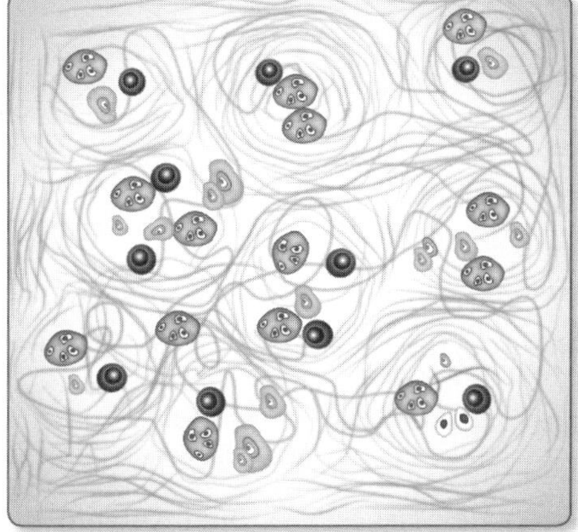

Fig. 13.11: Lymphocyte-depleted classical Hodgkin lymphoma with the pleomorphic variant of RS cells surrounded by fibrous tissue

Nodular Lymphocyte Predominant Hodgkin Lymphoma (NLPHL)

- **Uncommon**—5% of all Hodgkin lymphomas.
- **Not associated** with **EBV**.
- Majority males, usually **30–50 year** of age.
- Involves mainly **cervical or axillary lymph nodes**.

Microscopy of NLPHL (Fig. 13.12)

- Loss of lymph node architecture.
- Nodular and/or diffuse infiltrate of **abundant small lymphocytes** with histiocytes and **scattered LP cells.**
- **Lymphocyte predominant cells** (LP cells)/"popcorn" cells (Fig. 13.12)
  - Specific to NLPHL.
  - Large with relatively abundant, pale cytoplasm.
  - Single large delicate **multilobulated** nucleus **or folded nuclei** resembling bubbly outlines of popcorn kernels.
  - One or more **inconspicuous nucleoli.**
- **Hodgkin and RS cell**s are not found.

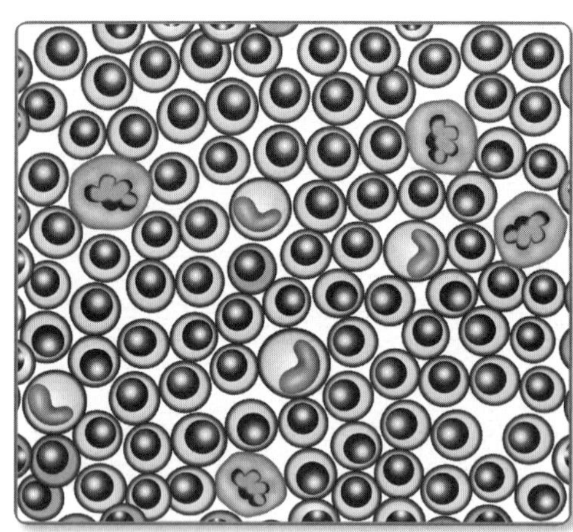

Fig. 13.12: Nodular lymphocyte predominant Hodgkin lymphoma with 'popcorn' cells in a background of reactive lymphocytes and few macrophages

Immunophenotype: LP cell are **CD20+, CD 45+** and **CD15–, C30– and EBV–ve.** Express BCL6.

Etiology and Pathogenesis of Hodgkin Lymphoma

- **EBV:** Previous EBV infection (infectious mononucleosis) ↑ risk of HL.
- **Genetic factors:** HLA-B18 higher in HL.
- **Immune status:** HL more frequent in immunocompromised patients and autoimmune diseases (e.g. rheumatoid arthritis).

Laboratory Findings

- **Peripheral smear:**
  - *RBCs:* Normocytic normochromic anemia.
  - *WBCs:* Leukocytosis occurs in 1/3rd of the patients. Eosinophilia is frequent.
  - *Platelets:* Normal or increased.

Fine Needle Aspiration Cytology (FNAC)

RS cells/its variants against a background of inflammatory cells (depending on the subtype).

Spread

- Mainly **by contiguity**
- First nodal disease → then splenic disease, hepatic disease → and finally marrow involvement and extranodal disease.

Staging of Hodgkin Lymphoma (Table 13.5)

Table 13.5: Clinical staging of Hodgkin lymphomas (Cotswold revision of Ann Arbor staging classification)

Stage	Definition
I	Involvement of a single lymph node region or lymphoid structure (e.g. spleen, Waldeyer ring, thymus)
II	Involvement of two or more lymph node regions on the same side of the diaphragm (the mediastinum is a single site; hilar lymph nodes are lateralized); the number of anatomic sites should be indicated by suffix (e.g. II_3)
III	Involvement of lymph node regions or structures on both sides of the diaphragm
	III_1 With or without splenic, hilar, celiac or portal nodes III_2 With para-aortic, iliac or mesenteric nodes
IV	Involvement of extranodal site(s) beyond those designated E

E—involvement of a single extranodal site, or contiguous or proximal to known nodal site of disease

Differences between Hodgkin Lymphoma and Non-Hodgkin Lymphoma

Q. List the differences between HL and NHL.

HL differs from NHL in several respects and their main differences are shown in Table 13.6.

Table 13.6: Differences between Hodgkin and non-Hodgkin lymphomas

Sl. No.	Characteristics	Hodgkin lymphoma	Non-Hodgkin lymphoma
1.	Site of involvement	Arises in a single node or chain of nodes (cervical, mediastinal, para-aortic)	Mainly involves multiple peripheral nodes
2.	Pattern of spread	Orderly spread by contiguity in a predictable fashion	Noncontiguous spread in an unpredictable fashion
3.	Mesenteric nodes and Waldeyer ring	Rarely involved	Commonly involved
4.	Extranodal involvement	Uncommon	Common
5.	Characteristic of neoplastic cells	Neoplastic cells—Hodgkin or Reed-Sternberg cells form minor tumor cell mass (1–5%)	Neoplastic cells form the major tumor cell mass

METASTATIC CARCINOMA (FIGS 13.13 AND 13.14)

Most common pathway of spread for carcinomas is spread through lymphatics. Once the tumor cells gain access into the lymphatic vessels, they are carried to the regional draining lymph nodes.

Pattern of lymph node involvement follows the natural routes of lymphatic drainage.

- **Sentinel lymph node** biopsy is done to know the presence or absence of metastatic lesions.
- **Skip metastasis**: When **local lymph nodes are bypassed** and **lymphatic metastases develop in lymph nodes distant from the site of the primary tumor**; these are called "skip metastasis". Example: **Abdominal cancers** may be **first detected by an enlarged supraclavicular node**.
- **Retrograde metastasis**: **Tumors spreading against the flow of lymphatics** may cause metastases at unusual sites. Example: Carcinoma prostate metastasizing to supraclavicular lymph node.

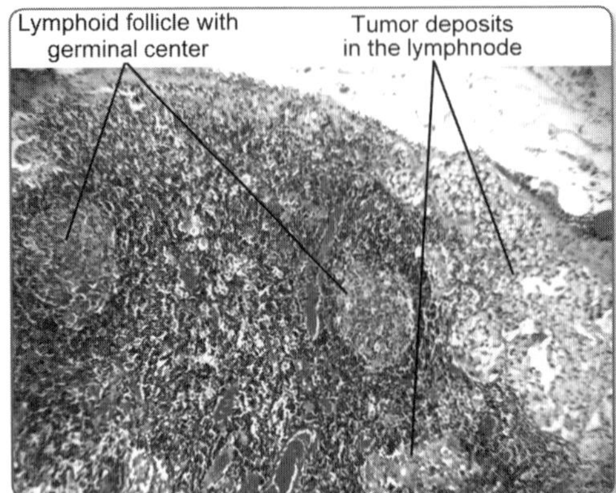

Fig. 13.13: Lymph node with metastasis from carcinoma

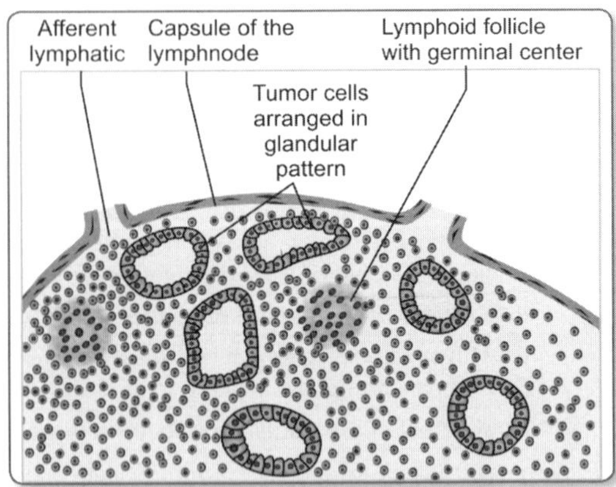

Fig. 13.14: Lymph node with secondaries from adenocarcinoma (diagrammatic)

Microscopic pattern of deposits:

- Initially, **tumor cells** are deposited in the **marginal sinus and later extend throughout the node**.
- **Micrometastases consist of single tumor cells or very small clusters.**

Significance of lymph node metastases: Prognostic value- e.g. in breast cancer, involvement of axillary lymph nodes is very important for assessing prognosis and for type of therapy.

Chapter 14

Oral Cavity

Chapter Outline
- Lichen planus
- Stomatitis
- Precancerous lesions of oral cavity
- Squamous cell carcinoma
- Odontogenic cysts
- Odontogenic tumors

LICHEN PLANUS

- Lichen planus is usually self-limited disease that involves both skin and mucosa.
- It most commonly resolves spontaneously 1 to 2 years after onset. Resolution often leaves a postinflammatory hyperpigmentation of the area involved.
- Oral lesions may persist for years. Squamous cell carcinoma may develop in chronic mucosal and paramucosal lesions of lichen planus.

Pathogenesis

The pathogenesis of lichen planus is not known. It appears that expression of altered antigens in basal epidermal cells or the dermoepidermal junction elicits a cell-mediated cytotoxic (CD8+) T cell response.

Morphology

- **Gross**
  - **Sites:** (1) Skin mainly of extremities (wrists and elbows), (2) glans penis in males, and (3) oral mucosa.
  - **Skin lesions**: They consist of itchy, violaceous, flat-topped papules that may coalesce focally to form plaques. These papules may be highlighted by white dots or lines called **Wickham striae**. Lesions are usually multiple and symmetrically distributed.
  - **Oral lesions:** In majority (70%) of patients, oral lesions are present as white, reticulated, or net-like areas involving the mucosa.
- **Microscopy:**
  - Dense, continuous infiltrate of lymphocytes along the dermoepidermal junction (**interface dermatitis**) producing on an angulated zigzag contour (sawtoothing).

- The lymphocytes are intimately associated with basal layer of epidermis, which show degeneration, necrosis the dermoepidermal interface.
- Anucleate, necrotic basal cells may be found among the inflammatory cells in the papillary dermis and are referred to as **colloid** or **Civatte bodies.**

STOMATITIS

Q. Write short note on Canker sores/aphthous ulcers.

- Stomatitis is the inflammation of the mucus membrane of the mouth.
- It can occur in several diseases.

Aphthous Ulcers (Canker Sores)

- Aphthous ulcers are **common, often recurrent**, exceedingly **painful,** superficial oral mucosal ulcerations.

Etiology: Unknown, but may be precipitated by emotional factors, stress, nutritional deficiency, hormonal imbalance etc. Aphthous ulcers may also be associated with immunologic disorders such as celiac disease, inflammatory bowel disease, and Behçet disease.

- They are most common in the first 2 decades of life.
- The lesions appear as single or multiple, shallow, hyperemic ulcers covered by a thin exudate and rimmed by a narrow zone of erythema.
- Initially, the inflammatory infiltrate is mononuclear, but secondary bacterial infection may result in a neutrophilic infiltrate.
- It usually resolves spontaneously in 7 to 10 days. Sometimes it may persist for weeks (e.g. in immunocompromised patients).

PRECANCEROUS LESIONS OF ORAL CAVITY

Q. Write short note on premalignant lesions of the oral cavity.

Leukoplakia and Erythroplakia

Leukoplakia

Q. Write short note on definition and morphology of leukoplakia.

Definition: It is defined as a **white patch or plaque, not less than 5 mm in diameter**, that cannot be removed (scraped off) by rubbing and cannot be classified as any other diagnosable disease.

If any white patches in the oral cavity can be given a specific diagnosis, it is not a leukoplakia.

- **Sites:** May be seen **anywhere in the oral cavity**. Most common sites are buccal mucosa, floor of the mouth, ventral surface of the tongue, palate, and gingiva.
- **Number**: It may be **single or multiple.**
- **Appearance: White patches or plaques** having **sharply defined borders**. Surface may be smooth or wrinkled.

Erythroplakia

- **Less common** and appears as a **red, velvety area within the oral cavity**.
- It remains level with or slightly depressed in relation to the surrounding mucosa.
- **Microscopically**, the **epithelium is atypical** and has an **increased risk of malignant transformation** than leukoplakia.

Intermediate forms, which have the characteristics of both leukoplakia and erythroplakia, are termed **speckled leukoerythroplakia**.

Features of Leukoplakia and Erythroplakia

Age and Gender

Q. List the differences between erythroplakia and leukoplakia.

Both leukoplakia and erythroplakia may be found in adults of any age, but they are usually seen between **40 to 70 years**. Male to female ratio is 2: 1.

Etiology

Q. Write short note on etiology and morphology of leukoplakia.

Both have **multifactorial** origin and are associated with use of **tobacco** (cigarettes, pipes, cigars, and chewing tobacco).

Microscopy

Leukoplakia:

- **Surface stratified squamous epithelium** show a spectrum of changes ranging from **hyperkeratosis and acanthosis** to lesions with **variable degree of dysplastic changes** (including carcinoma in situ).
- **Subepithelial region** shows **inflammatory infiltrate of lymphocytes and macrophages**, the intensity of which is proportional to the degree of dysplasia.

Erythroplakia:

- **Epithelium shows erosions with dysplasia, carcinoma in situ, or frank carcinoma.**
- **Subepithelial region** shows **intense inflammatory reaction** and **vascular dilatation, which is responsible for the reddish clinical appearance.**

Hairy Leukoplakia

- Hairy leukoplakia is a **distinctive oral lesion** and is **seen in immunocompromised patients.**
- About 80% of patients with hairy leukoplakia are infected with the human immunodeficiency virus (**HIV**) and remaining 20% are seen in patients who are immunocompromised for other reasons (e.g. cancer therapy or transplant immunosuppression).

Etiology: It is due to **Epstein–Barr virus (EBV) infection**.

Site: Located mostly on the **lateral edges/border of the tongue**.

Morphology

- **Gross: White, confluent patches of fluffy ("hairy") thickenings**, which cannot be scraped off.
- **Microscopy:** It shows **hyperparakeratosis and acanthosis** with "**balloon cells**" in the **upper spinous layer** of the epithelium.

SQUAMOUS CELL CARCINOMA

In India, oral cavity cancer is the most common malignant tumor.

Etiology

Q. Write short note on etiology of squamous cell carcinoma of oral cavity.

Squamous cell carcinoma (SCC) of oral cavity is **multifactorial disease** usually seen in middle-aged men.

Risk Factors

1. **Tobacco products and smoking**: Any irritating smoked product increases the risk for tumors of the oral cavity. Nicotine in tobacco and other tobacco leaf components cause cancer. **Carcinogens in tobacco can act as initiators, as well as promoters.** Risk increases with amount and duration of tobacco use. Tobacco may be used either for **smoking** or as **smokeless tobacco**.
   a. **Smoking:** It may be in the form of cigarette, beedi, cigar, or pipe smoking, or reverse smoking (smoking a cheroot with the burning end inside the mouth is practiced in certain regions of India). Regular marijuana use has also been associated with oropharyngeal cancer.
   b. **Smokeless tobacco:** It is in the form of **betel quid**/pan that contains several ingredients such as areca nut, slaked lime, and tobacco, which are wrapped in a betel leaf. It is commonly used in India and Southeast Asia, and is associated with marked increase in oral cancer. **Betel quid appears to be the major carcinogen**. However, it may also be related to slaked lime and the areca nut. Other methods of tobacco consumption include snuff dipping and tobacco chewing.

   Oral cancers are found on the **buccal and gingival** surfaces in the sites **where tobacco products** are held in **contact** with the mucosa for long periods.
2. **Alcohol consumption**: It is another important etiologic factor and act synergistically with tobacco as either a cocarcinogen (increasing the risk) or a promoter (decreasing the lag time). The risk of oral SCC is magnified in individuals who smoke as well as consume alcohol.
3. **Other risk factors:**
   - Radiation exposure and solar actinic radiation (sunlight).
   - Welding, metal refining, diesel exhaust, wood stove, and asbestos exposure.
   - Chronic irritation of the mucosa: It may be due to ill-fitting dentures, jagged teeth, or chronic infections.
   - Vitamin A deficiency and immunosuppression.
   - Poor nutrition.

Role of Oncogenic HPV Virus Infection

High-risk HPV types 16 and 18 and, less commonly low-risk HPV types 6 and 11 have been found in oral carcinomas.

Inherited Genomic Instability

Family history of head and neck cancer is a risk factor, and is thought to be due to inherited genomic instability.

Pathogenesis

Q. Write short note on etiology and morphology of oral cancer.

The development of squamous cell carcinoma is a **multi-step process**. It involves sequential activation of oncogenes and inactivation of tumor suppressor genes in a clonal population of cells.

- **Inactivation of the *p16* gene** (about 80% of the cases) → stratified squamous epithelium undergoes hyperplasia/hyperkeratosis.
- **Mutation of the *p53* tumor suppressor gene** is associated with progression of hyperplasia/hyperkeratosis to dysplasia.
- **Amplification and overexpression of the** *cyclin D1 gene* constitutively activates cell cycle progression.

Morphology

Site

- Anywhere in the oral cavity. Common sites are **lower lip, the ventral surface of the tongue, floor of the mouth**, buccal mucosa, soft palate, and gingiva.

Gross

- **Early stages**: It appears either as raised, firm, pearly plaques or as irregular, roughened, or verrucous areas of mucosal thickening. May be superimposed on a leukoplakia or erythroplakia.
- **Later**: It may appear as **ulcerated and protruding gray white** masses with **irregular and indurated** (rolled) **borders.**

Microscopy

- Squamous cell carcinomas (Figs 14.1A and B) range from well-differentiated keratinizing neoplasms to poorly differentiated/anaplastic tumors. However, the histological grading does not correlate with behavior.

Spread

1. **Local:** Tissue involved depends on the primary site.
2. **Lymph node:** The involved site of lymph node depends on the location of the primary tumor. The more anterior the tumor, more is the spread to the cervical nodes. Carcinomas of the base of the tongue and oropharynx metastasize to the deep retropharyngeal lymph nodes.
3. **Blood spread**: It spreads to lungs, liver, and bones.

Verrucous Carcinoma

Verrucous carcinoma (Ackerman tumor) is **a variant of well-differentiated squamous cell carcinoma**.

Site: Most common in the buccal mucosa and lower gingiva.

Age and gender: Most are elderly males.

Etiology: Tobacco, especially chewing or snuff dipping and HPV infection.

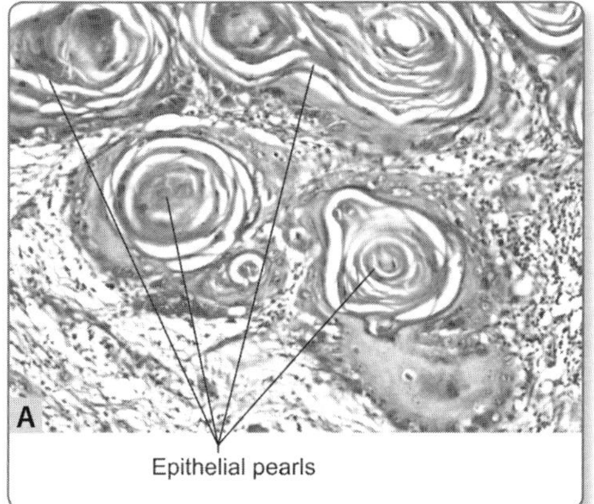

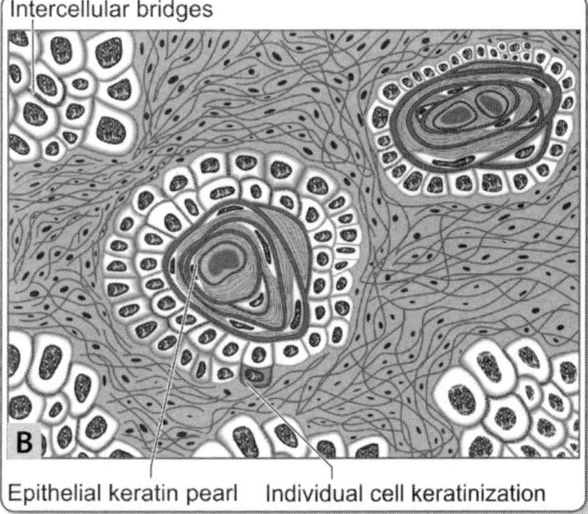

Figs 14.1A and B: Well-differentiated squamous cell carcinoma microscopic appearance. A. H and E staining; B. Diagrammatic

Morphology

Gross: Large, fungating, soft papillary growth.

Microscopy: The surface epithelium shows hyperkeratosis, acanthosis, and benign-appearing papillomatosis. Rete pegs are swollen and voluminous and extend into the deeper tissues.

Spread: May infiltrate the soft tissues of the cheek, mandible or maxilla, and invade perineurial spaces. **Regional lymph node metastases are exceedingly rare**, and **distant metastases have not been reported**.

ODONTOGENIC CYSTS

- **Majority of odontogenic cysts are derived from remnants of odontogenic epithelium present within the jaws.**
- Epithelial-lined cysts are quite common in the jaws.

Dentigerous (Follicular) Cyst

- **Definition**: It is a cyst that originates around the crown of an unerupted tooth and is thought to be due to the accumulation of fluid between the developing tooth and the dental follicle.
- **Radiography**: They are unilocular lesions most often associated with impacted third molar (wisdom) teeth.
- **Microscopy**: They are lined by a thin layer of stratified squamous epithelium. Dense chronic inflammatory cell infiltrate is seen in the connective tissue stroma.
- **Treatment**: Complete removal of the cyst is curative.

Odontogenic Keratocyst (OKC)

- Also called as keratocystic odontogenic tumor.
- It must be differentiated from other odontogenic cysts because of its aggressive behavior.
- Can be seen at any age but are most often between ages 10 and 40.
- Occur most commonly in males within the posterior mandible.
- Majority are solitary.
- Radiography: Well-defined unilocular or multilocular radiolucencies.
- Microscopy: The cyst is lined by a thin layer of keratinized stratified squamous epithelium with a prominent basal cell layer. It has a corrugated epithelial surface.
- OKCs are locally aggressive and recurrence rates are high.

ODONTOGENIC TUMORS

- Odontogenic tumors constitute a group of lesions having diverse histologic appearances and clinical behavior. Some are true neoplasms (both benign and malignant), while others are likely to be hamartomas.
- Odontogenic tumors are derived from odontogenic epithelium, ectomesenchyme, or both. Ameloblastoma is the most common and clinically significant tumor.

Ameloblastoma

Q. Write short note on pathology of ameloblastoma.

Q. Write short note on ameloblastoma.

- Most common slow growing, benign but locally invasive epithelial odontogenic tumor. It has an indolent course in most cases.

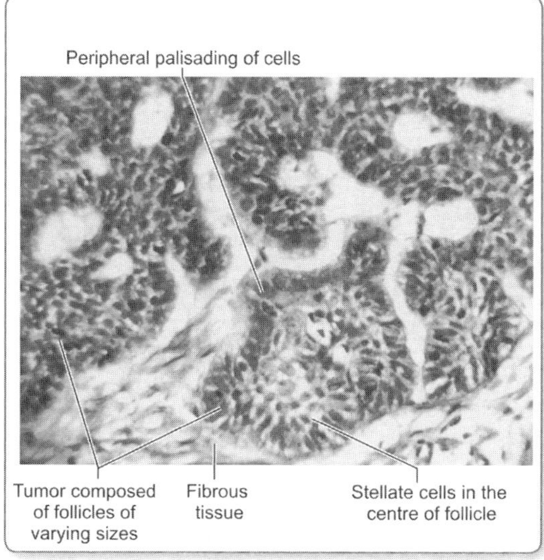

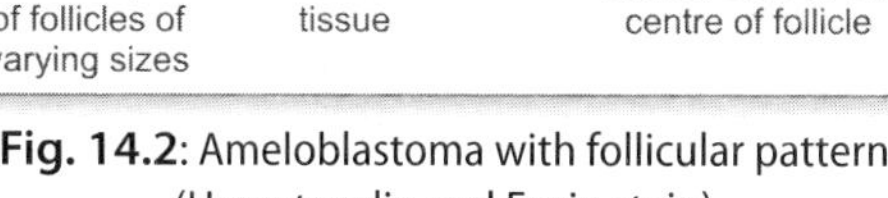

Fig. 14.2: Ameloblastoma with follicular pattern (Hematoxylin and Eosin stain)

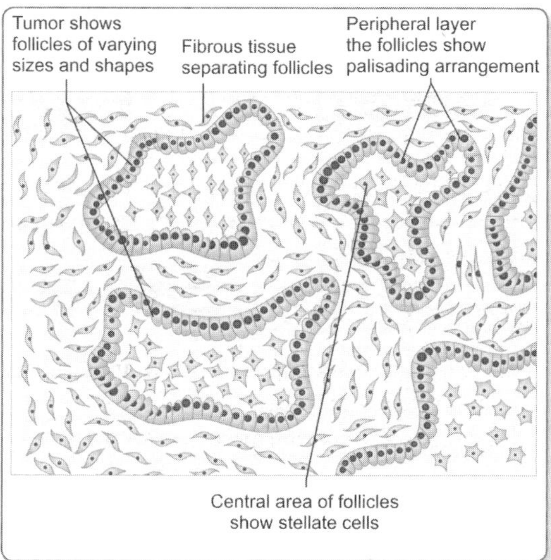

Fig. 14.3: Ameloblastoma with follicular pattern (diagrammatic)

- **Age:** Most often seen during 3rd to 5th decades of life.
- **Sites**: Commonly arises in the molar ramus and the maxilla.
- **Origin**: Arises from odontogenic epithelium and shows *no* ectomesenchymal differentiation.
- **Radiology**: Shows multilocular destruction of the involved bone.
- **Gross:** It is grey-white, commonly cystic, replaces and expands the involved bone.
- **Microscopy**: It can show various patterns:
  - **Follicular pattern** (Figs 14.2 and 14.3): It is the most common pattern. Tumor shows follicles of varying sizes and shapes separated by fibrous tissue. The follicles appear similar to the enamel organ and consist of central area of stellate cells resembling stellate reticulum. The central area may show cystic changes. The peripheral layer of these follicles is cuboidal to columnar and appears to have palisading arrangement.
  - **Plexiform pattern**: The tumor cells form irregular plexiform masses or network of strands. The stroma is scanty and may show microcyst formation.
  - **Acanthomatous pattern**: Islands of tumor cells show squamous metaplasia.
  - **Basal cell pattern**: Appear similar o basal cell carcinoma of skin.
  - **Granular cell pattern**: Tumor cells have acidophilic granular cytoplasm.
- **Treatment:** Wide surgical resection to prevent recurrences.

Chapter 15

Salivary Glands

Chapter Outline

- Salivary glands
- Salivary gland neoplasms
- Pleomorphic adenoma
- Warthin tumor
- Mucoepidermoid carcinoma

SALIVARY GLANDS

Normal Structure

Groups of Salivary Glands

- **Major salivary glands**: There are three major paired salivary glands namely parotid, submandibular, and sublingual.
  - The main duct of parotid gland opens into the oral cavity, opposite the second maxillary molar.
  - The ducts of submandibular and sublingual glands opens into the floor of the mouth.
- **Minor salivary glands:** There are many minor salivary glands widely distributed throughout the mucosa of the oral cavity.

Histology

- **Salivary glands**:
  - They are tubuloalveolar glands.
  - The secretory acini may contain mucus cells, serous cells or both.
    - **Parotid gland: Purely serous**
    - **Submandibular gland: Mixed type but is predominantly serous.**
    - **Sublingual gland: Mixed type but is predominantly mucus.**
    - **Minor salivary glands: Serous, mucus or mixed type.**
- **Salivary duct**: The secretory acini of major glands are drained by ducts. They are lined by:
  - Low cuboidal epithelium in the intercalated portion.
  - Tall columnar epithelium in the intralobular ducts.
  - Simpler epithelium in the secretory ducts.

Saliva: Salivary glands secrete saliva. It acts as a lubricant during swallowing and speech, contains enzyme amylase and has antibacterial properties.
Salivary gland may develop inflammatory or neoplastic disease.

Sialadenitis

- Sialadenitis is **inflammation of the salivary gland.**
- **Types:** Acute or chronic (more common).

Etiology

It may be caused by trauma, viral or bacterial infection, or autoimmune disease.

Viral infections

1. **Mumps** is the most common cause of **viral** sialadenitis in school children. Mumps involves **the major salivary glands, particularly the parotids.** Mumps may also involve other glands such as testis (orchitis)/ovary (oophoritis) and pancreas (pancreatitis). Involvement of testis can result in testicular atrophy and infertility.
2. **Other:** Cytomegalovirus infection is rare.

Bacterial and Fungal Infection

Bacterial infections of the salivary gland cause acute sialadenitis and recurrent attacks of acute sialadenitis can lead to chronic sialadenitis. Nonspecific bacterial sialadenitis is a common especially in submandibular glands. It usually secondary to ductal obstruction caused by stones *(sialolithiasis)*.The common organisms are *S. aureus* and *Streptococcus viridans*. The stone formation may due to obstruction of the orifices of the salivary glands by impacted food debris or by edema about the orifice after injury.

Causes of Acute Sialadenitis

It may occur in acute infectious fevers. Decreased salivary secretions caused by dehydration may lead to the development of acute bacterial suppurative parotitis in elderly patients with a recent history of major thoracic or abdominal surgery. It is due to ascend of infection from mouth into parotid duct.

Causes of Chronic Sialadenitis:

- **Recurrent obstructive type:** Recurrent obstruction of ducts due to calculi (sialolithiasis), stricture, injury, surgery etc. may cause recurrent attacks of acute sialadenitis due to ascending infections. These acute attacks may result in chronic sialadenitis.
- **Recurrent non-obstructive type:** Decreased secretory function or reduced salivary secretion may also predispose to secondary bacterial invasion. This may occur in patients receiving drugs (e.g. antihistamines, antihypertensives, antidepressants, and phenothiazines), irradiation or congenital malformations of duct system.
- **Chronic inflammatory diseases:** E.g. tuberculosis, actinomycosis and fungal infections can rarely cause chronic sialadenitis.
- **Autoimmune diseases:** Sialadenitis is observed in two autoimmune diseases
  1. **Sjögren syndrome**: It is characterized by widespread inflammation of the salivary glands and the mucus-secreting glands of the mucosa which induces dry mouth (xerostomia). Concomitant involvement of the lacrimal glands in Sjögren syndrome may also produce dry eyes (*keratoconjunctivitis sicca)*.
  2. **Mikulicz's syndrome**: It is characterized by inflammatory enlargement of salivary and lacrimal glands.
- Frequently, no underlying cause can be detected.

Morphology

Gross

Irrespective of the etiological agent, the salivary glands are swollen. Acute sialadenitis produce local redness, painful enlargement and tenderness. The ducts opening in the mouth may show purulent discharge. Chronic sialadenitis may show firm swelling of the involved gland.

Microscopy

- **Acute viral sialadenitis in mumps:** Swelling and vacuolation of cytoplasm of acinar epithelial cells. Interstitial edema, fibrinoid degeneration of collagen, and dense infiltration by lymphocytes, macrophages and plasma cells.
- **Acute bacterial sialadenitis:** It is usually unilateral and involved a single gland. Whatever, the origin, the obstructive process and bacterial invasion lead to a nonspecific inflammation of the affected glands. The inflammation may be largely interstitial. If it caused by staphylococcal or other pyogens, it may be associated with suppurative necrosis and abscess formation.
- **Chronic and recurrent sialadenitis:** Increased lymphoid tissue in the interstitium, progressive loss of secretory epithelial tissue and fibrosis at a later stage.

SALIVARY GLAND NEOPLASMS

Salivary gland neoplasms are relatively uncommon.

Incidence

- Parotid gland—65% to 80% and ~ 15% to 30% parotid tumors are malignant.
- Submandibular gland—10% and ~ 40% are malignant.
- Minor salivary glands including the sublingual glands—10%. About 50% of minor salivary gland and 70% to 90% of sublingual tumors are malignant.
- Malignancy in salivary gland is inversely proportional to the size of the gland.

Classification of Salivary Glands Tumors (Table 15.1)

Q. Classify salivary gland tumors.

- **Age:** Benign tumors occur in the fifth to seventh decades of life. The malignant tumors appear later.
- **Sex: Slight female predominance**, except **Warthin tumor, which occur often in males than in females.**

Clinical Presentation

- Parotid gland neoplasms produce swellings in front of and below the ear.
- Both benign and malignant tumors range in size from 4 to 6 cm in diameter.
- Most tumors are mobile except advanced malignant tumors.

Table 15.1: Classification of tumors of the salivary glands

Benign	Malignant
Pleomorphic adenoma (mixed tumor)	Mucoepidermoid carcinoma
Warthin tumor	Adenocarcinoma
Oncocytoma	Acinic cell carcinoma
Basal cell adenoma	Adenoid cystic carcinoma
	Malignant mixed tumor

PLEOMORPHIC ADENOMA

Q. Write short note on pleomorphic adenoma.

Pleomorphic adenoma is a **most common benign tumor of the salivary glands,** characterized by an **admixture of epithelial and stromal elements**, and is also called **mixed tumors.**

Age: It occurs usually during **third to fifth decade** of life (middle-age).

Sex: It is most frequent in **females.**

Site

- **Major salivary gland**: Common site and constitute about 60% of tumors in the parotid. Usually arise in the **superficial lobe of the parotid**. Less common in the submandibular glands and very rare in the sublingual gland.
- **Minor salivary gland**: Its involvement is relatively rare.

Etiology

Not known. Exposure to radiation increases the risk.

- **Nature:** It is a benign tumor.
- **Cell of origin**: Histogenesis uncertain. **It was called as mixed tumor**, because of the mixture of epithelial and mesenchymal components. However, it is now considered that the tumor neoplastic cells (epithelial and those which appear mesenchymal), are of either **myoepithelial or ductal reserve cell origin.**

Q. Write short note on gross and microscopy of pleomorphic adenoma.

Morphology

Gross

- **Shape**: Round
- **Size:** Ranges from **2.5 to 6 cm in diameter.**
- **Consistency**: It depends on the relative amount of epithelial cells and stroma. **Usually rubbery,** resilient mass with a **bosselated surface.**
- **Well-circumscribed/capsulated**: In some, the capsule is not fully developed, and small extensions can be seen protruding into the surrounding salivary gland. This makes enucleation of the tumor difficult.
- **Cut surface**: It shows **gray-white** with **myxoid and blue glistening, translucent chondroid** (cartilage-like).

Microscopy (Figs 15.1 and 15.2)

Characteristic feature is the **pleomorphic appearance.** Neoplastic cells show varying **mixture of epithelial tissue** component intermingled with **cells showing mesenchymal differentiation.**

- **Epithelial element**: This component consists of **ductal cells and myoepithelial cells.**
  - **Epithelial elements** are arranged in the form of **ducts, acini and irregular tubules**. The ducts are lined by both epithelial (cuboidal to columnar) cells and **surrounded by myoepithelial components** (a layer of deeply chromatic, small myoepithelial cells).
  - May show **strands or sheets** of plasmacytoid or spindled **myoepithelial cells.**
  - Islands of well-differentiated squamous epithelium may also be seen.
- **Mesenchymal-like elements:** The epithelial elements are dispersed within a varying amount of mesenchyme-like background of loose **myxoid tissue, islands of hyaline, chondroid (cartilaginous), and mucoid matrix.**

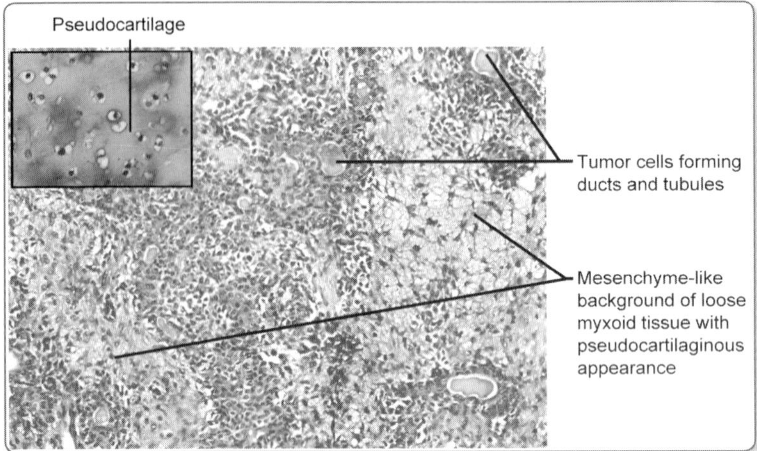

Fig. 15.1: Pleomorphic adenoma showing epithelial cells and myoepithelial cells separated by chondroid matrix. Inset shows pseudocartilage

(For color version, see Plate 13)

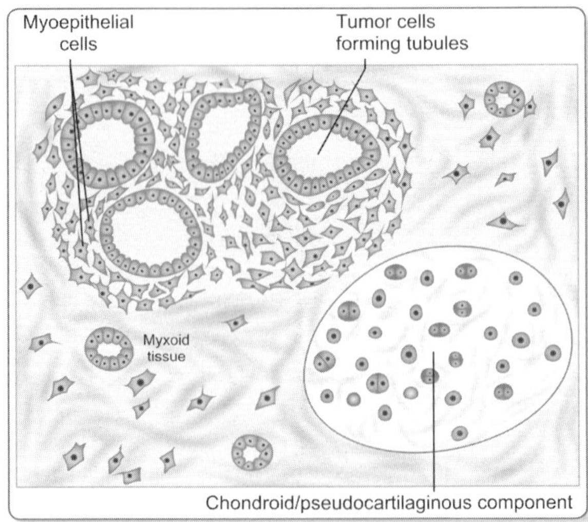

Fig. 15.2: Microscopic features of pleomorphic adenoma of salivary gland (diagrammatic)

(For color version, see Plate 13)

Clinical Features

- Pleomorphic adenomas present as **painless, slow-growing, mobile, discrete** tumors in the **parotid or submandibular** areas or in the buccal cavity.
- The tumors tend to protrude focally from the main tumor into adjacent tissues.
- Failure to recognize these minute protrusions at surgery is responsible for recurrence of these tumors.

Carcinoma Ex Pleomorphic Adenoma

- Rarely, a carcinoma may arise in pleomorphic adenomas—referred to as a **carcinoma ex pleomorphic adenoma or a malignant mixed tumor**.

- Incidence of carcinoma increases with the duration of the tumor.
- **Microscopy**: These tumors show poorly differentiated adenocarcinoma or undifferentiated carcinoma in an otherwise benign pleomorphic adenoma.

WARTHIN TUMOR

Q. Write short note on Warthin tumor.

Warthin tumor (**papillary cystadenoma lymphomatosum, adenolymphoma**) is a **benign** and the **second most common** salivary gland neoplasm.

- **Site**: It almost **exclusively** arises in the **parotid gland**.
- **Sex:** It is the only salivary glands tumor that is more **common in males** than in females.
- **Age:** It usually occur between **fifth to seventh** decades of life.
- **Predisposing factor**: **Smokers** have eight times the risk of nonsmokers.

Morphology

Gross

- **Shape:** It is round to oval, **encapsulated masses.**
- **Size:** It ranges from **2 to 5 cm** in diameter.
- Usually arises in the **superficial parotid gland** and are readily palpable.
- About 10% are multifocal and 10% bilateral.
- **Cut section**: It is **pale gray** tumor punctuated by narrow cystic or cleft-like spaces filled with a mucinous or serous secretion or even resemble used (dark) motor oil.

Microscopy (Figs 15.3 and 15.4)

Tumors consist of cystic glandular spaces embedded in dense lymphoid stromal tissue.

- **Cystic spaces:**
  - Cystic glandular spaces show **papillary or polypoid projections.**
  - **Cystic spaces** are lined by a distinctive **double layer of neoplastic epithelial cells** consisting of:
    - **Surface superficial layer of columnar cells** with **abundant, finely granular, eosinophilic cytoplasm** (oncocytes). Oncocytes have **abundant mitochondria** → responsible for the **granular appearance** to the cytoplasm.
    - **Second layer** below the superficial layer consisting of **cuboidal to polygonal cells.**
- **Lymphoid stromal tissue:** Cystic spaces are embedded in a dense lymphoid stroma which **closely resembles a normal lymph node.** The lymphoid tissue is prominent with germinal centers and is composed of B and few T cells.

Histogenesis: Warthin tumor may represent an aberrant incorporation of lymphoid tissue in the parotids.

Behavior: It is **benign**, and about 2% may recur.

MUCOEPIDERMOID CARCINOMA

Most common primary malignant tumor of the salivary glands.

Incidence

- Constitute about 15% of all salivary gland tumors.
- Occur mainly (60–70%) in the parotids.
- Account for a major fraction of the minor salivary gland tumors.

Q. Write short note on gross and microscopy of Warthin tumor.

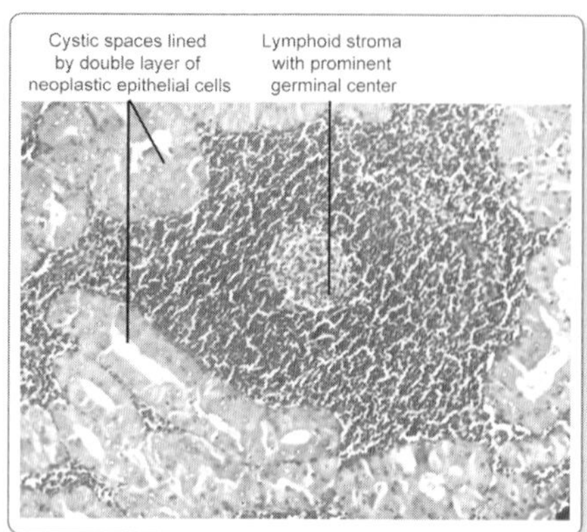

Fig. 15.3: Warthin tumor showing epithelial and lymphoid elements. Note the follicular germinal center in the center. The cystic spaces are lined by double layer of eosinophilic epithelial cells separated by reactive lymphoid stroma

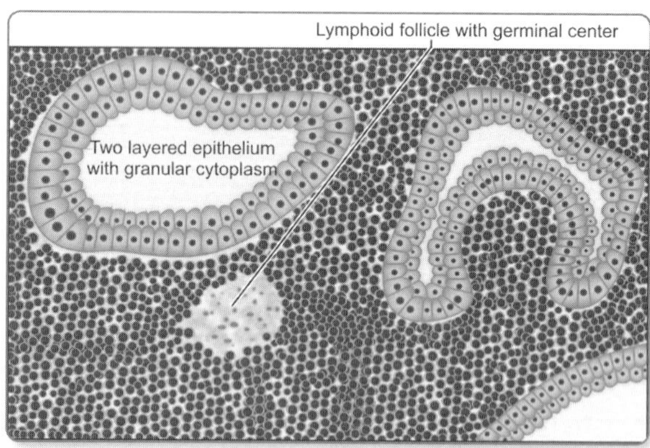

Fig. 15.4: Warthin tumor showing epithelial and lymphoid elements (diagrammatic)

Etiology

In about one-third of cases, it is associated with a distinctive balanced (11;19) (q21;p13) chromosomal translocation. This creates a fusion gene composed of portions of the *CRTC1* (formerly known as *MECT1*) and *MAML2* genes.

The translocation results in activation of the Notch pathway.

Morphology

Gross:

- **Size:** It can grow as large as 8 cm in diameter.
- **Appear circumscribed**, but do not show well-defined capsules and are often infiltrative at the margins.
- **Cut section:** It is **pale and gray-white** and frequently contain small, mucin-containing **cysts.**

Microscopy (Fig. 15.5)

Composed of variable mixtures of:

1. Squamous cells
2. Mucus-secreting cells
3. Intermediate cells.

These tumor cells are arranged in cords, sheets, or cystic structures. The intermediate cells have squamous features, with small to large mucus-filled vacuoles. The mucus stains positive with mucin stains. The tumor cells may appear regular and benign or highly anaplastic and malignant.

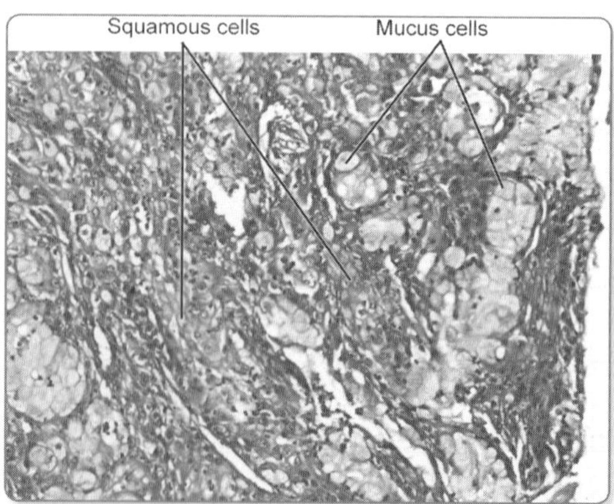

Fig. 15.5: Mucoepidermoid carcinoma composed of squamous cells as well as clear vacuolated cells containing mucin

Grading: These tumors are graded as low, intermediate or high grade. Clinical features and prognosis depends on the grade of the neoplasm.

Chapter 16

Bone

Chapter Outline
- Infections—osteomyelitis
- Osteoporosis
- Bone tumors

INFECTIONS—OSTEOMYELITIS

Q. Write short note on etiology of osteomyelitis.

Definition: Osteomyelitis is defined as inflammation of the bone and marrow.

Classification

- **Primary:** Where bone is the primary solitary focus of disease.
- **Secondary**: Develops as a complication of any systemic infection.

Any infection (bacteria, viruses, parasites, fungi) may cause osteomyelitis, but infections by certain pyogenic bacteria and mycobacteria are the most common.

Pyogenic Osteomyelitis

Q. Write short note on morphology of pyogenic osteomyelitis.

Etiology

It is **usually caused by bacteria**.

- Most common pathogens are *Staphylococcus* **species** (*aureus* in 80–90% of the cases).
- **Other organisms**:
  - *Escherichia coli, Pseudomonas, Klebsiella, Neisseria gonorrhoeae, Haemophilus influenzae* and *Salmonella* species.
  - *Escherichia coli* in patients with genitourinary tract infections or intravenous drug abusers.
  - **Neonatal period**: *Haemophilus influenzae* and group B streptococci.
  - **Patients with sickle cell disease**: *Salmonella* infection.
- **Mixed bacterial infections**: It is due to direct spread or surgery or open fractures.
- In about 50%, no organisms can be isolated.

Portal of Entry of Organism

Causative organisms may reach the bone through the **bloodstream, directly** or extend **from a contiguous site**.

1. **Hematogenous spread**:
   - Source of organisms may be a **focus of infection anywhere in the body** (e.g. skin pustule or infected teeth and gums, intestinal mucosa).
   - **Minor injuries** to the mucosa (vigorous chewing of hard foods, brushing of teeth), or minor infections of the skin, **release these organisms** into the blood → causing temporary **bacteremia → reach the bone.**
   - In **children** (5 to 15 years) and **drug addicts** (infected needles), it develops in the long bones.
2. **Direct implantation:** Organisms may enter into bone by penetrating wounds, open fractures, or surgical procedures (staphylococci, streptococci, anaerobic organisms).
3. **Spread from adjacent (contiguous) site**: e.g. infections of the feet may spread into the bone in diabetics.

Location of infection: It **varies** with age.

- **Children** with hematogenous spread: **Metaphysis of long bones** (knee, ankle, and hip).
- Neonate: **Metaphysis, epiphysis, or both.**
- **Adult: Epiphysis and subchondral regions.**

Pathogenesis and Morphology (Figs 16.1A to D)

Q. Write short note on pathogenesis and morphology of pyogenic osteomyelitis.

The sequence of events and morphological features in osteomyelitis are described together.

- **Transient bacteremia**: Mild injury or trauma can initiate bacteremia by organisms (e.g. *Staphylococcus aureus*).
- **Infection reaches metaphysis long bone:** Because in the metaphysis capillaries form loop → which slows the blood flow → provides time for bacteria to penetrate blood vessel walls and establish infective foci within the marrow.
- **Inflammatory reaction**: Once in bone, the bacteria grow and induce an **acute inflammatory reaction with exudates.**
- **Necrosis of bone: Exudate increases the pressure** on the adjacent vessels and further **decreases the blood supply** → produces **bone necrosis**. The necrotic areas coalesce and allow **further bacterial proliferation.**
- **Formation of sequestrum:**
  - Bacterial **infections and pus spreads into cortex** and collect beneath the periosteum → may **lift the periosteum → reduces the blood supply** to the affected region → results in **segmental necrosis of the bone** due to both suppuration and ischemia.
  - The fragment of **dead necrotic piece of bone**, which is embedded in the pus, is known as a **sequestrum.**
- **Draining sinus**

Q. Write short note on sequestrum.

  - The **pus penetrates the periosteum** and leads to a **soft-tissue abscess** → may penetrate the skin → form a **draining sinus. Hole formed in the bone** during the formation of a draining sinus is known as **cloaca.**
  - The sinus tract may become epithelialized and may remain open, continually draining pus, necrotic bone, and bacteria.

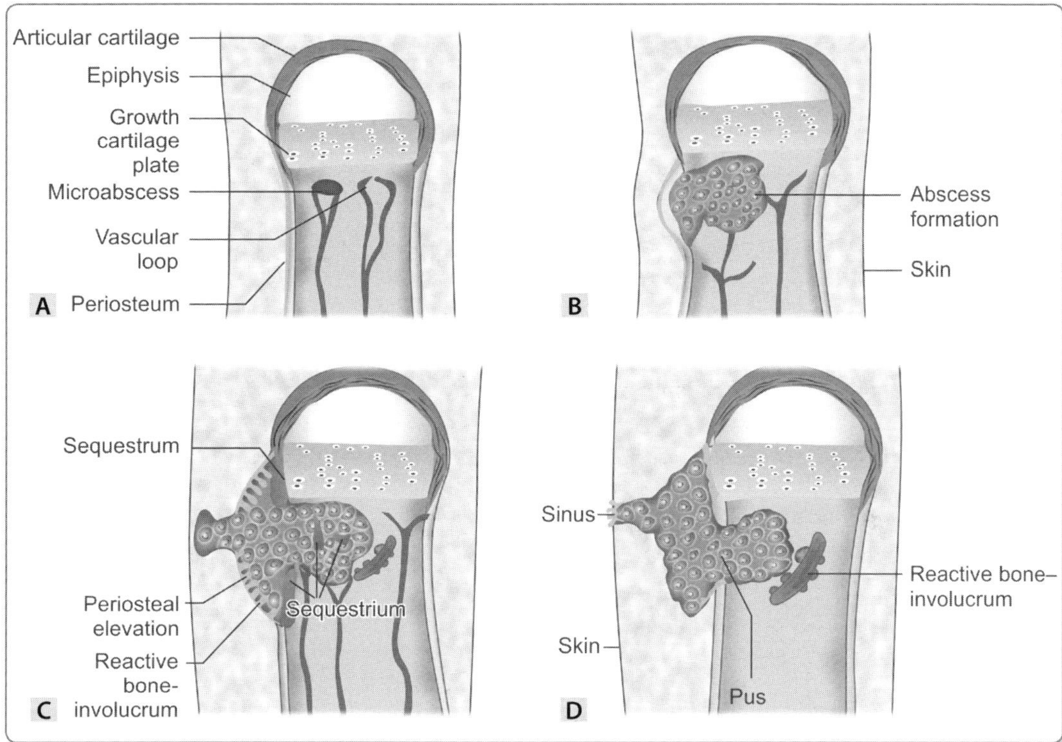

Figs 16.1A to D: Pathogenesis of hematogenous osteomyelitis. A. A small, septic microabscess is formed at the capillary loop; B. Expansion of the septic focus stimulates resorption of adjacent bony trabeculae. The abscess expands and stimulates reactive bone formation by the periosteum; C. The abscess, which continues to expand through the cortex into the subperiosteal tissue; D. The extension of this process into the skin produces a draining sinus. The necrotic bone is called a sequestrum. The viable bone surrounding a sequestrum is termed the involucrum

- **Involucrum**: After first week, chronic inflammatory cells become more numerous and the cytokines released stimulates osteoclastic bone resorption and **deposition of reactive bone in the periphery**. Reactive new bone forms a sheath around the necrotic (segment of devitalized infected bone) sequestrum. This **reactive new bone formed is known as involucrum**.

Morphology

The morphologic features **depend on the stage** (acute, subacute, or chronic) and location of the infection.

- **Gross:** Sequestrum appears as a fragment of bone with ragged brownish to black colored margins.
- **Microscopy:**
  - In the **initial stages**, only the **neutrophils** are seen. As the diseases becomes chronic, neutrophils admixed with chronic inflammatory cells (lymphocytes and plasma cells) are seen.
  - Sequestrum does not show osteocytes and have empty lacunae.

Morphologic Variants of Osteomyelitis

- **Brodie abscess:** It is a distinctive form of **subacute pyogenic osteomyelitis**.
  - It appears as a **small, solitary, intraosseous abscess localized to the metaphysis** and is surrounded by reactive bone.
  - It may be **due to inadequate treatment of infection by less virulent organisms**.

- **Sclerosing osteomyelitis of Garré**: It is characterized by **extensive new bone formation**, which obscures the underlying structure of the bone and **typically develops in the jaw**.

Complications

Q. Write short note on complications of pyogenic osteomyelitis.

- **Septicemia**: From infection in the bone, organisms may disseminate through the bloodstream and cause septicemia.
- **Acute suppurative arthritis**: Infection may spread through the articular surface into a joint → producing suppurative arthritis → may lead to destruction of the articular cartilage and permanent disability. It is more common in infants.
- **Pathologic fractures**.
- **Squamous cell carcinoma:** It may arise from the epithelialized sinus tract, rarely sarcoma of bone may develop.
- **Secondary amyloidosis**.
- **Chronic osteomyelitis:** It may develop due to delay in diagnosis, extensive bone necrosis, and inadequate therapy.

Clinical Course

- Present with malaise**, fever, chills, leukocytosis**, and **throbbing pain over the affected region**.
- **Diagnosis:**
  - **Radiography:** Lytic focus of bone destruction surrounded by a zone of sclerosis.
  - **Blood cultures** are positive.
  - **Biopsy** and bone cultures.

Tuberculous Osteomyelitis

Q. Write short note on tuberculous osteomyelitis.

Tuberculous osteomyelitis is **usually solitary** but in patients with acquired immunodeficiency syndrome, it is frequently multifocal. It tends to be **more destructive and resistant to control** than pyogenic osteomyelitis.

- **Age**: Usually **adolescents or young adults** in developing countries.
- **Source of infection: Pulmonary or extrapulmonary** tuberculosis.
- **Predisposing factors:** Diabetes, elderly, immune compromised states and general debility
- **Route of infection:**
  - **Blood borne**: Usually blood borne infection, which is from a focus of **active pulmonary or extrapulmonary disease**.
  - **Direct extension**: From
    - **Lung into a rib**
    - **Tracheobronchial nodes into adjacent vertebrae.**
- **Sites:**
  - **Spine** (thoracic and lumbar vertebrae) commonly known as **Pott disease.** The **infection breaks through intervertebral discs** to involve multiple vertebrae and **extends down into the soft tissues** forming abscesses (**cold abscess-psoas abscess**).
  - **Knees and hips**.

Microscopy

It shows dead bone surrounded by **tuberculous granuloma**. The granuloma consists of central area of caseous necrosis surrounded by epithelioid cells and Langhans giant cells, which in turn is surrounded by lymphocytes (see Fig. 6.3). The epithelioid cells have a pale pink granular cytoplasm with indistinct cell boundaries, often appearing to merge into one another. The nucleus is oval or elongate.

Clinical Course

- Low-grade fever with evening rise of temperature
- Pain on motion, localized tenderness
- Weight loss.

Complications

- **Spine:**
  - **Destruction of vertebrae**: Causes severe **scoliosis or kyphosis a**nd neurologic deficits due to spinal cord and nerve compression.
  - **Psoas abscess:** Infection from spine may rupture into the soft tissue anteriorly and pus and necrotic debris may drain along the spinal ligaments and form a **cold abscess, i.e. an abscess lacking acute inflammation. Psoas abscess** is the condition in which infection from lower lumbar vertebrae dissects along the pelvis, and appears as a draining sinus of the skin in the inguinal region. It may be the first manifestation of tuberculous spondylitis.
- **Tuberculous arthritis**
- **Sinus tract formation**
- **Amyloidosis.**

OSTEOPOROSIS

Osteoporosis is a disease of bone characterized by **low bone mass** (quantitative reduction) which leads to porosity of bones.

Types: Osteoporosis may be:

- **Localized:** It is usually due to disuse and is seen as a complication of some other disease. For example, local immobilization following fracture due to other causes.
- **Generalized:** Involves the entire skeleton. It may be **primary or secondary**.
  - **Primary** osteoporosis occurs without any known cause. These include senile and postmenopausal.
  - **Secondary** osteoporosis develops due to a large variety of conditions. These include **endocrine disorders** (hyperparathyroidism, hyperthyroidism, etc.), **gastrointestinal disorders** (e.g. malabsorption, vitamin D deficiency, malnutrition), **drugs** (e.g. corticosteroids), **tumors** (multiple myeloma) **reduced physical activity, hormonal disturbances** and other causes (e.g. immobilization).

Etiology and Pathogenesis

Age: Peak bone mass is achieved between 25 and 35 years of age and gradually declines from the age of 50 years onwards.

Sex: It is generally seen in **elderly and women. Genetic/hereditary factors** also play an important role.

Pathogenesis: In normal bone, there is balance between bone formation and resorption. In osteoporosis, the balance is upset due to diminished bone formation, excessive bone resorption or both.

Morphology (Fig. 16.2)

Entire skeleton is involved in postmenopausal and senile osteoporosis but certain regions are more severely involved than others. The **involved bones are thin and brittle**. Microscopically, it is composed of the **lamellar bone** which is discontinuous and has **thin trabeculae**.

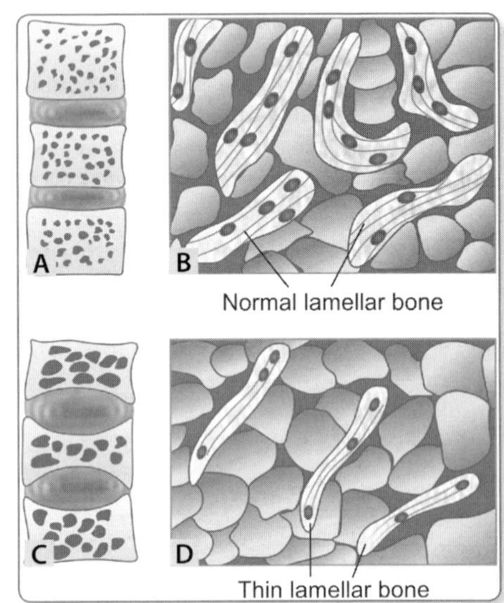

Fig. 16.2: (A) Normal gross appearance of bone-vertebral column. (B) Normal microscopic appearance of trabecular bone and fatty marrow. The trabecular bone is lamellar and contains evenly distributed osteocytes. (C) Gross appearance of osteoporosis. (D) Microscopic appearance of osteoporosis composed of the lamellar bone which are discontinuous and have thin trabeculae

Clinical Features

Depend on the bones involved. Loss of bone mass **predisposes** the bone **to fracture** which results in bone pain. Fractures are most common in the vertebra in the thoracic and lumbar region, neck of the femur and Colles' fracture (fracture of distal radius).

Complications

- Pulmonary embolism and pneumonia as a complication of fractures of the femoral neck, pelvis or spine.
- When fractures of vertebra are multiple, it may lead to lumbar lordosis and kyphoscoliosis (forward bending).

Diagnosis

- **Plain X-ray:** Not reliable till 30 – 40% of the bone mass is lost.
- **Dual-energy X-ray absorptiometry** and **quantitative computed tomography.**
- **Bone biopsy.**

Rickets and osteomalacia are discussed in chapter 8.

BONE TUMORS

Q. Classify bone tumors.

Fibrous Dysplasia

- Fibrous dysplasia is a benign tumor. It is a localized developmental arrest in which all of the components of normal bone are present, but they do not differentiate into mature structures.

Types of Fibrous Dysplasia

It arises during skeletal development. There are several distinctive types sometimes with overlapping clinical patterns:

- **Monostotic**: Affects a single bone and most common type (~70%).
- **Polyostotic**: Affects multiple bones and constitutes 25% of cases.
- ***Mazabraud syndrome***: Characterized by fibrous dysplasia (usually polyostotic) and soft tissue myxomas.
- ***McCune-Albright syndrome***: It is a polyostotic disease, associated with café-au-lait skin pigmentations and endocrine abnormalities (e.g. precocious puberty).

Pathogenesis

- Fibrous dysplasia is due to somatic gain-of-function mutation during development in *GNAS1*, the gene. The mutations produce a constitutively active Gs-protein that promotes cellular proliferation.

Morphology

- Gross: The lesions are well-circumscribed, intramedullary, and vary greatly in size (2 to 5 cms). Larger lesions expand and distort the bone. The lesion is tan-white and gritty.
- Microscopy (Fig. 16.3): It is composed of curvilinear trabeculae of woven bone (non-lamellar) surrounded by a moderately cellular fibroblastic tissue. The **curvilinear shapes of the trabeculae mimic Chinese characters**, and the bone **lacks prominent osteoblastic rimming.**

Clinical Course

- **Monostotic fibrous dysplasia:** Most patients are between 20 to 30 years of age and occurs equally in boys and girls. It often stops enlarging at the time of growth plate closure. It commonly affects femur, tibia, ribs, jawbones, calvarium, and humerus. It is usually asymptomatic and discovered incidentally. Radiologically, it has typical ground-glass appearance and well-defined margins. Symptomatic lesions are cured by curettage.
- **Polyostotic fibrous dysplasia:** It manifests at a slightly earlier age than the monostotic type. The bones affected, in descending order of frequency, are the femur, skull, tibia,

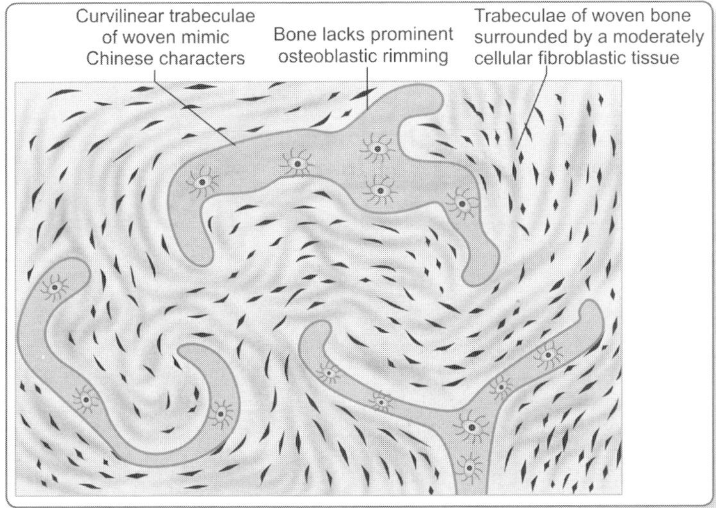

Fig. 16.3: Fibrous dysplasia composed of curvilinear trabeculae of woven bone (non-lamellar) surrounded by a moderately cellular fibroblastic tissue (To be drawn)

humerus, ribs, fibula, radius, ulna, mandible, and vertebrae. Polyostotic disease results in severe, progressive disease including crippling deformities and fractures. Rarely, it may be complicated by malignant transformation into a sarcoma.

- ***Mazabraud syndrome:*** It presents with skeletal features with multiple skeletal deformities during childhood. The intramuscular myxomas often develops in the same anatomic region as existing fibrous dysplasia.
- ***McCune-Albright syndrome:*** Most common presentation is precocious sexual development, which occurs most often in girls. The bone lesions are usually unilateral, and the skin pigmentation is usually limited to the same side of the body. The skin macules are large; dark to café-au-lait in color; have irregular serpiginous borders. They are found usually on the neck, chest, back, shoulder, and pelvic region.

Aneurysmal Bone Cyst

Aneurysmal bone cyst (ABC) is a tumor characterized by multiloculated blood-filled cystic spaces.

- Age: ABC affects all age groups but usually manifests during the first 2 decades of life and has no sex predilection.
- Site: Most frequently involves metaphysis of long bones and the posterior elements of vertebral bodies.

Clinical features: Most commonly presents with pain and swelling. ABC of the vertebrae can compress nerves and produce neurologic symptoms.

Radiography: ABC is usually an eccentric, expansile lesion with well-defined margins. They are mostly osteolytic lesions and contain a thin shell of reactive bone at the periphery. Computed tomography and magnetic resonance imaging may show internal septa and characteristic fluid-fluid levels.

Microscopy (Fig. 16.4):

- Aneurysmal bone cyst shows multiple blood-filled cystic spaces separated by thin, tan-white septa.

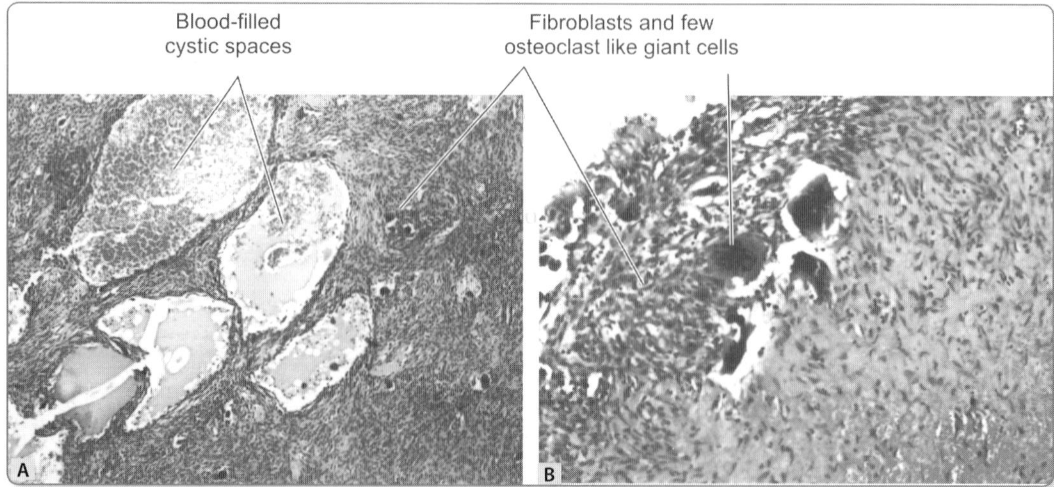

Fig 16.4: Aneurysmal Bone cyst. A. Low power shows many blood-filled cystic spaces surrounded by fibroblasts and few osteoclast like giant cells. B. High power shows cyst wall showing osteoclast-type giant cells

- The septa consists of plump uniform fibroblasts, multinucleated osteoclast-like giant cells, and reactive woven bone.
- The bone is lined by osteoblasts.

Clinical course: The treatment is surgical, usually curettage or, in certain cases, en bloc resection. The recurrence rate is low.

Classification of Bone Tumors (Table 16.1)

Table 16.1: Major primary tumors of bone

Histologic type	Benign	Malignant
Osteogenic/bone forming	Osteoma Osteoid osteoma Osteoblastoma	Osteosarcoma (primary/secondary)
Chondrogenic/cartilaginous	Osteochondroma Chondroma Chondroblastoma	Chondrosarcoma Dedifferentiated chondrosarcoma
Hematopoietic		Myeloma Malignant lymphoma
Unknown origin	Giant-cell tumor Unicameral cyst Aneurysmal bone cyst	
Neuroectodermal		Ewing sarcoma

Osteosarcoma

Q. Write short note on osteosarcoma.

- Osteosarcoma (osteogenic sarcoma-OS) is the **most common (20%) primary malignant bone tumor**, excluding of myeloma and lymphoma.

Definition: Osteosarcoma is a **highly malignant bone tumor** characterized by formation of **bone matrix or osteoid** (unmineralized bone) **by malignant tumor cells.**

- **Age group**: Osteosarcoma has a **bimodal age distribution.**
  - Three-fourth occur in between **10 and 20 years age.**
  - **Secondary** osteosarcoma (following **Paget disease, bone infarcts, irradiation**, etc.) develop in **elderly after 40 years of age.**
- **Sex:** Affects boys more commonly than girls (2:1).

Pathogenesis

Based on the pathogenesis, OS is divided into primary and secondary.

Primary Osteosarcomas

In this type, the underlying bone is unremarkable. About 70% of osteosarcomas have acquired genetic abnormalities such as **ploidy changes** and **chromosomal aberrations.**

- **Mutations in tumor suppressor gene**:
  a. ***RB*, the retinoblastoma gene** (a cell cycle regulator) mutations is associated with 1000-fold increased risk of osteosarcoma and its mutation is found in about two-thirds of patients.
  b. **Patients with Li-Fraumeni syndrome (germline *p53* mutations)** have a greater incidence of osteosarcoma.

Secondary Osteosarcoma

Osteosarcomas in older persons almost always develop in association with pre-existing bone disorders. These include:

- **Paget disease of bone**.
- **Radiation exposure**
- **Chemotherapy**: Children treated with **alkylating agents** (other malignancies) have an increased risk.
- **Pre-existing benign bone lesions**: e.g. **fibrous dysplasia, osteomyelitis**, and bone marrow infarcts. Trauma may call attention to an existing osteosarcoma rather than causing the tumor.

Classification

Q. Write short note on morphology and radiological appearance of osteosarcoma.

It can be classified in different ways:

1. **Anatomic site of origin**
    - **Conventional** (classical, medullary, intramedullary, textbook)
    - **Intracortical**
    - **Surface osteosarcoma**
        - Parosteal (juxtacortical): They arise on the surface of the cortex.
        - Periosteal: They arise on the surface of periosteum.
2. **Degree of differentiation:**
    - Well-differentiated
    - Moderately differentiated
    - Poorly differentiated.
3. **Number of tumors**
    - **Solitary**
    - **Multicentric**
        - Synchronous
        - Metachronous.
4. **Pathogenesis** (described above)
    - **Primary**
    - **Secondary** to pre-existing disorders.
5. **Histologic features** (described below).

Morphology

Most Common Subtype

- Primary
- Solitary
- Conventional/intramedullary
- Poorly differentiated.
- **Location:** Usually arise in the **metaphyseal region of the long bones** of the extremities.
- **Sites:** It usually arises near the knee or shoulder. The common site is:
    - Lower femur
    - Upper tibia, or fibula
    - Proximal humerus.

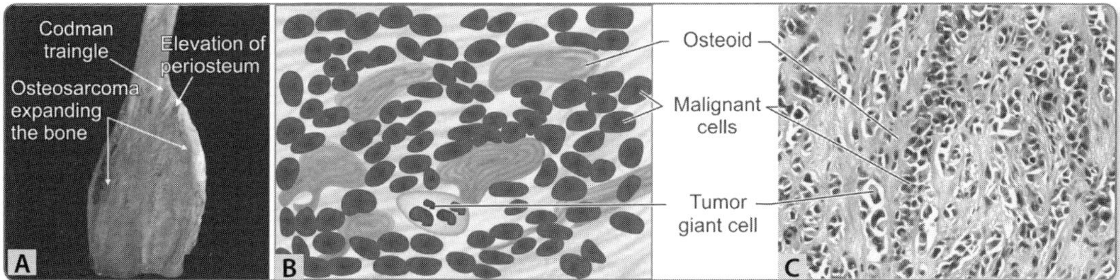

Figs 16.5A to C: A. Gross appearance of osteosarcoma of the lower part of distal femur showing a tan-white tumor filling most of the medullary cavity of the metaphysis and proximal diaphysis. The tumor has infiltrated through the cortex, lifted the periosteum and this region on X-ray appears as Codman triangle; B. Diagrammatic and C. Photomicrograph of microscopy of osteosarcoma composed of pleomorphic tumor cells separated by osteoid

(For color version, see Plate 14)

Gross (Fig. 16.5):
- Gross appearance **varies depending on the proportions of bone, cartilage, stroma and blood vessels.**
- **Size:** Usually **big bulky tumors.**
- **Cut surface**: **Gray-white** in color, **gritty**, shows **areas of hemorrhage and cystic degeneration.**

Microscopy (Fig. 16.5)
- **Malignant tumor cells**:
  - **Tumor cells vary in size and shape.**
  - **Nucleus:** Usually show **large hyperchromatic** nuclei and **often shows mitotic figures.**
  - **Bizarre tumor giant cells** are common.
- **Matrix component: Production** of **osteoid** (unmineralized/noncalcified) **or bone** (calcified osteoid) **by malignant tumor cells** is the single **diagnostic feature** of conventional OS.
  - **Osteoid:** It appears as a **dense, uniform, eosinophilic glassy intercellular material.**
  - **Neoplastic bone:** It usually has a coarse, lace-like architecture.
- **Histological subtype**: Most tumors contain a **mixture of cells with varying amounts matrices** mentioned below. **Depending on the one predominant matrix**, conventional OS is **divided into**:
  - **Osteoblastic: Large amount of osteoid and bony trabeculae.**
  - **Chondroblastic: Abundant malignant cartilage.**
  - **Fibroblastic/fibrohistiocytic**: They appear **similar to malignant fibrous histiocytoma.**
  - **Telangiectatic: Large cavernous dilated vascular channels** and it is **more aggressive.**
  - **Small cell:** The tumor **cells are small in size, uniform** and simulate the appearance of Ewing's sarcoma and malignant lymphoma.
  - **Giant cell:** This subtype contains **numerous giant cells.**
- Vascular invasion and necrotic area may be conspicuous.
- **Immunohistochemistry**: The malignant tumor cells **stain prominently for alkaline phosphatase** and **osteonectin.**

Clinical Course

- Usually present as **painful, progressively enlarging masses** around the knee or other involved site.
- The involved area is **swollen and tender** and the function adjacent joint become reduced.
- **Serum alkaline phosphatase is increased**.

Radiological Appearance

- OS shows a **large destructive, mixed lytic** (bone destruction) and **blastic mass** (neoplastic bone formation) with infiltrative margins.

- **Codman triangle**:
  - The tumor frequently **infiltrates the cortex and lifts the periosteum,** and produces a **space between the cortex and lifted ends of periosteum.** Radiologically, this space appears as **triangular shadow** and is known as **Codman triangle (characteristic but not diagnostic** of this tumor).
  - The **space** mainly contains **reactive new bone, which is arranged perpendicular to the bone surface,** but it may also contain malignant tumor.
- **Sunburst appearance**: **When** the malignant **tumor extends into soft tissue, parallel lines of mineral deposition** in the **periosteal region** gives an appearance of rays of sun → called as "sunburst" appearance (Fig. 16.6).

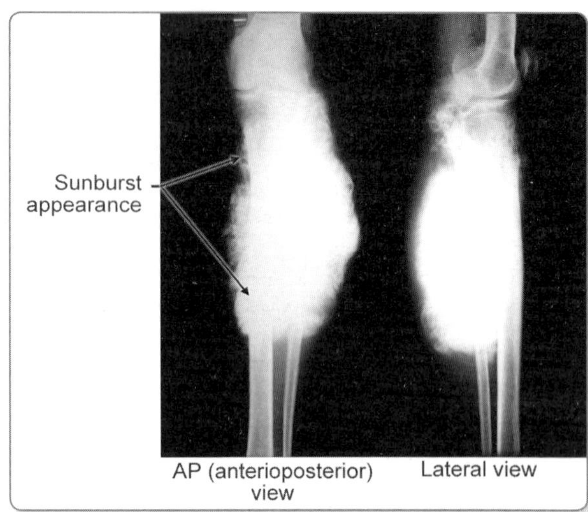

Fig. 16.6: X-ray of the knee joint. Osteosarcoma of proximal tibia extending into the soft tissue with parallel lines of mineral deposition giving rise to sunburst appearance

Spread

- **Local spread**:
  - **Invasion of the adjacent cortex** and destroys the nearby cortex.
  - **Elevation or perforation of the periosteum** by tumor tissue.
  - **Spread along the** medullary (**marrow**) **cavity**.
  - **Extension into the epiphysis**:
    - **Articular end of the bone is generally not involved in the initial stage.**
    - **Later, it may infiltrate the epiphyseal plate and may even involve the joint space.**
  - **Extension into the soft tissues** and may involve skin.
- **Blood spread**: It is an aggressive tumor, which may spread through the bloodstream to the **lungs.** Less commonly, it may metastasize to other bones, the pleura, brain, and the heart.

Giant-Cell Tumor

Q. Write short note on giant cell tumor/osteoclastoma.

Definition: Giant-cell tumor (GCT synonym **osteoclastoma**) is characterized by **multinucleated osteoclast-type giant cells randomly and uniformly distributed in a background of mononuclear cells.**

- Giant cell tumor is a **relatively uncommon, locally aggressive** and **potentially malignant neoplasm.**
- **Age**: Usually seen between **20 to 40 years**. In elderly, it may be secondary to irradiation.
- **Sex**: Slight predilection for women.
- **Cell of origin**: Primitive stromal cells.

Q. Write short note on morphology of osteoclastoma.

Morphology

- **Site**: Giant-cell tumors in adults involve **both the epiphyses and the metaphyses** of a **long bone**, but **in adolescents, they are limited to the metaphysis.**
- **Bones involved:**
  - Knee area: Distal femur and proximal tibia.
  - Lower end of radius, humerus and fibula.
- **Gross (Fig. 16.7 A):** Large tumor, clearly circumscribed.
  - **Cut surface**
    - **Soft and red-brown** without bone or calcification
    - **Numerous hemorrhagic areas** give an **appearance of a sponge** full of blood.

Microscopy (Figs 16.7 B and C)

Two types of cells

1. **Mononuclear (stromal) cells**: They are of two types.
   - **Neoplastic mononuclear cells:** They are **uniform oval and plump** with **large nuclei** and **scanty cytoplasm**. Tumor mostly consists of these neoplastic cells. Mitotic activity is common in these cells but not found in the giant cells. **Diagnosis of malignancy depends upon the morphology of the mononuclear cells rather than that of the multinucleated giant cells.**
   - **Non-neoplastic:** These are mononuclear cells derived from macrophage-monocyte.
2. **Multinucleated (osteoclastic) giant cells**:
   - The **background** shows **numerous large osteoclast-type giant cells** throughout the richly vascularized stroma.
   - These **cells have 100 or more nuclei**, which resemble those of the mononuclear cells.

Area of cystic degeneration and necrosis.

Secondary features: These include areas of **hemorrhage, necrosis**, hemosiderin deposition, and reactive bone formation.

Radiological Appearance

Q. Write short note on clinical features, radiological findings and morphology of oseoclastoma

- It produces a **lytic lesion** and **grows slowly, expands the bone** and **destroys the overlying cortex**.

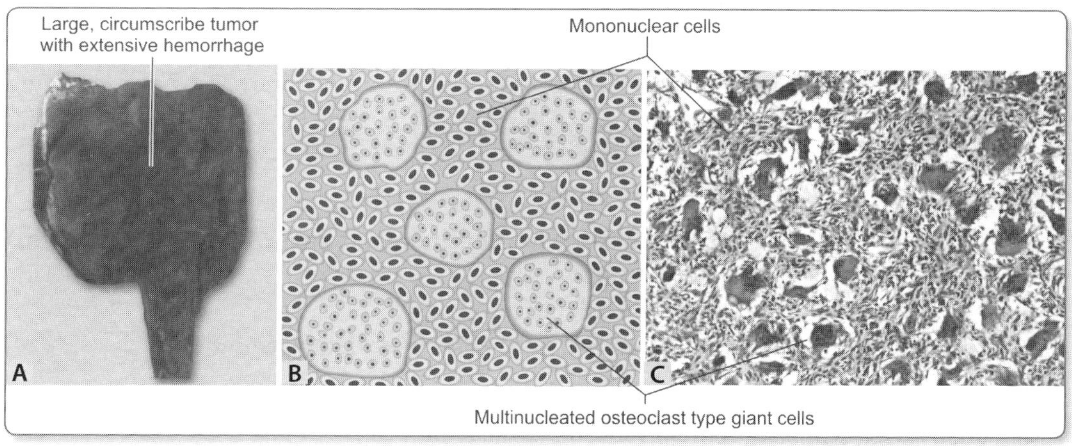

Figs 16.7A to C: Giant-cell tumor of bone. A. Grossly shows a circumscribed tumor with hemorrhage in the upper end of tibia. Microscopically; B. Diagrammatic and C. Photomicrograph, shows numerous multinucleated giant cells. The background shows mononuclear stromal cells

(For color version, see Plate 14)

- The tumor produces a bulging **soft tissue mass surrounded by a thin, shell of reactive bone** due to periosteal reaction. This on radiology has multiloculated or **soap bubble** appearance (Fig. 16.8).

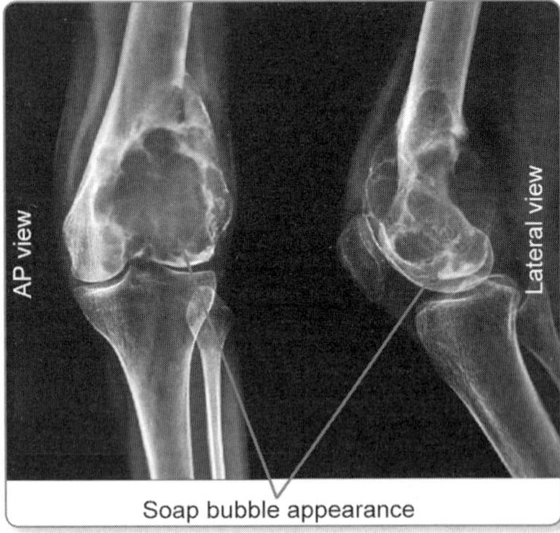

Fig. 16.8: X-ray of the knee joint. Giant cell tumor of distal femur showing soap bubble appearance

Clinical Course

- Commonly seen near knee joints.
- Pain (usually in the joint adjacent to the tumor) and arthritis-like symptoms.
- Microfractures and pathologic fractures may develop due to thinning of the cortex.

Biologic Behavior

- Majority of GCTs behaves in a **benign fashion**, but **locally aggressive tumors may locally recur**.
- However, **all GCTs** must be **considered as potentially malignant**, because they may metastasize.

Spread

- **Local spread**: Tumor is usually restricted within the involved bone surrounded by periosteum.
  - Aggressive tumors may penetrate the cortex and the periosteum, and may involve the joint capsule and the synovial membrane.
- **Hematogenous spread:** Common site is lung.

Ewing Sarcoma/Primitive Neuroectodermal Tumor

Q. Write short note on Ewing sarcoma.

Definition: Ewing sarcoma family of tumors is **primary malignant small round-cell tumors of bone and soft tissue**.

- **Uncommon** tumors and constitute ~ 6–10% of primary malignant bone tumors.
- **Age:** Mostly seen between **10 to 15 years** of age, and about 80% are seen in patients younger than 20 years. In children, it is second most common group of bone sarcomas, first being osteosarcoma.
- **Sex**: More frequent in **boys** than girls (2:1).

Categories

- It consists of **two tumors that differ only in their degree of neural differentiation**. This distinction has no clinical significance.
  1. **Ewing sarcoma** (EWS): **Undifferentiated** tumors.
  2. **Primitive neuroectodermal tumor** (PNET): With **neural differentiation**.

Etiology and Pathogenesis

- **Origin:** It arises from **multipotent mesenchymal stem cell**.
- **Chromosomal abnormalities**.
  - **Translocation of *EWS* gene on chromosome 22 (22q12)** with a gene encoding an ETS family transcription factor (*FLI-1 or ERG gene).*

- The **fusion of the *EWS1* gene to *FLI-1* gene** (more common) resulting in fusion protein, EWS/FLI-1 → produces chimeric/aberrant transcription factors → **activation of C-myc promoter** → abnormal cell proliferation and survival.
- A less common translocation produces *EWS/ERG* fusion gene → produces a variant of EWS with a significantly worse prognosis.

Q. Write short note on morphology of Ewing sarcoma.

Morphology

- **Location**: Arise in the **diaphysis of the medullary cavity of long bones.**
- **Site:** Ewing sarcoma and PNET involve the **long tubular bones in childhood.**
  - **Long bones: Humerus, tibia** and **femur**.
  - **Flat bones**: Pelvis.
- **Gross:**
  - Arise in the **diaphysis** and **may infiltrate the medullary spaces** without destroying the bony trabeculae.
  - **Diffusely infiltrate the cortex** and the tumor **may also penetrate the periosteum** and spread into the soft tissues.
  - **Soft, grayish white/tan-white**, and frequently show areas of **hemorrhage and necrosis.**
- Microscopy (Fig. 16.9):
  - **Tumor cells**: They are **uniform, small and round.**
    - **Size:** Tumor cells are about **twice the size of a lymphocyte.**
    - **Cytoplasm: Scant or little** and **appears clear** because it is **rich in glycogen,** which is an important diagnostic feature. This **stains positive** with the **periodic acid-Schiff (PAS) stain.**
  - **Arrangement: Closely packed sheets** of cells.
  - **Homer-Wright rosettes:** They may be seen. They consist of **tumor cells arranged in a circle about a central fibrillary space.** This is **indicative of neural differentiation.**
  - **Mitoses are infrequent** even though the tumor is highly cellular.
  - **Interstitial stroma: Little or absent** and the fibrous strands separate the sheets of tumor cells into irregular **nests or sheets. Necrosis** may be prominent.
  - **Immunohistochemistry: EWS cells express characteristic antigens**, some of which are part of the translocation product (e.g. **FLI-1 and CD99**).

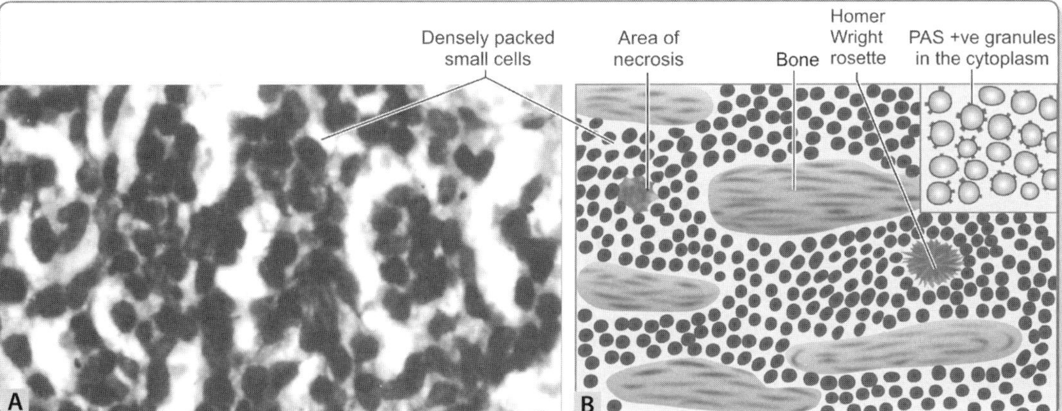

Figs 16.9A and B: A. Photomicrograph; and B. Diagrammatic; Ewing sarcoma composed of sheets of closely packed uniform small round cells with scanty cytoplasm. The inset of B shows PAS positive granules in the cytoplasm **(For color version, see Plate 14)**

Radiographic Appearance

- It produces **destructive lytic lesion** in which the border between normal bone and the tumor is indistinct. The tumor may extend into the surrounding soft tissues.
- Characteristic circumferential, **discontinuous layers of periosteal new bone formation** produces **onion-skin pattern** (Fig. 16.10).

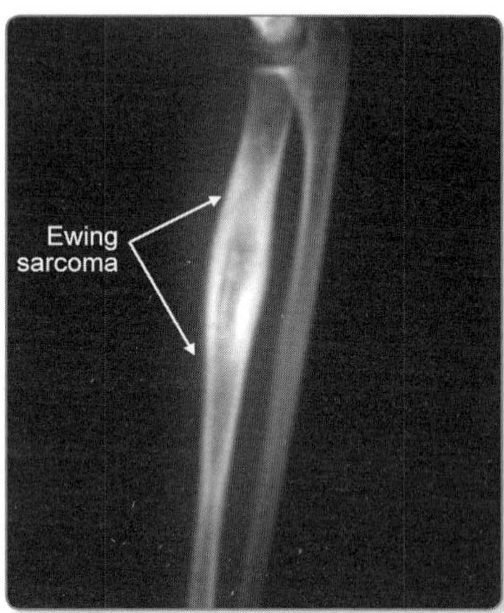

Fig. 16.10: X-ray of Ewing sarcoma involving the diaphysis of tibia

Clinical Features

- **Painful enlarging masses** and the affected site is **tender, warm, and swollen**.
- **Systemic features**: It may develop in some and **mistaken for infection like osteomyelitis**.
  - Fever, weakness, and bone pain.
  - Hematological findings: Anemia, leukocytosis, and raised erythrocyte sedimentation rate.

Spread

- **Local spread:** It may spread from medullary cavity **into cortex, periosteum and surrounding soft tissue**.
- **Blood spread:** Lungs, brain and other bones (skull).

Treatment includes chemotherapy and surgical excision with or without irradiation.

Chapter 17

Cardiovascular System

Chapter Outline

- Congenital heart disease
- Left-to-right shunts
- Right-to-left shunts
- Heart failure
- Infective endocarditis
- Atherosclerosis
- Ischemic heart disease
- Angina pectoris
- Myocardial infarction (MI)

CONGENITAL HEART DISEASE

Congenital heart disease (CHD) is the **abnormalities of the heart or great vessels** that are **present from birth**.

Incidence

Congenital heart diseases are the **most important and common type of heart disease in children**.

Etiology and Pathogenesis

Most CHD arise from defective embryogenesis during 3 to 8 weeks of gestation, when major cardiovascular structures form and begin to function. Two factors that are involved in CHD are:

1. **Genetic factors**: The main causes of congenital heart disease are sporadic genetic abnormalities. The most common genetic cause of congenital heart disease is **trisomy 21 (Down syndrome)**.
2. **Environmental factors:** These factors may be the primary cause congenital heart disease. **Examples:**
   - **Congenital rubella infection**
   - **Gestational diabetes**
   - **Exposure to teratogens** (including drugs)
   - **Nutritional factors: During pregnancy**, consumption of multivitamin containing **folate may reduce the risk**, whereas heavy consumption of **alcohol increases the risk** of congenital heart defects.

3. **Multifactorial:** Majority of CHD may be due to combination environmental and with genetic factors.

Clinical Features

- **Severe** congenital heart diseases result in **intrauterine death**.
- Some congenital heart diseases produce clinical manifestations soon after birth, but some may not be evident until adulthood (e.g. ASD).

Classification (Table 17.1)

The structural anomalies in congenital heart disease may be divided into four major categories: (1) right-to-left shunt, (2) left-to-right shunt, (3) an obstruction and (4) malposition of heart.

1. Left-to-right Shunt

These are characterized by the flow of blood from the left (systemic) side to the right (pulmonary) side of the circulation.

Consequences

- Left-to-right shunt causes **increased pulmonary blood flow** and initially does not produce cyanosis.
- But increased pulmonary blood flow **increases the volumes and pressures** in pulmonary circulation → results in **pulmonary hypertension** → causes **right ventricular hypertrophy**.
- Later, when the **pressure in right ventricle reaches systemic levels**, the shunt changes to a new **right-to-left,** which diverts the unoxygenated blood into the systemic circulation → results in cyanosis, and hence these CHD are known as **late cyanotic congenital heart disease, or Eisenmenger syndrome**.
- When the pulmonary hypertension becomes irreversible, the structural defects of congenital heart disease become irreparable.

Table 17.1: Classification of congenital heart diseases

Type of CHD
1. **Left-to-right shunt**
– Ventricular septal defect
– Atrial septal defect
– Patent ductus arteriosus
2. **Right-to-left shunt**
– Tetralogy of Fallot
– Transposition of the great arteries
– Persistent truncus arteriosus
– Tricuspid atresia
– Total anomalous pulmonary venous connection
3. **Obstructive congenital heart disease**
– Coarctation of the aorta
– Aortic stenosis
– Pulmonary stenosis
4. **Malposition of heart**—very rare
– Dextrocardia

2. Right-to-left Shunt

If the pressure in the right side rises more than that in left, the blood flows from the right to left side (right-to-left shunt) → results in hypoxemia and **cyanosis** (blue discoloration of the skin and mucous membranes) due to the mixing of poorly oxygenated venous blood with systemic arterial blood (called **cyanotic congenital heart disease**).

- **Clubbing and polycythemia:** Severe, long-standing cyanosis causes clubbing of the tips of the fingers and toes (called **hypertrophic osteoarthropathy**) and **polycythemia**.

3. Obstructive Congenital Heart Disease

These are characterized by abnormal narrowing of chambers, valves, or blood vessels. **If the obstruction is complete**, it is called an **atresia**.

In some CHD, there may be coexistence of (e.g. Tetralogy of Fallot), both obstruction (pulmonary stenosis) and a shunt (right-to-left through a VSD).

Malposition of heart are very rare type of congenital heart diseases.

LEFT-TO-RIGHT SHUNTS

The common left-to-right shunt include ventricular septal defects (VSDs), patent ductus arteriosus (PDA), and atrioventricular septal defects (ASDs).

Atrial Septal Defect

An atrial septal defect (ASD) is an abnormal, fixed opening in the atrial septum. It is due to incomplete formation of tissue in the atrial septum, which allows flow of blood between the left and right atria. ASDs are **usually asymptomatic till adulthood**.

Morphology

Classification: It is classified into three major types according to their location as: Secundum, primum, and sinus venosus.

- **Secundum ASDs** (90%): These result from a deficient or fenestrated oval fossa near the center of the atrial septum. The size varies, and may be single or multiple, or be fenestrated.
- **Primum** anomalies (5%) occur near the AV valves.
- **Sinus venosus** defects (5%) develop near the entrance of the superior vena cava.

Clinical Features

- ASDs cause a left-to-right shunt and results in increased pulmonary blood flow by about two to four times normal. Consequences of atrial septal defect are presented in Figure 17.1.
- A murmur may be heard due to increased blood flow through the pulmonary valve.
- ASDs usually do not produce symptoms before 30 years of age.

Complications: (1) heart failure, (2) paradoxical embolization, and (3) irreversible pulmonary vascular disease.

Prognosis: Mortality is low.

Ventricular Septal Defect (VSD)

- Incomplete closure of the ventricular septum is known as ventricular septal defect (VSD), is the **most common form of congenital cardiac anomaly**.

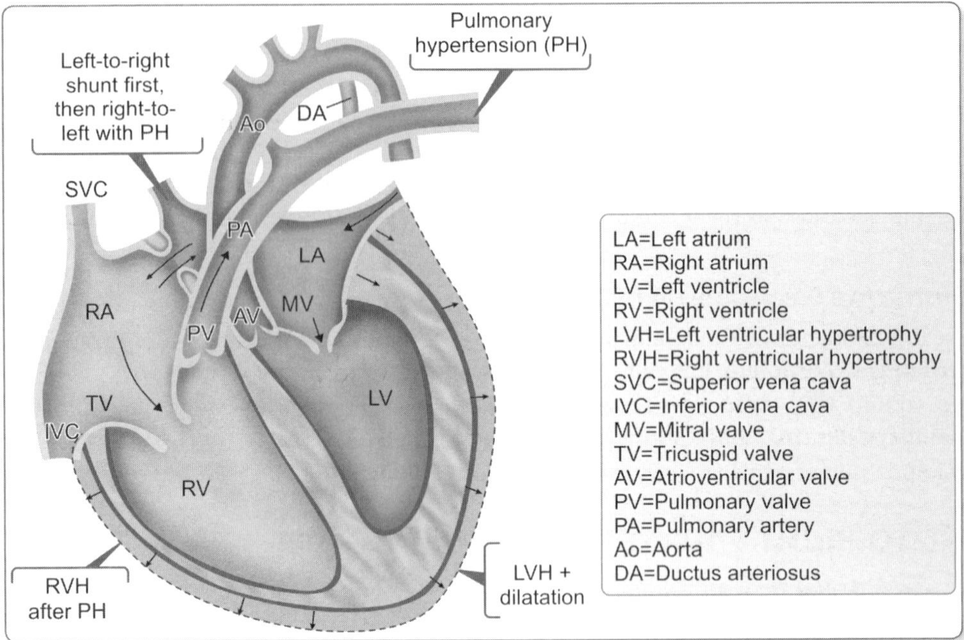

Fig. 17.1: Consequences of atrial septal defect

- Most (70–80%) VSDs are associated with other congenital cardiac anomalies (e.g. tetralogy of Fallot).
- Cause free blood flow from the left-to-right ventricles.

Classification

VSDs are classified according to their size and location.

- **Membranous VSD (90%):** They involve the membranous region of interventricular septum.
- **Infundibular VSD (10%):** They lie below the pulmonary valve or within the muscular part of the interventricular septum.

Clinical Features

The clinical features depend on the size of the defect.

- **Large VSDs**
  - Usually **membranous or infundibular type** and manifest from birth.
  - Cause **left-to-right shunt** → leading to right ventricular hypertrophy and pulmonary hypertension.
  - Irreversible pulmonary vascular disease develops later, in all patients resulting **reversal of shunt, cyanosis, and death**.
- **Small VSDs**:
  - May not be recognized until adult life.
  - About 50% of small muscular VSDs may close spontaneously.

Consequences of ventricular septal defect are presented in Figure 17.2.

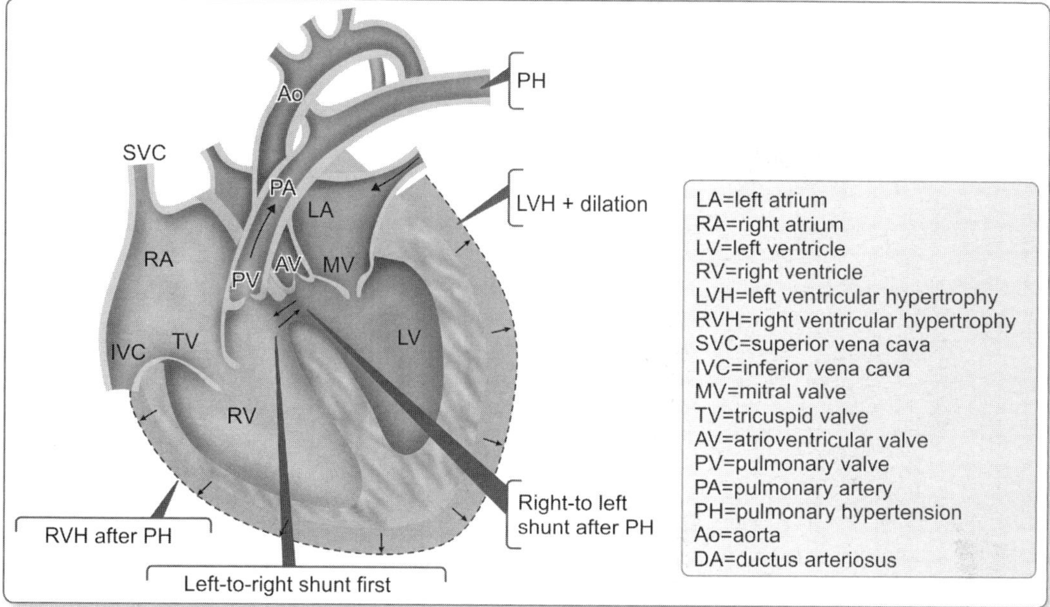

Fig. 17.2: Consequences of ventricular septal defect

Patent Ductus Arteriosus

Normal Function of Ductus Arteriosus

In the fetus, it is an essential structure that carries the blood from the pulmonary artery to the aorta, thus bypasses the flow of blood to lungs (like the patent foramen ovale). After birth, it normally spontaneously closes and the blood from pulmonary artery flows to the lung.

Patent (Persistent) Ductus Arteriosus (PDA)

It is a congenital anomaly in which the **ductus arteriosus remains open after birth (Fig. 17.3)**. PDAs may occur as an **isolated anomaly** (about 90%), **or associated with VSD, coarctation of the aorta, or pulmonary or aortic valve stenosis**. PDA produces a **characteristic continuous harsh murmur known as "machinery-like"**.

Clinical Features

Depends on diameter of PDA and the cardiovascular status of the patient. PDA is usually asymptomatic at birth, and a narrow PDA may not affect the child's growth and development. First, the shunt is from left-to-right and there is no cyanosis. But additional volume and pressure overload produces obstructive changes in small pulmonary arteries, leading to reversal of flow and its associated consequences.

PDA may be **either life Threatening or lifesaving.**

Preservation of ductal patency (by administering prostaglandin E) is essential for survival of infants with congenital malformations that obstruct the pulmonary or systemic blood flow tracts. For example, in aortic valve atresia, preserved PDA supplies the major blood into the systemic circulation. Consequences of patent ductus arteriosus are presented in Figure 17.3.

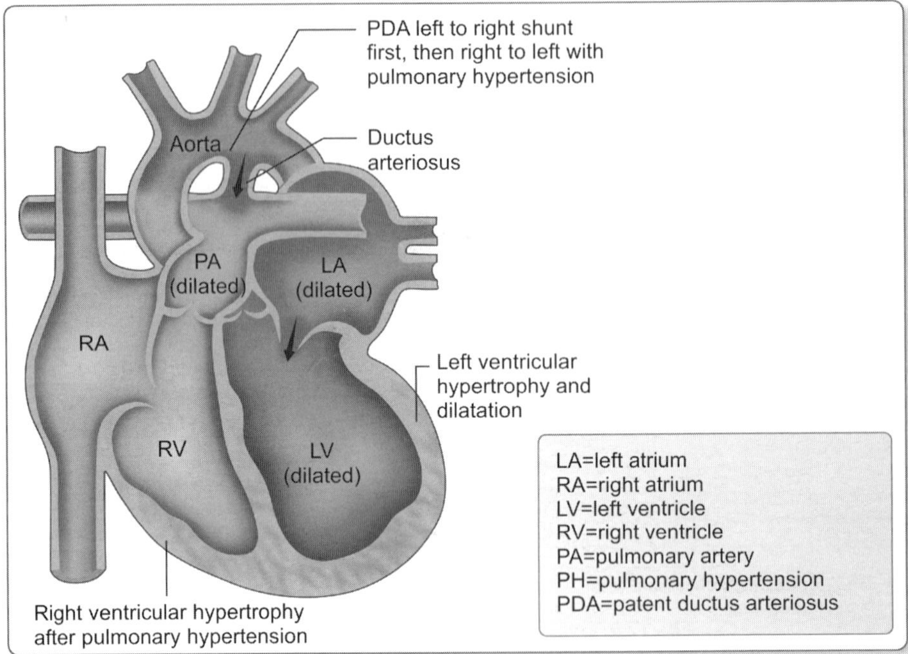

Fig. 17.3: Patent ductus arteriosus

RIGHT-TO-LEFT SHUNTS

These congenital diseases cause **cyanosis early in postnatal life** (cyanotic congenital heart disease). Tetralogy of Fallot, the most common, and others include transposition of the great arteries, persistent truncus arteriosus, tricuspid atresia, and total anomalous pulmonary venous connection.

Tetralogy of Fallot

Q. Write short note on tetralogy of Fallot.

Components (Fig. 17.4): The **four main features** of the tetralogy of Fallot (TOF) are:

1. **Ventricular septal defect (VSD):** Usually large.
2. **Subpulmonic stenosis/pulmonary valvular stenosis:** It causes obstruction of the right ventricular outflow tract.
3. **Aorta overriding the VSD** and both ventricular chambers.
4. **Right ventricular hypertrophy:** It is due to the obstruction to right ventricular outflow.

Morphology

Heart is enlarged and may be **"boot-shaped"** due to marked right ventricular hypertrophy, particularly of the apical region.

Clinical Features

Clinical features depend mainly on the severity of the subpulmonary stenosis, because this decides the direction of blood flow.

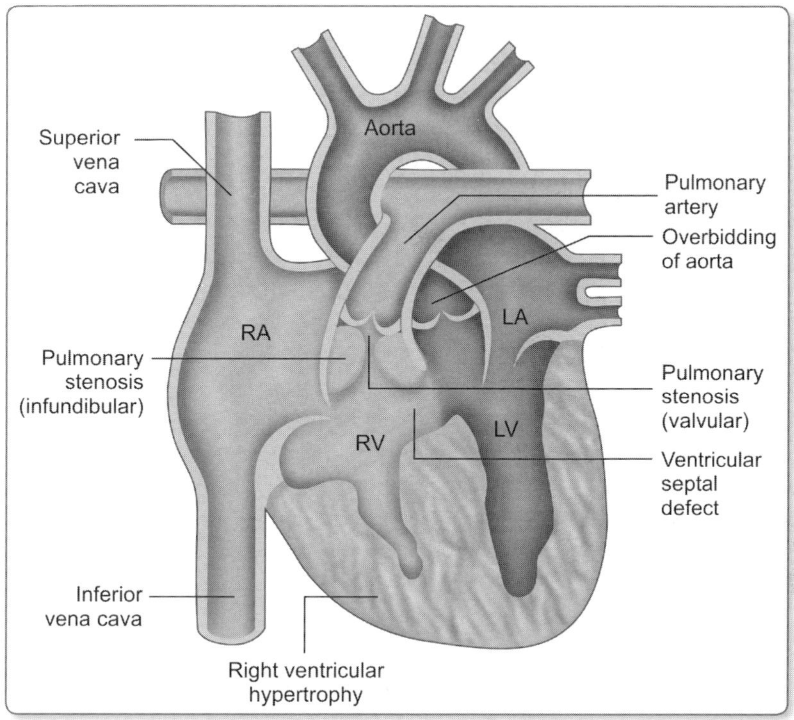

Fig. 17.4: Diagrammatic representation of tetralogy of Fallot. Four components are: (1) ventricular septal defect, (2) subpulmonic stenosis/pulmonary valvular stenosis, (3) aorta overriding the VSD and (4) right ventricular hypertrophy

- **Mild subpulmonary stenosis:** It clinically resembles an isolated VSD, and the shunt may be from left-to-right, **without cyanosis** (so-called pink tetralogy).
- **Moderate subpulmonary stenosis:** It produces increased resistance to right ventricular outflow. When the right-sided pressures approach or exceed that of left-sided pressures → right-to-left shunt develops → **producing cyanosis** (classic TOF).
- **Severe subpulmonary stenosis:**
  - Pulmonary arteries become progressively hypoplastic with small and thin walled.
  - Aorta becomes progressively larger in diameter.
  - As the child grows, the size of heart increases, but pulmonary orifice does not expand proportionally. This results in progressive worsening of the obstruction.
  - **Majority of infants with TOF have cyanosis from birth or soon thereafter**.

HEART FAILURE

Definition: It is a pathophysiological state in which impaired cardiac function fails to maintain a circulation adequate for the metabolic needs of the body despite an adequate blood volume.

- Types of heart failure: It may be acute or chronic, and may affect the left ventricle, right ventricle or both.

Causes of Heart Failure

- **Acute heart failure**: More frequent in myocardial infarction, and arrhythmias.
- **Chronic heart failure**: It is often called *congestive heart failure (CHF).* Chronic heart failure is the end-result of various forms of heart diseases. It occurs when the heart is unable to pump blood at a rate sufficient to meet the metabolic demands of the tissues. It is the common end stage of many forms of chronic heart disease. It often develops slowly from the cumulative effects of chronic work overload (e.g. in valve disease or hypertension) or ischemic heart disease (e.g. following myocardial infarction with heart damage).

Heart failure may also be divided into left ventricular failure or right ventricular failure. Their causes are mentioned in Table 17.2.

Table 17.2: Causes of heart failure

Left ventricle	Right ventricle
Myocardial injury: Myocardial infarction, myocarditis	Increased workload: Pulmonary hypertension (e.g. chronic lung disease, pulmonary and tricuspid valvular diseases)
Increased workload: Systemic hypertension, aortic and mitral valvular diseases, increased cardiac output (anemia, thyrotoxicosis)	Myocardial injury: Myocardial infarction, myocarditis

Clinical Consequences:

- The clinical spectrum ranges from asymptomatic to symptoms and signs of heart failure occurs at rest.
  - Asymptomatic phase: The cardiac dysfunction may produce reduced exercise tolerance, in which compensatory mechanism maintain tissue perfusion. The compensatory mechanisms include ventricular hypertrophy, peripheral vasoconstriction, salt and water retention.
  - Symptomatic phase: In this phase, the compensatory mechanisms are exhausted and symptoms and signs of heart failure occurs at rest. Inadequate tissue perfusion leads to breathlessness, fatigue, peripheral and pulmonary edema. Multiorgan involvement leads to renal impairment, skeletal muscle dysfunction, impaired pulmonary and peripheral gas exchange, and hepatic dysfunction.

INFECTIVE ENDOCARDITIS

Q. Describe heart in infective endocarditis.

Definition: Infective endocarditis (IE) is defined as an **infection** (usually bacterial) **of the endocardium of heart valves or the mural endocardium**. It results in focal area of colonization or invasion by microbial agents.

- **Sites of colonization by microbial agents:**
  1. **Heart valves**
  2. Mural endocardium
  3. Congenital defect (e.g. patent ductus arteriosus or coarctation of the aorta)
  4. Other less common sites: (i) aorta, (ii) aneurysmal sacs, (iii) other blood vessels, and (iv) prosthetic devices.
- **Lesions produced**:
  1. **Vegetations**: These are lesions seen at the site of colonization or invasion. Composed of thrombotic debris and organisms.
  2. **Destruction** of the underlying cardiac tissues/site of colonization is often observed.

- **Microbes responsible:**
  1. **Bacterial infections** (bacterial endocarditis) in most of the cases.
  2. **Other microbes:** Fungi, *Chlamydia, Rickettsiae* and microorganisms.

Classification

A. **According to the clinical course (Table 17.3): Acute or subacute** endocarditis. The clinical course depends on the virulence of the infecting microorganism and whether any underlying cardiac disease is present.

1. **Acute infective endocarditis:** The characteristic features are:
   - **Acute** in onset
   - Infection of **normal heart/cardiac valve**
   - **Caused by highly virulent (suppurative) organism**. Mainly by ***Staphylococcus aureus*** and ***S. pyogenes***
   - **Affected valve is rapidly destroyed** by necrotizing, ulcerative valvular lesions
   - **Death within 6 weeks in many patients**, due to complications like acute heart failure or overwhelming sepsis.
2. **Subacute infective endocarditis**: The characteristic features are:
   - **Insidious** in onset
   - It **involves structurally abnormal/deformed valves** (e.g. rheumatic heart disease or congenital heart disease)
   - **Caused by organisms are of lower virulence** (e.g. ***Streptococcus viridans* or *Staphylococcus epidermidis***)
   - The lesions are **less destructive**
   - Pursue a **protracted course of weeks to months** and typically survive for 6 months or more. Mostly cured with antibiotics
   - Infectious **complications are uncommon**.

B. **According to anatomic location and causative microbes:** The clinical presentations described above are unusual today because of advance in antimicrobial therapy. So, IE is now classified according to the anatomical location and the offending organism, e.g. infective endocarditis of mitral valve due to *Staphylococcus aureus*.

Table 17.3: Differences between acute and subacute endocarditis

Characteristic	Acute infective endocarditis	Subacute infective endocarditis
Onset	Acute	Insidious
Condition of valve	Infection of normal heart/cardiac valve	Infection of structurally abnormal/deformed valves
Virulence of organisms	Highly virulent (suppurative)	Low virulent
Lesions	Affected valve is rapidly destroyed	Less destructive
Clinical features	Of acute infection	Of complications
Course	Death within 6 weeks	Protracted course of weeks
Complications	Acute heart failure or overwhelming sepsis	Infectious complications are uncommon

Etiology

Causative Organism

Q. Describe the etiology and pathogenesis of infective endocarditis.

Many organisms can cause endocarditis, most originate from the normal flora of the body surfaces, and enter into the bloodstream in a variety of different ways. More than 90% of IE is caused by streptococci and staphylococci.

- ***Staphylococcus aureus:*** It is **virulent organisms** commonly found on the skin. It can infect either **healthy or deformed** valves. It is the major organism responsible for IE in **intravenous drug abusers**.
- ***Streptococcus viridans:*** It is present in the **normal flora of the oral cavity**. It is the most commonly causes endocarditis of previously **damaged** or **abnormal valves**.
- **Coagulase-negative staphylococci** (e.g. *S. epidermidis*): It is the most common cause for **prosthetic valve** endocarditis.
- **Other bacteria** commensals in the oral cavity:
  - **HACEK** group (*Haemophilus, Actinobacillus, Cardiobacterium, Eikenella,* and *Kingella*)
  - Enterococci.
- **Other agents**: It includes gram-negative bacilli and fungi.
- **Culture-negative endocarditis**: They constitutes 10 to 15% of cases in which no organism can be isolated from the blood.

Predisposing Factors

Three main factors which may predispose to IE are: (1) conditions that lead to bacteremia, (2) underlying heart disease, and (3) impaired host defense mechanism.

1. **Conditions with bacteremia**: Most important predisposing factors to the development of endocarditis are conditions that lead to bacteremia.

   Sources of microbes: **Transient bacteremia** from any cause may lead to infective endocarditis.
2. **Underlying heart disease:** IE may involve either normal or damaged heart/valve. IE on previously normal valves develop usually with high virulent organisms. Underlying heart disease is one of the predisposing factors for IE. These diseases include:
   - **Congenital heart disease**: Unrepaired and repaired congenital defects—most common predisposing condition (e.g. valvular or septal defect).
   - **Mitral valve prolapse** (MVP) in adults.
   - **Chronic rheumatic heart disease (**mitral valve in over 85% of cases, and the aortic valve is involved in 50%).
   - **Degenerative calcific valvular diseases** (mainly in elderly).
   - Bicuspid aortic valve.
   - **Iatrogenic**
     - Artificial (prosthetic) valves
     - Indwelling vascular catheters.
3. **Impaired host defense mechanism:** It may occur in:
   - Diabetes mellitus
   - Malignancies: Leukemia and lymphomas
   - Cytotoxic therapy
   - Neutropenia.

Prevention of IE in patients with predisposing factors: Prophylaxis with antibiotics.

Pathogenesis

Mechanism by which virulent organisms infect apparently normal valves is poorly understood.

The probable sequence of events (Fig. 17.5), which occur with the infection of a damaged valve by less-virulent organisms is as follows:

1. **Endocardial damage and denudation**: Development of the infective endocarditis follows a predictable sequence. Damaged valve or a congenital defect creates abnormal high-velocity blood flow at the center and turbulent flow at the periphery → cause endocardial damage and denudation of endothelial surfaces.
2. **Formation of sterile thrombus (Fig. 17.5A)**: Damaged endothelial surface → attracts focal deposition of platelets and fibrin → aggregation of platelets and fibrin → formation of small sterile vegetations (sterile thrombi).
3. **Adherence of the microorganisms (Fig. 17.5B)**: Transient bacteremia → microorganisms gain access to the circulation → adherence deposition to the sterile vegetations (infection of thrombi).
4. **Proliferation of microorganisms within vegetations (Fig. 17.5C):** On the deposited microorganisms, further platelets and fibrin are laid down, which separates them from the bloodstream. Microorganisms proliferate within the vegetations and form colonies.
5. **Formation of emboli (Fig. 17.5D):** The vegetation may get detached and form infective emboli → cause spread of infection to visceral organs and brain.

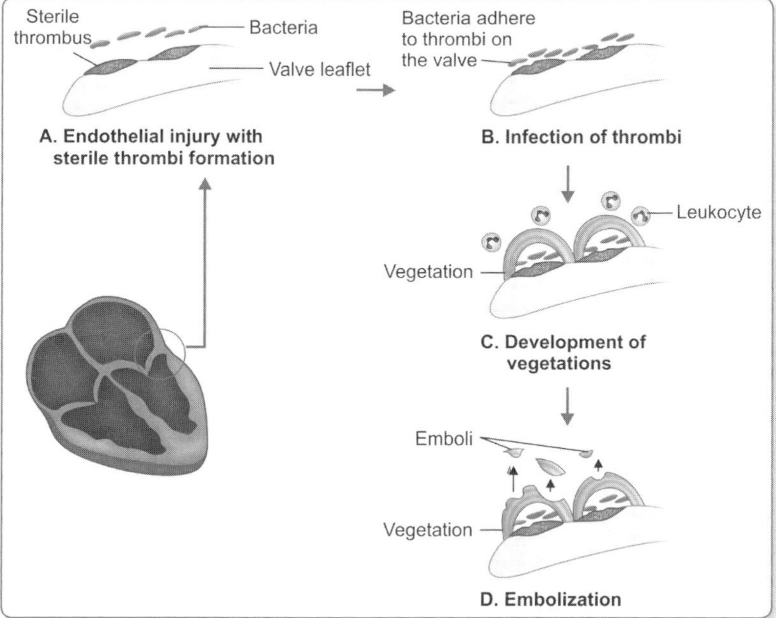

Figs 17.5A to D: Pathogenesis of vegetation on a valve leaflet in infective endocarditis. A. Focal endothelial injury of a valve leaflet is covered with tiny deposits of platelets and fibrin to form a thrombus; B. Circulating microorganisms colonize the platelet thrombus; C. Further platelets and fibrin are laid down and the microorganisms proliferate slowly; D. Vegetations fragment and form emboli

Q. Describe the morphology of infective endocarditis.

Q. Describe heart in infective endocarditis.

Morphology

Gross (Figs 17.6 and 17.7):

Valves affected: Aortic and mitral valves (most common) and **valves of the right heart (especially tricuspid) in intravenous drug abusers.**

Vegetations: These are **hallmark/pathognomonic of IE** which have following features:

- **Appearance: Friable, bulky, potentially destructive vegetations** (less destructive in subacute than in acute endocarditis).
- **Number:** They may be **single or multiple** and may involve **one or more than one valve.**
- **Size:** Lesions **vary in size** from a small, superficial deposit to bulky, exuberant vegetations.
- **Changes in the involved valve: Edema and inflammation** and in severe cases, leaflet may perforate causing regurgitation.
- **Sites:** Vegetations form on:
  1. **Atrial side of the atrioventricular valves.**
  2. **Ventricular side of the semilunar valves.**
  3. **Points of closure of the leaflets or cusps.**

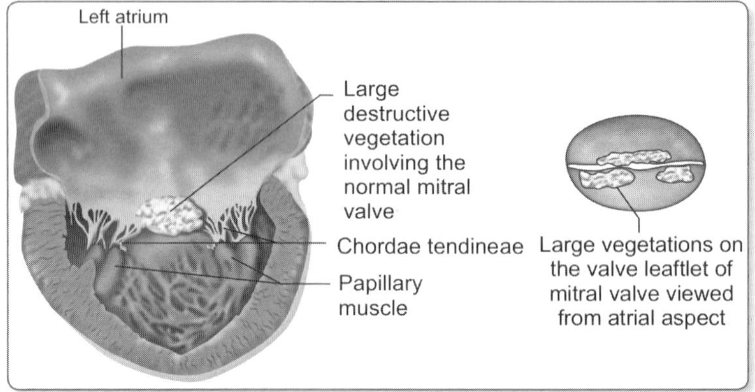

Fig. 17.6: Acute bacterial endocarditis. Mitral valve shows large friable vegetations

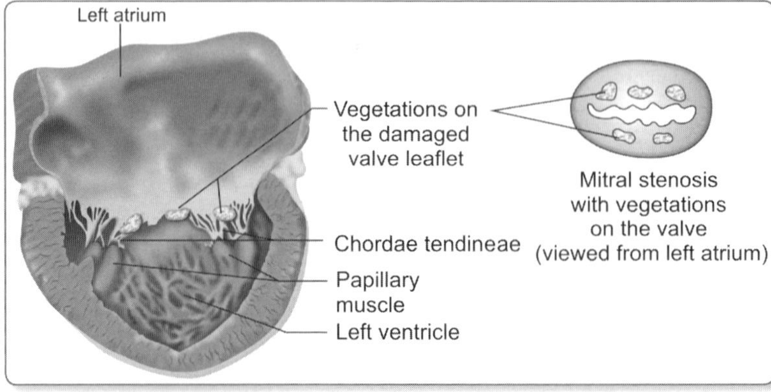

Fig. 17.7: Subacute bacterial endocarditis. Mitral valve shows vegetations

Microscopy

- Vegetations are composed of platelets, fibrin, cell debris, inflammatory cells, and masses of (bacteria or other organisms).
- Vegetations of subacute IE may show granulation tissue at their bases indicative of healing. Later, it may show fibrosis, calcification, and chronic inflammatory infiltrate.

Complications of IE

Q. Describe the complications of infective endocarditis.

These may be divided into cardiac and extracardiac.

A. Cardiac Complications

These are **due to direct valvular damage** and **consequences of local invasion**. The infection may spread locally from valve into the valve ring, adjacent mural endocardium or chordae tendineae.

1. **Ring abscess**: Vegetations may erode the **underlying myocardium** and produce an **abscess** which is known as ring abscess.
2. **Perforation and rupture**: May involve valve leaflets, aorta or interventricular septa (depending on the site of infection).
3. **Myocardial abscess.**
4. **Suppurative pericarditis.**
5. **Valvular dysfunction**: Stenosis or insufficiency.

B. Extracardiac Complications

Q. Extracardiac complications of subacute bacterial endocarditis.

Vegetations are usually friable and likely to be break, detach and cause embolism.

1. **Embolic complications (due to septic emboli)**: Emboli contain large numbers of virulent organisms → **abscesses develop at the sites of arrest** of the emboli.
   - **Septic emboli from left side of the heart**: They enter systemic circulation and its consequences are:
     - **Septic infarcts (e.g. spleen, kidney or brain)**
     - **Mycotic aneurysms**
     - **Small emboli (microthromboemboli) may produce tiny hemorrhagic lesions namely, (1) splinter or subungual hemorrhages** and **(2) Janeway lesions** which are small erythematous or hemorrhagic nontender, macular, lesions **on the palms or soles.**
   - **Septic emboli from right side of the heart**: They enter pulmonary circulation → lead to **pulmonary abscess.**
2. **Immunological phenomena**
   - **Focal segmental glomerulonephritis: Develop due to deposition of antigen-antibody complexes** in glomeruli. Grossly, the **outer surface of kidney** develops a **flea-bitten** appearance due to patchy hemorrhagic foci involving the glomeruli.
   - **Osler nodes**: They are small, **tender subcutaneous nodules in the pulp of the digits** and persist for hours to several days.
   - **Roth spots** are **retinal hemorrhages** with white or pale centers composed of fibrin.

Clinical Features

- Symptoms:
  - **Fever** is the most common feature of IE.
  - Acute IE develops rapidly presenting with fever, chills, weakness, and lassitude.
- Clinical examination:
  - Murmurs may be heard either due to new valvular defect or a pre-existing cardiac disease.

ATHEROSCLEROSIS

Definition: Atherosclerosis is primarily a progressive **disease of intima involving large and medium-sized elastic and muscular arteries**. It is characterized by **focal lipid-rich** intimal lesions called **atheromas** (atheromatous or atherosclerotic plaques).

Epidemiology: Atherosclerosis is a worldwide disease seen in both developed and developing countries.

Risk Factors for Atherosclerosis

- They were identified through several studies most important being the Framingham Heart Study and Atherosclerosis Risk in Communities Study.
- **Classification of risk factors:** The risk factors may be broadly classified as modifiable, nonmodifiable and additional (Table 17.4).

Table 17.4: Risk factors for atherosclerosis

A. Modifiable major risk factors	
• Hyperlipidemia • Hypertension	• Cigarette smoking • Diabetes mellitus
B. Nonmodifiable risk factors	
• Increasing age • Male gender	• Family history • Genetic abnormalities
C. Additional risk factors	
• Inflammation • CRP level • Hyperhomocystinemia • Metabolic syndrome • Lipoprotein (a)	• Raised procoagulant levels • Inadequate physical activity • Stressful lifestyle • Obesity • Alcohol

Modifiable Risk Factors in IHD

Q. Write short note on risk factors for atherosclerosis.

These are **four** in number namely, 1) hyperlipidemia, 2) hypertension, 3) cigarette smoking, and 4) diabetes.

1. **Hyperlipidemia: Increase in the serum lipids** mainly cholesterol (**hypercholesterolemia**) is a major modifiable risk factor. The major components of lipids in the blood:
   - **Low-density lipoprotein (LDL)** known as **"bad cholesterol"** is one of the components of serum lipid and its **higher level** is associated with **increased risk of atherosclerosis**.
   - **High-density lipoprotein (HDL)** known as **"good cholesterol"** and its **higher levels are associated with decreased risk**.

- **Serum cholesterol level**: Normal range is 140 to 240 mg/dL. Serum cholesterol is **strongly related to the dietary intake of saturated fat** (in the absence of genetic disorders of lipid metabolism). Risk of atherosclerosis increases with increasing serum cholesterol concentrations and lowering serum cholesterol concentrations reduces the risk. The risk of atherosclerosis can be reduced by lowering LDL or total plasma cholesterol, and/or raising serum HDL. This can be achieved either by dietary modification or by treatment with cholesterol-lowering drugs.
  - **Diet which raises blood cholesterol:**
    - **Diet high in cholesterol and saturated fats** (e.g. egg yolks, animal fats, and butter). Transunsaturated fats produced by artificial hydrogenation of polyunsaturated oils (used in baked goods and margarine).
    - **Diet which lower blood cholesterol:** Diets low in cholesterol and/or with higher ratios of **polyunsaturated fats**.
    - **Omega-3 fatty acids** (high in fish and fish oils).
  - **Cholesterol-lowering drug:** For example, statins.

2. **Hypertension:** It is one of the major risk factor.
   - Incidence of atherosclerosis increases as BP rises, and this excess risk **is related to both systolic and diastolic levels of blood pressure.**
   - Control of hypertension with antihypertensive therapy reduces the risk of myocardial infarction and stroke.
3. **Cigarette smoking:** It is the **most important avoidable cause** of atherosclerosis.
   - Atherosclerosis is **more severe and extensive among smokers than in nonsmokers.** This may be the reason for the increased incidence and severity of atherosclerosis in men compared to women. **There is a strong dose-linked relationship between cigarette smoking and ischemic heart disease. Cessation of smoking reduces the risk.**
4. **Diabetes mellitus:** It is a potent risk factor for atherosclerosis.
   - Diabetes is associated with hypercholesterolemia → increases the risk of atherosclerosis. The incidence of myocardial infarction and other atherosclerotic vascular diseases (strokes, gangrene of the lower extremities) is more in diabetics than in nondiabetics.

Nonmodifiable/Constitutional Risk Factors

1. **Increasing age***:* Age is the most powerful independent risk factor. Clinical manifestation of atherosclerosis is usually observed after middle age and the lesions progressively rise with each decade.
2. **Sex: Premenopausal women have lower incidence** of atherosclerosis-related diseases compared to males of the same age group. However, after menopause this sex difference disappears. This may be due to protective role of estrogen. However, hormone replacement therapy has no role in the prevention of coronary heart disease.
3. **Family history**: **Atherosclerotic disease often runs in families.** Familial predisposition is usually multifactorial, due to genetic, environmental and lifestyle factors.
4. **Genetic abnormalities:** Most common inherited modifiable risk factors (hypertension, hyperlipidemia, and diabetes mellitus) are polygenic. Mendelian disorders, such as **familial hypercholesterolemia** are associated with atherosclerosis.

Additional Risk Factors

1. **Inflammation:** It plays a role in atherogenesis and may be a risk factor.
2. **C-reactive protein** (CRP) **level**: It is a marker of systemic inflammation and **predicts the risk** of atherosclerosis related diseases.
3. **Hyperhomocysteinemia:** It is a rare autosomal recessive inborn error and results in elevated circulating homocysteine → premature and severe atherosclerosis.
4. **Metabolic syndrome**: It is associated with central obesity, insulin resistance and is known risk factors for atherosclerosis.
5. **Increased Lipoprotein (a) Lp(a) levels**: It is an altered form of LDL and is associated with increased risk. Lp(a) has structural similarity to plasminogen. It competes with plasminogen in clots and decreases the ability to form and clear clots. Increased Lp(a) levels are associated with higher risk of atherosclerosis, independent of total cholesterol or LDL levels.
6. **Raised procoagulant levels:** These procoagulants include: thrombin (procoagulant and proinflammatory action), platelet activation and raised fibrinogen → increased risk.
7. **Inadequate physical activity:** Lack of exercise doubles the risk.
8. **Stressful lifestyle**: Certain personality associated with competitive, stressful life ("type A" personality) is associated with an increased risk of coronary disease.
9. **Obesity**: It is often associated with hypertension, diabetes mellitus, hypertriglyceridemia, decreased HDL and physical inactivity.
10. **Alcohol consumption:** It is **associated with reduced rates of coronary artery disease**.

Pathogenesis of Atherosclerosis

Q. Write short note on pathogenesis of atherosclerosis.

There are several theories proposed for pathogenesis of atherosclerosis and few of them are:

A. **Insudation hypothesis**: According to this, the focal accumulation of lipid in a vessel wall is due to insudation (transport) of plasma lipoproteins across an intact endothelium.
B. **Encrustation hypothesis**: This hypothesis states that small mural thrombi are formed at the site of endothelial damage. These thrombi become organized and form plaque.
C. **Monoclonal hypothesis**: The monoclonal concept postulates that single clone (monoclonal) of smooth muscle migrate from the underlying media into the intima and then proliferate. The stimulus for monoclonal proliferation may be metabolites of cholesterol.
D. **Response-to-injury hypothesis**: This is the currently favored hypothesis.

Response-to-Injury Hypothesis (Fig. 17.8)

Q. Write short note on reaction-to-injury hypothesis of atherosclerogenesis.

According to this theory, **atherosclerosis develops as a chronic** (inflammatory and healing) **response of the arterial wall to the endothelial injury**. The **sequence of pathogenic events** (Fig. 17.9) is as follows:

1. **Endothelial injury and dysfunction:**
   - **Causes of endothelial injury/dysfunction**:
     - **Hemodynamic disturbances:** Plaques develop in regions having disturbed blood flow such as origin or ostia of vessels, branching points of vessel and along the posterior wall of the abdominal aorta.

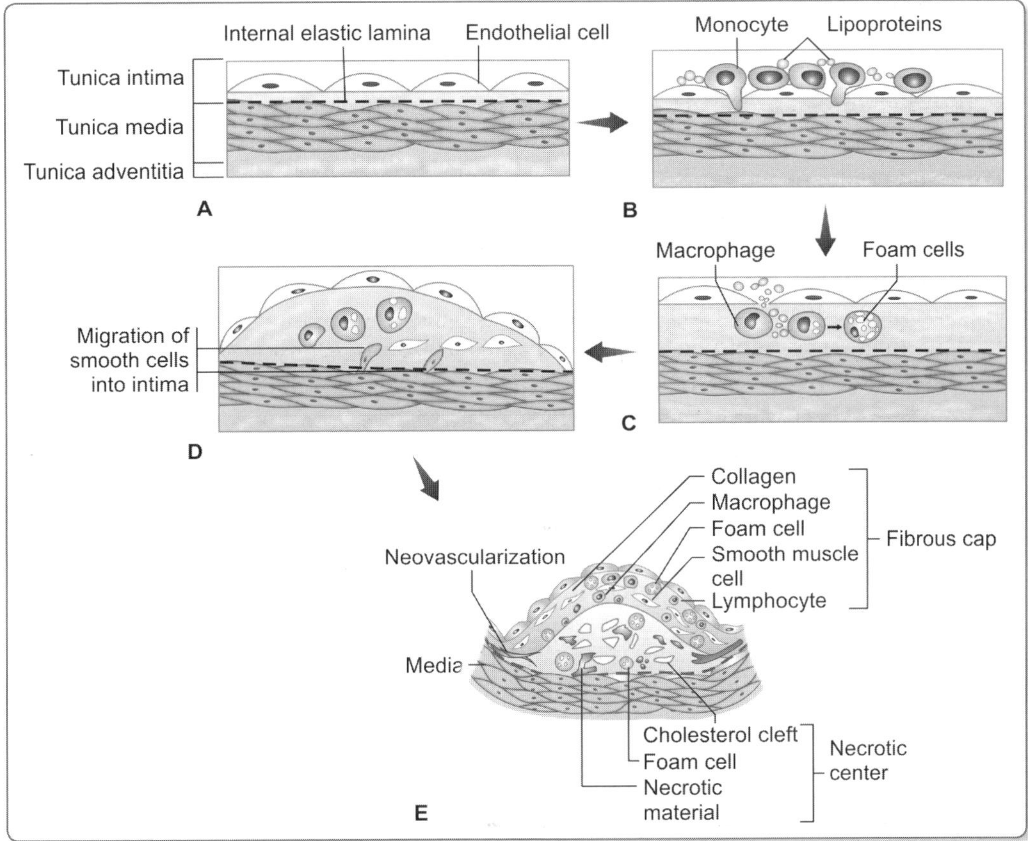

Figs 17.8A to E: Various steps in response to injury hypothesis of atherogenesis. A. Normal; B. Endothelial injury/dysfunction with adhesion of monocytes; C. Migration of monocytes into the arterial intima and are transformed into macrophages. They engulf lipoproteins and oxidized LDL to form foam cells; D. Migration of smooth muscle followed by their proliferation in the intima; E. Fully developed atheromatous plaque

  - **Risk factors: Hyperlipidemia, hypertension, toxins from cigarette smoke,** and advanced glycation end products in **diabetes** can **produce endothelial injury/dysfunction**.
- **Effect of endothelial injury or dysfunction**:
  - **Leukocyte (mainly monocyte) adhesion** to endothelium
  - **Increased vascular permeability**
  - **Platelet adhesion and thrombosis**
  - **Movement of low-density lipoproteins (LDLs) across the endothelium into the intima**.

2. **Migration of monocytes into the intima:**
   - The **leukocytes,** which adhere at the site of endothelial injury/dysfunction, are **mainly monocytes and T lymphocytes**. Accumulation of leukocytes **initiates the atheroma formation**.
   - Locally produced **chemokines allows penetration of the endothelial layer by monocytes and lymphocytes.** The **monocytes migrate into the intima** where they are **transformed into macrophages**.

3. **Lipid accumulation in the intima:**
   - Endothelial dysfunction also allows **penetration of endothelium by lipoproteins (mainly LDL)** from blood → **LDLs accumulate within the intima** of the vessel.
   - **LDL is oxidized** by the action of oxygen free radicals produced locally by monocytes/ macrophages and dysfunctional endothelial cells.
4. **Formation of foam cells and activation of macrophages:**
   - **Macrophage engulfs lipoproteins** and **oxidized LDL** from the extracellular space in the intima. Their cytoplasm becomes foamy and these cells are called as **foam cells.**
   - Some **foam cells may undergo apoptosis** → **release lipids** → form lipid-rich center, often called the necrotic core in atheromatous plaques.
   - **Oxidized LDL is cytotoxic to endothelial cells and smooth muscle** cells and can cause endothelial dysfunction.
   - **Oxidized LDL causes activation of macrophages.**
5. **Migration of smooth muscle cells into the intima:**
   - Growth factor (e.g. platelet-derived growth factor) from activated platelets, macrophages, and endothelial cells causes migration of smooth muscle cells **either from the arterial media or from circulating precursors.**
6. **Smooth muscle cell proliferation in the intima and ECM production:**
   - Many **growth factors** can **cause smooth muscle cell proliferation.** These includes: PDGF, fibroblast growth factor (FGF) and transforming growth factor α (TGF-α).
   - Smooth muscle cell **may also engulf oxidized LDL and form foam cells.**
7. **Lipid accumulation**
   - Occurs both **intracellularly** (within macrophages and smooth muscle cells) and **extracellularly.**
   - **Extracellular lipid** is derived **from insudation** from the vessel lumen (mainly in the presence of hypercholesterolemia) and also from **necrotic foam cells.**
   - Cholesterol in the plaque is also due to an **imbalance between influx and efflux.** High-density lipoprotein (HDL) probably transfers cholesterol from these lesions and leads to its excretion by liver.

Q. Write short note on gross and microscopic features of atherosclerosis.

Q. Write short note on aortic lesions in atherosclerosis.

Morphology

Fatty Streaks: They may be the earliest or precursor lesions of atherosclerosis. They are found in young children (older than 10 years) as well as in adults.

- **Gross: Multiple small (~1 mm) flat yellow lesions in the intima,** which **may coalesce to form long streaks 1 cm or more in length.** They may be mildly elevated above intima without disturbing the blood flow.
- **Microscopy:** Consist of **lipid-filled foamy macrophages** in the intima.

Atherosclerotic Plaque

Gross (Fig. 17.9):

- **Sites:** Major vessels involved in atherosclerosis in descending order are:
  - **Lower abdominal aorta** (abdominal aorta more than the thoracic aorta)
  - **Coronary arteries**
  - **Popliteal arteries**
  - **Internal carotid arteries**
  - **Vessels of the circle of Willis.**

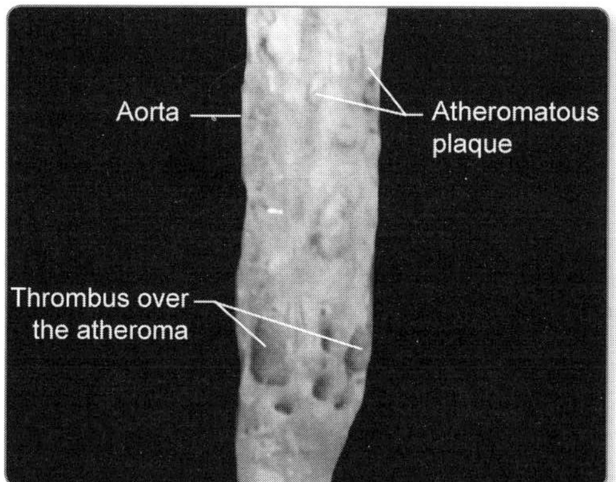

Fig. 17.9A: Atheromatous plaques on the intimal surface of aorta. Lower region shows thrombus over the plaque

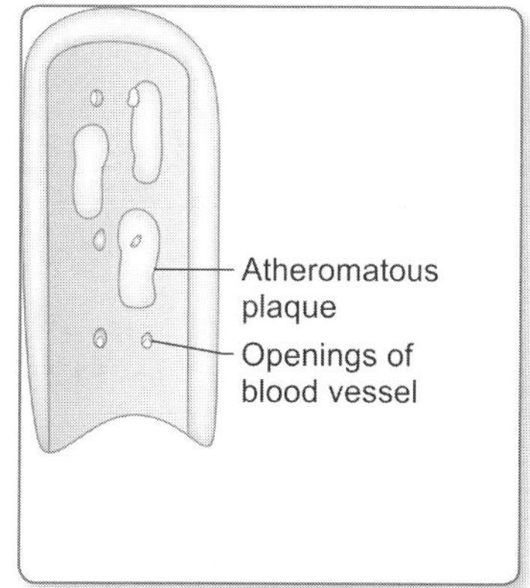

Fig. 17.9B: Diagrammatic gross appearance of atheromas

- **Color: White to yellow**. If superimposed by a thrombus → red-brown.
- **Size:** Range **from 0.3 to 1.5 cm in diameter**. Can coalesce to form larger masses. **Advanced lesions** are oval and range from **8 to 12 cm in diameter.**
- **Shape: Irregular with well-defined borders.**
- **Distribution: Patchy (focal)** and usually involve only a portion of the involved arterial wall. On cross-section → appears as an **eccentric** lesion.
- **Composition**: Soft, yellow, grumous core of lipid covered by a white fibrous cap.

Microscopy (Fig. 17.8E)

Three main components in varying proportions in different lesions:

1. **Cells: Smooth muscle cells, macrophages, and T cells.**
2. **Extracellular matrix (ECM): Collagen, elastic fibers, and proteoglycans.**
3. **Lipid: Both intracellular and extracellular lipid.**

These components occur in three regions:

- **Superficial fibrous cap:** Composed of **smooth muscle cells and collagen.**
- **Necrotic core:** It is seen deep to the fibrous cap and contains:
  - Lipid: Typical atheroma contains **abundant lipid, mainly cholesterol and cholesterol esters**, which is seen as empty needle, shaped cleft-like spaces.
  - Debris from dead cells.
  - **Foam cells** (lipid-laden macrophages and smooth muscle cells).
  - Others: Fibrin, organized thrombus, and plasma proteins.
- **Shoulder**: It is the peripheral region beneath and to the side of the cap. It is more cellular and contains macrophages, smooth muscle cells, and T cells.

Neovascularization (proliferating small blood vessels): It may be seen at the periphery of the lesions near the shoulder.

Major clinical consequences of atherosclerosis are shown in Fig 17.10.

Complicated plaques: Atherosclerotic plaques can undergo the following clinically important changes:

Q. Write short note on complications of atherosclerosis.

1. **Rupture, ulceration, or erosion:** Plaque protrudes into the lumen and can disturb the blood flow → resulting in turbulent flow of blood → which can damage the endothelium → cause rupture, ulceration or erosion of the intimal surface of plaques.

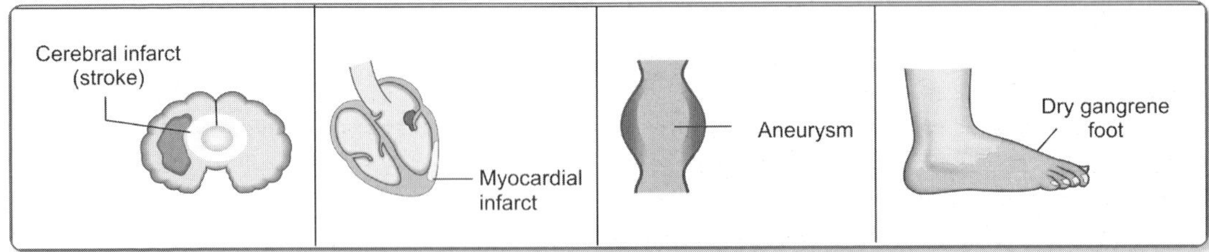

Fig. 17.10: Major clinical consequences of atherosclerosis

2. **Hemorrhage into a plaque:** It may occur due to rupture of the fibrous cap of the plaque or of the thin-walled vessels formed due to neovascularization.
3. **Thrombosis and embolism:** Ulceration/erosion/rupture of endothelial surface → exposes the blood to highly thrombogenic subendothelial collagen → favors **thrombus formation** → can partially or completely occlude the lumen (depending on the size of the lumen) → lead to ischemia. The thrombus may become organized or fragment to form thromboemboli.
4. **Atheroembolism:** Plaque rupture → discharge atherosclerotic debris into the bloodstream → results in atheroemboli.
5. **Aneurysm formation (Fig 17.12):** Atherosclerosis even though an intimal disease may cause pressure or ischemic atrophy of the underlying media. It may also damage the elastic tissue and cause weakening the wall → result in aneurysmal dilation → which may rupture.
6. **Calcification:** It may occur in the central necrotic area of the plaque (dystrophic calcification).

ISCHEMIC HEART DISEASE

Definition: Ischemic heart disease (IHD) is a group of heart diseases in which there is an **inadequate supply of blood and oxygen to a portion of the myocardium**. Typically it occurs when there is an imbalance between the demand and supply (perfusion) of oxygenated blood.

List of diseases includes under ischemic heart disease is presented in Table 17.5.

Epidemiology: IHD is the **leading cause of death** in both males and females.

Table 17.5: List of ischemic heart diseases

1. Myocardial infarction (ischemia causes the necrosis of heart muscle)
2. Angina pectoris (ischemia is less severe to cause frank necrosis)
a. Stable angina
b. Prinzmetal variant angina
c. Unstable angina
3. Chronic IHD with heart failure
4. Sudden cardiac death due to fatal ventricular arrhythmia

Etiology and Pathogenesis of IHD

Ischemic heart disease is caused by an imbalance between the demand and supply of oxygenated blood to myocardium.

Decreased/Impaired Coronary Blood Flow

Coronary arterial occlusion is the main cause of myocardial ischemia.

1. Coronary Atherosclerosis

It narrows one or more of the epicardial coronary arteries → decreases the coronary blood flow in about 90% of cases. Hence, **IHD is often known as coronary artery disease** (CAD) or **coronary heart disease. Risk of IHD depends on:** (a) **extent and severity of** pre-existing (fixed) **atherosclerotic occlusion** and (b) **sudden/dynamic morphological changes** in the atheromatous plaque.

a. **Extent and severity of pre-existing (fixed) atherosclerotic occlusion**
   - **Number of coronaries affected/involved**: Atherosclerosis may affect **one, two or all three coronaries.**
   - **Structure of plaque (Fig. 17.11):** Plaques can be divided into stable and vulnerable (unstable) plaques:
     - **Stable plaques:** They have **dense collagenous and thick fibrous caps** with **minimal inflammation** and negligible underlying atheromatous **necrotic core.** These are **less likely to undergo rupture.**
     - **Vulnerable plaque**: They have **core with many foam cells** and **abundant extracellular lipid.** The **fibrous cap is thin** with few smooth muscle cells or groups of inflammatory cells and **increased inflammation.** These are **likely to undergo rupture.**
   - **Degree/extent of stenosis (obstruction) by atheromatous plaques**:
   - **Rate of development of occlusion**:
     - **Slow progressive occlusion** allows time to **develop collateral circulation** to **prevent infarction.**
     - **Acute blockage—no time for collateral flow → infarction.**

b. **Sudden morphological changes in atheromatous plaque:** It is known as **acute plaque change** and is followed by **thrombosis,** produces **unstable angina, myocardial infarction and sudden cardiac death** in most of the patients. Hence, termed **acute coronary syndrome.** This is discussed under pathogenesis of myocardial infarction.

2. Other Causes of Coronary Artery Occlusion **Coronary emboli** from thrombi in left side of the heart

- **Coronary vasospasm**
- **Diminished availability of blood or oxygen**:
  - Lowered systemic blood pressure (e.g. shock)
  - Hypoxemia.

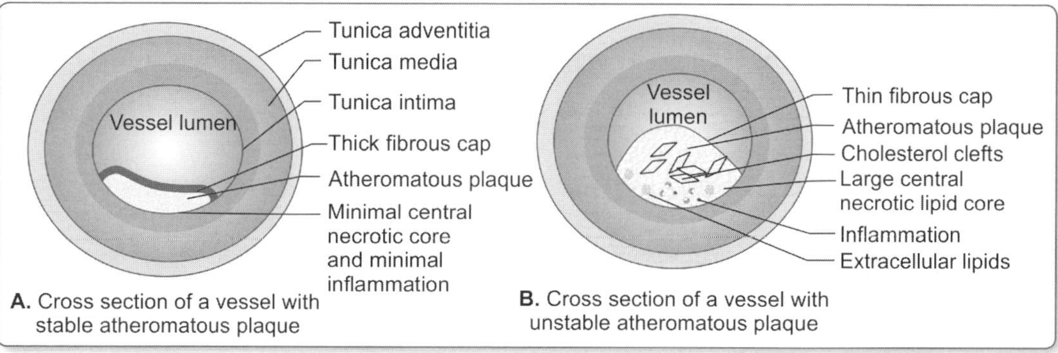

Figs 17.11A and B: A. Diagrammatic appearance of stable, and B. Vulnerable plaque

Increased Myocardial Demand

It occurs:
- With **myocardial hypertrophy**
- Increased heart rate (**tachycardia**).

ANGINA PECTORIS

Definition: Angina pectoris clinically present as **paroxysmal** and **recurrent attacks of substernal or precordial chest discomfort** due to **transient myocardial ischemia**, which falls short of inducing necrosis of myocardial cell.

Variants of Angina Pectoris

Stable Angina

It is the **most common** and is also known as **typical angina pectoris**.
- **Cause**: **Coronary atherosclerosis** and it develops when myocardial oxygen demand increases with **increased physical activity or emotional excitement**.
- **Pain:**
  - **Duration**: It ranges from **1 to 15 minutes**.
  - **Characteristics: Pain is relieved by rest** (which decreases demand) or **by sublingual nitroglycerin**, a strong vasodilator (which increases perfusion).

Prinzmetal Variant Angina

It is an **uncommon atypical from** of angina.
- **Cause:** Due to **spasm of coronary artery having atherosclerosis**. It is **not related to physical activity, heart rate, or blood pressure**.
- **Characteristics: Occurs at rest** and responds promptly to vasodilators.

Unstable or Crescendo Angina

- **Cause**: It is caused by the **disruption/rupture of an atherosclerotic plaque** complicated by **thrombosis/embolization/vasospasm/vasoconstriction**.
- **Characteristics:** It is of **prolonged duration and occurs with minimal physical activity or even at rest.**
- **Consequence**: **May progress to myocardial infarction** and is also referred to as **preinfarction angina**.

MYOCARDIAL INFARCTION (MI)

Definition: Myocardial infarction is a **coagulative type of necrosis of cardiac muscle** and is **due to prolonged severe ischemia**.

Risk Factors

- **Race**: Any race can be affected; whites are affected more than blacks. Indians are also having high-risk of IHD.
- **Age**: Its frequency **rises progressively with age** and peak is between 40 to 65 years of age. It can develop at younger age in patients with major risk factors of atherosclerosis (hyperlipidemia, hypertension, diabetes and cigarette smoking).

- **Sex:** Males have significantly higher risk than females mainly during the reproductive period. However, after menopause the risk is similar to that of males. The protective effect may be due to estrogen.
- **Other risk factors**: Refer under risk factors for atherosclerosis.

Etiology

Q. Discuss etiopathogenesis of myocardial infarction.

Common etiological factor discussed under IHD.

Coronary Atherosclerosis

Coronary artery occlusion in 90% of cases, myocardial infarction is due to atherosclerotic narrowing of one or more coronary arteries.

Nonatheromatous Causes

In about 10% of cases, MI occurs without atherosclerosis of the coronary vessels. It may be due to:

- **Vasospasm without coronary atherosclerosis**
- **Emboli:** The source of which may be:
  - Left-sided mural thrombus
  - Vegetations of infective endocarditis
- **Ischemia due to other causes**: Vasculitis, Hematologic disorders like sickle cell disease.

Pathogenesis of MI

In **coronary arteries with pre-existing (fixed) atherosclerotic occlusion, inadequate coronary perfusion** may occur due to a **new superimposed thrombosis and/or coronary vasospasm**. Thrombus formation is due to acute plaque change.

Sequence of events in a typical case of MI (Fig. 17.12) is as follows:

1. **Acute plaque change: It is the sudden change/event occurring in an atheromatous plaque.** The initial event in pathogenesis of myocardial infarction is sudden change in the atheromatous plaques. These as a**cute plaque changes convert partially occlusive** atherosclerotic **plaque to produce sudden ischemia**. These changes are divided into three categories:
   i. **Rupture**, **fissuring** of plaque → exposes highly thrombogenic plaque constituents → sudden **thrombus formation** → **sudden occlusion of lumen.**
   ii. **Erosion/ulceration of plaque**
      - Exposes highly thrombogenic subendothelial basement membrane
      - Sudden **thrombus formation**
      - **Sudden occlusion of lumen**.
   iii. **Hemorrhage into the central core of plaque** → increases the plaque size → sudden **occlusion of lumen**.
2. **Formation of microthrombi:** Acute plaque changes exposes thrombogenic subendothelial collagen → platelets adhere to the site → platelet activation and aggregation → formation of microthrombi on the atheromatous plaque → **partial or complete occlusion of the affected coronary artery**.
3. **Vasospasm**: **Activated platelets, endothelial cell and inflammatory cells release mediators** → cause **vasospasm** at the sites of atheroma → further narrowing of the lumen.
4. **Activation of the coagulation pathway**: Tissue factor released at the site of acute plaque change → activates coagulation system → **increase the size of the thrombus**.

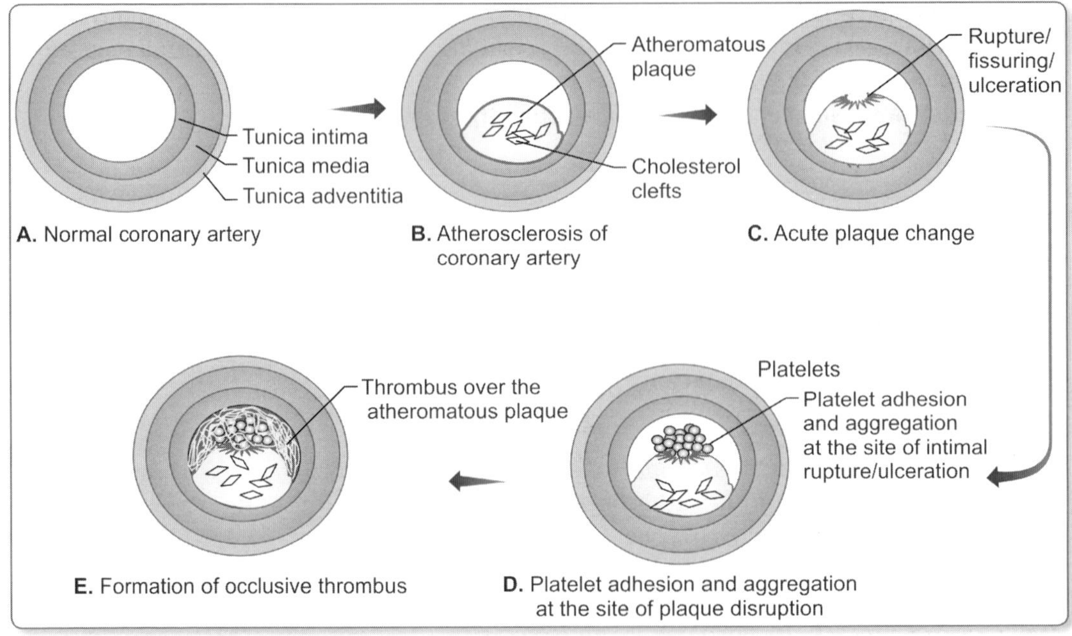

Fig. 17.12: Sequential changes in coronary artery atherosclerosis causing occlusion of lumen in ischemic heart disease

5. **Complete occlusion of vessel:** Within minutes, the thrombus may completely occlude the lumen of the vessel.
6. **Myocardial necrosis**: Complete occlusion → results in **ischemic coagulative necrosis of the area supplied** by the particular coronary artery.

Consequence of Myocardial Ischemia

These include functional, biochemical and morphological changes. Morphological changes can be divided into reversible and irreversible damage/injury.

A. **Reversible injury:** These changes are potentially reversible and include:
   1. **Biochemical changes: Cessation of aerobic glycolysis** occurs within seconds of myocardial ischemia → **decreased production of ATP** (adenosine triphosphate) → **accumulation of** potentially **toxic metabolites** (such as lactic acid).
   2. **Functional disturbances: Loss of contractility** within 60 seconds → can precipitate acute heart failure.
   3. **Morphological changes**: They are seen at ultrastructural level such as **mitochondrial swelling, glycogen depletion and myofibrillar relaxation**. They also develop within a few minutes.

B. **Irreversible injury:** A develops only after prolonged, severe myocardial ischemia of more than 20 to 40 minutes
   - **Biochemical changes:** They cause **leakage of cytoplasmic proteins into the blood.** In the early phases of myocardial cell necrosis, there is breakdown of the sarcolemmal membrane → leakage of intracellular proteins (such as **myoglobin, LDH, CK, and troponins I and T**) into the blood. The levels of these leaked myocardial proteins in the blood is **used for the diagnosis as well as management of MI.**

- **Functional disturbances:** Arrhythmias.
- **Morphological changes: Coagulative necrosis** of cardiac muscle fibers usually complete within 6 hours of the onset of myocardial ischemia.

  Zones damaged: First necrosis in the subendocardial zone → later transmural infarct.

Classification of Myocardial Infarct

Q. Classify myocardial infarction.

A. **Depending on the thickness of myocardium involved:**
   1. **Transmural**: Ischemic necrosis of the **entire thickness of the ventricular wall.**
   2. **Subendocardial (nontransmural)**: Ischemic necrosis of **inner one-third to one-half of the ventricular wall.**

B. **Depending on the age of the infarct: Recent (fresh) or old (healed).**

Q. Describe the sequential changes seen in myocardial infarction.

Q. Describe the morphological changes occurring in myocardial infarction.

Morphology

General features:

- **Most of transmural infarcts** (>50%) involve at **least a portion of the left ventricle** and/or **interventricular septum.**
- ~ 15 to 30% of MI, which involve posterior or posteroseptal wall also extend to involve right ventricle.
- **Isolated infarction of the right ventricle** and **infarction of the atria are rare.**

Pattern of left ventricular infarcts (Fig. 17.13):

1. **Left anterior descending (LAD) coronary artery occlusion** (40–50%): Infarcts involve:
   a. **Anterior wall of left ventricle near the** apex
   b. **Anterior portion of ventricular septum**
   c. Apex circumferentially.
2. **Right coronary artery occlusion (30–40%)**: Infarcts involves:
   a. **Region of the inferior/posterior wall of left ventricle**
   b. **Posterior portion of interventricular** septum (inferior infarct)
   c. Inferior/posterior right ventricular free wall (in some).
3. **Left circumflex coronary artery occlusion** (15–20%): Infarcts involve the **lateral wall of left ventricle** except at the apex.

The sequences of the morphologic changes in acute MI and subsequent healing are summarized in Table 17.6.

Gross (Table 17.6)

- **Within first 12 hours: No identifiable/apparent gross changes** are seen. **Triphenyltetrazolium chloride (a histochemical stain)** can grossly identify infarct within 2 to 3 hours after onset.
  - **Noninfarcted myocardium appears brick-red** (lactate dehydrogenase activity is preserved).
  - **Infarcted area** remains **unstained pale** (loss of dehydrogenases).
- **By 12 to 24 hours (Fig. 17.14A): Grossly identifiable.** Appears **pale reddish-blue area** (due to stagnated, trapped blood) → progressively becomes **sharply defined, yellow-tan, and soft.**
- **After 3 to 5 days:** Mottled with a **central pale, yellowish, necrotic region** with well-demarcated border of **hyperemic zone** (due to granulation tissue).
- **By 10 days to 2 weeks**: Appears **soft and rimmed by a hyperemic zone** of highly vascularized granulation tissue.
- **After 2 weeks:** Older, healed infarcts appear **firm, pale gray and contracted** → develops into a **fibrous scar (Fig. 17.14B).**

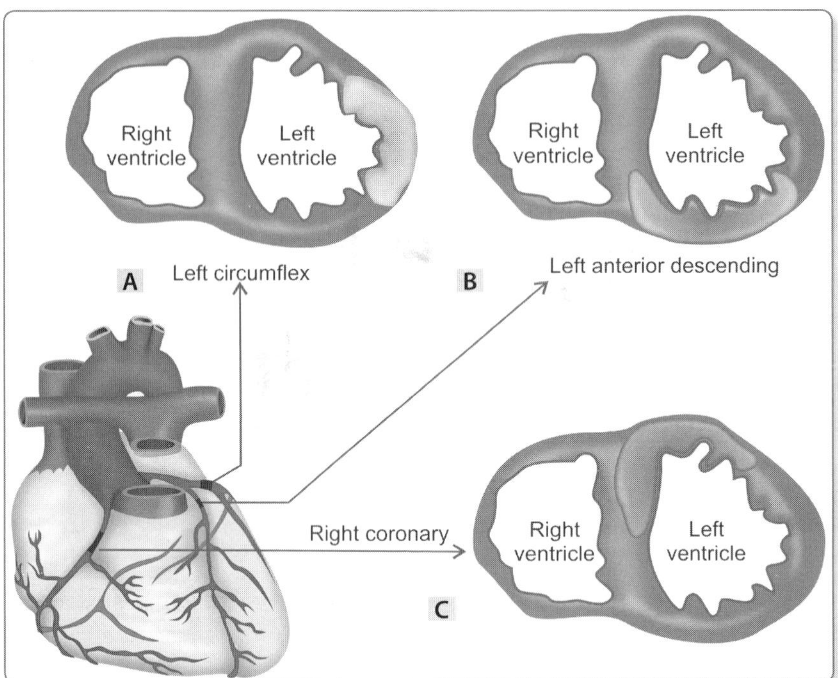

Figs 17.13A to C: Pattern of left ventricular infarcts resulting from occlusion of each of the three main coronary arteries. A. Posterolateral infarct develops following occlusion of the left circumflex artery; B. Anterior infarct develops following occlusion of the anterior descending branch of left coronary. The infarct is located in the anterior wall of left ventricle and adjacent two-thirds of the interventricular (AV) septum; C. Posterior infarct results from occlusion of the right coronary artery and involves the posterior wall, including the posterior third of the AV septum

Table 17.6: Sequence of morphologic changes in myocardial infarction

Duration	Gross changes	Light microscopic changes
Reversible injury		
0–½ hour	None	None (electron microscope—relaxation of myofibrils; glycogen loss; mitochondrial swelling)
Irreversible injury		
½–6 hours	None	Usually none; variable waviness of fibers at border (electron microscopy: sarcolemmal disruption; mitochondrial amorphous densities)
6–12 hours	Dark mottling (occasional)	Early coagulative necrosis; edema; hemorrhage
12–24 hours	Dark mottling	Progression of coagulation necrosis; pyknotic nuclei; increased eosinophilia of cytoplasm; contraction band necrosis at margins; beginning of neutrophilic infiltrate
1–3 days	Mottling with yellow-tan infarct center	Coagulation necrosis, with loss of nuclei and striations; increased interstitial infiltration of neutrophils
3–7 days	Hyperemic border; central yellow-tan softening	Beginning disintegration of dead myocardial cells, with dying neutrophils; early phagocytosis of dead cells by macrophages at infarct border
7–10 days	Maximally yellow-tan and soft, with depressed red-tan margins	Well-developed phagocytosis of dead cells; formation of fibrovascular granulation tissue at margins
10–14 days	Red-gray depressed infarct borders	Well-established granulation tissue with new blood vessels and collagen deposition
2–8 weeks	Gray-white scar, progressive from border toward core of infarct	Increased collagen deposition, with decreased cellularity
>2 months	Scarring complete	Dense collagenous scar

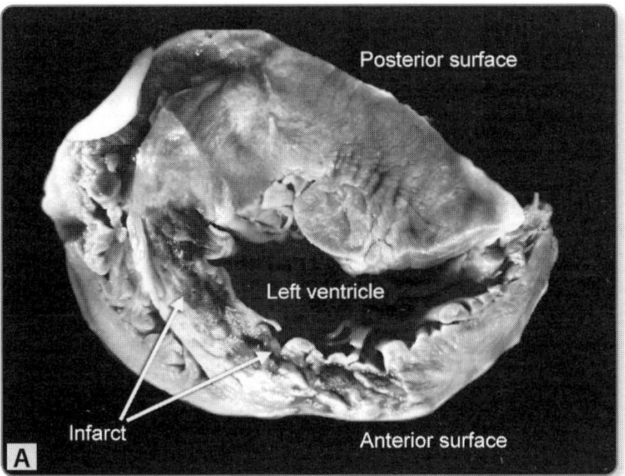

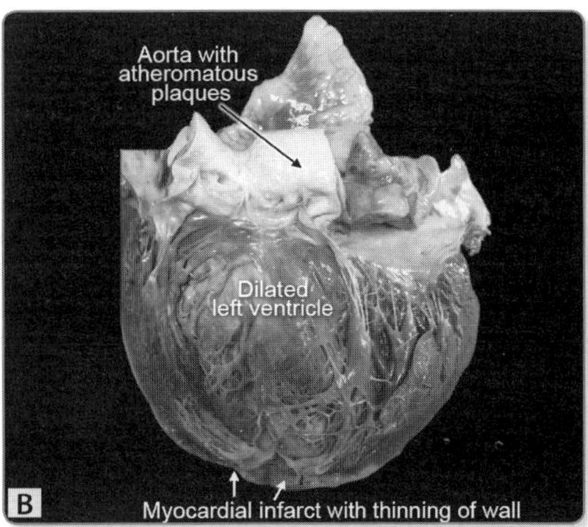

Figs 17.14A and B: A. Coronal section of left ventricle with acute myocardial infarct (12–24 hours old) involving anterior wall of left ventricle and anterior portion of interventricular septum; B. Myocardial infarct at the apex of heart

Microscopy (Fig. 17.15 and Table 17.6)

- **First 6 hours**: Earliest changes can be detected only by electron microscopy (ultrastructural changes)
  - **Reversible injury (0–1½ hours): Relaxation of myofibrils, loss of glycogen, and mitochondrial swelling.**
  - **Irreversible injury** (½–6 hours): Develops after 30 to 60 minutes of ischemia. The changes include **mitochondrial amorphous matrix densities, focal disruption of sarcolemma and clumping and margination of nuclear chromatin.**
- **6 to 12 hours**: Coagulative necrosis begins and shows edema and hemorrhage.
- **12 to 24 hours (Figs 17.15B and F)**: Characteristic changes of **coagulation necrosis** appear. These include: (1) **preserved cell outlines of myocardial cell**, (2) **deeply eosinophilic cytoplasm** and (3) **pyknotic nuclei**.
- **1 to 2 days:**
  - **Acute inflammatory reaction** characterized by accumulation of polymorphonuclear leukocytes **(Fig. 17.15C) at the periphery/borders of infarct.**
  - **Continuation of coagulation necrosis: Nuclei disappear**, and **striations become less prominent. Margins show contraction band necrosis.**
- **3 to 7 days:**
  - **Appearance of macrophages**: The polymorphonuclear leukocytes are replaced by macrophages. **Macrophages phagocytose** and remove the necrotic myocardial cells and neutrophil fragments at the border of infarct.
  - **Granulation tissue**: Appears **at the periphery of infarct**, and gradually extends toward the center.
- **1 to 2 weeks: Process of healing starts from its margins** toward its center which is responsible for most advanced healing at the periphery.
  - **Well-established highly vascularized granulation tissue,** which consists of proliferating capillaries and fibroblasts.
  - **Fibroblasts proliferate** and **collagen deposition** proceeds.
- **2 to 8 weeks (Fig. 17.15D): Increased collagen deposition and less cellularity**.
- **>2 months (Fig. 17.15E):** Dense collagenous **scar**. In a completely healed infarct, it is not possible to determine its age.

Diagnosis of MI

It is based on (1) clinical symptoms, (2) electrocardiographic changes and (3) laboratory findings.

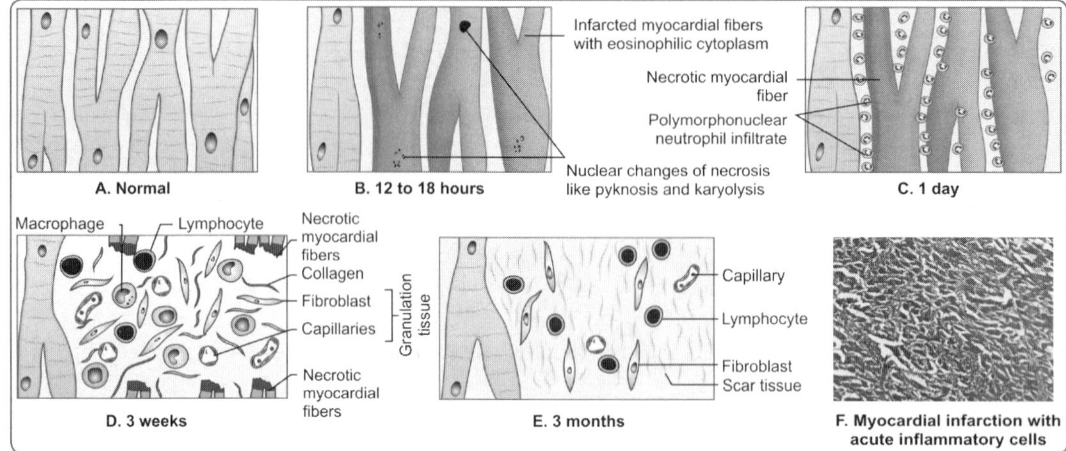

Figs 17.15A to F: Microscopic changes observed during development of a myocardial infarct. A. Normal myocardium; B. After about 12 to 18 hours, the infarcted myocardium shows myocardial fibers with eosinophilia; C. About 24 hours after the onset of infarction, polymorphonuclear neutrophils infiltrate at the periphery of infarcted area; D. After about 3 weeks, the infarcted area consists of granulation tissue infiltrated by lymphocytes and macrophages. E. After 3 months or more, the infarcted region is replaced by collagenous tissue; F. Photomicrograph of acute myocardial infarction showing coagulative necrosis with acute inflammatory infiltrate

Clinical Symptoms

1. **Severe, retrosternal chest pain** that can radiate to neck, jaw, epigastrium or left arm.
2. Rapid, weak pulse.
3. Profuse sweating (diaphoresis).
4. Dyspnea due to impaired contraction of the ischemic myocardium and the resultant pulmonary edema.

Electrocardiographic Changes

1. **Q waves.**
2. **ST segment changes.**
3. **T wave inversions.**

Laboratory Findings

Q. Laboratory diagnosis of myocardial infarction.

These findings are mainly, due to **leakage of proteins from the necrotic myocardial cells into the blood circulation**:

1. **Cardiac troponins**: These are proteins involved in heart muscle contraction. **Increased plasma levels establish the diagnosis of myocardial infarction.**
   - **Cardiac-specific proteins are of two types: Troponins I (TnI) and T (TnT).** They are **most sensitive and specific markers** of myocardial infarction. Levels begin to **rise at 2 to 4 hours** and **peaks at 48 hours**. The elevated troponin levels may **remain for 7 to 10 days** after acute MI.
2. **Cardiac creatine phosphokinase (CK):** It is a **nonspecific enzyme marker** and it is present in brain, myocardium, and skeletal muscle. It has two isoforms designated "M" and "B". **MB heterodimers chiefly in cardiac** muscle (lesser amounts in skeletal muscle).

Table 17.7: Laboratory markers of myocardial infarction`

Marker	Onset	Peak	Normalization	Significance
Troponins T and I	2 to 4 hours	48 hours	7 to 10 days	Most sensitive and specific marker
CK-MB	2 to 4 hours	24 hours	72 hours	Sensitive but not specific
LDH	24 to 48 hours	Many days	7 to 14 days	Not specific marker
Myoglobin	1 to 3 hours	8 to 12 hours	24 to 36 hours	Earliest marker

- **MB form of creatine kinase (CK-MB)** is **sensitive but not specific**, because it is also raised with skeletal muscle injury.
- CK-MB levels **rise within 2 to 4 hours** of the onset of MI, **peaks at 24 hours**, and returns to **normal within 72 hours.**

3. **Lactate dehydrogenase (LDH): It not specific marker**. It **starts rising** after **24 to 48 hours.** It remains **for many days** and **returns to normal in 7 to 14 days**.
4. **Myoglobin**: It is an oxygen-carrying respiratory protein found only in skeletal and cardiac muscle. It is an **earliest marker of MI**, the level rises within 1 to 3 hours, **peaks in about 8 to 12 hours** and **return to normal in about 24 to 36 hours**.

   Various laboratory markers of MI are presented in Table 17.7.

Complications of Myocardial Infarction

Q. Mention the complications of myocardial infarction.

The risk of complications depends on: (1) infarct size, (2) location, and (3) thickness of myocardium involved (subendocardial or transmural).

1. **Left ventricular failure and cardiogenic shock**: MI produces contractile functional abnormalities of left ventricle and is roughly proportional to the size of infarct.
   - **Mild dysfunction**: → left ventricular failure → **pulmonary edema.**
   - **Cardiogenic shock:** Severe "pump failure" occurs with a **large infarct** (>40% of the left ventricle) → cardiogenic shock → **fatal**.
2. **Arrhythmias**: Almost most MI patients develop **abnormal cardiac rhythm** → myocardial irritability and/or conduction disturbances → arrhythmias. These include **sinus bradycardia, tachycardia, ventricular tachycardia, and ventricular fibrillation**. In inferoseptal infarcts → **partial or complete heart block**.
3. **Myocardial rupture***:* Necrosis and neutrophilic infiltration → causes softening and weakening of myocardium → lead to cardiac rupture. **Most frequent during 3 to 7 days after transmural infarcts**.
   - **Rupture of the ventricular free wall (Fig. 17.16A)**: It is most common → result in **hemopericardium and cardiac tamponade.**
   - **Rupture of the ventricular septum (Fig. 17.16B)**: It is less common → lead to an **acute VSD and left-to-right shunt.**
   - **Rupture of papillary muscle (Fig. 17.16C):** It is least common → leads to acute severe mitral regurgitation.
4. **Dilatation of ventricular chamber**: Area of infarct being weak region may be disproportionately stretched → dilation of the infarct region (especially with anteroseptal infarcts) not severe enough to cause aneurysm described below.

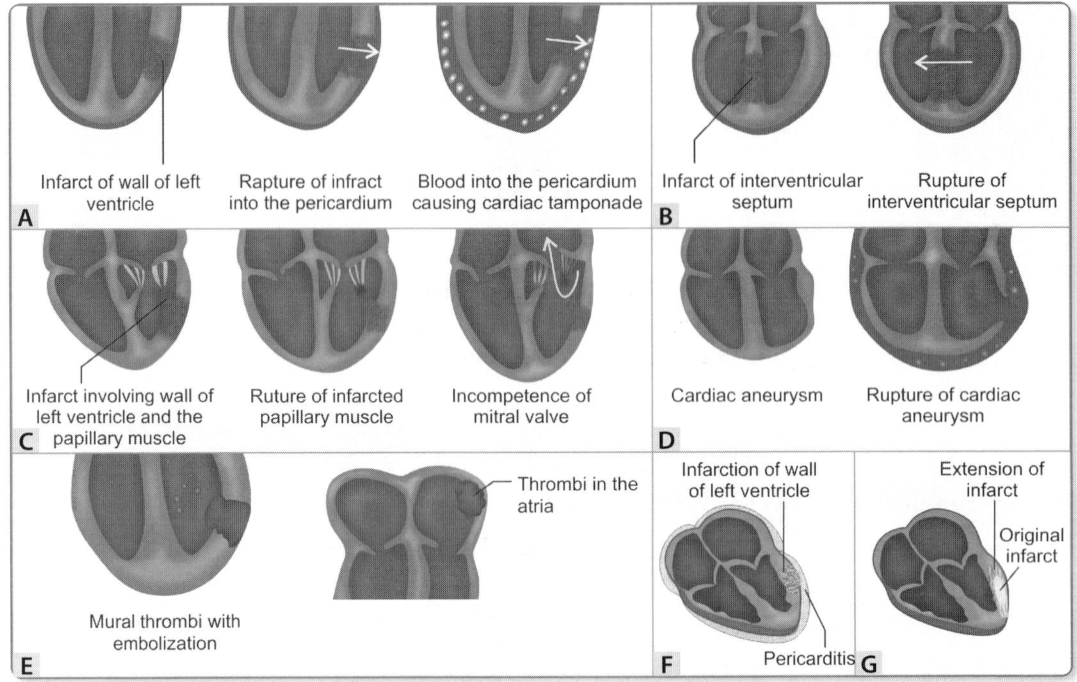

Figs 17.16A to G: Various complications of MI

5. **Ventricular aneurysm (Figs 17.16D)**: After acute transmural infarction, the affected ventricular wall may bulge outward during systole resulting ventricular aneurysm. It develops as a late complication of large transmural infarcts.
6. **Mural thrombus (Figs 17.16E)**: Infarct → causes local abnormality in myocardial contractility (causing stasis) and endocardial damage (creating a thrombogenic surface) → favor **mural thrombosis** → left-sided **thromboembolism**. They may also develop **within ventricular aneurysms**.
7. **Pericarditis:**
   - **Early pericarditis**: A transmural myocardial infarct → can involve the pericardium → cause **fibrinous or fibrinohemorrhagic** pericarditis (Fig. 17.16F). Usually develops on **second or third day**.
   - **Delayed form of pericarditis (postmyocardial infarction syndrome**/Dressler syndrome): Develops 2 to 10 weeks after infarction—**probably immunologically mediated**.
8. **Extension of infarct (Fig. 17.16):**
   - New areas of repeated necrosis can occur adjacent to an existing myocardial infarct causing extension of infarct.
   - In extended infarct, healing is more advanced in the central zone than the periphery of the infarct. This is in contrast with that simple infarct, in which the healing is more advanced at the periphery.
9. **Infarction of right ventricle**: It is **unusual**. However, part of right ventricular myocardium may be involved with infarction of adjacent posterior left ventricle and ventricular septum → venous circulation pooling → systemic hypotension.
10. **Progressive late heart failure** (chronic IHD): Usually develops due to the functional decompensation of hypertrophied noninfarcted myocardium.

Section 2

Practicals

Chapter 18

Urine Analysis

Chapter Outline

- Introduction
- Physical Examination
- Chemical Examination

INTRODUCTION

Urine analysis (urinalysis) reflects the state of function of the kidneys and urinary tract. It provides information about metabolic or systemic (nonrenal) disorders. Urine examination should precede all other invasive/noninvasive diagnostic investigations for renal function.

Examination of Urine

Urine examination consists of: (1) physical examination, (2) chemical examination and (3) microscopic examination.

PHYSICAL EXAMINATION

Volume

A healthy adult excretes about 600 to 2000 mL. of urine in 24 hours. In infants, the volume is 300-600 mL/day.

Polyuria

Increased urine output (more than 2 liters in 24 hours).

Causes

- **Physiological:** Increased fluid intake
- **Pathological**
  - Diabetes mellitus (polydipsia—excessive intake of water)
  - Chronic renal diseases
  - Diuretic therapy
  - Diabetes insipidus
  - Primary aldosteronism.

Oliguria

Decreased urinary output (less than 500 mL in 24 hours).

Causes

- Restricted intake of fluid
- Excessive loss of fluid, e.g. in hemorrhage, burns, dehydration and shock
- Renal diseases
  - Acute glomerulonephritis
  - Nephrotic syndrome
  - Acute tubular necrosis as in shock, burns, crush syndrome, incompatible blood transfusion and heavy metal poisoning
- Addison's disease.

Reaction (pH)

Normal urine is usually acidic with pH varying from 4.6 to 8. Urinary pH is measured as given below.

- **Litmus paper**

  Technique: The reaction of urine is determined with blue and red litmus paper. The urine when examined must be fresh as it turns alkaline on standing due to bacterial decomposition
  - **Acidic urine** turns blue litmus paper red
  - **Alkaline urine** turns red litmus paper blue
  - Both blue and red litmus papers turn reddish purple when the urine is faintly on the acid side (pH 7.0) or neutral.
- **pH indicator paper strips/strip multistix method** uses a methyl red and bromothymol blue double indicator system which can measure a pH from 5 to 9.

Specific Gravity

It is used as a measure of the concentrating power of the kidney. Normal specific gravity of a 24-hour urine sample is 1.003 to 1.035, average being 1.016. Specific gravity (SG) is measured by: (1) urinometer, (2) refractometer and, (3) dipstick method.

Urinometer and refractometer methods are more accurate as compared to the dipstick method.

Urinometer Method

Urinometer (Fig. 18.1) is a specialized hydrometer. It consists of a weighted glass cylinder which floats in urine and has a calibrated stem to measure specific gravity at a given temperature. The scale in many urinometers read in small divisions from 1.000 to 1060. It is usually calibrated in the range of 15° to 20°C (depends on the manufacturer). As the specific gravity varies with temperature, the reading obtained should be corrected to the room temperature by applying temperature correction.

- **Temperature correction:** For **every 3°C rise** in room temperature beyond the calibrated temperature (15°C), **add 0.001** to the recorded reading; and **subtract 0.001** for every 3°C fall in temperature.

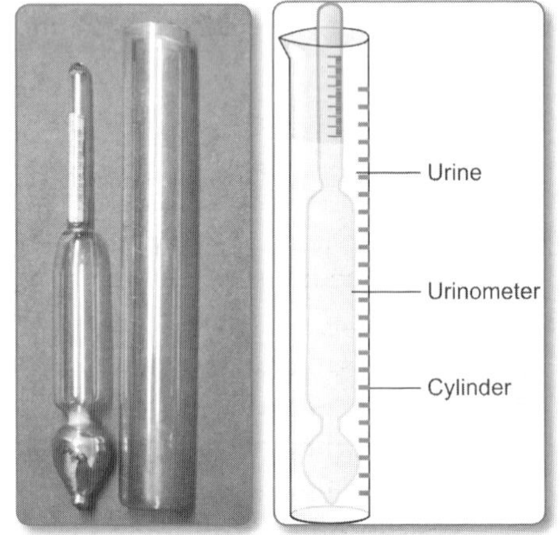

Fig. 18.1: Urinometer for specific gravity measurement

Technique

The urine is poured into a wide necked vessel (cylinder), and the urinometer is floated, so that it does not touch the sides of the container. The specific gravity is read from the graduations which lie at level with the true surface of the urine (lower meniscus). Observe the temperature of the urine. Check the temperature at which the urinometer is calibrated.

Refractometer Method

It is based on refractive index of urine and has the advantage of requiring only a few drops of urine.

Dipstick Method

SG is recorded by change of color on the strip and compared with the color chart on the multistix bottle.

Causes

- **Increased** specific gravity
  - Glycosuria
  - Dehydration: Restricted fluid intake, diarrhea, vomiting, fever, and excessive sweating.
- **Decreased** specific gravity
  - Excessive fluid intake
  - Diabetes insipidus
  - End stage kidney
- **Low and fixed** specific gravity: When **specific gravity is fixed** at 1.010, this is known as **isosthenuria.** It is indicative of severe renal damage (chronic renal failure) with disturbance of both the concentrating and diluting abilities of the kidney.

CHEMICAL EXAMINATION

Proteinuria

The presence of detectable protein in the urine is known as **proteinuria**. It indicates glomerular injury.

Heat and Acetic Acid Test

- ***Procedure* (Fig. 18.2):**
  - Fill three-fourth of a test tube with clear urine.
  - **Heat the upper part (1/3) of the urine** (the lower part of the urine acts as a control for checking turbidity in the heated upper part). **Do not boil the urine**, as it causes mixing of the upper and lower parts of urine and traces of proteins cannot be appreciated. The development of **turbidity may be due to coagulation of proteins or due to phosphates.**
  - Add a few (3–5) drops of 10% glacial acetic acid and if turbidity persists it is due to proteins (phosphates will dissolve).
- ***Interpretation:*** Depending on the amount of precipitate, results are interpreted as shown in Table 18.1.

Sulfosalicylic Acid Test

This test **detects all types of proteins** (albumin, globulin, glycoproteins and Bence Jones proteins).

- ***Procedure***
  - Take 2.5 mL of urine in a small test tube.
  - Slowly pour 2.5 mL of sulfosalicylic acid. Wait for 5 minutes.

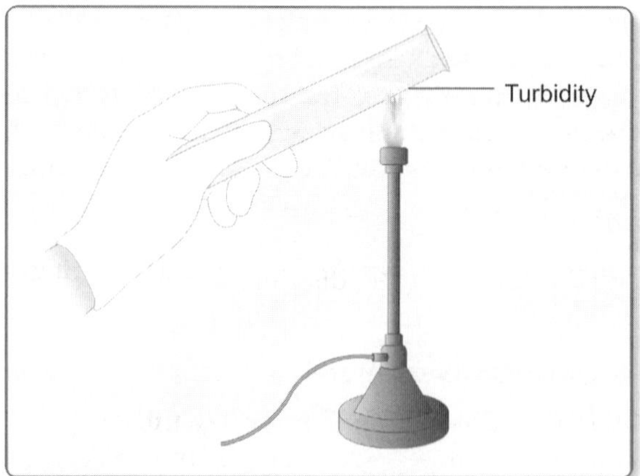

Fig. 18.2: Method of performing heat and acetic acid test

Table 18.1: Interpretation of heat and acetic acid test

Description	Result	Approximate protein concentration
No cloudiness/precipitate	Negative	–
White cloudiness	+	<100 mg/dL
Granular white precipitate	++	100 to 250 mg/dL
Floccular precipitate	+++	250 to 500 mg/dL
Thick opaque precipitate	++++	500 mg/dL

- ***Interpretation:*** Presence of a **cloudy precipitate** indicates the presence of proteins in urine. However, it also precipitates mucus and Bence Jones proteins.

Heller's Test

- ***Procedure:*** Take 5 mL of urine in a test tube and add a few drops of concentrated nitric acid.
- ***Interpretation:*** Presence of proteins is indicated by a **white ring** at the junction of urine and acid.

Dipstick Method

- ***Principle:*** The test is based on the protein error of pH indicators. At a constant pH any color change in the indicator is due to protein. The reagent strip is impregnated with an indicator tetrabromophenol blue or tetrachlorophenol-tetrabromosulfophthalein buffered to pH 3.0. At this pH, it is yellow in the absence of protein. If urine contains protein (which will elicit a pH change), it forms a complex with the indicator turning its color to green or bluish green.
- ***Interpretation:*** The strip is yellow in the absence of protein and variable shades of green develop depending on the type and concentration of protein present.

Quantitative Estimation of Proteins in Urine

Protein excretion in a 24-hour urine sample is required in suspected cases of nephrotic syndrome (>3.5 g/24 hours) and orthostatic/postural proteinuria. This may be carried out by **Esbach's albuminometer** (Fig. 18.3) **method.**

- ***Procedure***
  - Fill the albuminometer with urine up to the mark U.
  - Add Esbach's reagent up to the mark R.

- Stopper the Esbach's albuminometer, mix and allow it to stand for 24 hours.
- Take the reading from the level of precipitation in the albuminometer and divide the value by 10 to get the percentage of total proteins.

- ***Precaution:*** The urine must be of acid reaction, clear and should not be concentrated, in which case it must be diluted with water making allowance for the dilution in the final calculation.

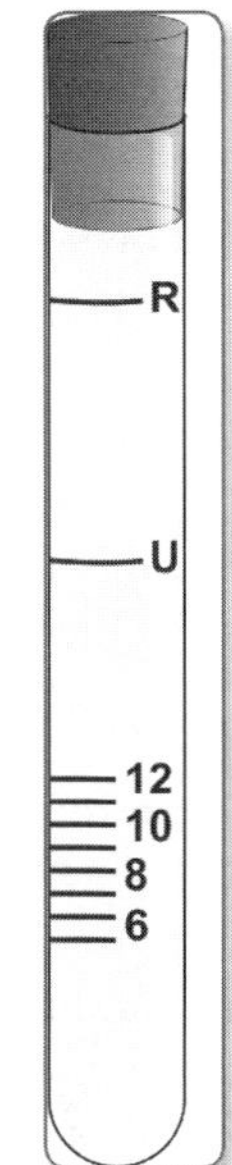

Fig. 18.3: Esbach's albuminometer used for quantitative measurement of proteins in urine

Causes of Proteinuria (albuminuria)

Proteinuria (Table 18.2) may be classified as **glomerular, tubular, lower urinary tract, prerenal and asymptomatic.** It may also be classified depending on the amount of protein as **heavy** (>4 g/day), **moderate** (1 to 4 g/day) and **mild** (less than 1 g/day) proteinuria.

Reducing Substances in Urine

Reducing substances are those compounds which reduce cupric ions (from copper sulfate in Benedict's reagent) in an alkaline solution to cuprous ions (cuprous oxide). Such substances may be sugar or nonsugar.

Table 18.2: Causes of proteinuria

Causes of proteinuria	Amount of proteinuria
Glomerular damage	
• Nephrotic syndrome	Heavy
• Acute glomerulonephritis	Mild-to-moderate
• Acute rapidly progressive glomerulonephritis	Moderate-to-heavy
• Chronic glomerulonephritis	Moderate-to-heavy
Tubular damage	
• Pyelonephritis	Mild
• Acute tubular necrosis	Mild
• Polycystic kidney disease	Mild
• Heavy metal and vitamin D intoxication	Moderate
• Hypokalemia	Mild
Prerenal	
• Multiple myeloma (Bence Jones protein).	Moderate
• Nephrosclerosis	Mild-to-moderate
• Malignant hypertension	Moderate-to-heavy
• Systemic lupus erythematosus	Moderate-to-heavy
• Congestive heart failure	Mild
• Dehydration	Mild
Asymptomatic proteinuria	
• After excessive exercise	Mild
• Postural (orthostatic) albuminuria	Mild

Sugar: These include: glucose, fructose, pentose, galactose, lactose, maltose and sucrose. Special tests are required to differentiate the sugar occurring in urine.

Nonsugar: Ascorbic acid, uric acid, urates, glucuronides, chloroform, formaldehyde, salicylates, streptomycin, phenol, PAS, homogentisic acid (alkaptonuria) and creatinine.

Blood glucose level varies between 70 to 120 mg/dL. This may increase to 120 to 160 mg/dL after a meal. Normally, all the glucose in the blood is filtered through glomerulus and reabsorbed at proximal tubules. If the renal threshold (the lowest blood glucose level that will result in glycosuria) is exceeded (usually greater than 180 to 200 mg/dL), the excess glucose will not be reabsorbed into the blood and will be eliminated in the urine as in cases of diabetes mellitus. The presence of detectable amounts of **glucose in urine** is termed **glycosuria**.

Benedict Qualitative test (semiquantitative)

- This test detects the presence of reducing substances in urine and is not specific for glucose.
- ***Principle of Benedict test:*** The copper sulfate present in the Benedict's reagent reacts with the **reducing substances** in the urine which **convert cupric sulfate to cuprous oxide** in hot alkaline media. Thus, this test is based on the reduction of cupric ions in Benedict's solution to cuprous ions. In the absence of reducing substances in urine, the color of the reagent remains blue.
- ***Procedure*** **(Fig. 18.4)**
  - Take **5 mL of Benedict's** (qualitative) reagent in a test tube.
  - Boil to exclude presence of reducing substance in reagent.
  - Add **8 drops (0.5 mL) of protein free urine.** Boil the mixture for 5 minutes and allow to cool.
  - Note the color of the precipitate which is cuprous oxide formed due to reduction of cupric sulfate of Benedict's reagent.
- ***Interpretation:*** The change of color from blue to green, yellow, and orange/red depends on the amount of sugar present (Fig. 18.4).

Dipstick Method

- ***Principle:*** Diastix/multistix/dipstix contains: (i) glucose oxidase (ii) peroxidase (iii) chromogen: O-toluidine (clinistix), potassium iodide (multistix/diastix).

  Glucose present in the urine is oxidized by atmospheric oxygen in the presence of glucose oxidase to gluconic acid and hydrogen peroxide. The hydrogen peroxide, in the presence of peroxidase, oxidizes the reduced chromogen present in the dipstick to various shades

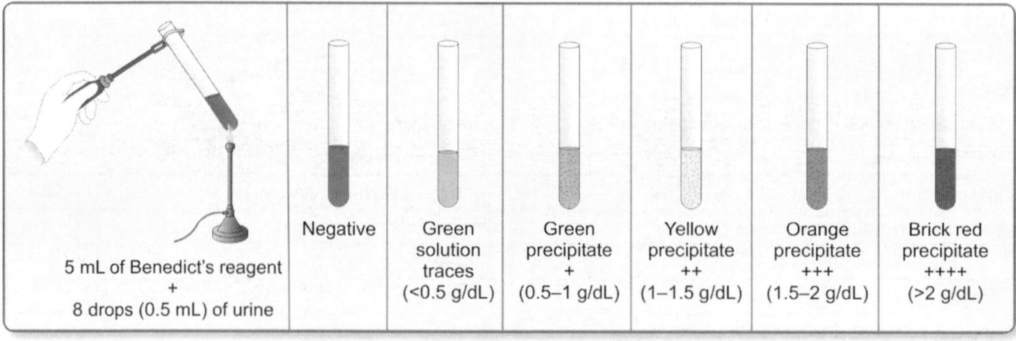

Fig. 18.4: Method and interpretation of Benedict's test

(For color version, see Plate 15)

of purple (oxidized chromogen). The color change depend on the amount of glucose (semi-quantitative) present in the urine.

Step 1:

$$\text{Glucose (in urine)} + \text{oxygen (from air)} \xrightarrow{\text{Glucose oxidase}} \text{Gluconic acid} + H_2O_2$$

Step 2:

$$H_2O_2 + \text{reduced chromogen} \xrightarrow{\text{Peroxidase}} \text{Oxidized chromogen} + H_2O$$

- ***Procedure***
  - The reagent area of the strip is completely immersed in fresh urine for 1–2 seconds. It is taken out and excess urine is drained off.
  - The change in color of the test area is compared with the color chart on the dipstick container exactly after 30 seconds (or as per manufacturer) after dipping the strip in the urine.

Cause of Glycosuria (Tables 18.3 and 18.4)

The substances which may give positive reaction with Benedict's test but negative with glucose oxidase strips are shown in Table 18.4.

Table 18.3: Causes of glycosuria

- Diabetes mellitus
- Pregnancy
- Renal glycosuria
- Alimentary glycosuria
- Endocrine disorders
  - Acromegaly
  - Cushings syndrome
  - Hyperadrenocorticism
  - Functioning α- or β-cell pancreatic tumors
  - Hyperthyroidism
  - Pheochromocytoma
- Increased intracranial tension (brain tumor or hemorrhage).

Table 18.4: Causes of false positivity by nonsugar reducing substances

- Ascorbic acid
- Glucuronic acid
- Homogentisic acid
- Salicylates
- Phenylketonuria
- Tyrosinemia

Ketone Bodies

The presence of ketone bodies in the urine is a measure of the metabolic rather than renal function. Whenever, there is a defect in carbohydrate metabolism, the fat is used as a source of energy. When increased quantities of fat are metabolized, there is increased production of ketone bodies which begin to accumulate in the blood and are subsequently excreted in the urine.

Ketone bodies are three metabolically related compounds:

- Acetoacetic (diacetic) acid
- β-hydroxybutyric acid
- Acetone.

If urine is left at room temperature, acetoacetic acid slowly converts into acetone.

Rothera's Test

- ***Procedure***
  - Take 4 mL of urine in a test tube.
  - Add a few crystals of sodium nitroprusside and saturate the urine with ammonium sulfate by mixing vigorously.
  - Overlay with few drops of liquor ammonia along the wall of the tube.
- ***Interpretation:*** Development of a **purple ring** (Fig. 18.5) indicates the presence of **acetoacetic acid/acetone** or both. A brown or red color is of no significance.

Gerhardt's Test (ferric chloride test)

This is neither a very specific nor a sensitive test. The test **detects acetoacetic acid.**

- ***Procedure***
  - Take 8 mL of urine in a test tube.
  - Add 10% ferric chloride solution drop by drop; a precipitate of ferric phosphate forms.
  - Add more ferric chloride solution till the ferric phosphate precipitate disappears.
  - Filter it and add excess of ferric chloride to the filtrate.
- ***Interpretation:*** A **red color** of the filtrate indicates positive test.

Dipstick Method

- ***Principle:*** Dipstick contains buffers and sodium nitroferricyanide, which react with acetoacetic acid in the urine to form a pink-maroon color in 15 seconds. The strips detect acetoacetic acid and not acetone. However, acetone can be detected if glycine is incorporated into it.

***Causes of ketonuria** (Table 18.5)*

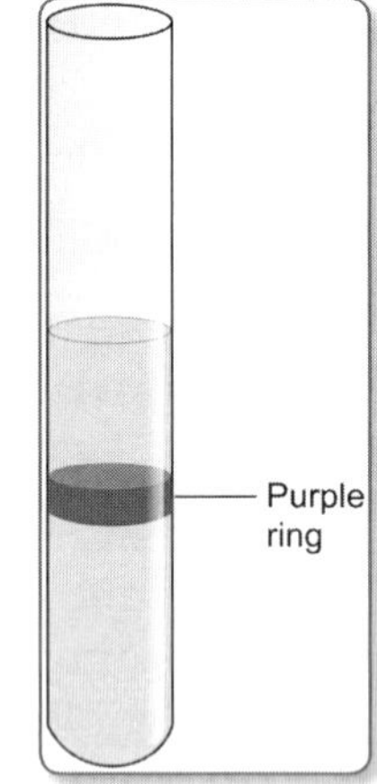

Fig. 18.5: Positive Rothera's test showing a purple ring

Table 18.5: Causes of ketonuria

- Diabetic ketoacidosis
- Starvation
- Prolonged vomiting or diarrhea
- Prolonged febrile illness
- von Gierke's disease
- Eclampsia

Bilirubin (bile pigment)

Tests for bilirubin in urine provide information concerning metabolic or systemic disorders, especially liver function. Bilirubin is a breakdown product of hemoglobin and is normally not present in urine. Even trace amounts are clinically significant and only conjugated bilirubin is found in urine. Bilirubinuria causes yellow-brown to greenish-brown urine and forms yellow foam on shaking. Bilirubin is found only in freshly voided urine which upon standing is oxidized to biliverdin.

Fouchet's Test

- ***Procedure***
  - Take 10 mL of urine in a test tube and add 3 mL of 10% barium chloride solution.
  - Mix the two and filter the mixture through a filter paper. Bilirubin along with barium salt remains on filter paper.
  - Add a few drops of Fouchet's reagent onto the filter paper.
- ***Interpretation:*** **Green** or **blue color** indicates bilirubinuria.

Note: Foam test is a simple test to detect bile pigments at the bed side. Take urine in a test tube and shake the urine. If bile pigments are present in the urine, the foam on top will be yellow in color.

Dipstick Method

- ***Principle:*** The test is **based on a diazo reaction.** Bilirubin in the urine couples with a diazotized dichloroaniline (content of strip) in a strongly acidic medium to form colored compound namely azobilirubin.

Causes of Bilirubinuria

- Obstructive jaundice: Urine shows bilirubin without urobilinogen
- Hepatocellular jaundice: Bilirubin is **absent** in urine of patients with **hemolytic jaundice.**

Urobilinogen

Urobilinogen is normally present in urine in trace amount (1–2 mg/dL) and is insufficient to cause a significant positive reaction. Whenever, the liver is unable to efficiently remove the reabsorbed urobilinogen from the portal circulation (e.g. liver diseases, hemolytic anemia) more urobilinogen than normal is routed through the kidney and hence excreted in the urine.

Ehrlich's Test

- ***Procedure***
  - Take 2.5 mL urine in a test tube.
  - Add 2.5 mL of Ehrlich's aldehyde reagent (paradimethyl amino benzaldehyde). Mix well by inversion.
  - Add 10 mL of saturated sodium acetate solution and mix.
- ***Interpretation:*** Pink to cherry red color indicates presence of urobilinogen.

Dipstick Method

- ***Principle:*** This method is based on the Ehrlich's test. The strip is coated with p-amino benzaldehyde with a color enhancer. It reacts with urobilinogen in a strongly acidic medium to produce a pink-red colored compound. The color is matched with the color chart on the container of the dipsticks.

Causes of Increased Urobilinogen in Urine

- Hemolytic anemias (without bilirubin in urine)
  - Thalassemia
  - Sickle cell anemia
  - Hereditary spherocytosis
- Liver diseases
  - Preicteric phase of infective hepatitis
  - Drugs or toxic hepatitis
  - Cirrhosis.

Causes of Decreased/Absent Urobilinogen in Urine

In **obstructive jaundice,** bilirubin does not reach the intestine and hence is not converted into urobilinogen.

Bile Salts

Bile salts are composed of mixture of bile acids and glycine or taurine. Two important bile salts are sodium and potassium salts of glycocholates and taurocholates. Normally, bile salts are not present in urine.

Hay's Sulfur Test

- ***Procedure:***
  - Take 10 mL urine in a wide bore test tube (2 cm diameter or more) or a small beaker.
  - Sprinkle sulfur powder over its surface, watch for 5 minutes.

- ***Interpretation:*** **Sulfur powder sinks to the bottom** of test tube (Fig. 18.6) in the presence of bile salts in urine.
- ***Precaution:*** Since soap can give false positive result, the test tube should be clean.

Causes: Hepatocellular and obstructive jaundice.

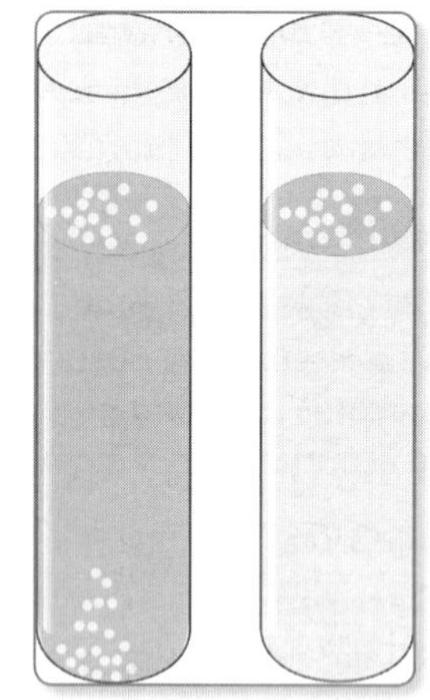

Fig. 18.6: Positive (left) and negative (right) Hay's test

Tests for Blood in Urine

These tests detect hematuria, hemoglobinuria or myoglobinuria.

Hematuria: Presence of red cells in urine, e.g. renal stones, renal cell carcinoma.

Hemoglobinuria: Presence of free hemoglobin in urine, e.g. intravascular hemolysis.

Myoglobinuria: Presence of myoglobin in urine, e.g. crush injury to muscle, strenuous exercise.

Benzidine Test

- ***Procedure:***
  - Dissolve a small amount (knife-point full) of benzidine in 2 mL of glacial acetic acid and add an equal volume of 3% hydrogen peroxide.
  - From the above, take 2 mL in another test tube and add 2 mL of previously boiled and cooled urine and mix.
- ***Control for the test:*** If the test is negative, add a drop of blood to the above test tube. It should give blue color. This is to confirm the potency of reagents especially hydrogen peroxide and excludes a false negative reaction.
- ***Interpretation:*** The appearance of **blue color** indicates the presence of blood.
- ***Precaution:*** Presence of hypochlorite (bleach) and microbial peroxidase can cause false positive results. **Benzidine is carcinogenic**.

Orthotoluidine Test

- ***Procedure:***
  - Take 2 mL of urine in a test tube.
  - Add 1 mL of orthotoluidine solution in glacial acetic acid.
  - Add few drops of hydrogen peroxide.
- ***Interpretation:*** The appearance of blue or green color indicates the presence of blood.

Dipstick Method

Very small amount of hemoglobin/RBCs are detected by dipstick method.

- ***Principle:*** The test is based on the **liberation of oxygen from peroxide in the reagent strip by peroxidase-like activity of heme** present in hemoglobin. The liberated oxygen changes the color of the chromogen. The reagent area is impregnated with organic peroxide and the chromogen is orthotoluidine/tetramethylbenzidine.

$$\text{Organic peroxide} \xrightarrow{\text{(peroxidase from Hb)}} H_2O + O$$

$$O + \text{chromogen} \xrightarrow{\text{(Orthotoludine)}} \text{Oxidized chromogen (colored compound)}$$

Causes of Hematuria

Urine is red colored in severe hematuria and smoky in mild hematuria. RBCs are demonstrable in urinary sediment. Causes of hematuria are shown in Table 18.6.

Table 18.6: Causes of hematuria

Renal diseases
• **Glomerular causes** – Acute glomerulonephritis – Renal infarct – Bacterial endocarditis with kidney involvement – Malignant hypertension
• **Nonglomerular causes** – Polycystic kidneys – Renal cell carcinoma – Renal stones (nephrolithiasis) – Trauma (including renal biopsy) – Renal tuberculosis – Hydronephrosis
Lower urinary tract/prostatic diseases
• Bladder stones (lithiasis) • Cystitis • Urethritis • Carcinoma bladder • Carcinoma prostate
Blood disorders
• Bleeding disorders: Coagulation disorders, severe thrombocytopenia • Acute leukemia • Sickle cell disease
Miscellaneous
• Instrumentation of urinary tract

Multistix Reagent Strips for Urine Testing

These have single/multiple discrete cellulose squares which are impregnated with reagents for testing glucose, protein, pH, specific gravity, hemoglobin, ketone bodies, bilirubin and urobilinogen. There are single test strips, e.g. diastix for glucose and multistix for multiple tests.

Automated Urinalysis

Fully automated urine analyzer provided with automatic functions are presently available, e.g. Uriplus.

Chapter 19

Hematology

Chapter Outline
- Hemoglobin estimation
- Cell count
- Hematocrit
- Erythrocyte sedimentation rate
- Blood grouping
- Peripheral smear staining

HEMOGLOBIN ESTIMATION

One of the important features of anemia is reduction in the red cell mass. Red cell mass can be estimated by measuring hemoglobin (Hb).

Methods of Hemoglobin Estimation

There are several methods for Hb estimation utilizing different principles (Table 19.1). The commonly used methods include colorimetric method, namely Sahli's and cyanmethemoglobin method.

Table 19.1: Methods of hemoglobin estimation

<table>
<tr><th>Method</th><th>Principle</th></tr>
<tr><td>Colorimetric method</td><td rowspan="2">These methods are based on measuring the color of hemoglobin or a hemoglobin derivative in the blood either visually or by photocolorimetry. The optical density of a colored solution is directly proportional to the concentration of the colored material in the solution</td></tr>
<tr><td>• Visual colorimetric method
– Sahli's method or acid hematin method
– Alkaline hematin method</td></tr>
<tr><td>• Photocolorimetric (photoelectric) method
– Cyanmethemoglobin (HiCN) method
– Automated analyzer
– Hemo-cue blood hemoglobin system
– Oxyhemoglobin method
– Haldane method</td><td></td></tr>
<tr><td>Physical method</td><td>Specific gravity</td></tr>
<tr><td>Chemical method</td><td>Iron content of hemoglobin</td></tr>
<tr><td>Gasometric method</td><td>Oxygen combining capacity of hemoglobin</td></tr>
</table>

Sahli's Method or Acid Hematin Method

This is the most popular colorimetric method.

Principle

When blood is added to N /10 HCl, **hemoglobin is converted into acid hematin.** The resulting brown color of acid hematin is matched against the standard brown color of the comparator. The intensity of the brown color depends on the amount of acid hematin produced, which in turn depends on the amount of hemoglobin in the blood sample.

Apparatus (Fig. 19.1)

It consists of:

- Hemoglobin pipette which has one mark of 0.02 mL (20 cu mm)
- A comparator which has a flat surface and a standard brown color
- A square/round tube with markings of hemoglobin percentage (100% = 14.5 g/dL) on one side and hemoglobin (in grams) on the other side
- Glass rod for mixing the blood in the square/round tube
- A dropper to take and transfer N/10 HCl and distilled water into the square tube.

Technique

- Take N/10 HCl with a dropper into the hemoglobinometer tube up to the lowest mark
- Draw blood up to 20 cu mm (0.02 mL) mark of Hb pipette and wipe off the excess blood at nozzle of the pipette with moist cotton. Blood may be taken either from a finger prick or an EDTA vial
- Blood in the Hb pipette is blown into the square tube of hemoglobinometer. Ensure that the entire blood inside the Hb pipette is transferred to the tube
- Wait for 10 minutes for the acid to act on the RBCs which causes lysis of RBCs liberating hemoglobin. The acid converts Hb to acid hematin (About 95% of Hb is converted at the end of 10 minutes, 98% of the color develops at the end of 20 minutes and the maximum color is reached after about 1 hour)
- With the help of a glass rod, mix the acid hematin
- Match the color of the solution in the tube with that of the comparator by holding against the natural light or fluorescent tube light

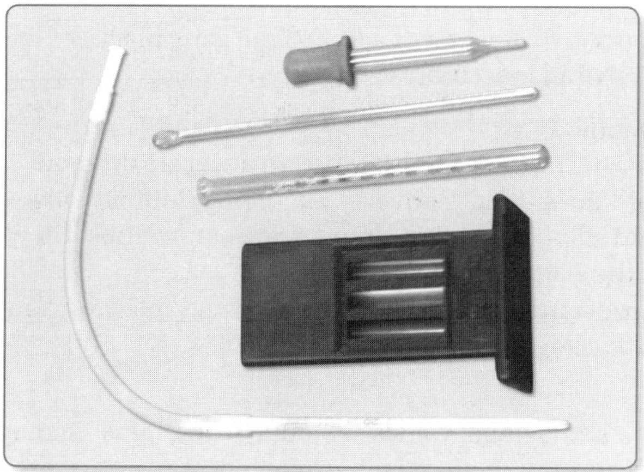

Fig. 19.1: Sahli's hemoglobinometer consisting of Hb pipette, comparator, round tube, glass rod and dropper

- Observe the following which interfere with matching and give wrong reading:
  - Remove the glass rod from the solution in the tube
  - Keep the tube inside the comparator in such a way that the markings do not interfere with the matching exercise
- If the solution in the tube is darker, add distilled water with a dropper and stir the solution with a glass rod. This process is continued till the color of the solution exactly matches the color of the comparator
- Take the tube out and remove the glass rod. Take the reading from the lower meniscus
- Hemoglobin is recorded as gram/dL (or g%).

Sources of error

*a. **Technical errors:*** These are errors inherent in handling the sample.

- **Improper collection:**
  - Improper venipuncture technique may produce hemoconcentration resulting in high hemoglobin value
  - In case of finger prick collection, improper technique or excessive squeezing results in tissue fluid contaminating capillary blood with corresponding error in the Hb value.
- **Improper mixing of blood sample:**
  - If blood is taken from EDTA vial it should be mixed properly before filling the pipette. If not, depending on whether the plasma or the sedimented RBCs have been aspirated in the Hb pipette, it may give rise to false low or high hemoglobin value.
- **Insufficient time for formation of hematin:** A minimum of 10 minutes is required for almost complete conversion of Hb to acid hematin. If reading is taken before, it can give false reading.
- **Time delay:** The brown color of acid hematin is not stable and the color gradually starts fading. Thus, undue delay in taking the reading results in errors.

b. Visual errors:

Comparison of colors is very subjective and can vary from person to person. Hence, the results may not be accurate.

c. Errors inherent in the equipment

- The accuracy of different equipments is not uniform. If Hb pipette has not been accurately calibrated at 0.02 mL it can give rise to wrong values. Calibration of pipettes will reduce the errors
- Color comparators can affect the reading. If the glass blocks of the comparators are old or faded, it may give an inaccurate value.

Disadvantages of the Method

- Apart from the above technical errors, it is **not an accurate method**
- Hydrochloric acid **does not convert all hemoglobins** (like carboxyhemoglobin, methemoglobin and sulphemoglobin) into acid hematin. Thus, Hb value obtained may be slightly lower than the actual Hb
- **Non-hemoglobin substances** such as protein, lipid and cell stroma **interfere** with the color of blood diluted with acid, and hence give false results.

Significance

- **Low Hb values:** Low hemoglobin values are found in **anemias.** Hemoglobin level is directly proportional to the severity of anemia. Morphological typing of the anemia can be done with the help of peripheral smear examination.

- **High Hb values:** High hemoglobin values (more than 18.5 g/dL in males and 16.5 g/dL in females) are seen in polycythemia.

Cyanmethemoglobin (Hemiglobincyanide; HiCN) Method

Cyanmethemoglobin method is the most accurate, convenient, readily available and preferred method for estimation of hemoglobin concentration. It is the standard method used in most of the centers.

Principle

Blood is diluted in a stable standard solution of potassium ferricyanide and potassium cyanide. **Hemoglobin is first oxidized to methemoglobin** (Hi) by the potassium ferricyanide. The cyanide ions (CN^-) of potassium cyanide convert **methemoglobin (Hi) to stable cyanmethemoglobin** (HiCN). The cyanmethemoglobin has a broad absorption, maximum being at a wavelength of 540 nm. Thus, the color of this solution is compared against a standard HiCN solution of known Hb value in a spectrophotometer or photoelectric colorimeter at 540 nm.

Reagents

The diluent is detergent-modified Drabkin solution, the composition of which is shown in Table 19.2.

Drabkin solution should be clear and pale yellow and when measured in the photoelectric colorimeter should give zero reading at 540 nm against water blank. The detergent enhances lysis of RBCs and decreases turbidity due to precipitation of proteins.

Advantages of the Method

- Hb value obtained is **accurate,** since almost all forms of hemoglobin (hemoglobin, oxyhemoglobin, methemoglobin, carboxyhemoglobin, but not sulphemoglobin) are converted into cyanmethemoglobin
- Being a colorimetric method there is direct comparison with HiCN Standard. Thus, **visual error** during matching the color like in Sahli's method is **eliminated**
- Cyanmethemoglobin is a stable compound and **color does not change with time.** So readings can be made at the operator's convenience
- **Easy** to perform the test
- The **standard is stable** and certified cyanmethemoglobin standards are available
- Reagents are readily available.

Disadvantages of the Method

- **Turbidity interferes with the reading:** Any turbidity due to abnormal plasma proteins, hyperlipidemia, high WBC count or fat droplets or in the Drabkin solution itself alters value, and therefore inaccurate Hb values are obtained.

Table 19.2: Constituents of Drabkin solution

Constituent	Quantity
Potassium ferricyanide	400 mg
Potassium cyanide (KCN)	100 mg
Potassium dihydrogen phosphate (anhydrous)	280 mg
Non-ionic detergent *(Sterox SE)*	1 mL
Distilled water	2 liters

- **Poisonous diluents:** Potassium cyanide in the solutions is poisonous, though it is present only in a very low concentration. Hence, the reagents should be handled carefully.
- **Explosive reagent:** Explosion can occur if undiluted reagents are poured in the sink. Hydrogen cyanide is released by acidification and the gas, if it accumulates, can result in explosion. Reagents and samples should be disposed off along with the running water in the sink.

Automated Analyzer (Cell Counter)

These instruments measure not only hemoglobin but also various parameters like cell counts, PCV and absolute values (MCV, MCH and MCHC).

CELL COUNT

Red blood cells, white blood cells and platelets are the formed elements of blood. Their counts are altered in various diseases and the estimation of their counts is a basic hematologic investigation.

Equipment

Hemocytometer: The hemocytometer (Fig. 19.2) is an instrument used for counting blood cells. The commonly used instrument is the improved Neubauer counting chamber.

- **RBC pipette**
- **WBC pipette**

  Note: Unopettes are self-contained diluting device that can eliminate pipetting errors or manual errors and can be used instead of RBC and WBC pipettes.

Uses of the (red/white) glass bead in the bulb of (RBC/WBC) pipette

  - **Identification** of pipette (red in RBC and white in WBC pipette)
  - Helps in **mixing blood** sample with diluting fluid
  - Ensures that the **pipette is dry.** If pipette is wet, the corresponding bead will be sticking to the wall of the pipette.

- **Improved Neubauer counting chamber (Fig. 19.3):** WBC count is performed in the four corner squares and RBC count in the middle square.

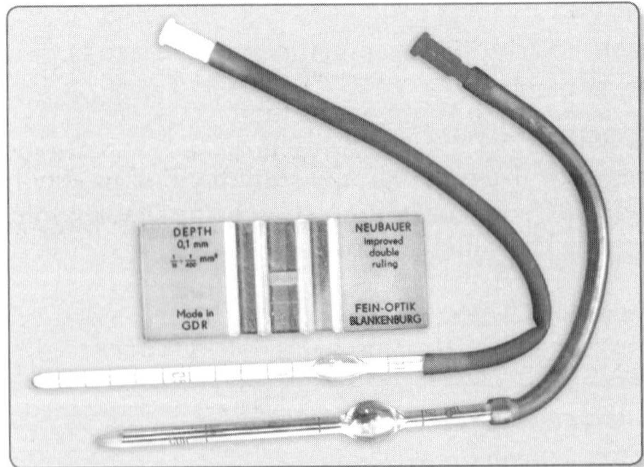

Fig. 19.2: Hemocytometer consisting of improved Neubauer counting chamber in the center with WBC (white bead) and RBC (red bead) pipette

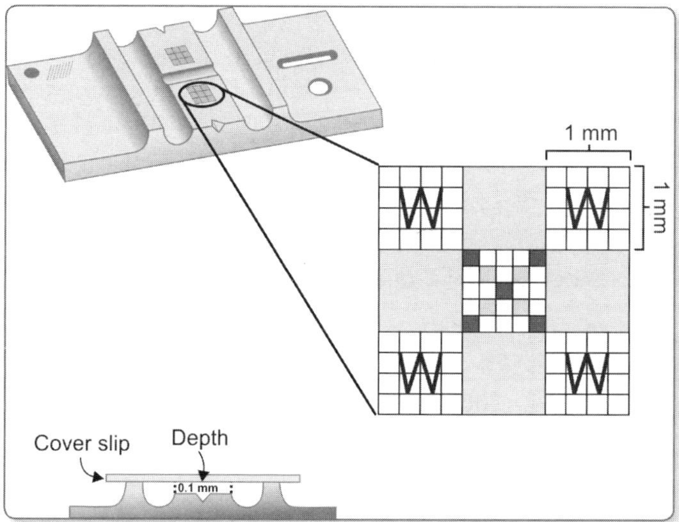

Fig. 19.3: Close-up view of improved Neubauer counting chamber. WBC counting areas marked W and RBC counting area in red square. The entire central square is used for platelet count

Red Blood Cell Count

It can be measured by manual method using an improved Neubauer counting chamber or by automated analyzer.

Manual Method

Equipment

- **Improved Neubauer counting chamber**
- **RBC** pipette (Thoma red cell pipette):
  - It consists of a graduated capillary tube divided into 10 parts marked 0.5 at the fifth mark and 1.0 at the tenth mark
  - The capillary tube opens into a mixing bulb containing a glass bead which facilitates mixing of the blood and the diluent
  - There is another short capillary tube above the bulb marked 101
  - Each pipette is provided with an aspirating tube
  - In the red cell pipette, blood is drawn up to the 0.5 mark and diluent up to the 101 mark. The resulting dilution is 1:200.

While loading the counting chamber, discard the first 2–3 drops since it contains only diluting fluid.

Principle

The blood is diluted with an isotonic solution and the erythrocytes in a portion of the diluted fluid are counted in a hemocytometer under a microscope.

RBC Diluting Fluids

Composition of two types of RBC diluting fluids is shown in Tables 19.3 and 19.4.

Table 19.3: Composition of Hayem's fluid

Constituents	Quantity	Action
Mercuric chloride	0.5 g	Prevents growth of bacteria
Sodium chloride	1.0 g	Provides iso-osmolarity
Sodium sulfate	5.0 g	
Distilled water	200 mL	

Table 19.4: Composition of Dacie's fluid (formal-citrate solution)

Constituents	Quantity	Action
Sodium citrate dihydrate	5.0 g	Anticoagulant
Formalin	1 mL	Fixation of cells, retards bacterial and fungal growth
Distilled water	100 mL	

Technique

- Gently mix the blood in the EDTA vial so that the cells mix well with plasma
- Draw the **blood upto 0.5 mark** of RBC pipette. Wipe off the excess blood from sides of the tip of the pipette
- Dip the tip of the pipette in the **RBC diluting fluid** and draw the fluid **upto mark 101**
- Holding the pipette horizontally in its long axis, rotate it slowly to ensure **thorough mixing of blood and diluent.** This is facilitated by the red bead in the bulb
- Place the cover slip on the ruled area of the chamber
- **Discard the first 2 to 3 drops** (since the fluid has not mixed with blood) of RBC fluid from the pipette
- **Charge the chamber** by placing the tip of the pipette just under the cover slip and allow the fluid to flow by capillary action till the counting chamber is just filled
- Wait for 2–5 minutes for the cells to settle in the chamber
- Examine the central ruled area for red cell counting by examining under low power objective
- **Count RBCs** using high power objective **in the 5 red squares** and total them together
- RBC count = counted cells × 10,000 per cu mm (mm^3) of blood.

Sources of Error

- **Equipment:** Inaccurate graduation of pipette and Neubauer chamber.
- **Improper technique:** Improper blood collection or improper mixing of blood sample.
- **Human errors:** Improper charging of Neubauer chamber.

Normal Range for RBC Count (Table 19.5)

Table 19.5: Normal range of RBC count

Adult male	4.4–6.0 million/cu mm (4.4–6.0 × 10^{12}/L) (4.4–6.0 × 10^6/μL)
Adult female	3.8–5.0 million/cu mm (3.8–5.0 × 10^{12}/L) (3.8–5.0 × 10^6/μL)
At birth	6.0–7.0 million/cu mm (6.0–7.0 × 10^{12}/L) (6.0–7.0 × 10^6/μL)

Note: RBC count is reported as red cells per cubic millimeter (cu mm/mm^3) or 10^{12}/L or 10^6/μL of blood.

Total WBC Count

Total leukocytes/WBC count (TLC) in the blood can be measured either by manual method using an improved Neubauer counting chamber or by automated analyzer.

Manual Method

Equipment

- **Improved Neubauer counting chamber**
- **WBC pipette**
  - The size of the pipette is smaller than that of RBC pipette and it has a white glass bead in the bulb which facilitates mixing of the blood and the diluent
  - It has 3 markings of 0.5, 1 and 11
  - In the white cell pipette, blood is drawn up to the 0.5 mark and diluent up to the 11.0 mark
  - The dilution in this case is 1:20.

Principle

Whole blood is diluted with WBC fluid and the glacial acetic acid in the fluid lyses the red cells. The nuclei of white blood cells are stained by gentian violet, which are counted in the WBC areas in the improved Neubauer counting chamber.

WBC Diluting Fluid

Composition of WBC diluting fluid is shown in Table 19.6.

Table 19.6: Composition of WBC diluting fluid (Turk's Fluid)

Constituents	Quantity	Action
Glacial acetic acid	2 mL	Lyses the RBCs
1% Gentian violet	5 drops	Stains nuclei of WBC
Add water	100 mL	Diluent

Technique

- Gently mix the blood in the EDTA vial, so that the cells mix well with plasma
- Draw the **blood in the WBC pipette upto 0.5 mark.** Wipe off the excess blood from sides of the tip of the pipette
- Dip the tip of the pipette in the **Turk's fluid** and draw the fluid **upto mark 11**
- Holding the pipette horizontally in its long axis, rotate it slowly to ensure thorough mixing of blood and diluent. This is facilitated by the white bead in the bulb
- Place the cover slip on the ruled area of the chamber
- Discard the first 2 to 3 drops (since the fluid has not mixed with blood) of WBC fluid from the pipette
- **Charge the chamber** by placing the tip of the pipette just under the cover slip and allow the fluid to flow by capillary action till the counting chamber is just filled
- Wait for 2–3 minutes for the cells to settle in the chamber
- Examine the ruled WBC areas under the microscope using a low power objective. White cells are identified because of their nuclei stained by gentian violet present in the Turk's fluid
- Count the total number of WBCs in the areas marked in the Fig. 41.2 (in big squares, each area is divided into 16 medium-sized squares)

- WBC count = counted cells × 50/cu mm of blood
- The result thus obtained is expressed as:
  Total WBC = per cu mm (mm^3) of blood.

Sources of Error

- **Equipment:** Inaccurate graduation of pipette and Neubauer chamber.
- **Improper technique**: Improper blood collection or improper mixing of blood sample.
- **Human errors**: Improper charging of Neubauer chamber.

Note:

- When there is marked leukopenia, it is advisable to use 1 in 10 dilutions for greater accuracy by taking blood up to mark 1 instead of 0.5
- In cases of very high WBC counts, a dilution of 1 in 100 or 1 in 200 using RBC pipette may be required for accurate count
- If nucleated red cells (nRBC) are present correction of WBC count should be done.

Uses

- Support diagnosis of various infections and inflammatory lesions
- Diagnosis of myeloproliferative neoplasms, myelodysplastic syndromes, leukemias and various other hematological disorders.

Normal Range for WBC Count (Table 19.7)

Note: Total WBC count is reported as white blood cells per/cubic millimeter (cu mm/mm^3)/ or 10^9/L or 10^3/μL of blood.

Table 19.7: Normal range of WBC count

Adults	4000-11000 cells/cu mm (4–11 × 10^9/L) (4–11 × 10^3/μL)
At birth	8000-22000 cells/cu mm (8–22 × 10^9/L) (8–22 × 10^3/μL)
Childhood	6000-15000 cells/cu mm (6–15 × 10^9 /L) (6–15 × 10^3/μL)

Platelet Count

Manual Method

Equipment

- Improved Neubauer counting chamber
- WBC pipette

Principle

Anticoagulated blood is diluted with a diluent that lyses the red cells (e.g. 1% ammonium oxalate) leaving visible platelets. Dacie's fluid and Rees-Ecker fluid can also be used for RBC count.

Platelet Diluting Fluids

- **These include Dacie's fluid** (Table 19.8, Rees-Ecker fluid and Brecher-Cronkite fluid).

Technique

- Gently mix the blood in the EDTA vial, so that the cells mix well with plasma
- Draw the **blood in the WBC pipette up to 0.5 mark.** Wipe off the excess blood from sides of the tip of the pipette

- Dip the tip of the pipette in 1% ammonium oxalate (Brecher-Cronkite fluid) and draw the **fluid up to mark 11**
- Holding the pipette horizontally in its long axis, rotate it slowly to ensure thorough mixing of blood and diluent. This is facilitated by the white bead in the bulb
- Place the cover slip on the ruled area of the chamber
- Discard the first 2 to 3 drops (since the fluid has not mixed with blood) of fluid from the pipette
- **Charge the chamber** by placing the tip of the pipette just under the cover slip and allow the fluid to flow by capillary action till the counting chamber is just filled
- Keep the charged chamber in a petri dish with wet filter paper at the bottom for 5 minutes for the platelets to settle down
- Platelets are counted in the entire central 1 × 1 mm square
- Platelets appear as highly refractile small structures. They are visualized easily with the following adjustments of the microscope:
  - Reducing the illumination by closure of the iris diaphragm
  - Lowering the condenser
  - Carefully altering the focus with fine adjustment
- Platelet count = Total counted platelets in the central square × 200 per cu mm of blood.

Automated Analyzer

RBC, WBC and platelet count can also be obtained by electronic particle counters.

Normal Range

- 1,50,000 to 4,50,000 platelets per cu mm (150–450 × 10^9/L) (150–450 × 10^3/μL)

Note: Platelet count is reported as number of platelets per cubic millimeter (cu mm/mm^3) or 10^9/L or × 10^3/μL of blood.

Decreased Platelet Count (thrombocytopenia): refer Table 12.30.

Table 19.8: Composition of Dacie's fluid

Constituents	Quantity	Actions
Sodium citrate dihydrate	5 g	Prevents coagulation
Formalin	1 mL	Fixation of cells, retards bacterial and fungal growth
0.2% brilliant cresyl blue	0.1 mL	Stains platelets
Distilled water	100 mL	

The above fluid is used as a stock solution, which is diluted 1 in 10 before use

HEMATOCRIT

Q. Write short note on packed cell volume/hematocrit.

Introduction: Hematocrit **(packed cell volume)** is the ratio of the volume of red cells to that of the whole blood. It indicates relative volume of red cells and plasma (*e.g.* in anemia red cells are reduced with corresponding reduction in the hematocrit).

Wintrobe Method

Wintrobe tube (Fig. 19.4): It is a special thick-walled glass tube measuring **11 cm in length** and an internal diameter of 2.5 mm, with a capacity of 1 mL. This is calibrated at 1 mm intervals up

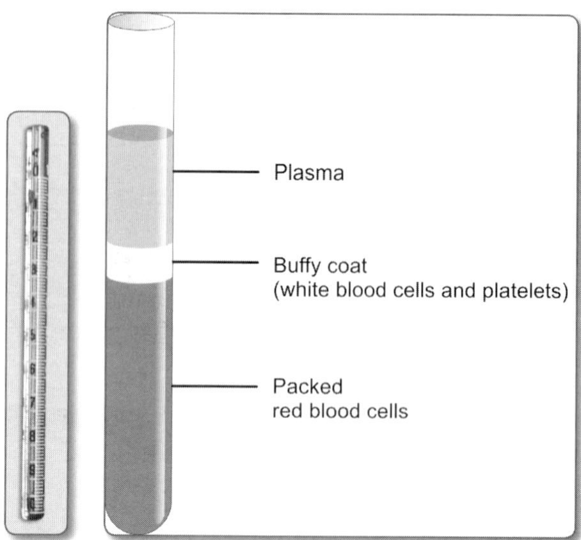

Fig. 19.4: Wintrobe tube (left) and different columns after the blood is centrifuged (right)

to 105–110 mm with bold markings from top as 0, 10, 20, 30,...100 for ESR and 100, 90, 80,...10, 0 for PCV. The markings are in descending order from the top for PCV estimation and markings in ascending order from the top for ESR determination.

Anticoagulants used: EDTA, dry heparin or double oxalate.

Principle

Anticoagulated whole blood is centrifuged at a standard speed (3500 RPM). RBCs which are heavier than white cells, platelets and plasma, sediment at the bottom and the volume of red cell mass denotes the hematocrit.

Method

- Collect the blood in an EDTA vial. Mix the blood sample properly so as to mix both plasma and cells
- With the help of a Pasteur's pipette (dropper with long, thin capillary tube like nozzle) draw the blood from the vial
- Place the nozzle of pipette at the bottom of dry and clean Wintrobe tube
- Slowly press the rubber teat of the pipette and fill the tube till the top mark of 100. Avoid any air bubble being trapped during filling of the tube
- Centrifuge the tube at 3500 RPM for half an hour
- Take the reading of packed red cells from bottom
- It is expressed as percentage.

Different Layers (Fig. 19.4)

- **Lower layer:** This consists of red blood cells (packed).
- **Middle layer:** It is also called buffy coat and is the thin red-gray layer between the red cells and plasma consisting of WBC and platelets.
- **Upper layer:** This layer is composed of the plasma which is normally clear or straw colored.
- Conditions causing changes in appearances of plasma are shown in Table 19.9.

Additional information from the Wintrobe method: PCV value is required to determine the red cell indices, namely MCV and MCHC.

Table 19.9: Interpretation of plasma column

Color	Condition
Clear/straw	Normal
Yellow (orange, green)	Jaundice
Opaque/turbid	Hyperlipidemia
Pink/red	Hemoglobinemia (hemolysis) as in PNH

Buffy coat gives an approximate indication of the number of WBCs (normally 0.1 mm of this layer = 1000 WBC/cu mm). Thickness of the buffy coat increases with marked leukocytosis, as in CML, CLL and acute leukemias. Absent or minimal buffy coat implies leukopenia.

Other uses of Buffy Coat

- Subleukemic leukemia—a smear made from the buffy coat has greater concentration of WBCs and identification of abnormal cells is easier
- LE cell test

Microhematocrit Method

A heparinized capillary tube is used and the blood is filled by capillary action. One end is sealed and it is centrifuged in a special centrifuge. As the tubes are not graduated, the PCV is measured using a special chart.

Advantages

- Easy
- Small quantity of blood is needed (useful in pediatric patients)
- Capillary blood is sufficient
- Less time
- Amount of plasma trapped in the red cell column is less, thereby minimizing the error.

Disadvantage

It requires a special (expensive) centrifuge.

Automated Analyzer

Nowadays, automated analyzers are available for estimation of hematocrit.

Normal range for PCV: Hematocrit is expressed as a percentage (e.g. 45%) or as a decimal fraction (e.g. 0.45). It is useful for evaluating absolute values like MCV and MCHC.

Males	40–50%
Females	36–46%
Infants	45–70% (cord blood)

ERYTHROCYTE SEDIMENTATION RATE

Q. Write short note on Erythrocyte sedimentation rate (ESR).

Erythrocyte sedimentation rate (ESR) estimation is a commonly used nonspecific test in routine clinical practice.

Principle: When anticoagulated blood is placed in a vertical tube and is allowed to stand, RBCs settle towards the bottom of the tube. The speed of sedimentation of red cells in plasma over a period of 1 hour is measured by the length of the sedimented RBC column and is expressed in millimeters. RBCs have net negative charge on their surface and tend to repel each other.

The repulsive forces are partially or totally counteracted if there is an increase in the positively charged plasma proteins.

Factors Affecting ESR

- **Plasma factors:** An accelerated ESR is favored by elevated levels of fibrinogen, globulins and cholesterol (which increase the positive charge of plasma) whereas albumin and lecithin retard ESR.
- **Red cell factors:** The sedimentation rate is directly proportional to the weight of the cell aggregates and inversely proportional to the surface area.
  - **Number:** Anemia increases the ESR and polycythemia decreases.
  - **Size:** Microcytes sediment slower than macrocytes.
  - **Rouleaux formation:** It accelerates the ESR.
  - Red cells with an **abnormal or irregular shape**, such as sickle cells or spherocytes, do not exhibit rouleaux formation and have low ESR.
- **Technical factors:** ESR tube must be kept vertical, otherwise it results in inaccurate ESR.

Stages of ESR

Sedimentation occurs in three stages:

- **Stage of aggregation/rouleaux formation**: In the initial 10 minutes, there is little sedimentation as rouleaux form and the size of the rouleaux formed influence the speed of sedimentation.
- **Stage of settling**: For about 40 minutes, settling occurs at a constant rate.
- **Stage of packing**: Packing of RBCs occurs in the final 10 minutes.

Methods

The two commonly employed methods are: Westergren and Wintrobe methods.

Westergren Method

Equipment (Fig. 19.5)

Westergren tube is a straight glass pipette (open at both ends) 30 cm in length, bore of 2.55 mm and calibrated in millimeters from 0–200. The capacity of tube is about 1 mL. The tube is vertically placed on the Westergren rack.

Anticoagulant used: 3.8% trisodium citrate

Ratio of blood and anticoagulant: 2 mL of whole blood in 0.5 mL of 3.8% trisodium citrate. Blood to anticoagulant ratio should be 4:1.

Procedure

- A Westergren pipette is filled upto the 0 mark and placed vertically in the Westergren rack at room temperature
- After 60 minutes, the distance between the top of the red cell column and 0 mark is noted in millimeters as ESR reading.

Result: ESR is expressed as mm at the end of one hour.

Advantage

This is a more sensitive and accurate method when compared to the Wintrobe method. This is because the column is longer, i.e. 200 mm.

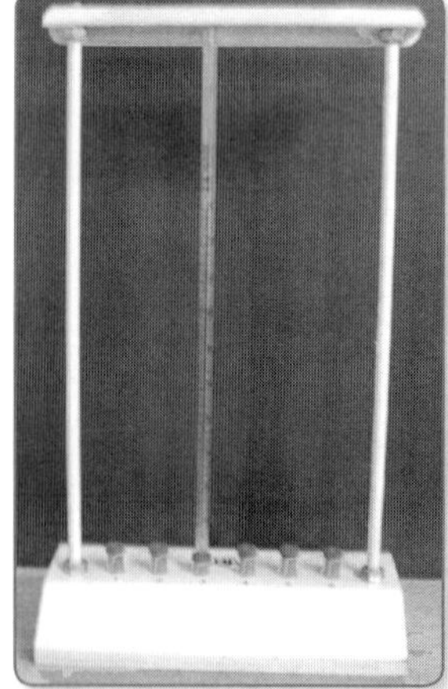

Fig. 19.5: Westergren pipette placed vertically in the rack

Disposable Methods

Disposable ESR kits are more convenient, where the ESR pipette sucks the blood to fill precisely to the zero mark. This eliminates risky mouth pipetting of blood.

Wintrobe Method

Wintrobe tube can be used first for estimation of ESR and then it is centrifuged for estimation of hematocrit.

Advantages

- It is simple and requires small amount of blood
- Same tube can be used for both ESR and PCV
- Buffy coat smear is useful in cases of leukopenia, subleukemic/aleukemic leukemia and for LE cell test.

Disadvantage

ESR value higher than PCV column can not be obtained by this method.

Alternative Methods

- Capillary method (micro ESR method) requires only 0.2 mL of blood, so it is useful in pediatric patients. The results are precise and reading time is 20 minutes
- Zeta Sedimentation Rate
- Automated ESR (e.g. Ves-Matic benchtop analyzer): Results are obtained within 30 minutes and are comparable with Westergren 1 hour reading.

Significance of ESR

ESR is a prognostic test rather than a diagnostic test. It is useful in monitoring disease activity. Note:

- ESR may be rarely normal in patients with neoplasms, connective tissue diseases and infections. A normal ESR cannot be used to exclude these diagnostic possibilities
- ESR is one of the Jones minor criteria for the diagnosis of rheumatic fever.

Causes of Increased ESR (Table 19.10)

Table 19.10: Causes of increased ESR

Markedly increased in:
• Multiple myeloma
• Macroglobulinemia
• Hyperfibrinogenemia
Moderately increased in:
• Infective diseases like tuberculosis
• Chronic inflammatory diseases
– Rheumatic fever
– Autoimmune diseases: Rheumatoid arthritis, SLE, etc.
• Neoplasia

BLOOD GROUPING

More than 400 red blood cell antigens have been identified, most of which are inherited in a Mendelian dominant fashion and only few are clinically important. These antigens form more than 20 genetically determined blood group systems.

The two most important blood group systems are ABO and Rh systems.

ABO Blood Group System

ABO Antigens

According to the ABO blood group system, there are four different kinds of blood groups: A, B, AB or O. The antigen on red cells may be A/B/AB or no antigen at all. There are two subgroups in group A, namely A_1 and A_2. A and B antigens are inherited as per the Mendelian laws. Each individual inherits two ABO genes, one from each parent and these genes determine the ABO antigens on their red blood cells. Absence of both antigens, A and B on the red cells is seen in blood group O.

ABO Antibodies

Natural ABO Antibodies

The serum contains naturally occurring antibodies against red cell A/B/AB antigens (Table 19.11). These are of IgM type and do not cross the placental barrier.

The serological typing indicates the phenotype and family studies indicate the genotype. Genotype refers to the genes present and the phenotype is the red cell antigen on the cell surface.

Table 19.11: ABO phenotypes ("blood groups") and genotype

Phenotype (blood group)	Antigens on RBCs	Antibodies in serum	Genotypes
A	A	Anti-B	AA or AO
B	B	Anti-A	BB or BO
AB	A and B	Neither	AB
O	Neither	Anti-A and Anti-B	OO

Acquired ABO Antibodies

- An individual lacking a particular antigen may develop an antibody after (acquired) exposure to red blood cells carrying the corresponding antigen.
- Exposure occurs due to parenteral introduction of red cell antigens. This may develop during:
  - Transfusion of red cells: These acquired antibodies cause hemolytic transfusion reaction.
  - Pregnancy: Passage of fetal red cells (having paternal antigens foreign to the mother) into the maternal circulation during pregnancy may result in mainly IgG type of antibodies. They can cross the placental barrier resulting in hemolytic disease of the newborn. The most important acquired *antibody* is anti-D, which is a major cause of hemolytic disease of the newborn.

H Genes and H Antigens

The expression of A and B antigens are dependent on the presence of H gene. Most of the individuals are homozygous for the H gene. The sequence of events in the formation of A and B red cell antigens is:

- A and B red cell antigens are glycoproteins and their formation starts with basic precursor substance (Fig. 19.6)
- Basic precursor substance is first converted into H substance (by transferase) under the influence of H gene.

Q. Write short note Bombay blood group.

- H substance is partially converted under the influence of A and B genes (and specific transferase) into A and B antigens. Some of the H substance remains unconverted
- Since O group individuals do not have A and B genes, neither A nor B antigen is formed and these have only H substance (H substance remains unchanged).

Note: A, B and H antigens may be detected in the saliva and other body fluids also. Such individuals are called **secretors,** while the remaining without it are **nonsecretors.**

Bombay Blood Group

In 1952, Bhende, Bhatia and Deshpande discovered a new blood group known as Bombay blood group (phenotype Oh). These individuals lack the H gene, and therefore the basic

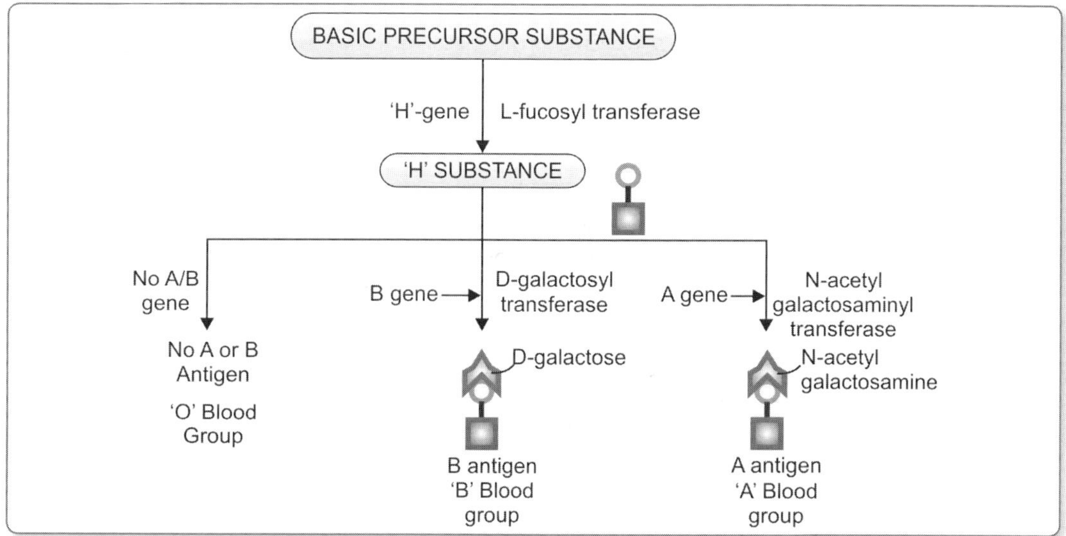

Fig. 19.6: Role of H gene in the formation of A and B antigens

precursor substance cannot be converted into H substance. This in turn results in failure to form A or B antigen. When their blood sample is tested for routine ABO grouping, they will be labeled as blood group O. However, their serum contains anti-A, anti-B and anti-H antibodies. These individuals, therefore, should be transfused with only Bombay blood group.

ABO Grouping Technique

ABO grouping is carried out by making a 2% saline suspension of red cells and adding anti-A, anti-B and anti-AB sera.

The different methods available are:

- Slide or tile technique
- Tube technique
- Microplate method
- Microtyping system
- Automated or semi-automated method.

The slide technique is easier to do and is described below.

Slide or Tile Technique

- Take a slide/white tile and mark it anti-A, anti-B and anti-AB
- Put one drop each of anti- A, anti-B and anti-AB sera on the marked slide
- Add one drop of washed 2% red cell suspension to each anti-sera
- Mix each one separately with clean applicator stick and spread the mixture over an area of 2 cm
- Rock the slide gently and look for "agglutination" within 5 minutes.

Interpretation: Blood group A, B, AB or O is interpreted depending on the agglutination in the anti-sera (Table 19.12 and Fig. 19.7).

Tube Technique

- Take 3 test tubes (75 × 10 mm size) and label them as anti-A, anti-B and anti-AB, respectively
- Add one drop each of the corresponding serum to each tube (i.e. anti-A, anti-B and anti-AB).

Table 19.12: Interpretation of ABO Grouping

	Antisera added		Interpretation
Anti-A	*Anti-B*	*Anti-AB*	*Blood group*
–	–	–	O
+	–	+	A
–	+	+	B
+	+	+	AB

+ = Agglutination; – = No agglutination

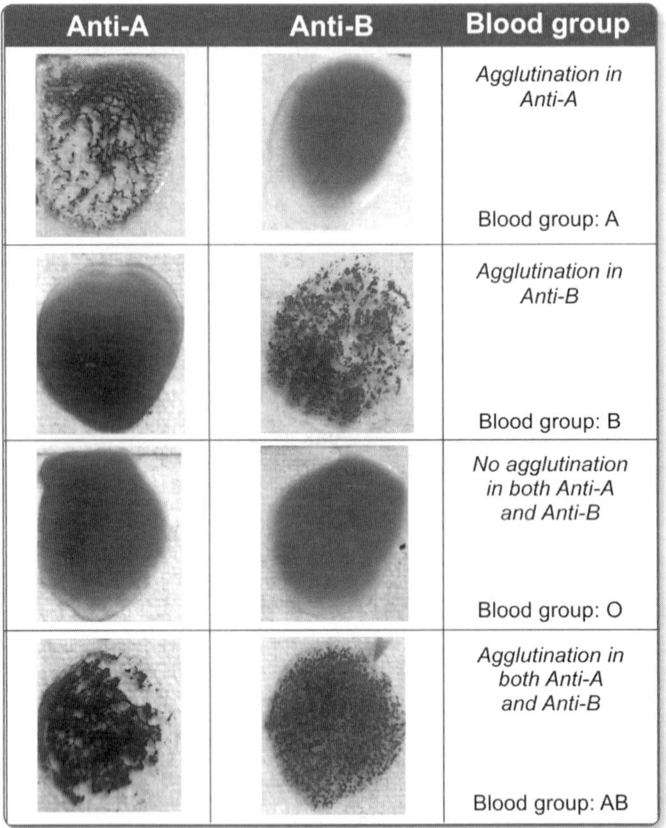

Fig. 19.7: Interpretation of blood group by slide method

- Add 1 drop of 2% red cells suspension to each one of the three test tubes and mix them gently
- Leave the tubes at room temperature for 90 minutes (or centrifuge for 15–20 minutes)
- Look for agglutination
- Transfer one drop of mixture from each tube onto a glass slide, using a thin bore Pasteur pipette. Spread the cells over an area of 2 × 1 cm, using the pipette
- Examine the slide under microscope for "agglutination".

Interpretation: Blood group is interpreted depending upon the agglutination in the anti-sera (Table 19.12).

Controls

Each blood group test should preferably have controls, both positive and negative.

Positive control: This is run by performing the above techniques by using cells of known groups A, B, AB and O. This is especially useful for testing the potency of anti-sera.

Negative control: Run the above tests by adding saline instead of anti-sera. If agglutination develops it indicates autoagglutination or pseudoagglutination.

Microplate Method

Microplate method is ideal for testing large number of blood samples and has replaced test tube method in many laboratories. Microplates are polystyrene plates having 96 small well. It saves time and cost.

Microtyping System (Gel Card)

Microtyping system (MTS) is a gel-based technology in which plastic cards contain microtubes filled with buffered dextran gel. The gel contains sodium azide (preservative) and group specific antisera (anti-A, anti-B, anti-AB, anti-D) or antiglobulin (for Coombs test). These constituents are incorporated into gel at the time of manufacture.

Rh Blood Group System

Rh blood group system is the second system of clinical significance in transfusion medicine. This is a complete system of antigens which are labeled as D, d, C, c, E and e. The D antigen is highly immunogenic. Cc *and Ee antigens* are weak antigens, and therefore risk of sensitization to these antigens is less than the risk of sensitization to D.

Rh (D) System

Rh Antigen

Rh positive (+ve)

Individuals who have D antigen on the red cell surface are Rh positive (+). This may be present as homozygous (DD) or heterozygous (Dd) state.

Rh negative (-ve)

Individuals who lack the D antigens are called as Rh-negative.

Rh Antibodies

- In contrast to ABO system, there are no naturally occurring antibodies against Rh antigens in Rh negative individuals
- Acquired (immune) antibodies: Rh antibodies develop after exposure to Rh antigens either following transfusion (Rh +ve blood given to Rh -ve patients) or pregnancy (Rh +ve fetus in an Rh -ve mother). These antibodies are of IgG type and do not bind complement. They can be detected by antiglobulin test (Coombs test).

Clinical Significance

- Rh incompatibility between donor and recipient results in hemolytic transfusion reactions
- Rh incompatibility between mother and fetus results in hemolytic disease of the newborn (HDN).

Rh (D) Typing Techniques

The different methods available are:

- Slide or tile technique
- Tube technique
- Microplate method
- Microtyping System
- Automated or semi-automated method.

Slide or Tile Techniques

- Place one drop of anti-Rh (D) reagent (should be monoclonal IgM type) on a slide/white tile
- Add 1 drop of 2% red cell suspension
- Mix them using a clean applicator stick
- Observe for agglutination after 2 minutes.

Interpretation: Presence of agglutination indicates that the blood sample is Rh +ve.

Tube Techniques

- Add one drop of anti-D to a small test tube (75 × 10 mm size)
- Add 1 drop of 2% saline red cell suspension
- Mix them and incubate at 37°C for 30 minutes or centrifuge for 15 to 20 seconds
- Look for agglutination
- Transfer one drop of the mixture onto a glass slide, using a thin bore Pasteur pipette. Spread the cells over an area of 2 × 1 cm using the pipette
- Examine the slide under microscope for "agglutination".

Interpretation: Presence of agglutination indicates Rh +ve blood group.

Controls

Known Rh +ve and Rh –ve samples should be run as positive and negative controls.

PERIPHERAL SMEAR STAINING

Peripheral smear (peripheral blood film) is the most important, valuable and frequently asked investigation in hematology laboratory. It provides the following information:

- **Red cell morphology:** Morphological features of RBCs are important for diagnosis of anemias and other hematologic disorders.
- **WBC disorders and differential leukocyte count** (DLC): Quantitative and qualitative changes in WBCs help in diagnosis of both hematologic and non-hematologic disorders.
- **Platelet number and morphology**: These features are useful in the diagnosis of bleeding disorders.
- **Cross check the CBC parameters:** It helps in cross-checking the complete blood count (CBC) parameters derived from automated cell counters.
- Detection of **blood parasites** (hemoparasites).

Stains for Blood Smear

- The blood cells contain cellular structures which vary in their reaction (pH), some are acidic and others being basic
- The aniline dyes used in staining blood smears are of two general classes: basic dyes, such as methylene blue, and acidic dyes, such as eosin

- All stains which are made of combinations of acidic and basic dyes are called **Romanowsky stains.** The differences between the various Romanowsky stains are mainly in the proportion of the reagents and in their preparation.

Romanowsky Stains

A mixture of methylene blue (basic stain) and eosin (acidic stain) was first prepared by Romanowsky in 1891 and employed on his work on malarial parasite. The action of these stains depends on compounds formed by the interaction of methylene blue and eosin. Methylene blue on oxidation produces colored compounds called azures that have the ability to combine with eosin. Oxidation is achieved during maturation/chemical treatment of the stain. The azures are responsible for different shades of staining in the smears.

- Nuclei and structures in the blood which are stained by the basic dyes are called basophilic
- Structures that take up only acidic dyes are called acidophilic or eosinophilic.

Romanowsky group includes the following stains:

- ***Leishman stain*** which contains Leishman powder and acetone free methyl alcohol (methanol).
  - Preparation of stain: Dissolve 1 g of Leishman powder in 500 mL of acetone free methyl alcohol in a conical flask. Warm it at 50^0C for 15 minutes. Keep it for ripening by exposing to sunlight for 2 days. **Acetone free methyl alcohol** acts as a **fixative**. Since acetone destroys the cells, methyl alcohol should be free from acetone.
- ***Giemsa stain*** contains Giemsa stain powder, glycerol and acetone free methyl alcohol.
- ***Wright stain***
- ***Jenner stain***
- ***Jenner-Giemsa stain***

Preparation of the Peripheral Blood Smear (Figs 19.8A to D)

- A drop of blood is placed on a clean grease free glass slide 1 cm away from one end
- Take a spreader (either another slide or a narrower piece of slide with smooth edge) and place its smooth edge over the drop of blood so as to spread the blood along its edge
- Place the slide at about 30° to 40° angle and make the smear with a smooth (not jerky) forward movement. The resulting ideal smear should be about 2.5 to 3.5 cm in length
- Allow it to dry at room temperature and label.

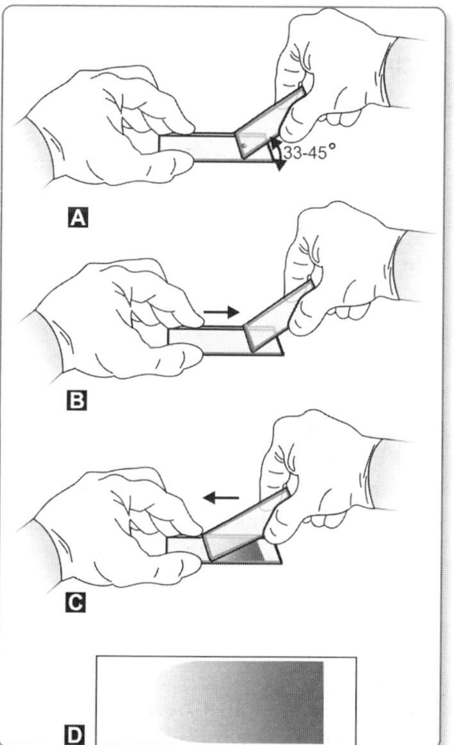

Figs 19.8A to D: Different steps in the preparation of peripheral blood smear and appearance of a well-made smear

Features of a Well-made Peripheral Smear

- Length: Smear should be 2/3 to 3/4 of the length of the slide.
- Shape: The smear should be either tongue or finger-shaped (smooth without any irregularities or holes).

Fixation of the Smear

- The blood smears should be fixed within 4 hours for good staining

- Blood films are 'fixed' by **acetone-free methyl alcohol** which is present in most of the commonly used stains, namely Leishman or Wright or Giemsa stain
- It can also be fixed by dipping the slide 8 to 10 times in a coplin jar with methyl alcohol.

Staining of the Smear

Staining of the smears is carried out using *Romanowsky stains* which stain red cells, white cells, platelets and parasites.

Procedure of Staining with Leishman Stain

- Keep the peripheral smear on the staining rack
- **Pour the undiluted stain** on the slide with a dropper so that stain covers the entire upper surface of slide
- Wait for **2 minutes** for the methyl alcohol to **fix the smear**. Then pour double the amount of buffer water on the slide. Gently mix using a dropper
- Wait for another **8–10 minutes** (time depends on the batch of stain) for **staining**. Look for greenish metallic scum to appear
- Displace the stain by pouring running water from one side of the slide so that the stain scum is drained off the slide and no more stain is left on the slide
  - Precaution: Do not discard the stain from slide by just tilting it, since it will result in stain precipitates over the smear.
- Remove the slide from staining rack and keep it in slanting position to dry it up
- Examine the slide under microscope.

Examination of A Peripheral Blood Smear

A well prepared peripheral smear usually has three parts namely, head, body and tail. The best area of the smear to study the morphology of cells is the body, where the cells are well separated out and touch one another without overlapping. Apply a thin layer of oil over the smear which makes the appearance of cells very clear.

First look under low power, followed by high power and oil immersion. Observe the following:

- The **quality of the film** and uniformity of staining
- **Red blood cells:** Select an area (best between tail and body of the smear) suitable for examination of red cells in the thin area of the smear where the red cells are evenly placed and just touch each other. Look for number, distribution and staining of the red cells, degree of rouleaux formation if present.
- **White blood cells:** Number and distribution of white cells
- **Platelets:** Number and distribution
- **Hemoparasites** (such as malaria, microfilaria)
- **Any abnormal cells.**

Red Blood Cells

Red cells are examined for: (1) size, (2) shape, (3) color, (4) inclusions, and (5) other abnormalities.

1. **Size:** In the peripheral smear, size of the red blood cells is compared with that of a small lymphocyte which has size of about 7-8 μm. The red cells are called microcytic if smaller than small lymphocyte and macrocytic if larger than 9 μm. Appearance of size variation and conditions responsible for these variations are shown in Fig. 19.9.

TERM	DESCRIPTION	APPEARANCE	CONDITION
Normocyte	• Normal RBC is biconcave, 7.2 μm in diameter	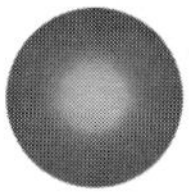	• Normal RBC • Normocytic normochromic anemia
Microcyte	• RBCs smaller than normal and less than 6 μm in diameter		• Iron deficiency anemia • Thalassemia
Macroovalocyte	• Larger than normal, more than 9 μm in diameter and also oval	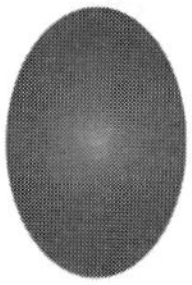	• Megaloblastic anemia due to vitamin B_{12} and folic acid deficiency
Anisocytosis	• Variation in size	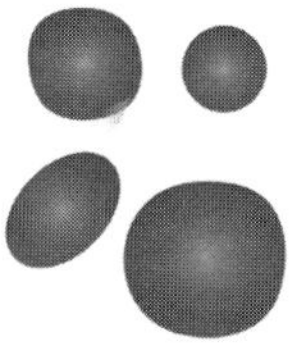	• Severe anemia of any type

Fig. 19.9: Variation in size of red blood cells and associated conditions

2. **Shape:** Variation in red cell shape and conditions responsible for these variations are shown in Figs 19.10.
3. **Color:** Variations in red cell color are depicted in Fig. 19.11.
   - Sometimes red cells appear to be hyperchromic without a central area of pallor. This is not actually due to an increase in the concentration of hemoglobin in the cell, but due to change in cell shape and increase in the thickness of the cell membrane in macrocytes.
4. **Inclusions in the red cells.**
5. **Other abnormalities:** Example, rouleaux formation.

White Blood Cells

White cells (leukocytes) are examined for the following features:

- **Number:** Note whether the number is decreased, normal or increased.
  - Assessment of approximate total white cell count: Observe at least 10 high power fields in the thick portion of the smear where red blood cells overlap. Estimate the approximate number of WBCs/high power filed. Each WBC/high power field is approximately equivalent to 2,000 WBC/cu mm.
- **Abnormal or immature forms**
- **Predominant cell type:** This is determined by performing the differential white cell count. At least 100 white cells should be counted. Normal range of differential leukocyte count is shown in Table 19.13
- Varous types of normal leukocytes in peripheral blood are shown in Fig. 19.12.

Platelets

They are examined for the following features under oil immersion. A single platelet under oil immersion is equivalent to 15,000 to 20,000 platelets/cu mm.

TERM	DESCRIPTION	APPEARANCE	CONDITION
Normal	• Biconcave, flattened on smear		• Normal
Poikilocytosis	• Variation in shape		• Severe anemia
Target cells or Leptocytes	• Only the periphery and the central regions of the cell appear hemoglobinized		• Thalassemia • Sickle cell anemia • Hemolytic anemia • Post splenectomy • Liver disease
Sickle cells	• Thin, elongated, slightly curved and have shape of a sickle		• Sickle cell anemia
Pencil-shaped cells	• Elongated thin cells (exaggerated ovalocytes)		• Iron deficiency anemia
Teardrop and pear-shaped cells	• RBCs have a teardrop or pear-like shape		• Myelofibrosis • Marrow infiltration

Fig. 19.10: Common Variation in shape of red blood cells and associated conditions

TERM	DESCRIPTION	APPEARANCE	CONDITION
Normochromic	Cell with central 1/3 pallor		• Normal RBC
Hypochromic	Central pallor more then 1/3		• Iron deficiency anemia • Thalassemia
Polychromasia	Cells stained purple and are larger than normal		• Hemolytic anemia • Response to therapy in deficiency anemia

Fig. 19.11: Variation in color of red blood cells

- **Number:** Normal/increased/decreased.
- **Form:** Note the size and shape.
- **Aggregation:** Smears made from finger-prick show aggregation of platelets or platelet clumps.

Table 19.13: Normal range of different leukocyte count (DLC)

Type of white blood cells	Normal range
Granulocytes	
• Neutrophil (polymorphonuclear leukocyte)	40–70% (2.0–7.0 × 10^9/L)
• Eosinophil	1–6% (0.02–0.5 × 10^9/L)
• Basophil	0–1% (0.02–0.1 × 10^9/L)
Lymphocytes	20–40% (1.0–3.0 × 10^9/L)
Monocyte	2–10% (0.2–1.0 × 10^9/L)

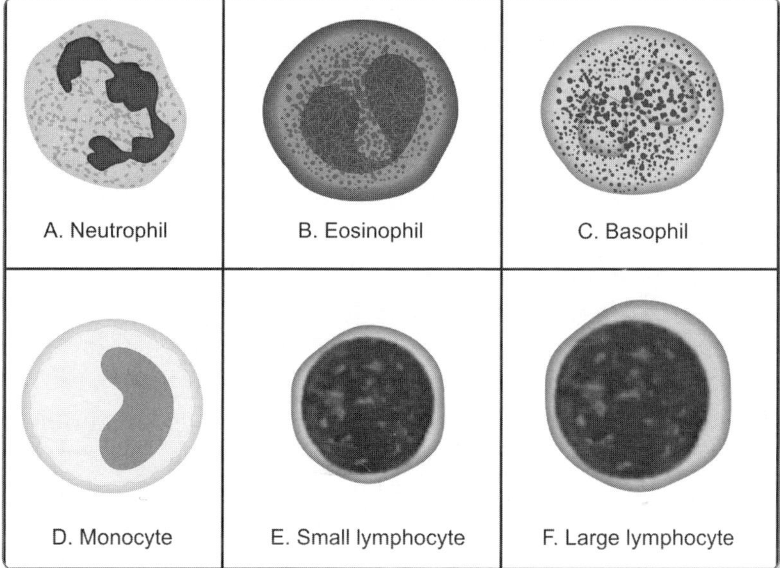

Fig. 19.12: Types of white blood cells

Hemoparasites

1. **Malaria:** Malarial parasites can be demonstrated in the peripheral smear; most common are *Plasmodium* vivax and *P. falciparum*.

   Plasmodium vivax: In the peripheral blood usually ring stage, the trophozoites schizonts and rarely gametocytes of *Plasmodium* vivax may be found.

   Plasmodium falciparum: In *falciparum* infections usually only ring stage and gametocytes may be demonstrated.
2. **Filariasis:** *Microfilaria* can also be demonstrated in peripheral blood.
3. **Trypanosomes:** These are motile flagellate protozoa.
4. ***Leishmania donovani:*** It causes **kala-azar,** amastigote forms known as LD bodies can be found in the reticuloendothelial cells of the bone marrow, spleen and buffy coat preparations of peripheral blood. LD bodies are small, round, 2 to 4 µm in diameter with a nucleus and a rod-shaped kinetoplast.
5. **Babesiosis:** It is a malaria like parasitic disease caused by babesia.

Table 19.14: Format for reporting peripheral blood smear

RBCs: Comment on the following features	
• Size	Normocytic (normal), microcytic or macrocytic (predominant feature to be mentioned)
• Chromasia	Normochromic (normal), hypochromic, absence of central pallor
• Anisocytosis	Present (slight /marked) or absent
• Poikilocytosis	Present (slight /marked) or absent
• Other abnormalities	Spherocytosis, sickle cells, target cells
• Polychromatophilia	Present or absent
• Nucleated red cells	Normoblasts—per 100 leukocytes
WBCs: Comment on total WBC count as normal/increased/decreased	
• Differential Count (on 100 cells)	
• Type of WBC (percentage) – Neutrophils – Eosinophils – Basophils – Lymphocytes – Monocytes – Immature leukocytes: Specify different cells	
Platelets: Approximate judgment on adequate/increased /reduced	
Hemoparasites	

Reporting of Peripheral Smear: Format for peripheral smear reporting is shown in Table 19.14.

Chapter 20

Tests for Bleeding Disorders

Chapter Outline
- Introduction
- Tests for bleeding disorders

INTRODUCTION

The clinical laboratory evaluation is an integral part of the diagnosis and management of patients with bleeding disorders. Laboratory tests for hemostatic disorders depend on the component of hemostasis that is involved (Table 20.1).

Most bleeding disorders are caused by one of three defects: (1) a defect in platelet number or function, (2) a defect in platelet -vessel wall interactions (i.e. an abnormality in the adhesive interactions between platelets and the vessel wall) or (3) a defect or deficiency in coagulation factor. The diagnosis of bleeding disorders requires a battery of tests (Table 20.2) which include screening tests done in all patients with history of bleeding, followed by specific tests to identify the exact nature of the disorder.

Table 20.1: Laboratory tests for hemostatic disorders depending on the component involved

Tests for bleeding disorders		
Platelet component	**Plate-vessel wall interaction**	**Coagulation component**
• Platelet count • Platelet aggregation test • Clot retraction test	• Capillary fragility test (tourniquet test) • Bleeding time	• Clotting time • Prothrombin time (PT) • Activated partial thromboplastin time (APTT) • Thrombin time (TT) • Prothrombin consumption time • Factor assay

Table 20.2: Laboratory tests in bleeding disorders

Screening tests	Accessory tests	Others
• Platelet count • Bleeding time • Prothrombin time (PT) • Activated partial thromboplastin time (APTT) • Thrombin time (TT)	• Capillary fragility test (tourniquet test) • Clotting time • Clot retraction test	• Prothrombin consumption time • Factor assay

TESTS FOR BLEEDING DISORDERS

Bleeding Time (BT)

Bleeding time is used as screening test for disorders of platelet-vessel wall interactions. It measures the time required for bleeding to stop after a standardized superficial cut of the skin capillary bed.

Template Method for BT

Template is a disposable blade fitted on to a holder made of plastic and is used for the test. The blade projects through the bottom so that the incision made through the slit is 9 mm long and 1 mm deep.

Principle: A small skin cut of a standard size and depth is made and the oozing blood is wiped with a filter paper. Bleeding stops when the capillaries contract and platelet plug seals the vessel.

Procedure (Fig. 20.1)

- Patient is made to sit on a chair with an arm rest, so that the forearm is steady and exposed.
- The skin of the forearm is cleaned with alcohol and allowed to dry.
- Sphygmomanometer cuff is tied to the upper arm and the cuff is inflated to 40 mm Hg.
- A site on the forearm is selected away from the superficial veins.
- Place the template 5 cm distal to antecubital crease (on volar surface).
- One cut is made using a smooth rapid movement with the template (in the *simplate/surgicutt* test, no pressure is applied to the device. On pressing the trigger an incision of 5 mm length and 1 mm depth develops).
- Immediately after the incision, a stop watch is started.

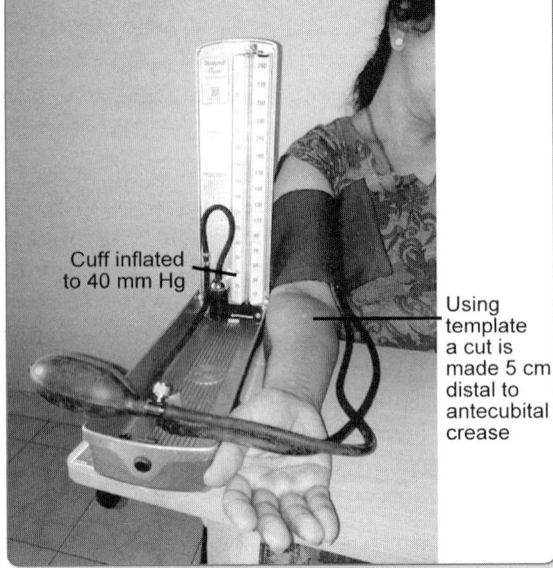

Fig. 20.1: Template method for bleeding time

- Another cut is made 1.5–2 cm away from the first one and another stop watch is started.
- The blood oozing from the sides of the cut is blotted with filter paper (Whatman No.1), every 30 seconds until bleeding stops. Do not touch the wound edges to avoid disturbing the clot as it is formed.
- Time at which bleeding stops is noted for both cuts.
- Place a butterfly adhesive bandage over the site of puncture to avoid scarring.
- Average of the two readings is the bleeding time for the patient.

Normal Range: 2–9 minutes.

Uses

- The test is prone to problems of reproducibility, sensitivity, and specificity. Though it is one of the screening tests, it is not recommended as routine preoperative screening test.
- This test evaluates the defects of primary hemostasis. Thus, bleeding time measures the platelet-vessel wall interactions (integrity of capillary and platelet function).

Note: The bleeding time usually is not prolonged in patients with coagulation factor deficiencies.

Interpretation

Prolonged bleeding time is found in:

- **Platelet disorders**
  - **Quantitative:** Thrombocytopenia. If platelet count is below 50,000/ mm^3, BT should not be performed as bleeding may be difficult to stop.
  - **Qualitative:** von Willebrand disease, Bernard-Soulier syndrome, Glanzmann's thrombasthenia.
- **Primary vascular disorders:** Ehlers- Danlos syndrome.
- **Platelet-vessel wall interactions:** von Willebrand disease.
- **Others:** Afibrinogenemia, severe hypofibrinogenemia, uremia, aspirin.

Coagulation or Clotting Time (Lee-White Method)

It measures the time taken for the fresh blood to clot.

Procedure

- Draw 3 mL of venous blood with aseptic precautions.
- Label 3 test tubes as No. 1, 2 and 3 and keep in a water bath at 37°C.
- Deliver 1 mL of blood into each of the above 3 test tubes and start the stop watch.
- After 3 minutes, take out tube No 1, tilt it every 30 seconds till a clot develops.
- Note the time when the tube can be inverted completely.
- Next examine the tube No 2 every 30 seconds, exactly the same way as tube No 1, till the clot forms and note the time.
- Finally, invert the third test tube as above till blood clots. Stop the watch.
- Record the time from the moment blood is delivered into the test tube to the complete clotting in the third tube.
- The clotting time of the third tube is reported as the clotting time.

Normal: 4–11 minutes.

Disadvantages

Not a sensitive test: It is one of the oldest tests and is not sensitive as it fails to detect mild/ moderate procoagulant defects. Hence, it is obsolete now and not recommended as a screening test. PTT is a more sensitive test for assessment of the coagulation cascade. Clotting time is prolonged only with severe deficiency of factor VIII, IX or fibrinogen (afibrinogenemia) and in heparin therapy.

Misleading: Normal value may be obtained in mild-to-moderately severe hemophilia A and B and it does not exclude major factor deficiency.

- **Other use:** Following the clotting time, the tubes can be left in the water-bath and examined after one hour for *clot retraction test.*

Quick's One Stage Prothrombin Time

Principle: Prothrombin time (PT) is the time taken by citrated plasma to clot after the addition of tissue thromboplastin and calcium. It tests ***extrinsic and common pathway*** of coagulation system.

Uses

- **Screening test to evaluate coagulation disorders:** It measures coagulation factor I, II, V, VII and X. Deficiency of any one of these factors leads to prolongation of PT. It should be used along with PTT.
- **To monitor oral anticoagulant therapy.**
- **To evaluate liver function:** Liver disease can result in deficiency of the coagulation factors. Hence, PT should be performed before a *liver biopsy* and *prolonged* PT is a contraindication for liver biopsy.

Normal Range: 11–16 seconds

Interpretation: **Prolonged PT is seen in:**

- Liver disease.
- Administration of oral anticoagulants like coumarin.
- Vitamin K deficiency
  - Obstructive jaundice.
  - Hemorrhagic disease of the newborn.
- Deficiency of factors I, II, V, VII and X.
- Disseminated intravascular coagulation (DIC).

Activated Partial Thromboplastin Time (Partial Thromboplastin Time)

Principle: Activated partial thromboplastin time (APTT) is the time taken for citrated plasma to clot in the presence of a surface activator (kaolin), phospholipid and calcium. Partial thromboplastin time (PTT) is a measure of the **intrinsic** and **common coagulation pathways.**

Uses

- Best single screening test for coagulation disorders. This test is abnormal with deficiencies of II, V, VIII, IX, X, XI and XII.
- For screening—hemophilia A and B.
- For detecting coagulation inhibitors.
- For monitoring anticoagulant therapy like heparin.

Normal Range: 30–40 seconds.

Interpretation

Common causes of a prolonged **APTT** are:

- Inherited coagulation disorders—deficiency of factor II, V, VIII, I X, X, XI, XII (e.g. hemophilia A, hemophilia B).
- von Willebrand disease.
- Disseminated intravascular coagulation.
- Liver disease.
- Heparin therapy.
- Vitamin K deficiency.
- Oral anticoagulant therapy.

Chapter 21

Histopathology

Chapter Outline

- Introduction
- Tissue processing and staining
- Frozen section techniques
- Histopathology slides

INTRODUCTION

- Histopathology is the study of microscopic changes or abnormalities in tissue that are caused by a disease.

TISSUE PROCESSING AND STAINING

The most commonly used method of examining tissues microscopically is by sectioning. Except for frozen sections of tissues, this requires the embedding of the tissues in a medium which will permit thin sections to be cut easily. The embedding media used for all routine purposes is paraffin wax and instrument used for cutting the sections for microscopy examination is called microtome.

Paraffin Embedding Technique

Fixation

For good histological preparations adequate and complete fixation of the tissue is important. Defects in fixation cannot be remedied at any later stage. It is essential that tissue be fixed as soon as possible. Fixation is required to prevent putrefaction and autolysis, to preserve cell architecture. Tissues selected for sectioning should be fixed in the desired fixatives for 12 to 24 hours. The commonly used fixatives for routine laboratory procedure are formal saline.

Dehydration

As paraffin does not mix with water, it is necessary to remove all traces of water before paraffin can permeate the tissue. This is achieved by immersion of tissues in increasing strengths of alcohol. For routine work, tissue is successively treated in 70%; 90% and absolute alcohol (at least two changes) for 2-4 hour in each.

Clearing

Since alcohol and wax are not miscible, the alcohol must be replaced by a wax solvent which at the same time clears the tissue and hence is known as clearing agent. The most common agents in use are xylene (xylol), benzene, chloroform and cedar wood oil. In routine procedures, tissue blocks after dehydration are immersed in Xylene for 1–2 hours with one change in half the time or till the tissue become transparent due to the permeation of xylene.

Nowadays, automatic tissue processors are readily available for processing the tissues.

Impregnation

By this process, the tissue is infiltrated with melted paraffin. The tissue on being cleared with xylene is transferred to a constant temperature paraffin bath of 58 to 60°C and is passed through at least two changes of paraffin of about 2–3 hours each.

Casting and Blocking

Tissue is now transferred from the final wax bath to a mould, filled with molten wax. The block is then quickly cooled and labeled.

Section Cutting

The paraffin block is trimmed and fixed to a block holder. This is then cut into thin sections of 3 to 5 μ thickness by a special instrument called microtome. Float sections in warm water at 45°C, prepare slides with a thin coating of equal parts of egg albumin and glycerin and mount sections on the prepared slides. Water is now drained off and the slide kept in an incubator before it is stained.

Staining of Paraffin Sections

For general purpose, it is usual to employ some form of hematoxylin as a nuclear stain and one of the acid aniline dyes such as eosin for the cytoplasm.

For deparaffinization heat section in a hot air oven till paraffin melts. Dip section in xylene 1–2 minutes and blot. Remove xylene with absolute alcohol and then 50% alcohol and finally wash in water.

Hematoxylin and Eosin (H and E) Stain

1. Stain section in hematoxylin for 30 minutes.
2. Wash in tap water and keep in running tap water for 5 minutes till color of tissue is blue.
3. Differentiate in acid alcohol (1% Hcl in 70% alcohol) for a few seconds and note the light pink color of the tissue section. Wash in tap water and examine under the low power of a microscope to ensure proper differentiation and leave the section in running water for 5–10 minutes till it develops deep blue color.
4. Counter stain in 1% aqueous eosin for 1–3 minutes.
5. Wash in tap water and dehydrate in two changes of absolute alcohol for 1–2 minutes. Clear in xylene and mount in D.P.X.

FROZEN SECTION TECHNIQUES

Frozen section diagnosis plays a vital role in the histopathology laboratory in intra-operative diagnosis.

Applications of Frozen Section

1. Rapid intraoperative diagnosis—to plan the ensuing surgery.
2. To study the resection margins (malignant tumors) for completeness of excision.
3. Stain for fat by Sudan IV, Sudan III, Oil Red-O or osmic acid. (Fat is removed by xylene during paraffin embedding).
4. Enzyme histochemistry: All enzymes are destroyed at temperatures above 56°C (required for paraffin embedding).
5. Immunohistochemistry and immunofluorescence.

Disadvantages

1. Serial sections cannot be obtained.
2. Lack of embedding media causes distortion of structural details during cutting and handling.
3. Unsatisfactory staining.

Frozen sections can be obtained by using either freezing microtome or cryostat. Nowadays cryostat is used.

Cryostat

It is a refrigerated cabinet, in which a modified microtome is housed. All the controls of the microtome are operated outside the cabinet. It has an open top giving direct control over the cutting operation. The temperature remains constant with the top open or closed. They are either mechanically driven or hand operated. The temperature of the cabinet is usually adjustable between 5° and 30°C. An operating temperature of 20°C is usually found to be suitable for most tissues. The tissue block, knife and section are maintained at the same temperature.

Advantages of the cryostat over the freezing microtome:

1. Thinner sections can be cut and the quality of the section is better in terms of staining.
2. Serial sections can be cut.

HISTOPATHOLOGY SLIDES

1. **Acute appendicitis:** It is one of the classical examples for acute inflammation.
   - **Gross**
     - Appendix with mesoappendix is swollen due to the edema of the wall.
     - Normal smooth, glistening, pale serosa is transformed into a dull, granular, red brown color due to engorgement (congestion) of the vessels and exudate over the serosa.
   - **Microscopy** (Fig. 21.1)
     - The histologic criterion for the diagnosis of acute appendicitis is neutrophilic infiltration of the muscularis propria. Normally neutrophils can be seen in both mucosa and submucosa.
     - Infiltration of the mucosa, submucosa, and muscularis propria (muscle layer) by neutrophils (acute inflammatory cells).
     - Subserosal vessels are congested, and often there is a modest perivascular neutrophilic infiltrate.

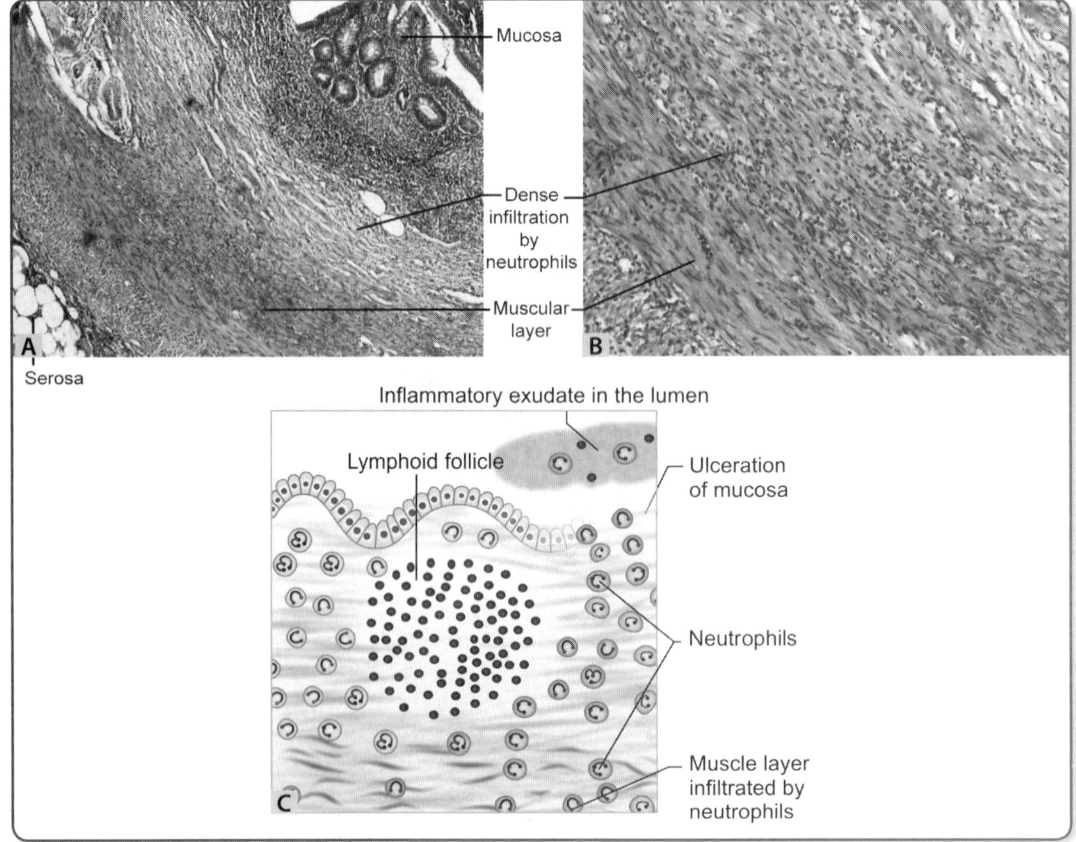

Fig. 21.1: A. Photomicrograph (low power) of acute appendicitis showing inflammation of mucosa, submucosa and muscular layer; B. (High power view) shows numerous neutrophils in the muscular layer; C. Diagrammatic appearance of acute appendicitis

(For color version, see Plate 15)

2. **Pneumonia:** It is also an example for acute inflammation. Pneumonia is inflammatory consolidation of lung. In this condition, the air in the alveoli are replaced by inflammatory exudate.
   - **Microscopy** (Fig. 21.2)
     - Congested blood vessels in the alveolar wall.
     - Alveolar spaces are packed with neutrophils and red cells.
     - Proteinaceous fluid (fluid exudates) with fibrin in the alveolar space.
3. **Granulation tissue**: It is called granulation tissue because of its pink granular appearance on the surface of healing wound.
   - **Microscopy** (see Fig. 4.3)
     - Numerous newly formed capillaries in transverse or longitudinal sections.
     - Abundant proliferation of fibroblasts.
     - Infiltration by polymorphonuclear leukocytes, macrophages, lymphocytes and plasma cells.

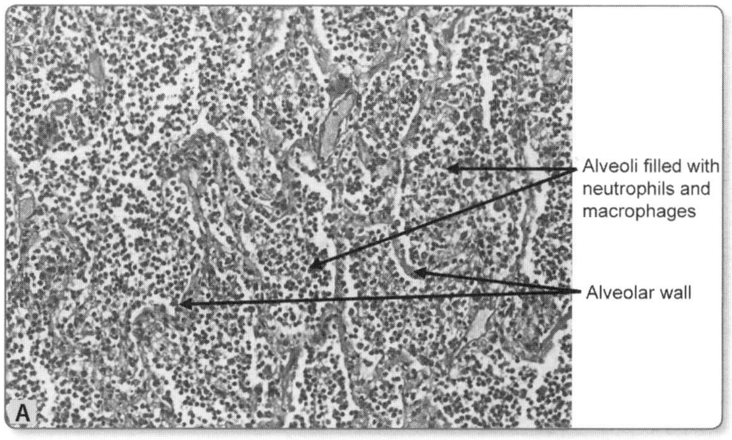

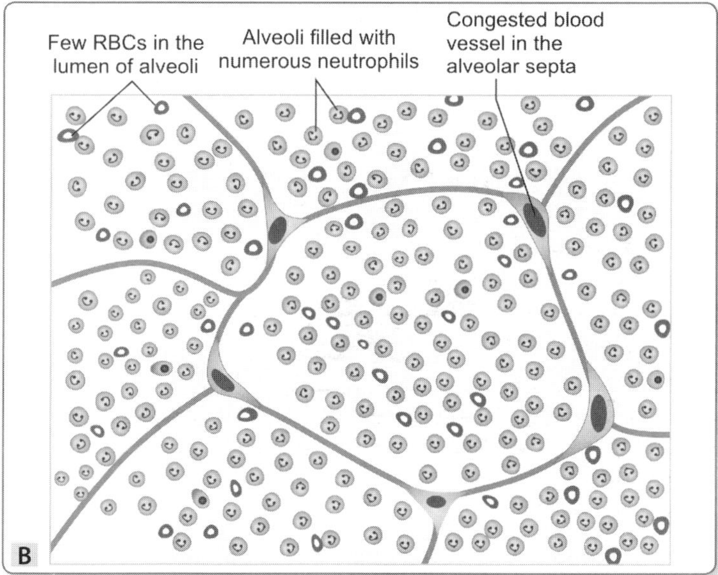

Figs 21.2A and B: Pneumonia A (H and E) and B (diagrammatic) shows alveoli filled with neutrophils

(For color version, see Plate 16)

4. **Fatty liver**
   - **Gross (see Fig. 2.13)**
     - Specimen of a portion of liver with sharp border
     - Cut surface and outer surface is yellowish, and greasy.
     - The capsule is stretched.
   - **Microscopy (see Fig. 2.14)**
     - Structure of liver.
     - Variable degree of vacuolation or clear spaces in the cytoplasm of hepatocytes.

Note: Intracellular accumulations of water or glycogen may also produce clear vacuoles. So, it is necessary to perform special techniques to distinguish these three types of clear vacuoles. Fat can be easily demonstrated by frozen section method and these sections may be then stained by Sudan III (gives orange color). Sudan IV or Oil Red O, both imparts orange red color.

5. **Chronic venous congestion liver (nutmeg liver)**
   - **Gross** (see Fig. 7.2)
     - Liver is enlarged.
     - Cut surface shows characteristic nutmeg appearance. The nutmeg appearance is due to alternate dark areas representing congested center of each lobule, and light areas being the peripheral part with fatty change (steatosis).
   - **Microscopy** (see Fig. 7.3)
     - Structure of liver.
     - Central congested area of the liver lobule appears darker than the pale peripheral portions.
     - Central hemorrhagic necrosis of the liver lobule with disappearance of the liver cells in the center of the lobule.
6. **Chronic venous congestion lung**
   - **Microscopy** (see Fig. 7.1)
     - Alveolar septa are widened due to distension of capillaries with blood. The septa show mild increase in the connective tissue.
     - The alveoli are filled with macrophages containing hemosiderin pigment (heart failure cells).
     - Special stain for demonstration of Hemosiderin pigment is Prussian blue reaction (Perl's stain) which gives blue color to hemosiderin pigment.
7. **Actinomycosis**
   - **Microscopy** (see Fig. 6.21)
     - Central abscess contains bacterial colony (sulfur granule) characterized by radiating filaments (was called as ray fungus) surrounded by hyaline, eosinophilic, club-like ends which represent immunoglobulins.
     - Periphery of the lesions shows chronic inflammatory cells, giant cells and fibroblasts.
8. **Rhinosporidiosis**: It is caused by *Rhinosporidium seeberi*. Usually, it occurs in nasopharynx but may also be observed in larynx and conjunctiva.
   - **Microscopy** (Figs 21.3A and B):
     - Structure of nasal mucosa.

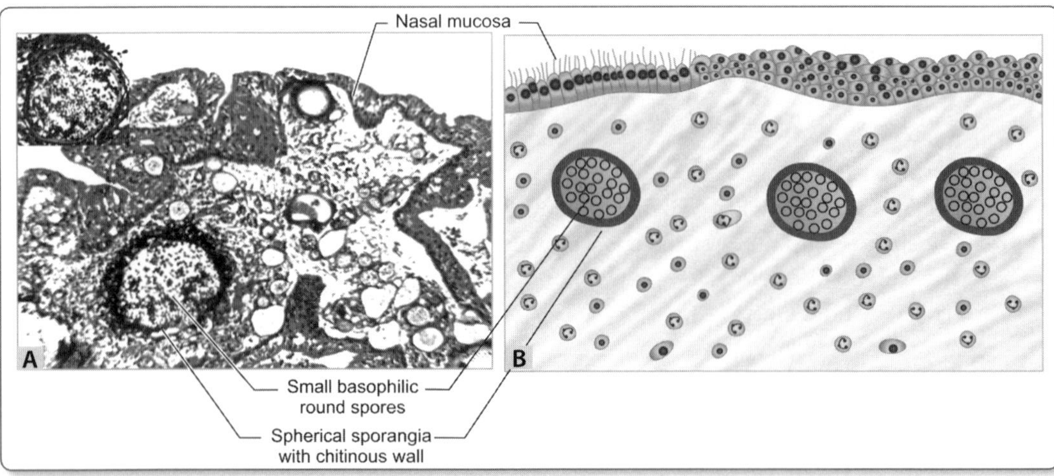

Figs 21.3A and B: Rhinosporidiosis of nasopharynx showing spherical sporangia A (H&E) and B (diagrammatic)

(For color version, see Plate 16)

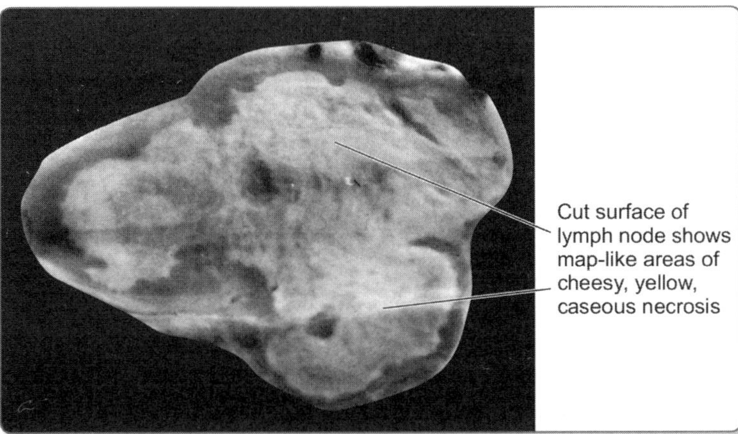

Fig. 21.4: Cut section of tuberculous lymphadenitis

- A number of spherical sporangia (with chitinous wall) containing small basophilic round spores.
- Chronic inflammatory infiltrate in the subepithelial layer.

9. **Tuberculosis of lung**
   - **Gross** (see Figs 6.2 and 6.4)
   - **Microscopy** (see Fig. 6.3)
     - Structure of lung with multiple granulomas.
     - Granulomas are composed of central area of caseation surrounded by epithelioid cells, Langhan's giant cells and lymphocytes.
10. **Tuberculosis lymph node**
    - **Gross** (Fig. 21.4):
      - Specimen of lymph node.
      - Cut surface shows map-like areas of cheesy yellow caseous necrosis.
    - **Microscopy** (see Fig. 3.11)
      - Structure of lymph node with multiple granulomas.
      - Granulomas are composed of central area of caseation surrounded by epithelioid cells, Langhan's giant cells and lymphocytes.
11. **Ameloblastoma**
    - **Microscopy** (see Figs 14.2 and 14.3): Follicular pattern is the most common pattern.
      - Tumor shows follicles of varying sizes and shapes separated by fibrous tissue.
      - The follicles consists of central area of stellate cells.
      - The peripheral layer of these follicles are cuboidal to columnar and appear to have palisading arrangement.
12. **Pleomorphic adenoma**
    - **Microscopy** (see Figs 15.1 and 15.2):
      - Neoplastic cells show varying mixture of epithelial tissue component intermingled with cells showing mesenchymal differentiation.

- Epithelial component consists of ductal cells and myoepithelial cells arranged in the form of ducts, acini and irregular tubules.
- Mesenchymal-like elements shows varying amount of mesenchyme-like background of loose myxoid tissue, islands of hyaline, chondroid (cartilaginous), and mucoid matrix.

13. Tubular adenoma of intestine

- **Microscopy:** Consists of closely packed small rounded or tubular glands (refer Fig.11.21C) embedded in a stroma (increase in the number of glands and cells per unit area compared to the normal mucosa). The cells lining the glands are crowded and contain enlarged hyperchromatic nuclei. May show variable degree of epithelial dysplasia.

14. Squamous papilloma

- **Microscopy** (see Figs 11.20 and 11.2B):
  - Papillary (finger like) proliferation of the squamous epithelia of the epidermis with intact basement membrane and the basal cells.
  - Central vascular connective tissue core.

15. Leiomyoma with hyaline change

- **Microscopy** (see Fig. 2.25):
  - Interlacing bundles of smooth muscle fibers.
  - Homogenous, glassy, pink material between the cells in many places.

16. Lipoma

- **Gross** (see Fig. 11.31)
  - Well encapsulated mass.
  - Cut surface shows yellow, greasy, with fibrous septae.
- **Microscopy** (see Fig. 11.4)
  - Fibrous capsule with septa containing blood vessels.
  - Numerous fat cells separated by fibrous septa.

17. Squamous cell carcinoma

- **Microscopy** (see Fig. 11.24):
  - Masses and groups of malignant squamous epithelial cells invading the dermis exhibiting pleomorphism, hyperchromasia and mitotic figures.
  - Epithelial pearls (concentrically laminated structures) in the midst of the invading masses of malignant cells.
  - Invasion/infiltration of underlying tissue.

18. Basal cell carcinoma (rodent ulcer) of skin

- **Microscopy** (see Fig. 11.25):
  - Groups and masses of darkly stained small epithelial cells (basaloid cells) with scanty cytoplasm invading the dermis from the basal layer of the epidermis.
  - Palisading of the peripheral layer of cells of the epithelial cell masses.

19. Malignant melanoma of skin

- **Gross** (see Fig. 11.26):
- **Microscopy** (see Fig. 11.27):
  - Structure of skin.
  - Malignant cells laden with brownish black pigment, growing down invading the dermis and subcutaneous fat.

20. Osteosarcoma

- **Gross** (see Fig. 16.5A):
- **Microscopy** (Figs 16.5 B and C)
  - Tumor consist of cells of varying size and shape with large hyperchromatic nuclei and little cytoplasm.
  - Formation of bone (osteoid matrix) by malignant cells.
  - Mitotic figures and bizarre tumor giant cells are very frequent.

21. Giant cell tumor/osteoclastoma

- **Gross** (see Fig. 16.7A)
- **Microscopy** (see Figs 16.7 B and C)
  - Tumor composed of uniform oval mononuclear cells with indistinct cell membranes arranged in syncytium.
  - Scattered within the background of such mononuclear cells are numerous uniformly placed multinucleated osteoclast-type of giant cells. These giant cells show 100 or more nuclei that are identical to those of the mononuclear cells.

22. Metastatic (secondaries) carcinoma in lymph node

- **Microscopy** (see Figs 13.13 and 13.14)
  - Structure of the lymph node.
  - Masses of malignant cells with nuclear pleomorphism and hyperchromasia.

Chapter 22

Blood Transfusion

Chapter Outline
- Blood transfusion
- Blood components
- Transfusion reactions

BLOOD TRANSFUSION

Blood transfusion is the process of transferring blood/blood products from donor into the circulating system of recipient. It is important to properly collect the blood from donor, prepare its components (if required) and store blood/components in a proper way and transfuse in such a way to avoid any risks or hazards.

Donor Selection

Donor selection is based on medical history and few routine physical examinations (weight, blood pressure, temperature, hemoglobin) are done to know whether donor is suitable for donating blood.

- Donor should be healthy. There are three types of donors, namely, voluntary (should be encouraged), replacement and professional
- It is important to know whether the patient has history of diseases like hepatitis, AIDS, syphilis and if so, blood should not be obtained from them. In the blood bank, blood is routinely screen for few common infections.

Anticoagulants used: The different anticoagulants—preservative solutions available are:
- Citrate phosphate dextrose (CPD)
- Citrate phosphate dextrose adenine (CPDA-1)
- Acid citrate dextrose (ACD) is not used nowadays.

Storage of blood: Blood is stored in a refrigerator at 2° to 6°C.

Predonation check-up

Donor Blood: The following tests are routinely carried out on donor's blood:
- ABO and Rh grouping

- Tests for:
  - HBsAg, anti-HCV, anti HIV-1 and HIV-2 and serum alanine aminotransferase (ALT)
  - Malaria and syphilis.

Recipient Blood: The recipient's ABO and Rh grouping is also carried out.

Compatibility Testing (Pretransfusion Testing)

Before transfusion of any blood or its components, it is essential to know whether they are compatible with the recipient's blood. This is achieved by performing a set of procedures known as compatibility testing. Sometimes, the term compatibility test and cross matching are used interchangeably, but cross-match is only a part of compatibility test.

Compatibility tests include:

- Review of patient's past blood bank history and records (if done earlier)
- ABO and Rh typing of the recipient and donor
- Antibody screening test of recipient's and donor's serum
- Cross-matching (Table 22.1). Cross-matching is very important before any blood transfusion.

Table 22.1: Types of cross-match

Type of cross-match	Donor's	Recipient's (patient's)
Major cross-match	Red cells	Serum
Minor cross-match	Serum	Red cells

BLOOD COMPONENTS (FIG. 22.1)

It is possible to separate different components of blood from a single unit of whole blood. These components can be used individually to help more than one patient with many purposes. Thus, red cells can be transfused to an anemic patient and plasma for a burns patient. This also ensures that only the required components are transfused.

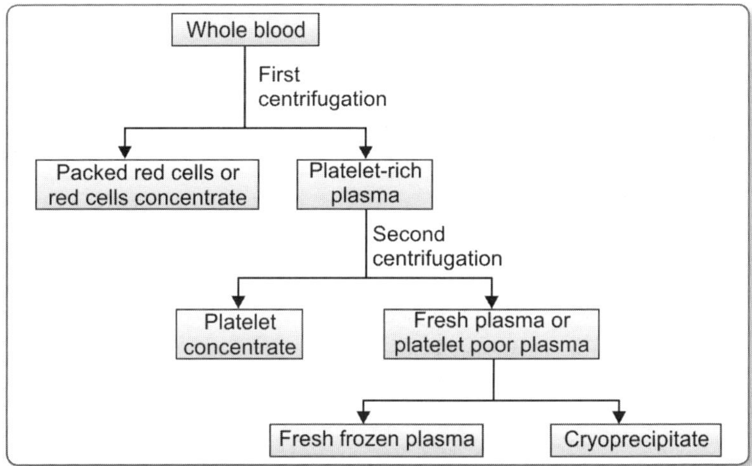

Fig. 22.1: Blood components

TRANSFUSION REACTIONS

Q. Write short note on transfusion reactions.

Blood transfusion is useful and life saving when performed with caution and with clear indication. Sometimes (about 2–4% of cases), unfavorable complications occur in spite of precaution and preventive measures, which are known as transfusion reactions. They may be broadly divided into infectious and non-infectious complications (Table 22.2).

Noninfectious Complications

Transfusion reactions may result from immune and nonimmune mechanisms.

Immune Mediated (Immediate and Delayed) Reactions

Acute hemolytic transfusion reaction

- ***ABO incompatibility*** between recipient and donor, resulting in destruction of donor cells. This is brought out by the naturally occurring (preformed) antibodies, namely, anti-A and anti-B (depending on the blood group).
  - **Massive intravascular hemolysis:** This is one of the serious complications which develop within 1 to 4 hours and with only a few milliliters of incompatible red cells. The preformed IgM antibodies (anti-A and anti-B) in the recipient coat transfused donor red cells and activate complement system to form membrane attack complex (C5-9). This results in intravascular destruction (hemolysis) of transfused donor red blood cells.
- ***Rh incompatibility:*** Because anti-Rh antibodies are not complement-fixing, in Rh incompatibility hemolysis develops in the extravascular compartment.

Table 22.2: Complications of blood transfusion

- **Noninfectious complications**
  - Immediate reactions
    - Immunological
      - Hemolytic transfusion reactions
      - Febrile nonhemolytic reaction
      - Allergic reaction
      - Anaphylactic
      - Transfusion-related acute lung injury (TRALI)
    - Nonimmunological
      - Circulatory overload
      - Air embolism
  - Delayed reactions
    - Immunological
      - Alloimmunization
      - Hemolytic transfusion reactions (mostly asymptomatic)
      - Transfusion associated graft versus host disease
    - Nonimmunological
      - Iron overload-transfusion hemosiderosis
      - Thrombophlebitis
- **Infectious complications**

  Few of the diseases transmitted by transfusion are:
  - Hepatitis (HBV, HCV and HDV)
  - HIV (AIDS)
  - Malaria
  - Cytomegalovirus
  - Syphilis

Delayed Hemolytic Transfusion Reaction

In the recipient, if antibody titer is too low and weak to be detected during cross-match, it may not cause immediate hemolysis at the time of transfusion. Instead, it may lead to a gradual increase in the antibody titer causing delayed, gradual lysis of donor red cells and is known as a delayed hemolytic transfusion reaction.

Febrile Nonhemolytic Reaction

Patient develops fever, chills, rigors and headache 30 to 60 minutes after transfusion. It is due to sensitization to leukocyte antigens.

Allergic Reaction

Allergic reaction manifests as urticaria (hives), fever, bronchospasm and rarely anaphylactic shock. It is due to exposure of allergens in donor's plasma to IgE antibodies in recipient's plasma, which activates mast cells and releases histamine/leukotrienes.

Transfusion Associated Graft Versus Host Disease (TA-GVHD)

Transfusion associated GVHD is a rare but potentially fatal complication of blood transfusion. This may develop 10 to 12 days after transfusion.

Transfusion-Related Acute Lung Injury (TRALI)

It is an uncommon complication of blood transfusion. It results from transfusion of donor plasma containing high levels of anti-HLA antibodies which bind to HLA of leukocytes of the recipient. These leukocytes aggregate in the pulmonary microcirculation and release mediators causing increased vascular permeability. This leads to acute pulmonary edema and signs and symptoms of acute respiratory failure.

Nonimmunological (Immediate and Delayed) Reactions

Circulatory Overload

Following whole blood transfusion, the blood volume and venous pressure also increases. This may be significant in the elderly, pregnant women and those with reduced cardiac function resulting in acute pulmonary edema. This can be avoided using blood components like packed red blood cells.

Air Embolism

This was common earlier when transfusion was given from the glass bottle. Presently, due to the use of plastic bags with closed tubing system, this complication does not develop.

Iron Overload (Transfusion Siderosis)

- This is seen in patients who receive multiple transfusions over a period of few years (e.g. thalassemia). The excess iron gets deposited in reticuloendothelial cells of spleen, bone marrow, liver, heart and endocrine glands.

Thrombophlebitis

Inflammation of vein may develop in patients with indwelling catheters.

Infectious Complications

Q. Write short note on infectious complications of blood transfusion.

Transfusion of infected blood may transmit few diseases like AIDS, hepatitis (HBV, HCV and HDV), HTLV-I and II, malaria and cytomegalovirus infection. This is prevented by screening the donors for these common and ominous infections.

APPENDICES

APPENDIX 1: TERMINOLOGIES

Abscess: Localized collection of pus formed as a result of inflammation often due to bacteria.

Acquired: Due to an event occurring after birth.

Acute: Appearing rapidly and has a short course, e.g. acute appendicitis.

Adenitis: It is the general term used for inflammation of a gland, e.g. lymphadenitis (lymph node), sialadenitis (salivary gland).

Adenocarcinoma: Malignant tumor of glandular or secretory epithelial cells forming glandular pattern.

Adenoma: Benign epithelial tumor in which the tumor cells form glands or benign tumors that are derived from glandular epithelium.

Allergy: Excessive and/or inappropriate immunological reaction to an allergen.

Amputation: Cutting off of a limb or part of a limb by trauma or surgery.

Amyloidosis: A disease is characterized by the extracellular accumulation of pink homogeneous substance called amyloid in various organs and tissues of the body.

Anaphylaxis: Acute multi-systemic, severe inappropriate type I hypersensitivity reaction to foreign protein.

Anaplasia: Lack of structural differentiation within a cell or group of cells often with increased capacity for multiplication, as in a malignant tumor.

Anasarca: Generalized accumulation of edema fluid within the subcutaneous connective tissue, resulting in generalized edema.

Anemia: Decrease in number of RBCs or less than the normal quantity of hemoglobin in the blood.

Aneurysm: Abnormal, permanent, localized dilation of the weakened wall of a blood vessel or part of a heart chamber.

Angina pectoris: Commonly known as angina, is characterized by severe chest pain due to lack of blood (oxygen) supply to the muscle of heart, usually due to obstruction or spasm of the coronary arteries.

Anoxia: Lack of oxygen.

Antibody: Class of immunoglobulins present in the blood or body fluids as a result of antigen stimulus or naturally.

Antigen: Substance when introduced into the body triggers the production of an antibody by the immune system.

Apoptosis: A type of normal or pathological individual cell death in which cells activate endogenous enzymes. These enzymes degrade the cell's own nuclear DNA and cytoplasmic proteins.

Ascites: An abnormal accumulation of fluid in the peritoneal cavity.

Atheroma: Lipid deposits in the intima of arteries producing yellow swelling on the endothelial surface. The lesion is seen in atherosclerosis.

Atherosclerosis: Atheroma causing hardening of arteries.

Atopy: Condition characterized by predisposition to allergic reactions.

Atrophy: Reduced size of an organ or tissue resulting from a decrease in cell size and number.

Atypia: State of being not typical. It is departure from the typical normal appearance usually, a histological term. The atypia may be either reactive or sometimes a feature of pre-neoplastic change.

Autoantibody: Antibody that reacts with body's own tissue.

Autoimmunity: Abnormal condition in which the body's immune system produces antibody against its own tissues.

Autolysis: Digestion/destruction of cells by the enzymes present within them.

Bacteremia: Presence of bacteria in the circulating blood.

Benign: Mild character of an illness or nonmalignant character of a tumor.

Biopsy: The process of removing tissue from living patients for diagnostic examination.

Blast cell: Any immature blood cell.

Bone marrow: Soft, fatty substance found in the medullary cavities of bones. The blood cells are produced in the bone marrow.

Bone marrow aspiration and biopsy: To study the marrow, it may be removed by aspiration or a needle biopsy under local anesthesia. These methods are often used together.

Cachexia: Extreme wasting of the body occurring in the course of chronic disease (e.g. cancer, AIDS) or emotional disturbances.

Calcification: Deposition of calcium salts, which may be physiological or pathological.

Callus: New immature bone formed during bone healing.

Cancer: A general term used for any malignant neoplasm. Most of these tumors invade surrounding tissues and metastasize to several sites.

Carcinogen: Any cancer-producing substance/agent.

Carcinogenesis: Mechanism of the causation of cancer.

Carcinoma: Malignant tumor derived from epithelial tissue in several sites.

Carcinoma in situ (CIS): An early form of cancer where the malignant epithelial cells are intraepithelial and there is absence of invasion of the surrounding tissue.

Caseation: A distinctive type of necrosis in which necrotic tissue resembles cheese, hence the name caseous (cheese-like) necrosis. It is characteristically seen in tuberculosis.

Cellulitis: Diffuse acute inflammation of skin and connective tissue caused by streptococcal infection.

Chemotaxis: Phenomenon in which migration of cells is induced by chemical influences.

Chromatin: The stained material that can be observed in interphase nuclei. It is composed of DNA, basic chromosomal proteins (histones), nonhistone chromosomal proteins, and small amounts of RNA.

Chromosome: Thread-like structures of chromatin containing genetic information (DNA) located in the cell nucleus.

Chronic: A disease of slow progress and long duration.

Complication: A negative pathologic process or event occurring during the course of a disease and usually aggravating the illness.

Congenital: Condition attributable to events before birth, need not be genetic or inherited.

Congestion: Engorgement with deoxygenated blood due to venous blockage.

Consolidation: Solidification of lung usually due to inflammatory exudates.

Cyst: A cavity with an epithelial lining containing usually a fluid or semisolid material.

Cytokines: Substances produced by one cell which influence the behavior of another cell.

Cytology: Study of the structure and function of the cell.

Degeneration: Retrogressive changes in cells short of necrosis; changes are reversible.

Deoxyribonucleic acid (DNA): The molecule containing the primary genetic information in the form of a linear sequence of nucleotides in groups of threes (triplets).

Diagnosis: Determination of the nature of a condition or disease.

Differentiation: Process by which a tissue develops its special characteristics. As a pathological process, it implies the extent to which the neoplasm resembles its parent tissue.

Dysplasia: Abnormal growth and differentiation of a tissue. It is a feature of early stages of neoplasia.

Ecchymosis: Any hemorrhagic patch larger than a petechiae on the skin.

Ectopic: Tissue or organ which is not in its proper position.

Edema: Abnormal accumulation of fluid in subcutaneous tissue or body cavities.

Effusion: Abnormal accumulation of fluid in a body cavity.

Embolus: An abnormal mass of undissolved material during life within the circulation and capable of blocking its lumen.

Endophytic: Tumor growing inwards from the surface.

Epithelioid: Histologically resembles epithelium. These are modified macrophages which resemble epithelial cells and are seen in granulomas.

Erosion: Loss of superficial layer of a surface.

Erythrocyte sedimentation rate (ESR): A non-specific test that measures settling of red blood cells per unit time in a column of fresh blood. It is not a diagnostic test but has prognostic value.

Etiology: Cause of disease.

Exophytic: Tumor growing outwards from a surface.

Exudate: Extravascular accumulation of protein-rich fluid due to increased vascular permeability.

Fat necrosis: It refers to focal areas of fat destruction, which affects adipose tissue. It is usually due to release of the enzyme lipase, from pancreas or follows trauma.

Focal: Localized abnormality.

Fracture: Break in a bone.

Free radical: It is a chemical radical characterized by unpaired electrons in the outer shell. They are highly reactive.

Frozen section: A method of rapid diagnosis performed during surgery in which tissue is rapidly frozen, and tissue sections are stained and examined under the microscope by the pathologist.

Fungating: Forming an elevated growth.

Gangrene: Massive necrosis with superadded putrefaction.

Giant cell: Abnormal large cells having more than one nucleus.

Glycosuria: Sugar in urine.

Grade: Degree of malignancy of a tumor judged by its histological features.

Granulation tissue: A specialized type characteristic of tissue repair. It appears pink, soft, granular on the surface of healing wounds. Microscopically, it consists of new small blood vessels and fibroblasts.

Granuloma: A distinctive type of chronic inflammation characterized by microscopic aggregation of macrophages that are transformed into epithelium-like (epithelioid) cells, surrounded by lymphocytes.

Gumma: Local necrotic lesion of tertiary syphilis with soft tumor-like formations made up of histiocytes.

Hamartoma: Tumor-like malformation consisting of jumbled tissue elements normally present in organ in which it arises.

Healing: Process of replacement of dead tissue by living tissue.

Hematocrit: Volume percentage of erythrocytes in whole blood.

Hematoma: Localized collection of extravasated blood or blood clot.

Hemophilia: A hereditary coagulation disorder due to deficiency of coagulation factor VIII/IX.

Hemosiderin: An iron-containing pigment which stains blue with Prussian blue stain.

Hemostasis: Natural process of arrest of bleeding.

Hereditary: Transmitted from parent to offspring.

Histiocyte: Large phagocytic cell (macrophage) of the reticuloendothelial system.

Homeostasis: The ability of an organism or cell to maintain internal equilibrium of temperature and fluid content by adjusting its physiological processes.

Hyaline: Refers to an alteration within cells or in the extracellular space which appears homogeneous, glassy and pink in routine histological sections.

Hyperemia: Increased blood flow to an organ or part due to arteriolar dilatation.

Hyperplasia: Increase in the size of an organ due to increase in the number of cells.

Hypersensitivity: Excessive or inappropriate reaction to an antigen, often immunologically mediated.

Hypertrophy: Increase in the size of an organ due to increase in the size of cells.

Hypoxia: Reduction of available oxygen.

Idiopathic: Cause not known.

Immunity: A body defense mechanism which has specificity and memory.

Infarction: A localized area of ischemic necrosis due to occlusion of the blood vessels. This may be due to either arterial supply or venous drainage.

Inflammation: It is a complex local response of the living vascularized tissues to injury. It mainly consists of responses of blood vessels and leukocytes.

Injury: Harm or damage.

Interstitial: Occurring in, or affecting spaces between cells.

Invasion: Spread of pathogenic microorganisms or local spread of a cancer by infiltration into the normal tissues.

Ischemia: A decrease in the blood supply to an organ or tissue.

Karyolysis: Disintegration of the nucleus.

Karyorrhexis: Nuclear fragmentation found in the nucleus of a necrotic cell.

Keloid: A raised fibrous scar tissue caused by excessive tissue repair in response to trauma or surgical incision.

Leiomyoma: Benign tumor arising from smooth muscle cells.

Lesion: A localized pathological change in an organ or tissue associated with injury or disease.

Leukemia: Malignant proliferation of white blood cells.

Leukemoid: Benign reaction which resembles leukemia. It is an extreme leukocytosis of normal cells.

Leukocytosis: Increase in the number of leukocytes (WBCs).

Leukopenia: Reduction in number of circulating leukocytes less than 4000 cells/cu mm of blood.

Lupus: Literally means wolf. An autoimmune disorder of skin with tissue destruction and sometimes systemic lesions of collagen.

Lymphadenitis: Inflammation of lymph nodes.

Lymphedema: Localized edema due to lymphatic obstruction.

Lymphoma: Primary malignant tumor of lymphoid tissue.

Lysis: The dissolution or destruction of cells, such as blood cells or bacteria.

Malformation: Abnormal or anomalous formation or structure; deformity.

Malignant: An abnormal growth which can invade the surrounding tissues or travel to other organs or tissues by the bloodstream or lymphatics ("metastasize").

Margination: Accumulation of leukocytes on the endothelial surface of blood vessels in acute inflammation.

Melanin: A brown-black endogenous pigment produced by melanocytes.

Metaplasia: It is a reversible process in which one adult type of cell is replaced by another adult type of cell.

Metastasis: Process by which a primary malignant tumor gives rise to secondary deposits in lymph nodes or other organs.

Miliary: Characterized by the presence of small lesions that have the size and appearance of millet seeds.

Mononuclear cells: Vague histological term for leukocytes other than polymorphonuclear leukocytes.

Morphology: Refers to the gross and microscopic structural changes in cells or tissues.

Mural: In the wall of a hollow structure.

Mutation: A permanent and heritable alteration in DNA sequence within a gene on chromosome.

Necrosis: Sum of morphological changes indicative of cell death in a living tissue following extremely harmful injury.

Needle aspiration: Method used by cytopathologists, using a needle and syringe, to obtain cells for microscopic examination and diagnosis of disease.

Neoplasm: Abnormal and uncoordinated growth of tissue persisting even after withdrawal of the initiating cause.

Oma: Suffix meaning tumor.

Oncogene: A gene that acts in a dominant fashion to unregulate cell growth and proliferation, resulting in tumor development.

Oncogenesis: Mechanism of causation of tumors.

Papanicolaou's smear (Pap smear): It is a type of preparation of cells on glass slides for microscopic examination. It is used most often for early detection of cancer of the cervix. The name is derived from Dr Papanicolaou, a Greek pathologist who developed the procedure.

Papillary: Descriptive term for a surface lesion composed of numerous finger-like projections.

Papilloma: Benign epithelial tumor consisting of finger-like projections.

Parenchyma: The morphologically and functionally specific cells of an organ, as distinguished from associated connective or supporting tissues.

Pathogenesis: Mechanism by which the causative factor of a disease produces structural and functional abnormalities, and hence symptoms and signs.

Pathognomonic: Pathological feature characteristic of a particular disease.

Pathologic calcification: Abnormal deposition of calcium salts in tissues other than osteoid or enamel.

Pathology: Scientific study of the nature of disease and its causes, processes, development and consequences.

Pedunculated: Having or growing on or from a peduncle or stalk.

Petechia: Pinpoint, non-raised, purplish-red spot caused by intradermal or subcutaneous hemorrhage (plural is petechiae).

Phagocytosis: Process by which a cell, such as a white blood cell, ingests microorganisms, other cells and foreign particles. The cell which engulfs or ingests is known as phagocyte.

Pleomorphism: Variation in size and shape, usually of nuclei and characteristic of cancer.

Polyp: Pedunculated or sessile growth arising from the body surface.

Polypoid: Like a polyp; projecting from a surface.

Prognosis: It forecasts or predicts the likely outcome of the disease, and therefore, the fate of the patient.

Pseudo: Prefix signifying false or non-identity.

Purpura: Small purplish spots or patches on the skin due to subcutaneous bleeding.

Pus: Creamy liquid material consisting of neutrophils, in various stages of disintegration and necrotic tissue. Usually results from acute inflammation.

Putrefaction: Decomposition or rotting of dead tissue by bacterial action, often accompanied by foul-smelling odor.

Pyemia: Septicemia caused by pyogenic microorganisms in the blood, often resulting in the formation of multiple abscesses.

Pyknosis: Shrinkage of nucleus appearing like an ink drop in necrotic cell.

Pyogenic: Inducing or forming pus.

Pyrexia: Fever, temperature above normal.

Radiation: Emission and propagation of energy in the form of rays or waves.

Recurrence: To happen, come up, or show up again or repeatedly.

Regeneration: Process in which lost tissue is replaced by tissue of similar type that was lost.

Repair: Process in which lost/damaged tissue is replaced by fibrous tissue or scar.

Resolution: Restoration of tissue to normal following acute inflammation.

Saponification: A chemical reaction in which hydrolysis of a fat or oil by alkali results in the formation of a soap and glycerol.

Sarcoma: Malignant tumor of mesenchyme (connective tissue), e.g. fibrosarcoma.

Scar: Mark left after a injury or wound has healed. It is remnant of the healing process.

Sepsis: Presence of bacteria (pathogenic organisms) or their toxins in the blood or tissues.

Serous membrane: Membrane lining the walls of the body cavities and enclosing the contained organs; it is mesothelial which secretes a watery serous fluid.

Sessile polyp: Polyp with a broad base without any stalk.

Shock: A state of cardiovascular collapse.

Signet ring cell: Neoplastic cell in which the nucleus is pushed to the periphery by the large globule of mucin in the cytoplasm.

Signs: Abnormalities of a disease found or observed on examination.

Sinus (pathological): Abnormal tract leading from an abscess to the skin surface and often discharging pus.

Splenomegaly: Enlargement of the spleen.

Stage: A recognizable phase of development or progression of a disease (usually a neoplasm).

Stasis: Stagnation of fluid often due to obstruction.

Steatorrhea: Excess of fat in stools.

Steatosis: Fatty change.

Stroma: The connective tissue framework of an organ or other structure.

Subcutaneous: Beneath the skin.

Suppuration: Formation of pus.

Symptom: The patient's complaints attributable to the presence of a particular disease.

Syndrome: A set of signs and symptoms characteristic of a particular disease, no one feature alone being diagnostic.

Telomere: End of a chromosome.

Teratoma: Germ cell neoplasm containing tissues representative of more than one germ cell layer, namely, ectoderm, mesoderm and ectoderm.

Thrombocytopenia: Decrease of circulating platelets below normal level in the blood.

Thrombus: Solid mass formed from the constituents of blood within the blood vessels or the heart, during life.

Transfusion: The transfer of whole blood or blood products from one individual to another.

Transudate: Abnormal collection of fluid of low protein content usually due to increased intravascular hydrostatic pressure.

Trauma: Injury.

Tumor: Abnormal swelling usually used for a neoplasm.

Ulcer: Lack of continuity of a mucous membrane or skin surface.

Vasodilator: An agent that causes dilatation of the blood vessels.

Virulence (microorganism): Relative ability to produce disease.

APPENDIX 2: STAGES OF ERYTHROPOIESIS

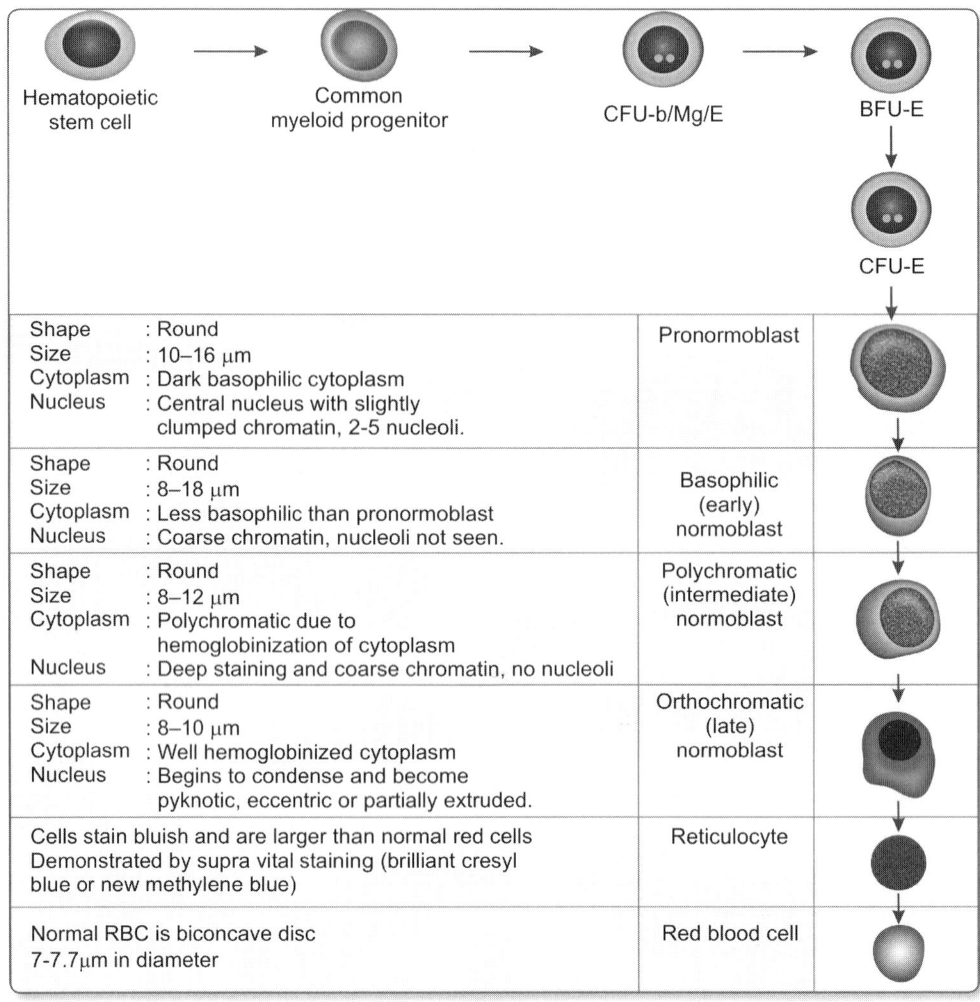

Shape : Round Size : 10–16 μm Cytoplasm : Dark basophilic cytoplasm Nucleus : Central nucleus with slightly clumped chromatin, 2-5 nucleoli.	Pronormoblast	
Shape : Round Size : 8–18 μm Cytoplasm : Less basophilic than pronormoblast Nucleus : Coarse chromatin, nucleoli not seen.	Basophilic (early) normoblast	
Shape : Round Size : 8–12 μm Cytoplasm : Polychromatic due to hemoglobinization of cytoplasm Nucleus : Deep staining and coarse chromatin, no nucleoli	Polychromatic (intermediate) normoblast	
Shape : Round Size : 8–10 μm Cytoplasm : Well hemoglobinized cytoplasm Nucleus : Begins to condense and become pyknotic, eccentric or partially extruded.	Orthochromatic (late) normoblast	
Cells stain bluish and are larger than normal red cells Demonstrated by supra vital staining (brilliant cresyl blue or new methylene blue)	Reticulocyte	
Normal RBC is biconcave disc 7-7.7μm in diameter	Red blood cell	

Fig. A-2.1: Stages of erythropoiesis

APPENDIX 3: STAGES OF MYELOPOIESIS

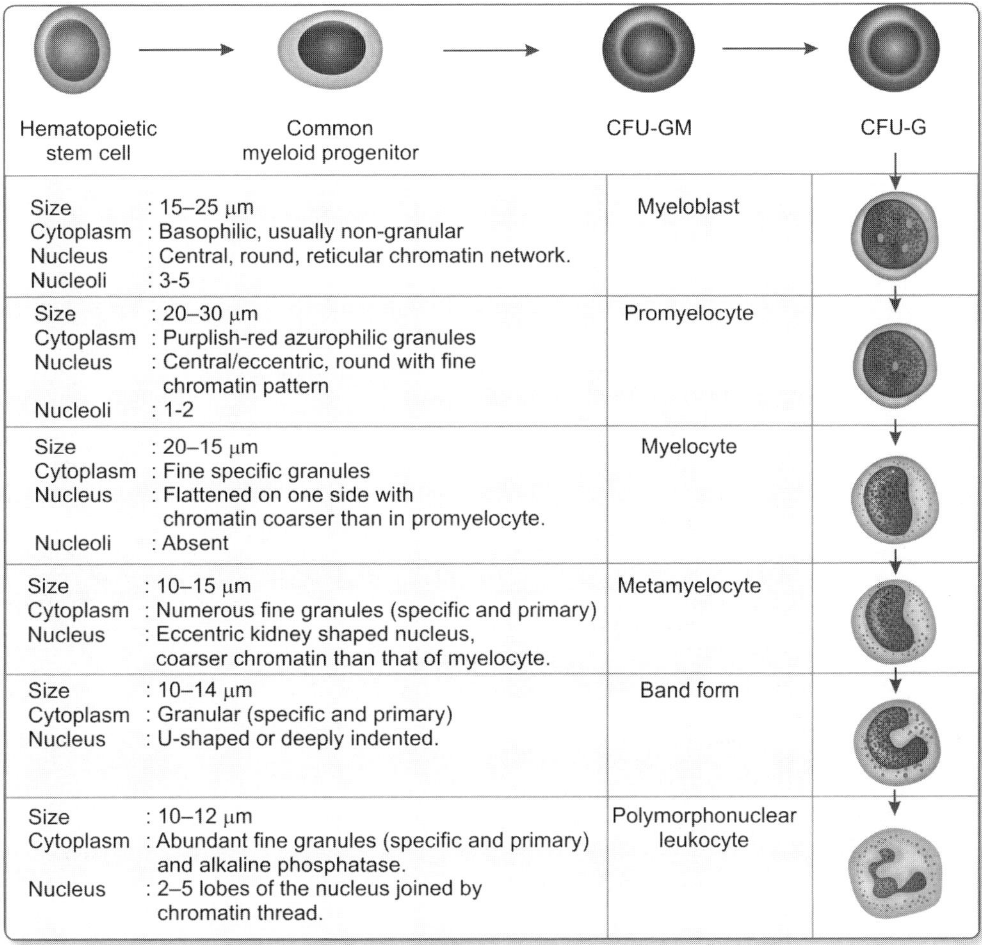

Fig. A-3.1: Stages of myelopoiesis

APPENDIX 4: STAGES OF MEGAKARYOPOIESIS

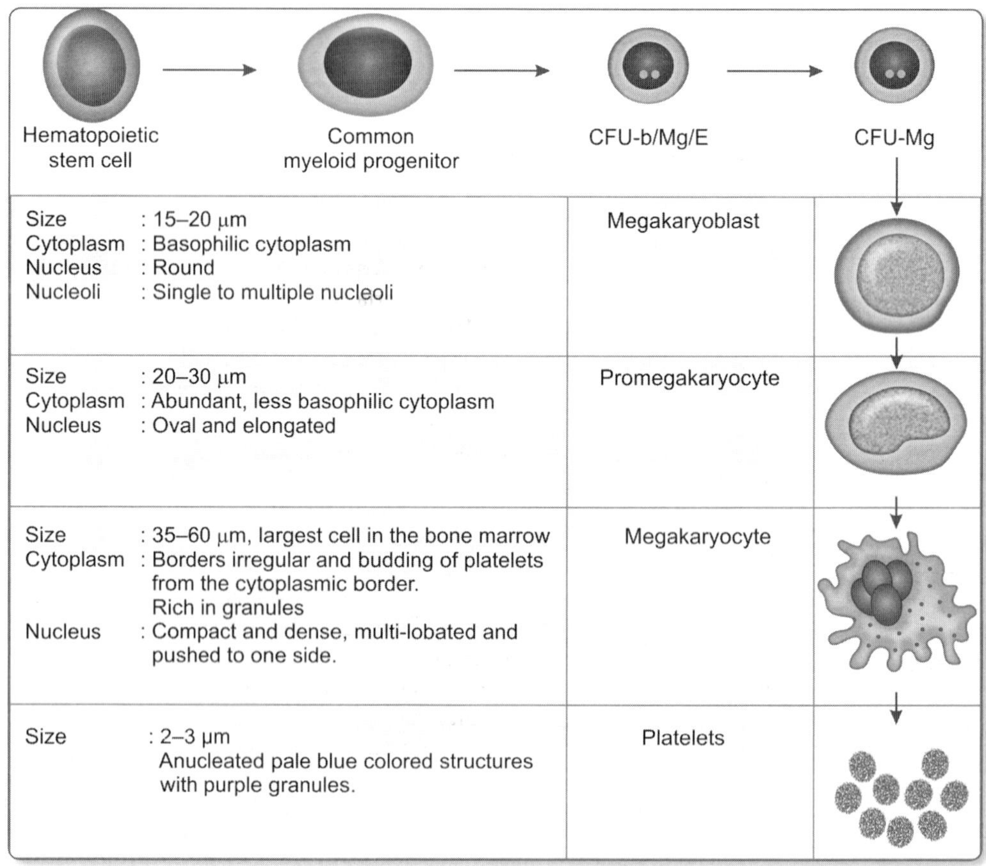

Fig. A-4.1: Stages of megakaryopoiesis

INDEX

Page numbers followed by *f* refer to figure and *t* refer to table.

A

B

C

D

E

G

H

M

N

O

P

R

S

T

U

V

W

X

Z